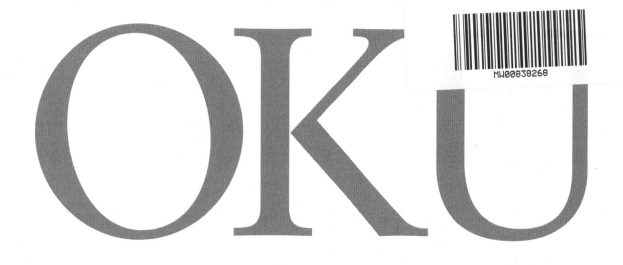

OKU
5

Orthopaedic
Knowledge
Update
Spine

AAOS
AMERICAN ACADEMY OF
ORTHOPAEDIC SURGEONS

OKU
5

Orthopaedic Knowledge Update

Spine

Eeric Truumees, MD
Professor
Department of Surgery
University of Texas at Austin, Dell Medical School
CEO, Seton Brain and Spine Institute
Austin, Texas

COEDITOR
Heidi Prather, DO
Professor
Vice Chair, Department of Orthopaedic Surgery
Division Chief, Physical Medicine and Rehabilitation
Departments of Orthopaedic Surgery and Neurology
Washington University School of Medicine
St. Louis, Missouri

Developed by the North American
Spine Society

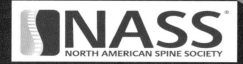

AMERICAN ACADEMY OF ORTHOPAEDIC SURGEONS

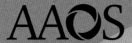

AMERICAN ACADEMY OF ORTHOPAEDIC SURGEONS

The material presented in the *Orthopaedic Knowledge Update: Spine 5* has been made available by the American Academy of Orthopaedic Surgeons for educational purposes only. This material is not intended to present the only, or necessarily best, methods or procedures for the medical situations discussed, but rather is intended to represent an approach, view, statement, or opinion of the author(s) or producer(s), which may be helpful to others who face similar situations.

Some drugs or medical devices demonstrated in Academy courses or described in Academy print or electronic publications have not been cleared by the Food and Drug Administration (FDA) or have been cleared for specific uses only. The FDA has stated that it is the responsibility of the physician to determine the FDA clearance status of each drug or device he or she wishes to use in clinical practice.

Furthermore, any statements about commercial products are solely the opinion(s) of the author(s) and do not represent an Academy endorsement or evaluation of these products. These statements may not be used in advertising or for any commercial purpose.

Published 2017 by the
American Academy of Orthopaedic Surgeons
9400 West Higgins Road
Rosemont, IL 60018

Copyright 2017
by the American Academy of Orthopaedic Surgeons

Library of Congress Control Number:
2017951329

ISBN 978-1-62552-694-6

Printed in the USA

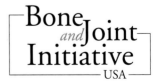

Acknowledgments

Editorial Board
Orthopaedic Knowledge Update: Spine 5

Eeric Truumees, MD
Professor
Department of Surgery
University of Texas at Austin, Dell Medical
  School
CEO, Seton Brain and Spine Institute
Austin, Texas

Heidi Prather, DO
Professor
Vice Chair, Department of Orthopaedic Surgery
Division Chief, Physical Medicine and
  Rehabilitation
Departments of Orthopaedic Surgery and
  Neurology
Washington University School of Medicine
St. Louis, Missouri

Christopher D. Chaput, MD
Chief of the Division of Spine Surgery
Department of Orthopedics
Baylor Scott and White Health, Central Texas
Temple, Texas

Charles H. Cho, MD, MBA
Interventional and Diagnostic Radiology
Department of Radiology
Brigham and Women's Hospital
Harvard Medical School
Boston, Massachusetts

Mitchel B. Harris, MD
Professor of Orthopaedics
Harvard Medical School
Department of Orthopaedic Surgery
Brigham and Women's Hospital
Boston, Massachusetts

Scott R. Laker, MD
Associate Professor
Department of Physical Medicine and
  Rehabilitation
University of Colorado Hospital
Aurora, Colorado

Ronald A. Lehman Jr, MD
Professor of Orthopaedic Surgery, Tenure
Chief, Degenerative, Minimally Invasive, and
  Robotic Spine Surgery
Director, Athletes Spine Center
Director, Spine Research
Co-Director, Adult and Pediatric Spine
  Fellowship
Advanced Pediatric and Adult Deformity
  Service
Department of Orthopaedic Surgery
Columbia University Medical Center
New York, New York

Charles A. Reitman, MD
Professor and Vice Chairman
Department of Orthopaedics
Medical University of South Carolina
Charleston, South Carolina

Andrew J. Schoenfeld, MD
Assistant Professor
Department of Orthopaedic Surgery
Harvard Medical School
Boston, Massachusetts

Jeffrey C. Wang, MD
Chief, Orthopaedic Spine Service
Co-Director, USC Spine Center
Professor of Orthopaedic Surgery and
  Neurosurgery
USC Spine Center
Los Angeles, California

Acknowledgments

**North American Spine Society
Board of Directors, 2016-2017**

F. Todd Wetzel, MD
President

Daniel K. Resnick, MD, MS
First Vice President

Jeffrey C. Wang, MD
Second Vice President

William J. Sullivan, MD
Secretary

Eeric Truumees, MD
Treasurer

Christopher M. Bono, MD
Past President

Edward Dohring, MD
Education Council Director

Alan S. Hilibrand, MD
Continuing Medical Education Chair

Donna Ohnmeiss, PhD
Education Publishing Chair

Zoher Ghogawala, MD, FACS
Research Council Director

Charles H. Cho, MD, MBA
Evidence Compilation & Analysis Chair

D. Scott Kreiner, MD
Clinical Research Development Chair

Charles A. Reitman, MD
*Administration & Development Council
   Director*

Jerome Schofferman MD
Ethics and Professionalism Committee Chair

Joseph S. Cheng, MD
Section Development Chair

Mitchel B. Harris, MD, FACS
Governance Committee Chair

David R. O'Brien Jr, MD
Health Policy Council Director

Mitchell F. Reiter, MD, PC
Payer Policy Review Committee Chair

John G. Finkenberg, MD
Advocacy Council Director

Norman B. Chutkan, MD
At-Large Member

Matthew Smuck, MD
At-Large Member

David Rothman, PhD
Ethicist

Eric J. Muehlbauer, MJ, CAE
Executive Director

Explore the full portfolio of AAOS educational programs and publications across the orthopaedic spectrum for every stage of an orthopaedic surgeon's career, at www.aaos.org/store. The AAOS, in partnership with Jones & Bartlett Learning, also offers a comprehensive collection of educational and training resources for emergency medical providers, from first responders to critical care transport paramedics. Learn more at www.aaos.org/ems.

Contributors

Oussama Abousamra, MD
Clinical Fellow
Department of Orthopaedic Surgery
Johns Hopkins Hospital
Baltimore, Maryland

Uzondu F. Agochukwu, MD
Assistant Professor
Department of Orthopaedic Surgery
Medical College of Georgia at Augusta
*   University*
Augusta, Georgia

Ilyas S. Aleem, MD, MSc, FRCSC
Assistant Professor
Department of Orthopaedic Surgery
University of Michigan
Ann Arbor, Michigan

Paul A. Anderson, MD
Professor, Orthopedic Surgery
Department of Orthopedic Surgery and
*   Rehabilitation*
University of Wisconsin
Madison, Wisconsin

Amandeep Bhalla, MD
Assistant Professor
Department of Orthopaedic Surgery
Harbor – UCLA Medical Center
David Geffen School of Medicine at UCLA
Torrance, California

Christopher M. Bono, MD
Chief, Orthopaedic Spine Service
Department of Orthopaedic Surgery
Brigham and Women's Hospital
Boston, Massachusetts

Étienne Bourassa-Moreau, MD, MSc
Fellow in Spine Surgery
Department of Orthopedic Surgery
University of British Columbia
Vancouver, British Columbia, Canada

Daniel Bouton, MD
Fellow
Department of Orthopaedic Surgery
Texas Scottish Rite Hospital for Children
Dallas, Texas

Joseph S. Butler, PhD, FRCS
Clinical Fellow
Rothman Institute
Thomas Jefferson University Hospitals
Philadelphia, Pennsylvania

Charles H. Cho, MD, MBA
Radiologist
Department of Radiology
Brigham and Women's Hospital, Harvard
*   Medical School*
Boston, Massachusetts

Norman B. Chutkan, MD, FACS
Executive Director
The Orthopedic and Spine Institute
Banner University Medical Center Phoenix
Phoenix, Arizona

Berdale Colorado, DO, MPH
Assistant Professor
Department of Orthopedic Surgery
Washington University School of Medicine
St. Louis, Missouri

John G. DeVine, MD
Professor
Department of Orthopaedic Surgery
Medical College of Georgia at Augusta
*   University*
Augusta, Georgia

Marco Ferrone, MD, FRCSC
Orthopaedic Spine & Oncology
Department of Orthopaedic Surgery
Brigham and Women's Hospital
Boston, Massachusetts

Jeffrey S. Fischgrund, MD
Chairman
Department of Orthopaedics
William Beaumont Hospital
Royal Oak, Michigan

Kenneth Foxx, MD
Spine Surgery Fellow
Department of Orthopedics
University of Rochester Medical Center
Rochester, New York

Jason Friedrich, MD
*Assistant Professor, Associate Fellowship
 Director*
*Department of Physical Medicine &
 Rehabilitation*
University of Colorado School of Medicine
Aurora, Colorado

Christopher G. Furey, MD
Chief, Spine Section
Henry Bohlman, MD Endowed Chair
Department of Orthopaedic Surgery
University Hospitals Cleveland Medical Center
Cleveland, Ohio

Michelle Gittler, MD
Medical Director, Chairperson
*Department of Physical Medicine and
 Rehabilitation*
Schwab Rehabilitation Hospital
Chicago, Illinois

John Glaser, MD
Professor
Department of Orthopaedic Surgery
Medical University of South Carolina
Charleston, South Carolina

S. Raymond Golish, MD, PhD, MBA
Medical Director of Spinal Surgery
Department of Surgery
Jupiter Medical Center
Palm Beach, Florida

Richard D. Guyer, MD
Texas Back Institute Fellowship Director
Associate Clinical Professor
Department of Orthopedics
*University of Texas Southwestern School
 of Medicine*
Dallas, Texas

Raymond J. Hah, MD
Assistant Professor
Department of Orthopaedic Surgery
Keck School of Medicine
University of Southern California
Los Angeles, California

Clifton W. Hancock, MD, MS, MBA
Texas Back Institute Fellow
Texas Back Institute
Plano, Texas

Colin B. Harris, MD
Assistant Professor
Department of Orthopaedics
Rutgers University – New Jersey Medical School
Newark, New Jersey

Alan S. Hilibrand, MD
*The Joseph and Marie Field Professor of Spinal
 Surgery*
Rothman Institute
Jefferson Medical College
Philadelphia, Pennsylvania

John A. Hipp, PhD
Chief Scientist
Medical Metrics, Inc.
Houston, Texas

Samantha R. Horn, BA
Research Fellow
NYU Hospital for Joint Diseases
NYU Langone Medical Center
New York, New York

Serena S. Hu, MD
Professor and Vice Chairman
Chief, Spine Surgery Service
Department of Orthopaedic Surgery
Professor of Neurological Surgery (by courtesy)
Stanford University School of Medicine
Stanford, California

Keith L. Jackson II, MD
Chief, Spine Surgery
Department of Orthopaedics and Rehabilitation
Womack Army Medical Center
Fort Bragg, North Carolina

M. Burhan Janjua, MD
Neurospine Fellow
NYU Hospital for Joint Diseases
NYU Langone Medical Center
New York, New York

Darnell T. Josiah, MD, MS
Clinical Instructor
Department of Neurosurgery
University of Wisconsin – Madison
Madison, Wisconsin

Brian J. Kelley, MD, PhD
Advanced Pediatric Spinal Deformity Fellow
Department of Pediatric Orthopedic Surgery
Morgan Stanley Children's Hospital
Columbia University Medical Center
New York, New York

Harish Kempegowda, MD
Spine Fellow
Department of Orthopaedics
MedStar Union Memorial Hospital
Baltimore, Maryland

Jad G. Khalil, MD
Assistant Professor
Department of Orthopaedic Surgery
Oakland University
William Beaumont Hospital
Royal Oak, Michigan

D. Scott Kreiner, MD
Partner
Ahwatukee Sports & Spine
Phoenix, Arizona

Mark F. Kurd, MD
Assistant Professor, Orthopaedic Surgery
The Rothman Institute
Thomas Jefferson University Hospitals
Philadelphia, Pennsylvania

Robert M. Kurtz, MD
Fellow
Department of Radiology
Brigham and Women's Hospital, Harvard
*   Medical School*
Boston, Massachusetts

Brian K. Kwon, MD, PhD, FRCSC
Professor and Canada Research Chair in SCI
Department of Orthopaedics
University of British Columbia
Vancouver, British Columbia, Canada

Hubert Labelle, MD
Professor of Surgery
University of Montreal
Montreal, Quebec, Canada

Adam LaBore, MD
Associate Professor
Physical Medicine and Rehabilitation
Department of Orthopaedic Surgery
Washington University School of Medicine
St. Louis, Missouri

John M. Lavelle, DO
Spine Physician
Department of Orthopaedics
Tennessee Orthopaedic Clinics
Knoxville, Tennessee

Ronald A. Lehman, Jr, MD
Professor of Orthopaedic Surgery, Tenure
Chief, Degenerative, Minimally Invasive, and
*   Robotic Spine Surgery*
Director, Athletes Spine Center
Director, Spine Research
Co-Director, Adult and Pediatric Spine
*   Fellowship*
Advanced Pediatric and Adult Deformity Service
The Spine Hospital - Columbia University
*   Medical Center*
New York, New York

Lawrence G. Lenke, MD
Professor of Orthopedic Surgery with Tenure
Department of Orthopedic Surgery
Columbia University Medical Center
New York, New York

Thomas J. Lotus, DC, FACO, Cert. MDT
President/Owner
Spine & Sports Center of Chicago
Chicago, Illinois

Jean-Marc Mac-Thiong, MD, PhD
Associate Professor
Department of Surgery
Université de Montréal
Montréal, Québec, Canada

Benjamin Marshall, DO
Fellow Physician
Department of Physical Medicine &
    Rehabilitation
University of Colorado School of Medicine
Aurora, Colorado

John P. Metzler, MD
Associate Professor
Department of Orthopaedic Surgery
Division of Physical Medicine and
    Rehabilitation
Washington University
St. Louis, Missouri

Patrick B. Morrissey, MD
Orthopaedic Spine Fellow
Rothman Institute
Philadelphia, Pennsylvania

Isaac L. Moss, MDCM, MASc, FRCSC
Assistant Professor
Department of Orthopaedic Surgery
University of Connecticut Health Center
Farmington, Connecticut

Ahmad Nassr, MD
Consultant
Associate Professor
Department of Orthopedic Surgery
Mayo Clinic
Rochester, Minnesota

Annie O'Connor, MSPT, OCS, Cert. MDT
Clinical Manager
River Forest Spine & Sport Center
Rehabilitation Institute of Chicago
Chicago, Illinois

Donna D. Ohnmeiss, DrMed
Texas Back Institute Research Foundation
Plano, Texas

Stefan Parent, MD, PhD
Associate Professor
Head, Paediatric Orthopaedic Surgery Service
Academic Chair in Pediatric Spinal Deformities
    of CHU Ste-Justine
Department of Surgery, CHU Ste-Justine
Université de Montréal
Montréal, Québec, Canada

Peter G. Passias, MD
Assistant Professor
NYU Hospital for Joint Diseases
NYU Langone Medical Center
New York, New York

Rakesh D. Patel, MD
Assistant Professor, Spine Service
Department of Orthopaedic Surgery
University of Michigan Health System
Ann Arbor, Michigan

Gregory W. Poorman, BA
Research Fellow
NYU Hospital for Joint Diseases
NYU Langone Medical Center
New York, New York

Michael L. Reed, DPT, OCS
President and CEO
Spine Trust
Palm Beach Gardens, Florida

Daniel K. Resnick, MD, MS
Professor
Department of Neurological Surgery
University of Wisconsin
Madison, Wisconsin

Richard V. Roberts, MD
Spine Research Fellow
Department of Orthopaedic Surgery
Beaumont Hospital
Royal Oak, Michigan

James O. Sanders, MD
Professor of Orthopaedics and Pediatrics
Department of Orthopaedics and Rehabilitation
University of Rochester
Rochester, New York

Timothy Sanford, MD
Physician
Physical Medicine and Rehabilitation
Ahwatukee Sports & Spine
Phoenix, Arizona

Zeeshan M. Sardar, MD, MSc
Assistant Professor
Department of Orthopaedic Surgery
Temple University
Philadelphia, Pennsylvania

Jerome Schofferman, MD
Founder and Member, Section on
Rehabilitation, Interventional and
Medical Spine
Chair, Committee on Ethics and Professionalism
North American Spine Society
Sausalito, California

Joseph H. Schwab, MD, MS
Assistant Professor
Department of Orthopaedic Surgery
Massachusetts General Hospital, Harvard
Medical School
Boston, Massachusetts

Paul Sponseller, MD, MBA
Professor and Head, Division of Pediatric
Orthopaedics
Department of Orthopaedic Surgery
Johns Hopkins Hospital
Baltimore, Maryland

Daniel J. Sucato, MD, MS
Chief of Staff
Texas Scottish Rite Hospital
Department of Orthopaedic Surgery
University of Texas at Southwestern Medical
Center
Dallas, Texas

Chi-Tsai Tang, MD
Assistant Professor
Department of Orthopaedic Surgery
Division of Physical Medicine and
Rehabilitation
Washington University School of Medicine
St. Louis, Missouri

P. Justin Tortolani, MD
Chief, Division of Spine Surgery
Director, Spinal Reconstructive Fellowship
Department of Orthopaedic Surgery
MedStar Union Memorial Hospital
Baltimore, Maryland

Michael G. Vitale, MD, MPH
Ana Lucia Professor of Pediatric Orthopaedic
Surgery
Columbia University Medical Center
Director, Division of Pediatric Orthopaedics
Chief, Pediatric Spine and Scoliosis Service
Morgan Stanley Children's Hospital of
New York - Presbyterian
New York, New York

Michael J. Vives, MD
Associate Professor
Department of Orthopaedics
Rutgers University – New Jersey Medical School
Newark, New Jersey

Gregory Whitcomb, DC
Assistant Professor
Department of Neurosurgery
Medical College of Wisconsin
Milwaukee, Wisconsin

Kirkham B. Wood, MD
Professor
Department of Orthopaedic Surgery
Stanford University
Palo Alto, California

Samuel A. Yoakum, DO
Non-Operative Spine Specialist
Department of Orthopaedics
Tennessee Orthopaedic Clinics
Knoxville, Tennessee

Haitao Zhou, MD
Acting Instructor
Orthopaedics and Sports Medicine
University of Washington
Harborview Medical Center
Seattle, Washington

Craig Ziegler, MD
Sports Medicine Fellow
Washington University Orthopedics
Washington University
St. Louis, Missouri

Preface

This fifth edition of *Orthopaedic Knowledge Update Spine* (*OKU Spine 5*) seeks to maintain the tradition of excellence fostered by previous editors and authors and recognize the rapidly changing world of spine care. Not only have the sources of data greatly increased in the 5 years since the publication of the prior edition of this work, but so have the means of accessing this information. Excellent research has emerged from throughout the world, including rapidly growing input from Asia. This research is often published in a host of new journals, and much of it is directly available on the Internet.

For both learners and specialists working to maintain up-to-date knowledge, the challenge is not finding information, but rather sifting through the mountains of available data. The editors of *OKU Spine 5* sought to address that challenge by assembling more than 80 experts from diverse backgrounds and regions and representing various disciplines and subspecialty interests. Together, we seek to provide concise answers to the questions "where are we in spine care?" and "where are we going"? Toward this end, the powerful OKU format allowed us to organize this information. Most topics begin with a review of critical background information, followed by an update of the literature from the past 5 years. Each chapter offers an annotated bibliography to guide the readers' further exploration of a topic.

Our thanks go to the project manager, Kim Hooker, and editorial team at the American Academy of Orthopaedic Surgeons (AAOS), including Lisa Claxton Moore, Kathleen Anderson, Laura Goetz, Steven Kellert, Genevieve Charet, and Rachel Winokur. To ensure timeliness, this book had very tight deadlines. The AAOS staff was instrumental in moving the project forward. They also hosted many conference calls during which the editors and section editors discussed concepts around section organization and author selection. These initial discussions led to a particularly engaged author group and strong content offering broad coverage of spine care with minimal redundancy.

Today, optimal spine care requires an interdisciplinary approach with invaluable input from our colleagues in physical medicine, rehabilitation, anesthesiology, radiology, neurology, neurosurgery, rheumatology, and internal medicine. That spectrum of caregivers is reflected in our selection of contributors to this work. As with previous editions of *OKU Spine*, this balance began with two book editors with different practices and training backgrounds and continued with a diverse group of section editors. We are indebted to the section editors—Chris Chaput, Charlie Cho, Mitchel Harris, Scott Laker, Ronald Lehman Jr, Charlie Reitman, Andrew Schoenfeld, and Jeffrey Wang—each a recognized expert in the field, for helping select topics and authors and for shepherding those chapters through to completion.

Although each chapter stands on its own, the book also is organized with a logic that allows it to be read cover to cover or section by section. *OKU Spine 5* begins with an overview of spine anatomy and physiology. This section is followed by a review of the assessment tools most useful to spine care providers. Approaches to management are grouped by type and disease state and include sections on medical and surgical management of spine disorders, spine deformity, spine trauma, neoplastic and inflammatory conditions, and the special populations affected by spine disorders.

For the first time, an *OKU Spine* update will be accompanied by section commentaries written by international spine experts; these commentaries will be available with the digital version of this work. The editors are indebted to these contributors for providing an international perspective that further emphasizes the wide-ranging approaches and viewpoints in current spine care.

We thank the North American Spine Society (NASS) and the AAOS for the honor of editing this book. We acknowledge our practices and our partners who have been very patient with our volunteer efforts and the time required for their completion. Finally, we thank our families for their patience while we attended those evening conference calls and weekends spent tapping away at the keyboard. With this done, we expect an increase in our exposure to those loved ones, the sun, and improvement in our vitamin D levels.

Eeric Truumees, MD
Editor
Heidi Prather, DO
Coeditor

Table of Contents

Section 5: Spine Deformity

Section 6: Trauma

Section 7: Neoplastic and Inflammatory Conditions

Section 8: Special Populations in Spine Care

Section Editor:
Andrew J. Schoenfeld, MD

Section 1

Spine Anatomy and Biomechanics

SECTION EDITOR:

Christopher D. Chaput, MD

Chapter 1

Musculoskeletal Anatomy and Physiology

Isaac L. Moss, MDCM, MASc, FRCSC

Abstract

The vertebral column is a complex three-dimensional structure whose function in health and disease is determined by the anatomy and physiology of the spine at its supporting structures, including the vertebrae, the disks, and the intimate connections with the surrounding soft tissues. To understand, diagnose, and safely treat patients with spinal pathology, it is helpful for surgeons to review the basic anatomy of the spine and be aware of recent developments in understanding how the anatomy of the vertebrae and the surrounding tissues affect function.

Keywords: anatomy; applied anatomy; vertebrae

Introduction

A detailed knowledge of spine anatomy is a prerequisite for safe and effective nonsurgical and surgical treatment of patients with spine pathology. The vertebrae, intervertebral disks, and surrounding ligaments and muscles are important determinants of spinal function, both in health and disease. The evolving body of knowledge on spine anatomy, function, and the complex interactions between the various elements that make up the spine allows a deeper understanding of the pathogenesis of disease and the potential development of future novel treatments.

Dr. Moss or an immediate family member is a member of a speakers' bureau or has made paid presentations on behalf of Pfizer; serves as a paid consultant to Atlas Spine, Avitus Orthopedics, Nuvasive, Spineart, and Stryker; has stock or stock options held in Orthozon LLC; and serves as a board member, owner, officer, or committee member of the North American Spine Society.

Basic Anatomy

The spinal column consists of 24 vertebral segments. Except for the first cervical level, all individual vertebrae share similar basic morphologic characteristics, including a vertebral body, pedicles, a lamina, and a variety of bony projections that serve as attachments for ligaments and muscles. The mobile spine is traditionally divided into three regions consisting of 7 cervical vertebrae, 12 thoracic vertebrae, and 5 lumbar vertebrae. The sacrum consists of five fused vertebrae, with no motion between the vertebrae. Despite important similarities, substantial anatomic variation exists between the vertebrae of each region, with the vertebrae being adapted to the varying functional demands throughout the spine. A thorough understanding of these variations is essential for the safe and effective management of spinal pathology.

The functional spinal unit consists of two adjacent vertebrae and their intervening intervertebral disk and facet joints. The facet joints are true synovial joints with characteristics similar to those of other synovial articulations in the body. The intervertebral disk, however, is the major load-bearing structure of the spine and has unique characteristics. Each intervertebral disk is composed of an inner gelatinous nucleus pulposus consisting primarily of type II collagen and proteoglycans and surrounded by a highly organized collagenous anulus fibrosus, which primarily consists of type I collagen in concentric lamellae, with fibers lying in alternating directions (**Figure 1**). These components are confined cranially and caudally by the vertebral end plates, resulting in a confined hydraulic system with biphasic viscoelastic biomechanical properties capable of withstanding considerable compressive loads.

Ligaments

The spine is stabilized by several ligamentous structures. The anterior longitudinal ligament (ALL) is found on the ventral aspect of the vertebral body, extending from the skull to the sacrum. The ALL has several layers, with its

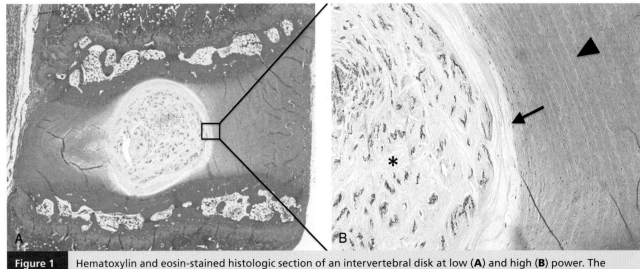

Figure 1   Hematoxylin and eosin-stained histologic section of an intervertebral disk at low (**A**) and high (**B**) power. The nucleus pulposus (*) is populated by clusters of cells within a gelatinous matrix. A clear border (arrow) between the nucleus pulposus and the anulus fibrosus is evident. The anulus fibrosus demonstrates organized fibrocartilage lamellae (arrow head). (Reproduced from Moss IL, An HS: Form and function of the intervertebral disc, in O'Keefe R, Jacobs JJ, Chu CR, Einhorn TA: *AAOS Orthopaedic Basic Science*, ed 4. Rosemont, IL, American Academy of Orthopaedic Surgeons, 2013, pp 253-260.)

deepest and strongest attachments being to the articular lip at the margins of each vertebra and its more superficial layers spanning multiple vertebrae. The posterior longitudinal ligament (PLL) also spans from the skull to the sacrum, but runs within the spinal canal on the dorsal aspect of the vertebral body. Unlike the ALL, the PLL has attachments only at the disk level, and it is bowstrung across the concavity of the vertebral bodies. The PLL can be elevated by pathologic processes, including disk herniations, hematomas, infections, and tumors. The location of the PLL reinforces the central anulus fibrosus, with most posterior disk herniations occurring at the lateral margin of the PLL. Because the ALL and PLL are innervated by the sinuvertebral nerves, which are branches from the spinal nerves near the origin of the anterior and posterior rami, they may be contributors to back pain.

The ligamentum flavum is an important anatomic structure to consider during surgical decompression because it is a major contributor to spinal canal stenosis. In contrast with the ALL and PLL, the ligamentum flavum is a noncontiguous structure, with attachments to the ventral surface of the cranial lamina and superior surface of the caudal lamina of each individual functional spinal unit. When entering the canal with a Kerrison rongeur or burr, surgeons often exploit the fact that the ligamentum flavum extends halfway to two-thirds up the ventral surface of the cephalad lamina because this natural anatomic barrier can help prevent inadvertent durotomy.[1]

Development

The spinal column is formed from the paraxial mesoderm in a process called somatogenesis.[2] As the body axis elongates, individual somites are added on either ventral portion of the somite, which becomes the mesenchymal sclerotome and is responsible for the formation of the vertebrae and the anulus fibrosus. The nucleus pulposus is formed from the remnant of the notochord and is populated by cells of notochordal origin in early life. These cells are subsequently replaced by chondrocyte-like cells by the end of the first decade of life. Each vertebra is formed by three primary ossification centers—the centrum, neural arch, and a costal element. Failure of one or more of these ossification centers to develop can result in the formation of a hemivertebra, which often causes substantial deformity (referred to as congenital deformity).[3] Failure of the somite to fully segment results in the formation of block vertebrae or unsegmented bars. The combination of a hemivertebra and a contralateral unsegmented bar leads to the most progressive form of congenital scoliosis.

Muscles

The paraspinal musculature plays an important role in stabilizing the spine and maintaining upright posture. In the cervical spine, the paraspinal muscles are divided into deep and superficial groups, with the deep musculature mainly responsible for spinal stability and the superficial musculature mainly responsible for movement (**Figure 2**). An increased cross-sectional area in the deep cervical extensor muscles is associated with a higher rate of bony union after

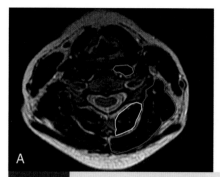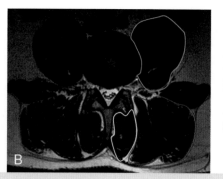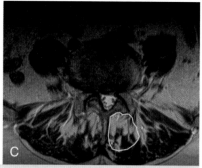

Figure 2 Axial T2-weighted magnetic resonance images of normal midcervical spine muscular. **A,** The anterior flexor longus collis (green), the deep extensors semispinalis cervicis and multifidus muscle (yellow), and the superficial extensors semispinalis capitus, splenius capitus, and longissimus muscles (red). **B,** Normal lumbar spine musculature at the L4-L5 disk space demonstrating the psoas muscle (green), the deep extensor multifidus muscle (yellow), and superficial erector spinae muscle (red). **C,** Lumbar spine musculature after open decompression shows substantial fatty atrophy of the multifidus muscle (yellow).

anterior cervical fusion.[4] In the thoracolumbar spine, the paraspinal musculature is generally divided into the deep multifidus muscles and the more superficial erector spinae muscles. The multifidus is considered the major posterior stabilizing muscle of the spine. Its large cross-sectional area and sarcomere orientation allow it to generate large forces with small changes in length.[5] The multifidus muscle originates from the spinous process of a single level and typically inserts three levels caudal (on the mammillary process in the lumbar spine). At each level, the multifidus is innervated by the medial branch nerve of the posterior ramus of the spinal nerve, which exits the spinal canal superolateral to the facet joint. Multifidus atrophy is seen after traditional open approaches to the spine and results from a combination of denervation, thermal injury, and pressure necrosis caused by prolonged retraction.[5] Medial branch nerve ablations, which are often performed to treat back pain, may lead to multifidus atrophy as well.[6]

Recently, the health and function of the paraspinal musculature has been investigated as it relates to back pain and surgical success.[7-9] Paraspinal muscle atrophy and fatty infiltration, most prominently affecting the multifidus, has been associated with chronic low back pain; however, it is unclear if this change is causative or related to disuse in patients with long-term pain.[7] Paraspinal atrophy and fatty infiltration also have been associated with an increased risk of adjacent-segment degeneration after lumbar fusion.[8] Many minimally invasive approaches to the lumbar spine have been designed to preserve the medial branch nerve and minimize trauma to the multifidus.[9]

Spinal Balance

Positioning of the C7 vertebrae over the sacrum is essential for the maintenance of upright posture and efficient locomotion. Proper positioning is achieved by balancing

the curvatures of the various anatomic regions of the spine, including lordosis of approximately 60° in the lumbar region and approximately 20° in the cervical region, and kyphosis of approximately 40° in the thoracic and sacral regions[10] (**Figure 3**).

The sagittal vertical axis is measured as the distance between the posterior corner of the S1 superior end plate and a vertical plumb line from the midpoint the C7 vertebral body. Increase in the sagittal vertical axis is linearly correlated with more pronounced symptoms and disability.[11] Lumbar lordosis is not evenly distributed, with two-thirds of overall lumbar lordosis contributed by L4-S1. Optimal lumbar lordosis is closely related to an individual's pelvic incidence, which is an important parameter to consider when planning corrective surgery for spine deformity. Recent evidence has shown that an individual's cervical lordosis is related to his or her cranial incidence, an anatomic parameter specific to an individual's skull[12] (**Figure 4**). Variation occurs in both sagittal balance and pelvic parameters as a result of shifting from a standing to a sitting position, with a reduction in both lumbar lordosis and thoracic kyphosis and a forward shift in the sagittal vertical axis.[13] The relevance of this information when planning spine deformity correction has yet to be determined. With aging, the regional curvatures often change, often with an increase in thoracic kyphosis. However, asymptomatic individuals may maintain a stable global balance by compensation in other areas of the spine.[14]

Applied Anatomy by Region

Cervical Spine

Occipitocervical Stability

The occipitocervical complex, which extends from the occiput to the C2-3 disk space, consists of specialized

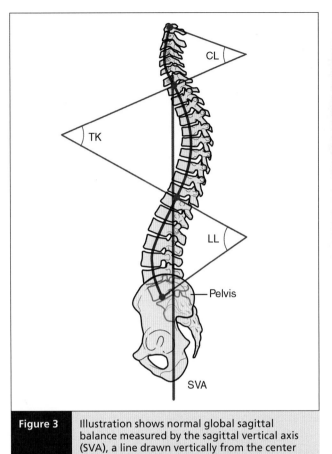

Figure 3 Illustration shows normal global sagittal balance measured by the sagittal vertical axis (SVA), a line drawn vertically from the center of the C7 vertebral body. Normal balance results from a balanced combination of cervical lordosis (CL), thoracic kyphosis (TK), and lumbar lordosis (LL).

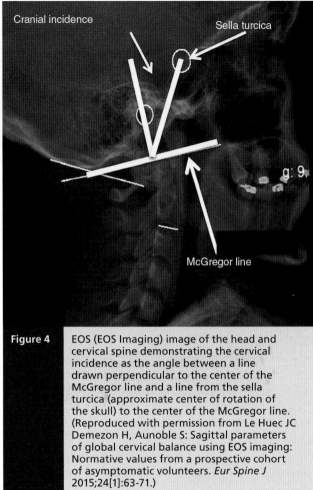

Figure 4 EOS (EOS Imaging) image of the head and cervical spine demonstrating the cervical incidence as the angle between a line drawn perpendicular to the center of the McGregor line and a line from the sella turcica (approximate center of rotation of the skull) to the center of the McGregor line. (Reproduced with permission from Le Huec JC Demezon H, Aunoble S: Sagittal parameters of global cervical balance using EOS imaging: Normative values from a prospective cohort of asymptomatic volunteers. *Eur Spine J* 2015;24[1]:63-71.)

bony and ligamentous structures to stabilize this area of vital anatomy while also acting as the major contributor to cervical range of motion. The tectorial membrane, once thought to be the primary stabilizer of the occipitoatlantal articulation, is an extension of the PLL and runs from the anterolateral edge of the foramen magnum to the posterior surface of the C2 body and odontoid process. A recent study performed using modern biomechanical techniques demonstrated that the primary stabilizers of the craniocervical junction are the transverse and alar ligaments.[15]

The cruciate ligament, the key structure in atlantoaxial stability, consists of vertical and transverse components, which stabilize the odontoid to the occiput and atlas, respectively (**Figure 5**). Disruption of the occipitocervical complex, which can result from high-energy trauma, can lead to occipitoatlantal or atlantoaxial dissociation. The sensitivity of plain radiography to detect these often-fatal injuries has been questioned. Efforts have been undertaken to define parameters predictive of ligamentous injury based on CT and MRI, which are commonly obtained imaging studies in trauma settings. On CT, a basion-dens interval of greater than 10 mm and a C1-C2 lateral mass interval of 4 mm or greater are highly sensitive measurements for the detection of occipitocervical complex instability.[16] MRI studies have defined two patterns of occipitocervical complex injury based on the integrity of the occipitoatlantal capsular ligaments.[17] Atlantoaxial dissociation occurs when occipitoatlantal capsular ligaments are preserved but the cruciate ligament is disrupted. In patients with combined occipitoatlantal and atlantoaxial dissociation, both the occipitoatlantal capsular ligaments and the cruciate ligaments are disrupted.[17] It may be easier to recognize a true dissociation by evaluating not only the midline structures (eg, basion-dens interval), but also the congruency and the displacement of the occiput-C1 articular surfaces.

Vertebral Artery

The foramen transversarium is a key distinguishing anatomic feature of the cervical vertebrae from C2-C7. The

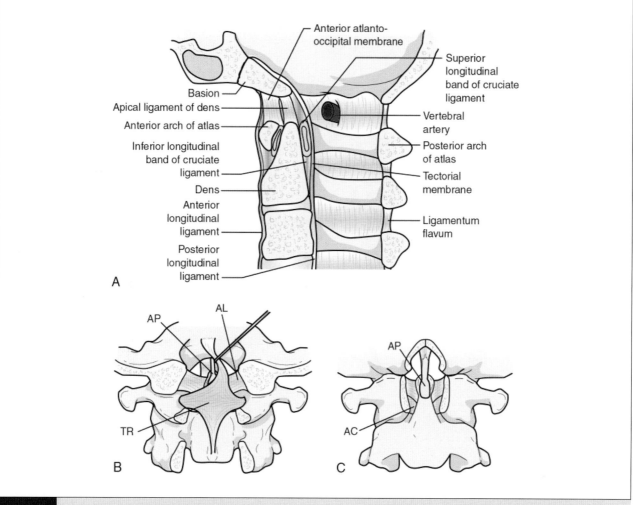

Figure 5 **A,** Illustration demonstrating the sagittal view of the occipitocervical articulation. Posterior (**B**) and anterior (**C**) illustrations of the atlantoaxial articulation. AC = accessory ligament, AL = alar ligament, AP = apical ligament, TR = transverse atlantal ligament.

vertebral artery, which is a branch of the subclavian artery, usually enters the foramen of C6, runs cranially to exit at C2, and then proceeds around the lateral mass of C1 to the superior surface of the posterior C1 arch and enters the foramen magnum (**Figure 6**). Frequent variations exist in the size and position of the foramen transversarium and the artery contained within.[18] In rare instances, the artery can run through the lateral aspect of the vertebral body and entirely outside the foramen. Thus, a careful review of axial imaging studies is essential when planning cervical instrumentation. The vertebral artery can be injured when using a burr to remove the uncovertebral joint. Fibrous bands, which connect the nerve root to the vertebral artery, can tear this vessel even when the burr remains medial. The vertebral artery is most at risk for injury during the posterior instrumentation of C1 and C2. In addition, a fine-cut CT scan or CT angiogram is

helpful when planning instrumentation at C1 and C2. The C2 pedicle has substantial anatomic variation in up to 18% of individuals, which can put the vertebral artery at risk for injury.[19] The Harms technique for C1-C2 fixation (with C1 lateral mass and C2 pedicle screws) has gained popularity over the Magerl transarticular screw technique because it provides greater freedom for screw trajectory and potentially reduces the risk of vertebral artery injury.[20]

Subaxial Cervical Spine

The subaxial cervical spine is most commonly instrumented from an anterior approach that takes advantage of an anatomic corridor to the spine and osseous anatomy for safe instrumentation. The cervical vertebrae and neural foramina of males are typically larger than those of females.[21] With advancing age, cervical vertebrae become

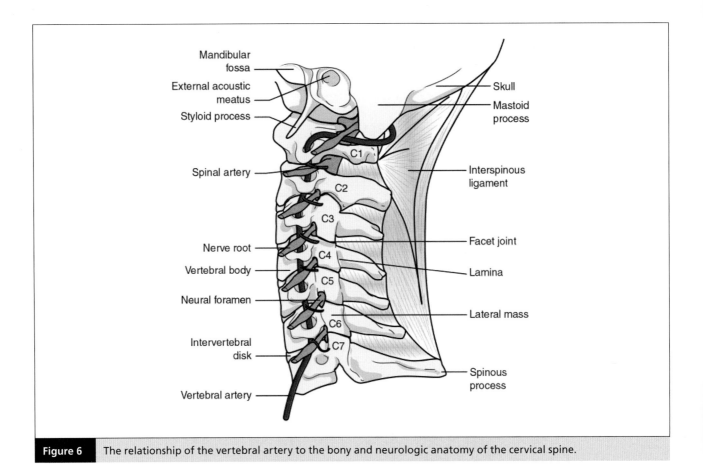

| Figure 6 | The relationship of the vertebral artery to the bony and neurologic anatomy of the cervical spine. |

wider and more elongated.[19] The average depth of the cervical vertebral bodies ranges from 15 to 17 mm and increases caudally. Subaxial cervical vertebrae have uncinate processes extending from the edges of the superior end plates, which form lateral borders of the intervertebral disk. The uncinate processes form an important landmark for the lateral extent of anterior decompression procedures. Posteriorly, the cervical vertebrae are characterized by bifid spinous processes and large lateral masses, but not the elongated transverse processes found in the thoracic and lumbar regions. Lateral mass instrumentation is most commonly used for posterior fixation from C3 through C6 because of its technical ease and safety.[22] The starting point for these screws is 1 mm medial to the center of the lateral mass. The screws are angulated approximately 15° cephalad and 30° lateral to limit the risk of injury to the vertebral artery and exiting nerve roots, although these parameters may change somewhat depending on the level instrumented and the amount of spinal degeneration.[23] Posterior instrumentation of subaxial cervical pedicles is possible; however, this is associated with a higher risk of neurologic and vascular complications compared with lateral mass

fixation.[24] Many surgeons limit the use of this technique to C7, where lateral mass fixation is poor and there is less risk of injury to the vertebral artery. The starting point for C7 pedicle screw instrumentation is the upper outer quadrant of the lateral mass. The screw trajectory angles medially 25° to 45°. A laminoforaminotomy to palpate the pedicle may improve the accuracy and safety of this procedure.

Thoracic Spine

Several unique anatomic characteristics are important to understand when assessing and treating thoracic spinal pathology. Each thoracic vertebra has a diarthrodial articulation with a rib on each side. This articulation adds to the inherent stability of the thoracic spine and is thought to be a major contributing factor to the decreased frequency of degenerative pathology in the thoracic region compared with the cervical and lumbar regions. The thoracic facet joints are oriented in the coronal plane to allow for axial rotation. The ratio of the canal to the spinal cord is relatively small in the thoracic spine, which increases the risk of neurologic injury even with small amounts of canal incursion.[25] Although the height of pedicles generally increases from cranial to caudal progression within thoracic vertebrae, CT-based studies have demonstrated that the pedicle width decreases from T1 (9.27 ± 1.01 mm) to T4 (4.5 ± 0.93 mm), and then subsequently increases to T12 (8.31 ± 1.83 mm).[26] As a result, a substantial portion of the pedicles in the midthoracic spine are not wide enough to accommodate a 4-mm screw with 1 mm of clearance, which is considered a satisfactory margin of safety. Close study of thoracic anatomy is mandatory before instrumentation in this region, and alternative techniques should be considered. Such techniques involve the use of hooks, translaminar screws, or an in-out-in trajectory in which the screw intentionally breaches the lateral pedicle wall and abuts the rib head for added stability.

Thoracic pedicles have been shown to expand in diameter to accommodate larger screws placed to maximize pullout strength.[27] Recent evidence shows that this expansion occurs primarily in the lateral direction; thus, the diameter of the spinal canal is not diminished and the risk of injury to the spinal cord is not increased.[28]

At T12, the entry point for pedicle screw insertions is the junction of the bisected transverse process and the lamina. Progressing cranially to the midthoracic spine, the starting point shifts to a more medial and cephalad position. In the cranial portion of the thoracic spine, the entry point is at a more cranial and lateral position[29] (**Figure 7**). Alternatively, the funnel and slide techniques can be used to identify the cancellous bone found within the pedicle in contrast to the cortical bone found on the anterior margin of the transverse process.[30] The transverse pedicle angle (TPA) decreases from cranial to caudal, requiring a more medialized trajectory in the proximal thoracic spine (TPA at T1 is approximately 35°) compared with distal vertebrae (TPA at T12 is approximately –10°).[25] Two techniques have been described with respect to sagittal plane angulation. The anatomic technique, with the screw angled caudally in line with the true pedicle anatomy, allows for placement of a longer screw but necessitates the use of a polyaxial screw, which can limit the success of deformity correction. The straightforward approach with the screw angled in line with the end plate, as opposed to the pedicle, has gained popularity because it allows placement of a fixed-angle screw to obtain more powerful deformity correction.[31]

The position of the great vessels with respect to the spine is an important consideration, especially when instrumenting thoracic vertebrae, because injury to the vessels can have catastrophic consequences. The aorta lies on the left anterolateral aspect of the vertebrae and follows the spine caudally, dividing into the common iliac arteries at or around the L4-L5 disk level. The distance

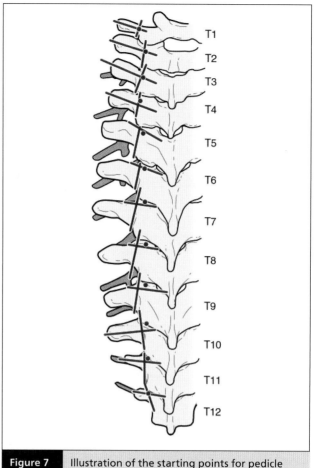

Figure 7 | Illustration of the starting points for pedicle screw instrumentation of the thoracic spine.

from the margin of the vertebrae to the aorta decreases from the cephalad to caudad thoracic spine (4.8 mm at T1, 1.2 mm at T12).[32] In patients with scoliosis, the relationship between the spine and aorta is altered as a result of both translation and rotation. The aorta is located more posterolateral and closer to the vertebrae at the levels above the apex of the curve. Below the apex of the curve, the aorta is located closer to the midline, which increases the risk of injury at the thoracolumbar junction in patients with Lenke type 1 curves.[33]

The use of navigation systems to improve the accuracy of pedicle screw placement is especially useful in the thoracic spine because the margin for error is small.[34]

Lumbosacral Spine
End Plate Anatomy and Biomechanics
Interbody fusion, including the application of interbody spacers, is used routinely in a stand-alone fashion or as an adjunct to traditional posterolateral fusion. This technique can restore disk height (which in turn provides indirect decompression of the neuroforamen and spinal

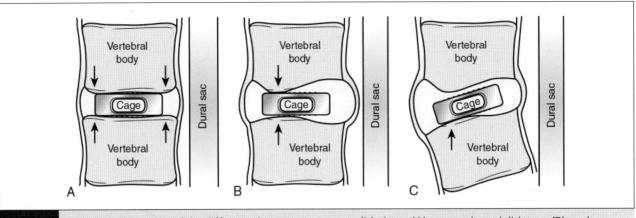

Figure 8 Schematic illustration of the difference between a common disk shape (**A**), a pear-shaped disk type (**B**), and a pear-shaped disk with greater disk angle type (**C**) regarding the stability of the cage. In the sagittal plane, the cage makes maximal contact with the end plates at all four corners of the interbody device, minimizing the risk for cage migration.

canal), restores segmental lordosis, and improves spinal alignment. The large surface area within the disk and the compressive environment also provide a favorable setting for bony fusion. The interbody space can be accessed with a variety of approaches, including posterolateral, anterior, or lateral.

Regardless of the approach used, an understanding of the anatomy and biomechanics of the vertebral end plates is essential for the success of the procedure. The bony end plate lies between a layer of hyaline cartilage adjacent to the intervertebral disk and the trabecular bone of the vertebral body. The strength and stiffness of the lumbar end plates increase in the more caudal vertebrae. Within an individual end plate, both strength and stiffness increase from the center to the periphery of the plate. Overall strength and stiffness of end plates decrease by up to 30% and 46%, respectively, at higher grades of disk degeneration, with the most substantial changes in the periphery of the end plates.[35] Injury to the end plates has been shown to reduce pressure within the adjacent nucleus pulposus and increase compressive stress concentration within the posterior anulus fibrosus.[36] This is thought to accelerate the degenerative cascade of the spinal motion segments. The motion segments above L4 and those in older patients are especially vulnerable to motion segment degeneration.[36] The end plates most commonly form a biconcave disk in the sagittal and coronal plane, with the apex of the concavity near the center of the disk. In some patients, a more dorsal apex of concavity is noted and has been associated with retropulsion of posteriorly inserted interbody devices[37] (**Figure 8**). Careful assessment of end plate morphology and the degree of degeneration are important for decreasing interbody cage subsidence and migration rates.

Instrumentation

Transpedicular screw fixation from an open posterior approach has become the standard technique for lumbar spine instrumentation because it provides increased strength and stiffness from three-column vertebral fixation. Recently, alternative methods of fixation have been described.[38,39] These methods attempt to decrease the morbidity associated with dissection of the paraspinal musculature required in traditional transpedicular fixation methods or to overcome problems associated with fixation in vertebrae with poor bone quality.

Cortical bone of the pars interarticularis and a medial-to-lateral trajectory can be used to obtain fixation while reducing the exposure required for instrumentation compared with a traditional trajectory. The starting point for the screws in a cortical bone trajectory is 2 to 3 mm medial to the lateral border of the pars interarticularis and caudal to the facet joint. After an initial pilot hole is made with a burr, the trajectory is drilled in an approximate 15° medial-to-lateral direction and a 20° to 25° caudal-to-cranial direction, generally under fluoroscopic guidance. The medial starting point and the medial-to-lateral trajectory limits the required dissection to an area no further than the lateral edge of the facet joint[38] (**Figure 9**). This can preserve innervation to the multifidus muscle and decrease intraoperative blood loss. The cortical bone trajectory also can minimize disruption of the facet joint immediately cranial to the fusion level. This trajectory can be used for all lumbar vertebrae; however, caution should be used at higher levels because the pars interarticularis becomes thinner and the pedicle diameter is smaller, which substantially increases the technical difficulty of screw placement and theoretically increases the risk of pars fracture or inadvertent cortical perforation.[38]

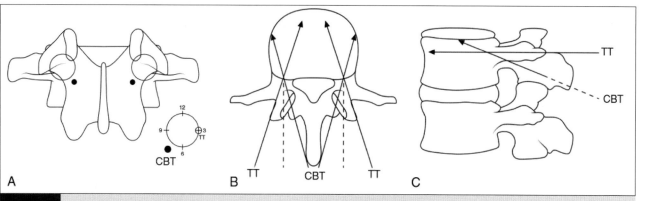

Figure 9 Axial (**A**) and sagittal (**B**) illustration demonstrating the trajectories for medial to lateral cortical bone trajectory (CBT) screws and traditional trajectory (TT) pedicle screws. (Reproduced from Tortolani PJ, Stroh DA: Cortical bone trajectory technique for posterior spinal instrumentation. *J Am Acad Orthop Surg* 2016;24[11]:755-761.)

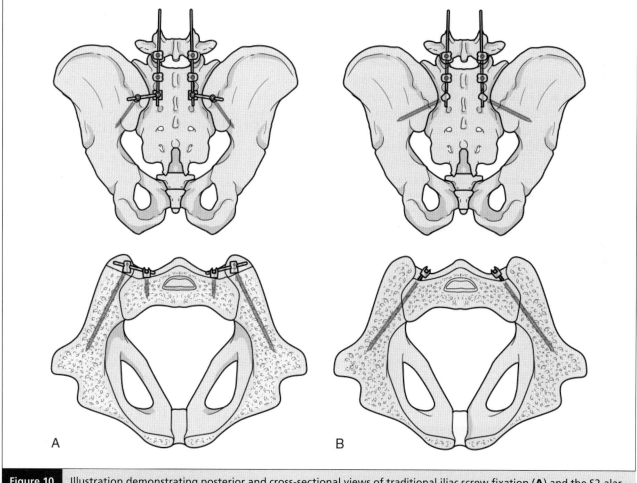

Figure 10 Illustration demonstrating posterior and cross-sectional views of traditional iliac screw fixation (**A**) and the S2-alar-iliac trajectory (**B**).

Techniques using facet and translaminar screws were originally described decades ago; however, the use of these techniques in posterior fixation has recently received renewed attention. Although facet and translaminar screws do not provide rigidity equivalent to that of pedicle screws, successful outcomes have been reported when these alternative screw techniques were used as adjuncts in anterior interbody fusion.[39]

1: Spine Anatomy and Biomechanics

Iliac Fixation

Obtaining stable fixation and successful fusion across the lumbosacral junction in long multilevel constructs historically has been challenging for spine surgeons because of the largely cancellous nature of the S1 and S2 pedicles and the substantial forces concentrated on the transition zone from the mobile spine to the relatively rigid pelvis. The addition of pelvic fixation overcomes this challenge by placing fixation across the center of rotation of the pelvis and out of the plane of the remainder of the instrumentation. Initially, the Galveston technique involved the placement of an L-shaped rod between the tables of the ilium.[40] With the advent of modern segmental instrumentation, the technique evolved to use screw fixation within the ilium.

Currently, multiple techniques are available to achieve fixation to the pelvis. Classic iliac fixation uses a starting point in or just medial to the posterior superior iliac spine. A long, large diameter screw is then inserted between the tables of the ilium in a caudal (20°-45°) and lateral (30°-45°) trajectory. Although this technique is relatively straightforward, it requires lateral connectors to join to the medial pedicle screw construct. Iliac screws are commonly removed because of symptomatic prominence. A more medial starting point on the posterior superior iliac spine can reduce implant prominence but makes connection of the remainder of the construct more difficult. Recently, an S2 starting point that is 2 to 4 mm lateral and 4 to 8 mm caudal to the S1 foramen and a trajectory proceeding through the sacral ala into the pelvis has gained popularity[41] (**Figure 10**). In this S2-alar-iliac technique, the screw tulips are aligned with the remainder of the construct and are unlikely to be symptomatically prominent; however, because the screws cross the sacroiliac joint, irritation or degeneration of the sacroiliac joint can result. Recent evidence suggests that the technique is associated with a lower revision rate.[42] Biomechanical evaluation of both traditional iliac fixation or S2-alar-iliac screw fixation has not demonstrated significant differences in stiffness or load to failure.[43]

Summary

Although the anatomy of the spine has not changed, the understanding of the relationships between the structures that make up the spine and the changes in these structures caused by aging, degeneration, and injury has advanced considerably in recent years. This understanding has implications in the diagnosis and treatment of spinal pathology and is essential knowledge for any surgeon treating patients with common and often debilitating spinal disorders and injuries.

Key Study Points

- A detailed knowledge of spine anatomy is a prerequisite for safe and effective nonsurgical and surgical treatment of patients with spine pathology.
- Growing evidence exists that the health and function of the multifidus muscles has an effect on clinical function in the lumbar spine.
- The freehand technique for thoracic pedicle screw instrumentation is safe and effective. In patients with spine deformity, the relationship of the great vessels to the spine may be altered.
- The morphology and degenerative state of the vertebral end plate is an important consideration when applying interbody instrumentation.
- Techniques for lumbar and lumbosacral instrumentation are evolving. Increasing evidence supports the safety and efficacy of the cortical bone screw trajectory and S2-alar-iliac fixation.

Annotated References

1. Abdel-Meguid EM: An anatomical study of the human lumbar ligamentum flavum. *Neurosciences (Riyadh)* 2008;13(1):11-16.

2. Scaal M: Early development of the vertebral column. *Semin Cell Dev Biol* 2016;49:83-91.

   The authors present a thorough and updated review of the embryology of the spine.

3. Johal J, Loukas M, Fisahn C, Chapman JR, Oskouian RJ, Tubbs RS: Hemivertebrae: A comprehensive review of embryology, imaging, classification, and management. *Childs Nerv Syst* 2016;32(11):2105-2109.

   A review on the development and classification of vertebral bony anomalies is presented.

4. Choi MK, Kim SB, Park CK, Lee SH, Jo DJ: Relation of deep paraspinal muscles' cross-sectional area of the cervical spine and bone union in anterior cervical decompression and fusion: A retrospective study. *World Neurosurg* 2016;96:91-100.

   This MRI study demonstrated that the increased cervical extensor cross-sectional area is associated with higher fusion rate after anterior cervical diskectomy and fusion.

5. Kim CW: Scientific basis of minimally invasive spine surgery: Prevention of multifidus muscle injury during posterior lumbar surgery. *Spine (Phila Pa 1976)* 2010;35(26suppl):S281-S286.

6. Smuck M, Crisostomo RA, Demirjian R, Fitch DS, Kennedy DJ, Geisser ME: Morphologic changes in the lumbar spine after lumbar medial branch radiofrequency neurotomy: A quantitative radiological study. *Spine J* 2015;15(6):1415-1421.

   This retrospective, MRI-based study demonstrated a significant increase in the severity of disk degeneration after radiofrequency medial branch neurotomy compared with degeneration at nonablated levels. No change in the multifidus cross-sectional area or facet deterioration was reported.

7. Goubert D, Oosterwijck JV, Meeus M, Danneels L: Structural changes of lumbar muscles in non-specific low back pain: A systematic review. *Pain Physician* 2016;19(7):E985-E1000.

   The cross-sectional area and fat content of paraspinal musculature in patients with chronic recurrent and acute low back pain was examined. The most consistent finding was paraspinal muscle atrophy (specifically in the multifidus) in patients with chronic low back pain.

8. Kim JY, Ryu DS, Paik HK, et al: Paraspinal muscle, facet joint, and disc problems: Risk factors for adjacent segment degeneration after lumbar fusion. *Spine J* 2016;16(7):867-875.

   This case-control study demonstrated that a higher body mass index, preexisting facet and intervertebral disk degeneration, paraspinal muscle atrophy, and fatty infiltration are risk factors for adjacent-segment degeneration.

9. Kim CW, Siemionow K, Anderson DG, Phillips FM: The current state of minimally invasive spine surgery. *Instr Course Lect* 2011;60:353-370.

   A review of the basis for and techniques used in minimally invasive spine surgery procedures is presented. Both potential advantages and limitations are addressed.

10. Kuntz C IV, Levin LS, Ondra SL, Shaffrey CI, Morgan CJ: Neutral upright sagittal spinal alignment from the occiput to the pelvis in asymptomatic adults: A review and resynthesis of the literature. *J Neurosurg Spine* 2007;6(2):104-112.

11. Glassman SD, Bridwell K, Dimar JR, Horton W, Berven S, Schwab F: The impact of positive sagittal balance in adult spinal deformity. *Spine (Phila Pa 1976)* 2005;30(18):2024-2029.

12. Le Huec JC, Demezon H, Aunoble S: Sagittal parameters of global cervical balance using EOS imaging: Normative values from a prospective cohort of asymptomatic volunteers. *Eur Spine J* 2015;24(1):63-71.

    This radiographic cohort study analyzed the sagittal balance of healthy volunteers and the relationship of cervical lordosis to newly defined cranial parameters, including the cranial incidence, which is analogous to pelvic incidence in the lumbosacral spine.

13. Hey HW, Teo AQ, Tan K-A, et al: How the spine differs in standing and in sitting: Important considerations for correction of spinal deformity. *Spine J* 2016;S1529-9430(16)30028-6.

    The authors compared sagittal alignment and pelvic parameters in 58 patients with back pain of less than 3 months' duration that resulted in no substantial deformity in the standing or sitting positions. When seated, there was a reduction in lumbar lordosis and thoracic kyphosis with forward displacement of the sagittal vertical axis and increased pelvic tilt and cervical lordosis compared with those parameters when standing.

14. Mac-Thiong J-M, Roussouly P, Berthonnaud E, Guigui P: Sagittal parameters of global spinal balance: Normative values from a prospective cohort of seven hundred nine Caucasian asymptomatic adults. *Spine (Phila Pa 1976)* 2010;35(22):E1193-E1198.

15. Radcliff KE, Hussain MM, Moldavsky M, et al: In vitro biomechanics of the craniocervical junction-a sequential sectioning of its stabilizing structures. *Spine J* 2015;15(7):1618-1628.

    Modern robotic testing with pure moments and six degrees of freedom were used during serial sectioning of the ligaments of the occipitocervical complex. Results emphasize the importance of the occipitoatlantal joint capsules in restraining occipitoatlantal motion and reaffirm the primary role of the cruciate ligament in atlantoaxial stability.

16. Chaput CD, Walgama J, Torres E, et al: Defining and detecting missed ligamentous injuries of the occipitocervical complex. *Spine (Phila Pa 1976)* 2011;36(9):709-714.

    The authors report on a retrospective CT-based study of occipitocervical complex injuries in patients with polytrauma at a level 1 trauma center. The injuries were not initially diagnosed on the neuroradiology report. It was determined that no injuries would be missed using the criteria of a basion-dens interval greater than 10 mm and a lateral mass interval of 4 mm or greater to define occipitocervical complex injuries.

17. Radcliff K, Kepler C, Reitman C, Harrop J, Vaccaro A: CT and MRI-based diagnosis of craniocervical dislocations: The role of the occipitoatlantal ligament. *Clin Orthop Relat Res* 2012;470(6):1602-1613.

    Using retrospective CT and MRI data, the authors defined two distinct atlantoaxial injury patterns: type I, isolated atlantoaxial injuries with an intact occipitoatlantal capsule and type II injuries, combined occipitoatlantal-atlantoaxial injuries, which are associated with a higher rate of complete spinal cord injury.

18. Zibis AH, Mitrousias V, Baxevanidou K, Hantes M, Karachalios T, Arvanitis D: Anatomical variations of the foramen transversarium in cervical vertebrae: Findings, review of the literature, and clinical significance during cervical spine surgery. *Eur Spine J* 2016;25(12):4132-4139.

    This anatomic study using cadaver skeletons demonstrated significant variation in the size and position of the foramen transversarium of the cervical spine.

1: Spine Anatomy and Biomechanics

19. Paramore CG, Dickman CA, Sonntag VK: The anatomical suitability of the C1-2 complex for transarticular screw fixation. *J Neurosurg* 1996;85(2):221-224.

20. Schulz R, Macchiavello N, Fernández E, et al: Harms C1-C2 instrumentation technique: Anatomo-surgical guide. *Spine (Phila Pa 1976)* 2011;36(12):945-950.

    Pertinent anatomy for C1-C2 posterior instrumentation using the Harms technique is reviewed.

21. Ezra D, Masharawi Y, Salame K, Slon V, Alperovitch-Najenson D, Hershkovitz I: Demographic aspects in cervical vertebral bodies' size and shape (C3-C7): A skeletal study. *Spine J* 2017;17(1):135-142.

    Results of a cross-sectional cadaver study to establish normative values for the size and shape of cervical vertebrae (C3-C7) are presented.

22. Katonis P, Papadakis SA, Galanakos S, et al: Lateral mass screw complications: Analysis of 1662 screws. *J Spinal Disord Tech* 2011;24(7):415-420.

    A retrospective review of 225 patients who underwent posterior cervical lateral mass instrumentation found that revision surgery was required in 6.2% of the patients because of nerve injury, hematoma formation, pseudarthrosis, or screw pullout.

23. Xu R, Haman SP, Ebraheim NA, Yeasting RA: The anatomic relation of lateral mass screws to the spinal nerves: A comparison of the Magerl, Anderson, and An techniques. *Spine (Phila Pa 1976)* 1999;24(19):2057-2061.

24. Yoshihara H, Passias PG, Errico TJ: Screw-related complications in the subaxial cervical spine with the use of lateral mass versus cervical pedicle screws: A systematic review. *J Neurosurg Spine* 2013;19(5):614-623.

    This systematic review of the literature compared the complications of posterior cervical lateral mass fixation and pedicle screw fixation. A low rate of vertebral artery injury was reported with pedicle screw fixation, but the rate was higher than that of lateral mass screw fixation.

25. Kaur K, Singh R, Prasath V, Magu S, Tanwar M: Computed tomographic-based morphometric study of thoracic spine and its relevance to anaesthetic and spinal surgical procedures. *J Clin Orthop Trauma* 2016;7(2):101-108.

    A CT-based study of 50 patients (600 thoracic vertebrae) without spine disorders was undertaken to determine normative anatomic data for pedicle width, length, and height; transverse pedicle angles; chord length; canal dimensions; body width and height; spinous process angle; and transverse process length.

26. Vaccaro AR, Rizzolo SJ, Allardyce TJ, et al: Placement of pedicle screws in the thoracic spine: Part I. Morphometric analysis of the thoracic vertebrae. *J Bone Joint Surg Am* 1995;77(8):1193-1199.

27. Misenhimer GR, Peek RD, Wiltse LL, Rothman SL, Widell EH Jr: Anatomic analysis of pedicle cortical and cancellous diameter as related to screw size. *Spine (Phila Pa 1976)* 1989;14(4):367-372.

28. Cho SK, Skovrlj B, Lu Y, Caridi JM, Lenke LG: The effect of increasing pedicle screw size on thoracic spinal canal dimensions: An anatomic study. *Spine (Phila Pa 1976)* 2014;39(20):E1195-E1200.

    This cadaver study of 162 pedicles from 81 fresh-frozen thoracic vertebrae demonstrated that, as pedicles expand with larger screws, expansion occurs in a lateral direction in 99.3% of vertebrae. This expansion does not affect spinal canal diameter.

29. Kim YJ, Lenke LG, Bridwell KH, Cho YS, Riew KD: Free hand pedicle screw placement in the thoracic spine: Is it safe? *Spine (Phila Pa 1976)* 2004;29(3):333-342, discussion 342.

30. Vialle R, Zeller R, Gaines RW: The "slide technique": An improvement on the "funnel technique" for safe pedicle screw placement in the thoracic spine. *Eur Spine J* 2014;23(suppl 4):S452-S456.

    The authors report on a freehand technique for thoracic pedicle instrumentation. This technique takes advantage of the contrast between the column of cancellous bone within the pedicle and the cortical anterior wall of the transverse process.

31. Rosner MK, Polly DW Jr, Kuklo TR, Ondra SL: Thoracic pedicle screw fixation for spinal deformity. *Neurosurg Focus* 2003;14(1):e7.

32. Sarlak AY, Buluç L, Sarisoy HT, Memişoğlu K, Tosun B: Placement of pedicle screws in thoracic idiopathic scoliosis: A magnetic resonance imaging analysis of screw placement relative to structures at risk. *Eur Spine J* 2008;17(5):657-662.

33. Bekki H, Harimaya K, Matsumoto Y, et al: The position of the aorta relative to the vertebrae in patients with Lenke type 1 adolescent idiopathic scoliosis. *Spine (Phila Pa 1976)* 2016;41(7):585-590.

    CT images were used to identify the position of the aorta relative to the spine in Lenke type 1 adolescent idiopathic scoliosis. Type 1A and 1C curves had a high risk of aortic injury at T11 when a 40-mm screw was used, even if angular error was less than 10°.

34. Tian N-F, Huang Q-S, Zhou P, et al: Pedicle screw insertion accuracy with different assisted methods: A systematic review and meta-analysis of comparative studies. *Eur Spine J* 2011;20(6):846-859.

    The results of systematic review of comparing accuracy of pedicle screw placement with and without the assistance of image guidance are presented. Image guidance improved the accuracy of screw placement. There was no strong evidence that any one specific navigation system was superior to another.

35. Liu J, Hao L, Suyou L, et al: Biomechanical properties of lumbar endplates and their correlation with MRI findings of lumbar degeneration. *J Biomech* 2016;49(4):586-593.

   This cadaver study demonstrated an increase in strength and stiffness of lumbar end plates from the center to the periphery, and in more caudal vertebrae. An inverse relationship between the grade of degeneration and end plate strength and stiffness was shown.

36. Dolan P, Luo J, Pollintine P, Landham PR, Stefanakis M, Adams MA: Intervertebral disc decompression following endplate damage: Implications for disc degeneration depend on spinal level and age. *Spine (Phila Pa 1976)* 2013;38(17):1473-1481.

   This cadaver study demonstrated that fracture of the end plate resulting from compressive overload leads to decreased nucleus pulposus pressures and increases stress in the posterior anulus. The effect was more severe at higher spinal levels and in older patients.

37. Kimura H, Shikata J, Odate S, Soeda T, Yamamura S: Risk factors for cage retropulsion after posterior lumbar interbody fusion: Analysis of 1070 cases. *Spine (Phila Pa 1976)* 2012;37(13):1164-1169.

   A retrospective review of 1,070 patients who underwent single- or multi-level posterior lumbar interbody fusion found that a pear-shaped disk space, inclusion of L5-S1, multilevel fusion, and a wide disk space with instability were risk factors for cage retropulsion.

38. Tortolani PJ, Stroh DA: Cortical bone trajectory technique for posterior spinal instrumentation. *J Am Acad Orthop Surg* 2016;24(11):755-761.

   A detailed review of the technique and current state of the evidence for the application of a cortical bone trajectory for posterior instrumentation of the lumbar spine is presented.

39. Verma K, Boniello A, Rihn J: Emerging techniques for posterior fixation of the lumbar spine. *J Am Acad Orthop Surg* 2016;24(6):357-364.

   The authors present a detailed review of the history, technique, and outcomes of various methods for posterior lumbar spine fixation, including pedicle, cortical, facet, and translaminar screws.

40. Allen BL Jr, Ferguson RL: The Galveston technique for L rod instrumentation of the scoliotic spine. *Spine (Phila Pa 1976)* 1982;7(3):276-284.

41. Kebaish KM: Sacropelvic fixation: Techniques and complications. *Spine (Phila Pa 1976)* 2010;35(25):2245-2251.

42. Elder BD, Ishida W, Lo SL, et al: Use of S2-alar-iliac screws associated with less complications than iliac screws in adult lumbosacropelvic fixation. *Spine (Phila Pa 1976)* 2017;42(3):E142-E149.

   This retrospective review of outcomes of patients treated using S2-alar-iliac fixation or traditional iliac screw fixation found that the S2-alar-iliac technique had lower rates of revision and surgical site infection than the traditional fixation technique. Similar clinical outcomes were reported for both techniques. Level of evidence: IV.

43. Burns CB, Dua K, Trasolini NA, Komatsu DE, Barsi JM: Biomechanical comparison of spinopelvic fixation constructs: Iliac screw versus S2-alar-iliac screw. *Spine Deform* 2016;4(1):10-15.

   This cadaver biomechanical study reported no statistical difference in stiffness and load-to-failure between S2-alar-iliac screws and traditional iliac screw fixation.

Chapter 2

Spine Neuroanatomy and Physiology

Joseph S. Butler, PhD, FRCS   Mark F. Kurd, MD

Abstract

A basic knowledge of spine neuroanatomy and physiology is required for the effective evaluation of spine pathology. It is helpful to be familiar with the applied neuroanatomy and physiology of the spine and understand the correlation of clinical signs and symptoms with relevant pathology. A stepwise approach to the diagnosis of spine pathology can aid in providing optimal patient care.

Keywords: neuroanatomy; neurophysiology; spinal cord; spine

Introduction

The spinal cord plays a fundamental role in sensory, motor, and autonomic control of the human body. Physicians who treat patients with spine disorders must have a basic understanding of the neuroanatomy and physiology of the spine to recognize, accurately diagnose, and manage pathologic spinal conditions.

Dr. Kurd or an immediate family member has served as a paid consultant to Stryker; has stock or stock options held in Duratap; has received research or institutional support from Innovative Surgical Designs; and serves as a board member, owner, officer, or committee member of the International Society for the Advancement of Spine Surgery. Neither Dr. Butler nor any immediate family member has received anything of value from or has stock or stock options held in a commercial company or institution related directly or indirectly to the subject of this chapter.

Spinal Cord Structure

The spinal cord provides both motor and sensory function. The cerebral cortex, internal capsule, corticospinal tracts, pyramidal tracts, and anterior horns cells control motor function. It is believed that 90% of the pyramidal tract crosses at the medulla to the contralateral lateral corticospinal fasciculus, where the tracts controlling the upper extremities lie medial to those controlling the lower extremities.[1] An understanding of this neuroanatomy has relevance for central cord syndrome, a clinical condition that predominantly affects the medial tracts of the lateral corticospinal fasciculus, which controls motor function to the upper extremities, with relative sparing of the most-lateral tracts, which primarily control motor function to the lower extremities.[1]

The posterior columns, the lateral spinothalamic fasciculus, and the anterior spinothalamic fasciculus control sensory function. The posterior columns are responsible for tactile discrimination, proprioception, and vibration sense. The sensory tracts decussate to the opposite side in the medulla oblongata on their pathway to the sensory cortex.

In anterior cord syndrome, posterior column function is preserved. The lateral spinothalamic fasciculus is responsible for temperature, light touch, and pain. Most fibers appear to decussate at the ventral commissure to the opposite side, ascending in the lateral spinothalamic tract. Brown-Séquard syndrome is a clinical condition associated with contralateral pain and loss of temperature sensation and ipsilateral proprioception. The anterior spinothalamic funiculus is responsible for crude touch, which is spared in the setting of posterior cord syndrome.[1]

The anterior and posterior spinal arteries provide vascularity to the spinal cord. The anterior spinal artery is the primary vessel supplying vascularity to the anterior and central aspects of the spinal cord in the cervical region.[1] At the brain stem, the vertebral arteries give rise to two medullary feeder vessels. The thoracolumbar region receives

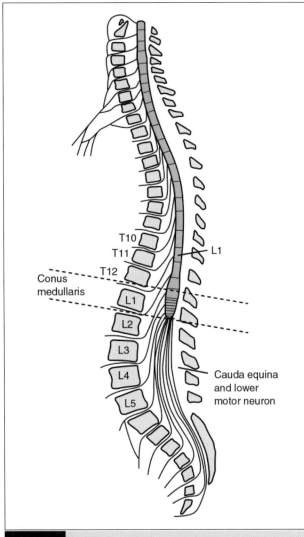

T10
T11
T12
Conus
medullaris
L1
L1
L2
L3
L4
L5
Cauda equina
and lower
motor neuron

Figure 1 Illustration of the spinal cord and nerve roots. The spinal cord emerges from the foramen magnum as a continuation of the medulla oblongata and ends in a cone-shaped structure known as the conus medullaris. The location of the conus medullaris is usually at the L1-2 intervertebral disk in adults.

spinal cord veins lie anterior and posterior to the cord. These vessels, in turn, drain into the extradural, valveless Batson venous plexus. This plexus plays an important role in the etiology of pyogenic spinal infection and the dissemination of metastatic disease.[1]

The termination of the spinal cord is at the L1-L2 level in the tapering conus medullaris (**Figure 1**). The spinal cord is 45 cm in length, with 25 cm of filum terminale.[1] It has a mean diameter of 10 mm and increases in length by approximately 10% with flexion. The spinal cord has two areas of enlargement—one area to supply innervation to the upper extremities and one area for the lower extremities.[3] It increases in size at each level caudal to C1 until approximately the level of C5, where it attains maximal cross-sectional area. At the thoracolumbar junction, it enlarges again before rapidly decreasing in size in the region of the conus medullaris.

The spinal cord is made of central gray matter and peripheral white matter (**Figure 2**). The gray matter comprises efferent neuron cell bodies. Somatosensory function is controlled by the posterior horns, somatomotor function is controlled by the anterior horns, and visceral function is controlled by the intermediolateral horns. The gray matter also acts as the center for somatic reflexes. The white matter contains nerve fibers and glia. The posterior column is composed of the fasciculus cuneatus and fasciculus gracilis; the lateral column consists of the descending motor lateral corticospinal and lateral spinothalamic fasciculi; and the anterior funiculus carries the ascending anterior spinothalamic tract and several descending tracts[1] (**Figure 3**).

Spinal Meninges

The outermost protective layer surrounding the spinal cord is the dura mater. The leptomeninx is made up of the pia mater and the arachnoid mater, which is a transparent sheet containing cerebrospinal fluid (**Figure 4**). The dentate ligaments connect the spinal cord to the dura. The space in the spinal canal between vertebral bone and dura mater is known as the epidural space. The diameter of this space is 2 mm at the level of L3-L4, 4 mm at L4-L5, and 6 mm at L5-S1.[1] The dura/arachnoid mater terminates between S1-S2 and S2-S3, where it surrounds the filum terminale and has a coccygeal attachment.

Spinal Nerves

There are 31 pairs of spinal nerves—8 in the cervical region, 12 in the thoracic region, 5 in the lumbar region, 5 in the sacrum, and 1 in the coccyx. The structure of

its vascular supply from the anterior spinal artery and two posterior spinal arteries.[2] In the cervicothoracic junction region, blood is supplied to the spinal cord by the superior intercostal artery, which is a feeder vessel of the deep cervical artery arising from the right subclavian artery.[2] Several segmental vessels provide a tenuous blood supply for the upper thoracic cord, with a watershed critical zone existing between T4 and T10.[1] One of these arteries, the artery of Adamkiewicz, arises from the left posterior intercostal artery at T10 in 80% of cases. In other cases, its origin ranges from T5 to L5.[1]

The azygous and hemiazygous venous systems provide the primary venous drainage for the spinal cord. The

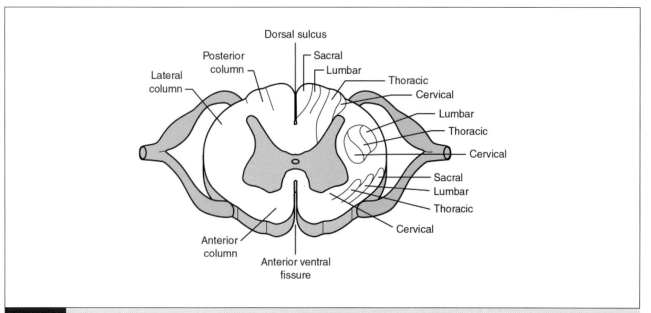

Figure 2   Cross-sectional illustration of the spinal cord with the outer white matter and the inner gray matter. The white matter of the spinal cord contains nerve fibers and glia and is divided into three columns: posterior, lateral, and anterior.

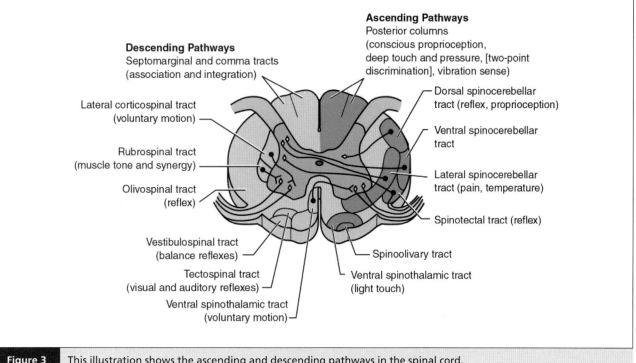

Figure 3   This illustration shows the ascending and descending pathways in the spinal cord.

each spinal root consists of motor and sensory rootlets, a dorsal root ganglion, and a spinal nerve. The sympathetic nervous system is supplied by myelinated preganglionic rami and unmyelinated postganglionic rami. Important branches of the spinal nerve include the sinuvertebral nerve, which supplies the anulus fibrosus of the intervertebral disk, and the dorsal ramus, which supplies the facet joints and posterior paraspinal musculature. The intervertebral disk in the lumbar region receives innervation from the sympathetic fibers anteriorly and the sinuvertebral

1: Spine Anatomy and Biomechanics

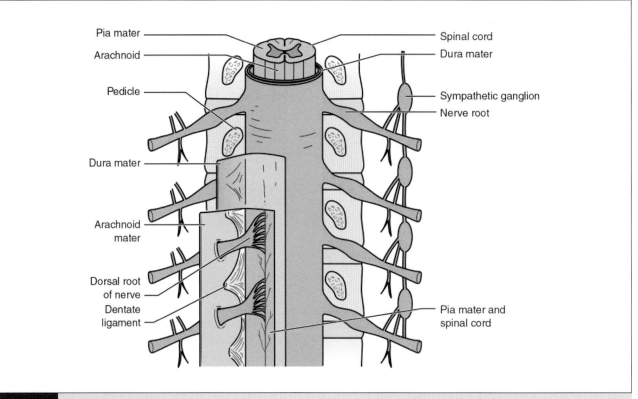

Pia mater — Spinal cord
Arachnoid — Dura mater
Pedicle — Sympathetic ganglion
— Nerve root
Dura mater —
Arachnoid mater —
Dorsal root of nerve —
Dentate ligament — Pia mater and spinal cord

Figure 4	Cross-sectional illustration of the spinal cord and meninges. The spinal cord is covered by the pia mater, which is the outer lining of the cord, and transparent arachnoid mater that contains the cerebrospinal fluid. The dura mater is the outer covering of the spinal cord. The spinal cord is anchored to the dura by the dentate ligaments that project laterally from the lateral side of the cord to the arachnoid and dura mater at points midway between exiting spinal nerves.

nerve posteriorly. The sinuvertebral nerves innervate the posterior longitudinal ligament, the posterior portion of the anulus fibrosus, the ventral aspect of the dura mater, and the superior portion of the intervertebral disk. The dorsal primary rami give off medial, lateral, and, occasionally, intermediate branches. The facets joints, interspinous ligaments, and segmental muscles are supplied by the medial branch, with the iliocostalis and longissimus muscles supplied by the lateral and intermediate branches, respectively.

When considering the anatomic pathway of the spinal nerves, it is important to be aware of regional variations. In the cervical spine, the C1 nerve arises above the C1 vertebra, whereas the C8 nerve arises above the T1 vertebra. Conversely, in the thoracic and lumbar spine, the spinal nerve passes under the pedicle of the same-numbered vertebra.[1] The spinal nerves emerge within the intervertebral foramina. In the cervical spine, no intervertebral foramina exist for C1 and C2; in the remaining subaxial spine, the C3-C8 nerve roots emerge through the corresponding intervertebral foramina to occupy approximately 75% of their respective

foramen.[2] Thoracic nerves are much smaller, occupying only 20% of their foramen. Lumbar spinal nerves are larger, occupying approximately 33% of the neural foramen, and emerge obliquely under their respective pedicles.[1] In the sacral region, the anterior and posterior rami exit the sacrum through their respective anterior and posterior foramina.[1]

The motor and sensory function of the spinal cord is distributed into distinct dermatomes (sensory) and myotomes (motor) (Figure 5). The C4 nerve supplies motor function to the muscles to allow spontaneous breathing and actions such as shoulder shrugging. C5 controls deltoid and biceps function, C6 wrist extension, C7 triceps and wrist flexion, C8 finger flexion, and T1 the hand intrinsic muscles. In the lumbar region, L2 controls iliopsoas function, L3 quadriceps function, L4 tibialis anterior function, and L5 extensor hallucis longus function. In the sacral region, S1 controls the gastrocnemius, S2 the bladder sphincter, and S3 the anal sphincter. When considering sensory function, C5 supplies the upper outer arm, C6 the thumb, C7 the long finger, C8 the little finger, T1 the medial forearm, T10 the

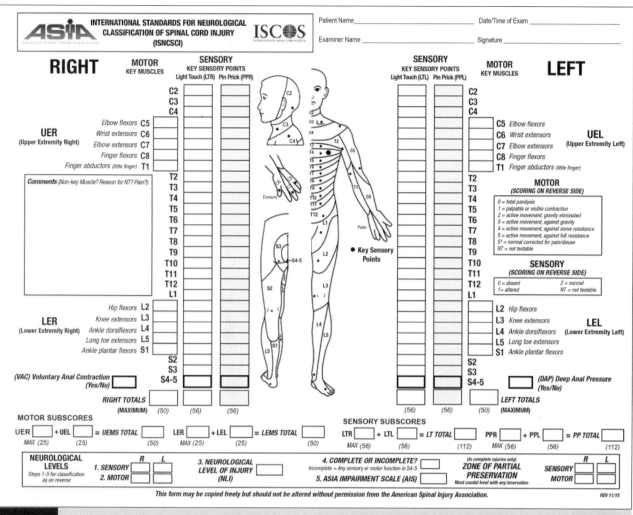

Figure 5 Illustration of the International Standards for Neurological Classification of Spinal Cord Injury and the American Spinal Injury Association (ASIA) Impairment Scale. ASIA scores provide a good format for dermatome and myotome assessment. (Reproduced with permission from the American Spinal Injury Association International Standards Committee: *International Standards for Neurological Classification of Spinal Cord Injury.* Available at: http://asia-spinalinjury.org/committees/international-standards/. Accessed June 1, 2017.)

periumbilical area, L1 the groin region, L2 the anterior thigh, L3 the knee, L4 the medial malleolus, L5 the great toe, S1 the small toe, S2 the posterior thigh, and S3-S5 the perianal region.

A variety of nerve root anomalies exist, and it is important to recognize them to avoid neural injury during surgery. These anomalies have been divided into type I, involving an intradural anastomosis; type II, involving an abnormal nerve root origin; type III, involving an extradural anastomosis; and type IV, involving an extradural division.[4]

Nerve root vascularization is a complex process. Both the proximal and distal radicular arteries anastomose at the proximal one-third of the spinal nerve root within the foramen, leading to a region of potential vascular insufficiency. Intrinsic vasculature includes interfascicular and intrafascicular vessels. The innermost pia mater permits exchange of metabolites within the cerebrospinal fluid. The mechanical compression of a nerve root can result in vascular compression, which can lead to the development of the classic symptoms of radiculopathy.

The cauda equina is an organized structure containing the lumbar and sacral nerve roots, and several of the spinal nerve roots are organized into plexus structures. The cervical plexus is composed of the ventral rami of C1-C4; the brachial plexus is formed by the anterior rami of C5-T1; and the sacral plexus is made up of the lumbosacral trunk (L4, L5) and the S1, S2, S3, and S4 anterior rami.[1]

Muscle Function Grading

0 = total paralysis

1 = palpable or visible contraction

2 = active movement, full range of motion (ROM) with gravity eliminated

3 = active movement, full ROM against gravity

4 = active movement, full ROM against gravity and moderate resistance in a muscle specific position

5 = (normal) active movement, full ROM against gravity and full resistance in a functional muscle position expected from an otherwise unimpaired person

5* = (normal) active movement, full ROM against gravity and sufficient resistance to be considered normal if identified inhibiting factors (i.e. pain, disuse) were not present

NT = not testable (i.e. due to immobilization, severe pain such that the patient cannot be graded, amputation of limb, or contracture of > 50% of the normal ROM)

Sensory Grading

0 = Absent

1 = Altered, either decreased/impaired sensation or hypersensitivity

2 = Normal

NT = Not testable

When to Test Non-Key Muscles:

In a patient with an apparent AIS B classification, non-key muscle functions more than 3 levels below the motor level on each side should be tested to most accurately classify the injury (differentiate between AIS B and C).

Movement	Root level
Shoulder: Flexion, extension, abduction, adduction, internal and external rotation **Elbow:** Supination	C5
Elbow: Pronation **Wrist:** Flexion	C6
Finger: Flexion at proximal joint, extension. **Thumb:** Flexion, extension and abduction in plane of thumb	C7
Finger: Flexion at MCP joint **Thumb:** Opposition, adduction and abduction perpendicular to palm	C8
Finger: Abduction of the index finger	T1
Hip: Adduction	L2
Hip: External rotation	L3
Hip: Extension, abduction, internal rotation **Knee:** Flexion **Ankle:** Inversion and eversion **Toe:** MP and IP extension	L4
Hallux and Toe: DIP and PIP flexion and abduction	L5
Hallux: Adduction	S1

ASIA Impairment Scale (AIS)

A = Complete. No sensory or motor function is preserved in the sacral segments S4-5.

B = Sensory Incomplete. Sensory but not motor function is preserved below the neurological level and includes the sacral segments S4-5 (light touch or pin prick at S4-5 or deep anal pressure) AND no motor function is preserved more than three levels below the motor level on either side of the body.

C = Motor Incomplete. Motor function is preserved at the most caudal sacral segments for voluntary anal contraction (VAC) OR the patient meets the criteria for sensory incomplete status (sensory function preserved at the most caudal sacral segments (S4-S5) by LT, PP or DAP), and has some sparing of motor function more than three levels below the ipsilateral motor level on either side of the body.
(This includes key or non-key muscle functions to determine motor incomplete status.) For AIS C – less than half of key muscle functions below the single NLI have a muscle grade ≥ 3.

D = Motor Incomplete. Motor incomplete status as defined above, with at least half (half or more) of key muscle functions below the single NLI having a muscle grade ≥ 3.

E = Normal. If sensation and motor function as tested with the ISNCSCI are graded as normal in all segments, and the patient had prior deficits, then the AIS grade is E. Someone without an initial SCI does not receive an AIS grade.

Using ND: To document the sensory, motor and NLI levels, the ASIA Impairment Scale grade, and/or the zone of partial preservation (ZPP) when they are unable to be determined based on the examination results.

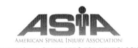

INTERNATIONAL STANDARDS FOR NEUROLOGICAL CLASSIFICATION OF SPINAL CORD INJURY

Steps in Classification

The following order is recommended for determining the classification of individuals with SCI.

1. Determine sensory levels for right and left sides.
The sensory level is the most caudal, intact dermatome for both pin prick and light touch sensation.

2. Determine motor levels for right and left sides.
Defined by the lowest key muscle function that has a grade of at least 3 (on supine testing), providing the key muscle functions represented by segments above that level are judged to be intact (graded as a 5).
Note: in regions where there is no myotome to test, the motor level is presumed to be the same as the sensory level, if testable motor function above that level is also normal.

3. Determine the neurological level of injury (NLI)
This refers to the most caudal segment of the cord with intact sensation and antigravity (3 or more) muscle function strength, provided that there is normal (intact) sensory and motor function rostrally respectively.
The NLI is the most cephalad of the sensory and motor levels determined in steps 1 and 2.

4. Determine whether the injury is Complete or Incomplete.
(i.e. absence or presence of sacral sparing)
If voluntary anal contraction = No AND all S4-5 sensory scores = 0 AND deep anal pressure = No, then injury is Complete. Otherwise, injury is Incomplete.

5. Determine ASIA Impairment Scale (AIS) Grade:

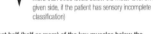

Is injury Complete? If YES, AIS=A and can record ZPP (lowest dermatome or myotome on each side with some preservation)

NO ↓

Is injury Motor Complete? If YES, AIS=B

NO ↓ (No=voluntary anal contraction OR motor function more than three levels below the motor level on a given side, if the patient has sensory incomplete classification)

Are at least half (half or more) of the key muscles below the neurological level of injury graded 3 or better?

NO ↓   YES ↓

AIS=C   AIS=D

If sensation and motor function is normal in all segments, AIS=E
Note: AIS E is used in follow-up testing when an individual with a documented SCI has recovered normal function. If at initial testing no deficits are found, the individual is neurologically intact; the ASIA Impairment Scale does not apply.

Figure 5 *(Continued)* Illustration of the International Standards for Neurological Classification of Spinal Cord Injury and the American Spinal Injury Association (ASIA) Impairment Scale. ASIA scores provide a good format for dermatome and myotome assessment. (Reproduced with permission from the American Spinal Injury Association International Standards Committee: *International Standards for Neurological Classification of Spinal Cord Injury*. Available at: http://asia-spinalinjury.org/committees/international-standards/. Accessed June 1, 2017.)

Autonomic Nervous System

The autonomic nervous system is divided into the sympathetic and parasympathetic systems. The preganglionic neurons of the sympathetic system are located between C8 and L4. The sympathetic centers control the cardiovascular and bronchopulmonary systems, sweat gland function, vasomotor activity, anorectal and bladder continence, and ejaculation. Horner syndrome is a clinical condition that can result from injury to the cervical or first thoracic sympathetic chain, which runs along the lateral borders of the vertebral body. Injury can lead to a combination of signs such as drooping of the upper eyelid (ptosis), contraction of the pupil (miosis), retraction of the eye (enophthalmos), and absence of sweating (anhidrosis). Hypogastric plexus injury (often where it lies anterior to the L1-S5 disk) can result in urogenital problems such as retrograde ejaculation. Autonomic dysreflexia results from spinal cord injury above the level of the sympathetic splanchnic outflow (T6) and leads to headache, sweating, flushing, and hypertension.

The parasympathetic nervous system controls a variety of visceral functions, including peristalsis and bladder wall contraction. The parasympathetic system also controls relaxation of certain smooth muscles such as those that regulate arterial blood flow and penile erection. Its cell bodies lie in the brainstem and sacral cord. Many visceral parasympathetic functions are carried through the vagus nerve and thus function unopposed by sympathetic outflow in cases of spinal cord injury. Disruption of the sacral signaling pathways can impair crucial autonomic functions such as bladder and defecation control and sexual arousal.[5]

Spinal Cord Tracts

The intrinsic pathways of the spinal cord establish connections between various neuronal groups and segments of the spinal cord and serve as relays between intrinsic spinal neurons and descending pathways.[5]

The ascending pathways of the spinal cord are formed by the axons of dorsal root ganglion cells, which enter the spinal cord through the dorsal roots. They subsequently enter an ascending fiber tract, such as the dorsal column pathways, which contain the fasciculus gracilis and fasciculus cuneatus. The fasciculus gracilis controls the lower trunk and lower limbs, whereas the fasciculus cuneatus controls the upper trunk and upper limbs. The dorsal pathways control a variety of discriminative sensory functions, including two-point discrimination, detection of speed, direction of movement, and assessment of cutaneous pressure.[5] Localization of pain and thermal stimuli are controlled by the spinothalamic tract. Its axons decussate to the ventrolateral column and terminate in the ventral posterolateral and central lateral nuclei of the thalamus.[5]

The corticospinal tract is the most developed tract of those in the descending pathways. It originates in the motor cortex, with its axons forming the pyramidal tract, and most of its fibers decussate in the lower medulla to form the lateral corticospinal tract. The remaining fibers remain in the ventral funiculus and subsequently decussate in the ventral commissure. The corticospinal tract exerts refined motor control through its influence on other descending spinal pathways.[6]

Spinal Cord Function

The spinal cord plays a central role in sensory, motor, and autonomic control. It controls the sensory processing of pain, temperature, touch, and proprioception. The peripheral sensory receptors are specialized sense organs that connect with axons from the dorsal root ganglion. They are called first-order neurons because they are directly linked with peripheral sensory receptors; their processing of sensory information is determined by their branching pattern (**Figure 6**). These neurons terminate and synapse on neurons in the substantia gelatinosa. In this part of the dorsal horn, the second-order neurons give rise to their processes, which carry signals to other areas of the brain and spinal cord.[2,5] Second-order neurons play an important role in processing sensory information within the spinal cord. Somatic afferent fibers, in addition to the

fibers controlling visceral sensation and pain, converge on the neurons of the substantia gelatinosa. Certain regions of the brain also supply substantial input to effect neuromodulation within the substantia gelatinosa.[7]

Specialized organs in the skin and connective tissue and free nerve endings in the dermis can sense light touch. These sense organs send signals along axons arising from the dorsal root ganglia. This signaling pathway conveying the sensation of touch is also responsible for controlling more sophisticated sensory functions such as proprioception and two-point discrimination.[5] Muscle spindles monitor muscle length, Golgi tendon organs monitor tendon stretch, and the Pacinian corpuscles monitor the pressure exerted on joints and bony structures.[5] The axons from muscle spindles, which send signals to the spinal cord, are among the largest and fastest conducting nerves in the nervous system. The central branch, making up the medial division of the dorsal root, splits after entering the spinal cord. These synapses with motor neurons allow monosynaptic reflex activity. These monosynaptic connections have a high degree of specificity, with muscle spindle afferents from a given muscle (in response to changes in muscle length and velocity) making contact only with motor neurons that innervate the muscle of origin of the afferent fiber. The monosynaptic stretch reflex is initiated by activation of the IA afferent fibers from the muscle spindle, which results in contraction of the synonymous muscle. Muscle contraction strength in response to the same stimulus is not always identical and is influenced by preceding activity of the spinal cord. The variability of reflex activity also is affected by temporal and spatial summation of excitatory inputs and inhibitory influences from other sources.

All other reflexes are considered polysynaptic, with each neuron involved in the reflex potentially contributing to the outcome, which is the motor response to a stimulus (**Figure 7**). Simple spinal reflexes demonstrate that neurons not only are excited but also can be inhibited by certain inputs. This inhibition can be postsynaptic or presynaptic. In postsynaptic inhibition, the membrane potential of the postsynaptic neuron increases, and the same excitatory input is unsuccessful in depolarizing the neuron sufficiently to initiate an action potential. In presynaptic inhibition, a reduced amount of excitatory transmitter is released from the presynaptic terminal.

Spinal Cord Lesions

When evaluating spinal cord lesions, it is important to classify the extent of the lesion. The term tetraplegia commonly refers to spinal cord injury at the cervical level, with a resultant neurologic deficit affecting the upper and

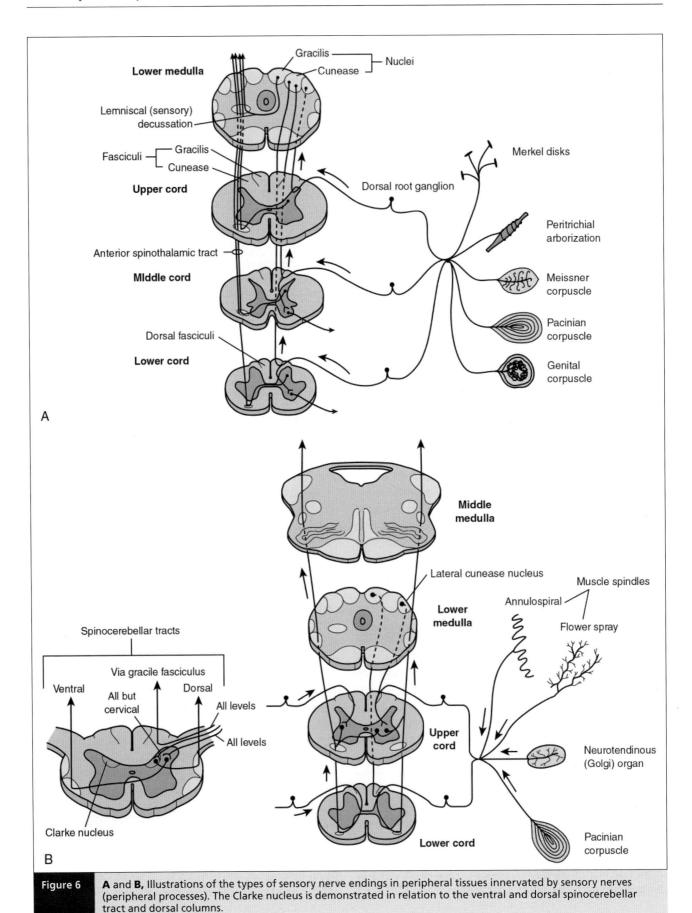

Figure 6   **A** and **B,** Illustrations of the types of sensory nerve endings in peripheral tissues innervated by sensory nerves (peripheral processes). The Clarke nucleus is demonstrated in relation to the ventral and dorsal spinocerebellar tract and dorsal columns.

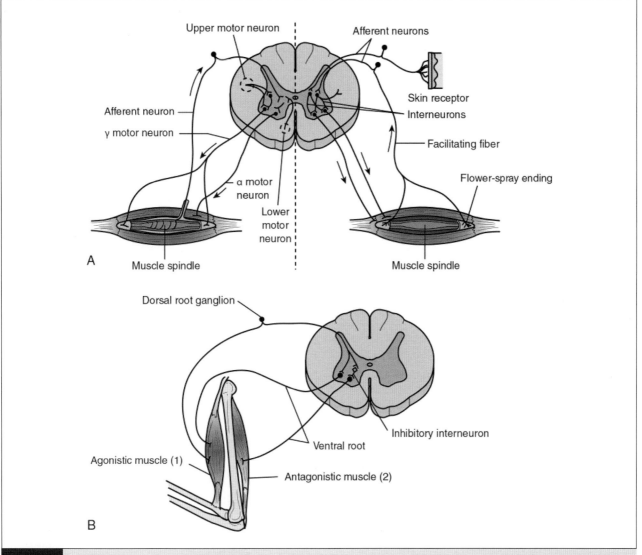

Figure 7 Illustrations show the sensory and motor innervation of muscles spindles along with a cross-section of the spinal cord with various inputs (**A**) and the reciprocal inhibition of antagonistic muscles during monosynaptic stretch reflex (**B**).

lower limbs, trunk, and pelvic organs. The term paraplegia refers to spinal cord injury at the thoracic, lumbar, or sacral levels, with a resultant neurologic deficit affecting the lower limbs and pelvic organs; upper limb function is preserved. A complete spinal cord injury indicates that there is no sparing of motor or sensory function below the affected level. In an incomplete injury, some motor or sensory function below the injury level is preserved.

Acute issues in spinal cord injury include both neurogenic and spinal shock. Neurogenic shock results in hypotension and relative bradycardia and can be fatal. It occurs as the result of circulatory collapse from loss of sympathetic tone and is attributable to disruption of the autonomic pathway within the spinal cord. This leads to lack of sympathetic tone, decreased systemic vascular resistance, pooling of blood in the limbs, and hypotension.

Spinal shock is a temporary loss of spinal cord function and reflex activity below the level of a spinal cord injury. It results in a flaccid areflexic paralysis, bradycardia, hypotension, and an absent bulbocavernosus reflex. Spinal shock occurs because of hyperpolarization of neurons that remain unresponsive to brain stimuli. It usually resolves within 48 hours.

A variety of incomplete spinal cord lesions can occur. Central cord syndrome is the most common and often affects elderly individuals who sustain a minor extension injury. It is caused by spinal cord compression and central cord edema and results in selective destruction of the white matter in the central area of the lateral corticospinal tract; the upper extremities are preferentially affected. Although central cord syndrome is associated with a good prognosis, complete functional recovery is rare.

Anterior cord syndrome presents as motor dysfunction and dissociated sensory deficit below the level of a spinal cord injury. Injury to the anterior spinal cord is often caused by direct osseous compression or damage to the anterior spinal artery. The lower extremity is affected more often than the upper extremity. Anterior cord syndrome carries the worst prognosis of all incomplete spinal cord lesions, and the effects are most likely to mimic those of a complete spinal cord injury.

Brown-Séquard syndrome results from spinal cord hemitransection, which often results from a penetrating injury. Hemitransection of the spinal cord leads to an ipsilateral deficit of the lateral corticospinal tract, which controls motor function, and a deficit in the dorsal columns, which control proprioception and vibration sense. A contralateral deficit in the lateral spinothalamic tract, which controls pain and temperature, also occurs. Brown-Séquard syndrome is associated with an excellent prognosis for functional improvement.

Posterior cord syndrome, which is very rare, results in loss of proprioception, with preservation of motor function, pain sensation, and light touch.

Summary

A thorough understanding of the basic principles of neuroanatomy and physiology is crucial for a better appreciation of the mechanisms that cause spine disorders. Knowledge of the anatomic and physiologic processes related to spinal pathology help facilitate an accurate diagnosis of spine disorders and optimal treatment for affected patients.

Key Study Points

- There are 31 pairs of spinal nerves, and the structure of each spinal root consists of motor and sensory rootlets, a dorsal root ganglion, and a spinal nerve.
- The intrinsic pathways of the spinal cord establish connections between various neuronal groups and segments of the spinal cord and serve as relays between intrinsic spinal neurons and descending pathways.
- The spinal cord plays a central role in sensory, motor, and autonomic control.

Annotated References

1. An H, Singh K: *Synopsis of Spine Surgery,* ed 2. New York, NY, Thieme Medical Publishing, 2008.

2. Jankowska E, Lundberg A: Interneurones in the spinal cord. *Trends Neurosci* 1981;4:230-233.

3. Ko HY, Park JH, Shin YB, Baek SY: Gross quantitative measurements of spinal cord segments in human. *Spinal Cord* 2004;42(1):35-40.

4. Kadish LJ, Simmons EH: Anomalies of the lumbosacral nerve roots: An anatomical investigation and myelographic study. *J Bone Joint Surg Br* 1984;66(3):411-416.

5. Nógrádi A, Vrbová G: Anatomy and physiology of the spinal cord. Madame Curie Bioscience Database 2000-2013. Available at https://www.ncbi.nlm.nih.gov/books/NBK6229/.

   This online database provides a good overview of the spinal cord, including anatomy, physiology, function, and the role of neurotransmitters and chemical messengers.

6. Kuypers HG: The descending pathways to the spinal cord, their anatomy and function. *Prog Brain Res* 1964;11:178-202.

7. Schomburg ED: Spinal sensorimotor systems and their supraspinal control. *Neurosci Res* 1990;7(4):265-340.

Chapter 3

Surgical Approaches to the Spine

Harish Kempegowda, MD   P. Justin Tortolani, MD

Abstract

Although conventional anterior and posterior surgical approaches to the spine are well established, spine surgeons are currently focusing more on minimally invasive muscle-sparing approaches to improve overall patient outcomes by limiting the morbidity associated with extensile surgical exposures. It is helpful to review conventional surgical approaches and to focus on recent developments such as lateral, oblique, and anterior approaches to the lumbar spine; minimally invasive posterior approaches to the cervical spine; and circumferential decompression of the thoracic spine through a single approach.

Keywords: complications; minimally invasive approach; patient positioning; surgical steps

Introduction

For every clinical scenario, the choice of surgical approach should be based on the underlying pathologic condition and its location. For example, if a neoplastic lesion corresponds to a vertebral body, an anterior approach may be preferred, whereas pathology affecting the posterior elements may be better treated through a posterior approach. Basic knowledge related to surgical approaches aids in

Dr. Tortolani or an immediate family member has received royalties from Globus Medical; serves as a paid consultant to Globus Medical, Innovasis, and Spineology; has received research or institutional support from Spineology; and serves as a board member, owner, officer, or committee member of MedStar Union Memorial Hospital. Neither Dr. Kempegowda nor any immediate family member has received anything of value from or has stock or stock options held in a commercial company or institution related directly or indirectly to the subject of this chapter.

performing various spinal procedures using conventional or minimally invasive techniques. Because every surgical approach to the spine has certain advantages and disadvantages, surgeons should be knowledgeable about various surgical exposures.

Anterior Smith-Robinson Approach for Cervical Spine Surgery

The anteromedial approach, which also is known as the Smith-Robinson approach, is the most common cervical approach because it allows tumor removal, abscess drainage, and performance of common procedures such as anterior cervical diskectomy and fusion, disk replacement, and corpectomy, all of which most frequently affect the subaxial spine (C3-C7).[1]

Preoperative and Positioning Consideration

An evaluation of the skin on the anterior and anterolateral aspect of the neck is strongly recommended along with an evaluation of the bilateral carotid arteries, previous incisions, and the thyroid gland. It is preferable that these evaluations be performed in the clinic for patients undergoing elective surgery. The anteromedial approach is performed with the patient supine, with his or her head slightly rotated in the direction opposite from the side of the approach. If additional extension is safe, a small bump may be placed between the patient's shoulder blades. The patient's arms are tucked to the sides of his or her body, and chin strap or cervical tong traction may be used. Although a left-sided approach is preferred, the decision regarding the side of the approach is critical only in patients in whom previous anterior cervical exposures have been performed. Although some surgeons prefer to use the previous scar tissue in all cases, if the recurrent laryngeal nerve was injured during initial surgery, use of the previous incision is strongly advocated to avoid contralateral recurrent laryngeal nerve injury.[2]

Surgical Steps

A 3-cm transverse skin incision, made from the midline, is centered over the affected vertebral level or, alternatively, over the skin crease nearest to the target vertebra.[3] Skin hooks are used to lift the incised edges, and the dermal and subcutaneous fat layers are then cut using electrocautery to reach the platysma. Skin flaps are created using Metzenbaum scissors. The platysma is divided in line with the skin incision, and a plane is then developed deep to the platysma, which helps define the medial border of the sternocleidomastoid muscle. The investing fascial layer is separated and then incised using scissors. The carotid artery is palpated, and an appendiceal retractor is placed medially to retract the trachea and the esophagus. The prevertebral fascia is thinned using two peanut dissectors on the anterior vertebral surface. A spinal needle is placed in the disk space, and a lateral radiograph is obtained to confirm the level. The medial surface of the longus colli is exposed, and a portion of the muscle corresponding to the target disk space is elevated using bipolar cautery. Horner syndrome is a rare complication that occurs secondary to a sympathetic plexus injury and can be avoided by keeping the dissection medial to the longus colli muscle.[4] A Caspar retractor is used for craniocaudal distraction of the disk space.

Complications

Complications related to the anteromedial surgical exposure include dysphagia, dysphonia (damage to the recurrent laryngeal nerve or the superior laryngeal nerve), hematoma, esophageal damage, Horner syndrome, and vascular injury.[5,6]

Anterior Exposure of the Upper Cervical Spine

The anterior exposure of the upper cervical spine (C1-C3) can be performed using the transoral approach or the anterior retropharyngeal approach.

Transoral Approach

The transoral approach provides direct access to C1 and C2.[7] The procedure is performed with the patient supine and his or her arms tucked at the sides. The elbows should be well padded. The table is placed in the Trendelenburg position to avoid aspiration of surgical debris. Endotracheal intubation is preferred over nasal intubation because the endotracheal tube can be easily moved laterally away from the operating field. Maintaining balloon integrity of the endotracheal tube is crucial. A self-retaining rectangular retractor that allows depression of the tongue and retraction of the uvula superiorly is used. Superiorly, the C1 anterior tubercle is palpated, and the level is confirmed fluoroscopically before an incision is made. A No. 10 blade is used to make an incision on the pharynx vertically, and the entire soft-tissue layer then is stripped off subperiosteally, including the anterior longitudinal ligament, until the lateral masses of C1 and C2 are evident. After the procedure has been completed, watertight closure of the soft tissues is performed in two layers.

Complications associated with the transoral approach include infection, aspiration, breakage of teeth, and laceration of the tongue or other soft-tissue structures.[7]

Anterior Retropharyngeal Approach

The anterior retropharyngeal approach, which provides access from the occiput to C3, is entirely extramucosal and confers less risk of wound infection. This approach also allows placement of bone graft, if required.[8-11] The procedure is performed with the patient supine with skeletal traction or chin strap traction. The skin incision extends from the mastoid process to the hyoid bone in the midline. Because the encountered neurovascular structures are symmetric, the side of the approach depends on surgeon preference and pathology. The platysma is identified and incised along the line of the skin incision. Deep to the platysma muscle, the parotid and submandibular glands are located. At this stage of the procedure, it is important to identify three important neurovascular structures—the marginal mandibular nerve, deep to the parotid gland; the retromandibular vein, at the middle portion of the parotid; and the common facial vein, at the angle of the jaw.[8] Both veins are ligated at their junctions with the internal jugular vein, and the dissection is deepened to define the medial border of the sternocleidomastoid. The submandibular gland is excised, and its duct is ligated to prevent fistula formation. The stylohyoid and the digastric muscles are identified and tagged and then detached from the hyoid bone, which helps in lateral retraction of the hyoid and the trachea/larynx. Care should be taken to avoid damage to the hypoglossal nerve, which lies deep to the detached muscles. The dissection is further deepened in the plane between the carotid sheath laterally and the esophagus/larynx medially. The following seven critical structures are identified and ligated in a cranial to caudal direction: the facial artery and vein, the ascending pharyngeal artery and vein, the superior laryngeal artery, and the superior thyroid artery and vein.[9,10] Peanut dissectors are used to thin the prevertebral fascia between the longus colli muscles. After performing the required procedures, the wound is closed over a drain and the digastric and stylohyoid tendons are repaired.

Possible complications of the anterior retropharyngeal approach include injury to the esophagus, hypopharynx, or the neurovascular structures previously mentioned.

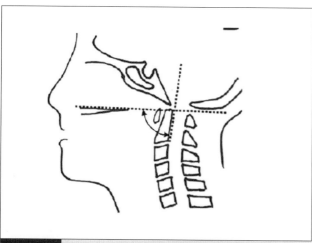

Figure 1 The angle of the craniocervical junction is made by drawing a line along the hard palate posteriorly to C2 and then placing a line along the posterior wall of C2. The mean measurement for this angle is approximately 100°. (Reproduced with permission from Takami T, Ichinose T, Ishibashi K, Goto T, Tsuyuguchi N, Ohata K: Importance of fixation angle in posterior instrumented occipitocervical fusion. *Neurol Med Chir (Tokyo)* 2008;48[6]:279-282.)

Posterior Occipitocervical Approach

The proximity of the vertebral arteries and the complex upper cervical vertebral anatomy make the posterior occipitocervical approach more challenging than most posterior approaches. This approach facilitates occiput to cervical and C1-C2 reconstruction procedures and is most commonly indicated for conditions such as trauma, rheumatoid arthritis, infections, and tumors.[12-14]

Surgical Steps

If there is no ligamentous distraction injury, Gardner-Wells tongs can be applied for traction. Some surgeons prefer to use the Mayfield head holder, whereas other surgeons prefer a moveable head holder that is available on Jackson frames or similar tables. Care should be taken to prevent fusion of the occipitocervical junction in a flexed or extended position because dysphagia, subaxial subluxation, and airway compromise can result. To assess the occipitocervical junction, the angle of the craniovertebral cervical junction provides a simple and reliable measurement (**Figure 1**). The mean angle of the craniovertebral cervical junction is 99°± 8°.[15]

The patient is turned prone on a frame with proper care and padding to avoid pressure on the eyes, face, and abdomen. The palpable landmarks, including the occipital protuberance and the C2 and C7 spinous process, are marked, and the correct level is confirmed under fluoroscopy. A midline incision is made extending from the occipital protuberance to the spinous process of C3. The superficial dissection is performed strictly in the midline to reach the ligamentum nuchae. To minimize bleeding, the ligamentum nuchae is split in the midline. The rectus capitis and oblique capitis are subperiosteally elevated from the spinous process and the lamina of C2, and attention is then turned to the occipital bone where subperiosteal dissection is performed from the midline along the inferior nuchal line. Exposure is maintained with right-angle cerebellar or Gelpi retractors proximally and distally.

The posterior tubercle of C1 is identified and subperiosteal exposure on both sides of the midline is performed using curets. The vertebral artery runs along the cranial surface of the lateral third of the posterior arch. To avoid injury to the vertebral vessels, it is necessary to stay 1 cm or less away from the midline as the superior aspect of the C1 arch is exposed.[14] In some complex clinical situations involving tumors, difficult anatomy, or C1 pedicle analog screw insertion, it may be necessary to expose the C1 arch more laterally. A study using CT angiography suggests that the vertebral artery intersects the outer cortex of the vertebral artery groove approximately 18 mm from the midline.[16] Preoperative CT angiography can help the surgeon plan for a safe amount of exposure for an individual patient. Meticulous surgical technique and avoidance of Bovie electrocautery and burring on the superior arch of C1 also are recommended. The exposure of the C1 lateral mass involves mobilizing the C2 dorsal nerve root caudally. Because this root, which lies at the junction of the posterior C1 arch and the lateral mass, is surrounded by an abundant perineural venous plexus, bleeding can make dissection in this area challenging. Bleeding usually can be controlled with the placement of small pieces of a gelatin sponge soaked with fibrin or slurry (made of gelatin powder and thrombin) along with a small cottonoid until bleeding stops; electrocautery usually is not as successful. In difficult cases, the C2 nerve root can be transected to dramatically improve visualization of the starting point on the C1 lateral mass, improve hemostasis, and allow formal débridement and packing of the C1-C2 articulation for arthrodesis[17] (**Figure 2**). Interestingly, not all patients report numbness after C2 transection. Without root transection, C2 neuralgia can occur after placement of C1 lateral mass screws in as many as 30% of cases. Alternatively, some surgeons use C1 pedicle screws with a starting point that lies on the posterior arch to avoid bleeding around and irritation of the greater occipital nerve that can result from lateral mass screw placement. Even more care and understanding of the proximity of the vertebral artery in relationship to the screw's starting point and trajectory is required.[16]

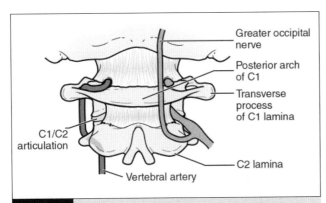

Greater occipital nerve

Posterior arch of C1

Transverse process of C1 lamina

C1/C2 articulation

C2 lamina

Vertebral artery

Figure 2 Schematic drawing depicting the posterior exposure of C1-C2. Note the position of the greater occipital nerve as it pierces the C1-C2 membrane and courses laterally and superiorly. Exposure of the C1-C2 articulation for bone grafting generally requires retraction or sectioning of this nerve. Note the position of the vertebral artery lateral to the C1-C2 articulation. Generally, the exposure does not need to be developed lateral to the lateral edge of the C2 lamina because this marks the lateral edge of the C1-C2 joint, and further lateral exposure puts the vertebral artery at risk.

Posterior Subaxial Cervical Approach in Laminoplasty and Laminectomy

The posterior approach to the subaxial cervical spine is commonly used in procedures such as laminectomy, laminoplasty, and lateral mass fixation. The patient is placed prone for the performance of laminoplasty or laminectomy. The patient's head is placed in tongs or a selected head holder is used. For patients with substantial cord compression, a slight flexion alignment is initially preferred. If fusion is to be performed, it is important to restore lordosis after decompression but before final implant tightening. The patient's arms are tucked to the sides of his or her body and wrapped in a sheet. Placing the knees in slight flexion can limit patient movement on the table.

Surgical Steps

The spinous processes of C2 and C7 are marked, and correct levels are identified using fluoroscopy. The skin and subcutaneous tissue can be infiltrated with a 1:500,000 epinephrine solution to help with hemostasis. The skin is incised in the midline corresponding to the levels of surgery. The dissection is then deepened, keeping strictly within the median raphe to avoid bleeding and muscle damage. After the spinous process is reached, further dissection is performed subperiosteally from distal to proximal using electrocautery; self-retaining retractors are then placed bilaterally. The lateral limit of dissection

is the lateral edge of the lateral mass. Depending on the pathology treated, a laminectomy is performed in a piece-meal or en bloc fashion.

Specific Instructions: Laminoplasty

When performing a laminoplasty, patient positioning, skin incision, and lamina exposure are like those of the conventional posterior approach, but care should be taken to preserve the C2 and C7 attachments.[18,19] The muscles attached to the C2 spinous process are the rectus major, inferior oblique, and semispinalis cervicis muscles. Preservation of the C2 and C7 muscle attachments theoretically reduces loss of lordosis and neck pain caused by mechanical instability after laminoplasty.[18] Technical goals of foraminotomy are similar to the goals of other posterior surgeries performed without fusion and include preservation of the joint capsules and avoidance of extensive facet resection.

Posterior Minimally Invasive Foraminotomy

The minimally invasive approach to the cervical spine has been shown to reduce the length of hospital stays and postoperative pain medication requirements. This approach is mainly useful in treating radiculopathy secondary to lateral disk herniation without instability and kyphotic deformity.[20-22]

Patient Position

A minimally invasive procedure can be performed with the patient prone or seated. A prone position with a slight reverse Trendelenburg position can reduce bleeding. The patient's arms are tucked to his or her sides and the shoulders are taped, which facilitates imaging when the procedure involves the lower cervical spine. When small incisions are planned, fluoroscopy is relatively more important for identification and confirmation of the target level before the incision is made.

Surgical Steps

A 3-cm midline skin incision is placed with the target disk level as the center. The superficial dissection is continued through the midline until the cervical fascia is encountered, which is divided longitudinally in the midline to expose the tips of the spinous process. Further dissection is performed subperiosteally elevating the paraspinal musculature from the lamina, spinous process, and facet joint using a Cobb elevator and electrocautery. At this stage, a self-retaining or handheld retractor is placed to reflect paraspinal muscles from the target interlaminar area. Decompression is performed under loupe or microscope magnification. A high-speed burr is used to remove the

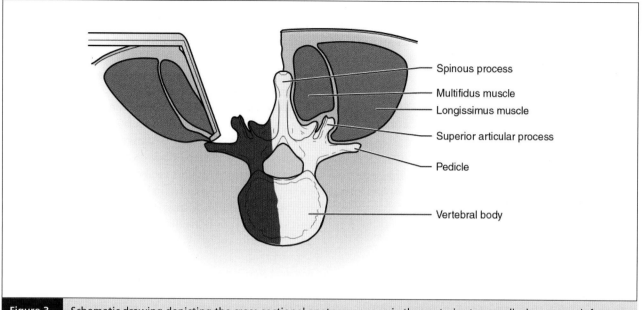

| Figure 3 | Schematic drawing depicting the cross-sectional anatomy as seen in the posterior transpedicular approach for exposure of the anterior column from a posterior incision. The shaded region of the lamina, facet region, pedicle, and vertebral body can be completely resected if a tumor or infection is present. The bilateral exposure allows for complete corpectomy, if needed. |

caudal edge of the upper lamina and the medial third of the facet. This resection may be completed with a small Kerrison rongeur, but no more than half of the facet should be resected. Next, the medial and cephalad portion of the caudal pedicle are located.[23] The root is typically mobilized in a cephalad direction; however, if root tension limits mobility, a small portion of the pedicle can be resected with a burr to facilitate exposure of the disk. Microscope magnification and protection of the nerve root with a small Penfield retractor is suggested. Bleeding from the perineural venous plexus can usually be controlled with hemostatic agents and cottonoid packing.

Circumferential Decompression of the Thoracic Spine Via a Posterolateral Transpedicular Approach

The posterolateral transpedicular approach is a single-stage approach used to reach the anterior and posterior aspect of the thoracic vertebral body (**Figure 3**). This approach is indicated in the treatment of tumors, infections, spine fractures, and spine dislocations.[24-27]

Surgical Steps

The procedure is performed with the patient under general anesthesia and positioned prone on a Wilson or Jackson frame. Intraoperative fluoroscopy or plain radiography is used to locate the intended surgical level. A posterior vertical midline incision is made, and the thoracolumbar fascia is divided in the midline.[25,26] The paraspinal muscles

are dissected using electrocautery and Cobb elevators. The muscles can then be retracted using self-retaining retractors. Total laminectomies of the affected levels are performed using a high-speed burr or Kerrison rongeurs. Next, complete facetectomy and pedicle resection are performed bilaterally. After the posterolateral decompression is completed, the disks corresponding to the upper and lower corpectomy levels are removed. The corpectomy is performed using curets, rongeurs, and osteotomes from the posterolateral corner through a transpedicular approach. The exiting nerve root often is transected to improve exposure; however, the T12 and T1 roots should be preserved whenever possible because of the potential for more important radicular sequelae. The posterior longitudinal ligament can be resected if needed, and the completeness of the corpectomy can be judged by direct visualization of the anterior longitudinal ligament. Care should be taken to preserve the bony end plates at the upper and lower levels of the corpectomy to avoid subsidence and enhance graft incorporation.[26,27] Preserving a thin bone wafer anteriorly may reduce the incidence of graft migration and provide another layer of protection between the instrumentation and the aorta.

Advantages

The advantages of the posterolateral transpedicular approach include circumferential decompression of the spinal cord and stabilization through a single skin incision. This approach obviates the need for single-lung ventilation and the lateral decubitus positioning required for standard anterior thoracic approaches.[25-27] This approach can sometimes be performed without the need for a postoperative chest tube if the pleural space is not entered.

Minimally Invasive Thoracotomy

Minimally invasive thoracotomy uses a smaller incision and generally smaller retractors compared with traditional open transthoracic exposures. Generally, a 5- to 6-cm skin incision is used to reach the anterior and lateral surface of the T5-T10 vertebral bodies.[28-30] This approach is indicated for thoracic disk herniations, infections, fractures, dislocations, and tumors.

Surgical Steps

Minimally invasive thoracotomy is performed with the patient placed in the right lateral decubitus position and under general anesthesia. Because this procedure requires single-lung ventilation, a double-lumen endotracheal tube is used. The intended spinal level is identified by counting the ribs and is confirmed with fluoroscopy. A 4- to 6-cm skin incision is made parallel to the rib. The serratus anterior muscle is separated along the direction of its fibers to expose the underlying rib and intercostal space. If the affected level is above T7, the ventral edge of the latissimus dorsi is retracted or incised.[30] The thoracotomy can be performed through a rib-sparing approach in which the intercostal spaces are elevated off the rib or by resecting a portion of the rib directly over the appropriate spinal level.[30] After rib resection or retraction, the pleura is incised and single-lung ventilation is initiated. The anesthesiologist generally reduces inspiration volume before the pleural incision to avoid inadvertent injury to the lung. Self-retaining rib retractors enable clear visualization of the lateral aspect of the spine. A spinal needle is inserted into the disk space and radiography is used to confirm the target spinal level. With this approach, the anterolateral circumference of the thoracic vertebra can be visualized. Segmental vessels can be ligated or clipped and cut if vertebral body access is needed. A radiolucent sponge is placed anterior to the spine to protect the aorta during the remainder of the surgical procedure.[29,30]

Advantages and Limitations

Minimally invasive thoracotomy is less technically demanding than closed thoracotomy and results in less blood loss and faster patient recovery compared with procedures using a larger thoracotomy incision. However, there is a substantial learning curve among surgeons not familiar with transthoracic approaches and those unaccustomed to working without the assistance of a thoracic surgeon. Also, some patients may be unable to tolerate single-lung ventilation.

Posterior Midline Approach to the Thoracolumbar Spine

The posterior midline approach is perhaps the most common approach used by spine surgeons in routine practice. This approach provides direct visualization of the spinous process, laminae, pars interarticularis, facet joints, transverse process, and pedicles. It can be used to perform diskectomy, direct decompression, osteotomies, and posterior interbody fusion and to place pedicle screws and cortical screws.

Patient Position

The posterior midline approach is performed with the patient prone on a spinal frame, with the abdomen hanging freely to decrease blood loss. Fluoroscopy can be used to mark the target level before the skin incision is made. The skin and subcutaneous tissue are infiltrated with 1:500,000 epinephrine, which may help in hemostasis.

Surgical Steps

A midline skin incision corresponding to the target vertebrae is performed, and further dissection down the midline is accomplished using electrocautery to reach thoracolumbar fascia, which are incised in line with the skin incision. Cerebellar or Gelpi retractors are used to help maintain sufficient tissue tension during exposure. The tendinous attachments of muscles over the spinous process are released, followed by subperiosteal exposure of the lamina of interest using a Cobb elevator. The procedure is repeated until all target vertebrae are exposed. This procedure can be performed unilaterally or bilaterally, depending on surgical indications. At this point in the procedure, the paraspinal muscles can be held laterally with self-retaining retractors. Exposure lateral to the facet joints can be accomplished if pedicle screws are planned or access to the intertransverse region is desired for bone graft placement. When using conventional pedicle screws, the multifidus tendons can be released from the lateral facet capsule with electrocautery. This facilitates gentle retraction of the muscles lying over the transverse processes, which can be elevated rather easily with a Cobb elevator. Care should be taken around the superior and inferior margins of the facet because arterial perforators can be a nuisance if not recognized and cauterized. For pedicle screw placement through the cortical bone trajectory, the exposure only needs to reach the lateral aspect of the pars interarticularis. This spares the muscle attachments along the lateral facet joint, which aids in achieving a minimally invasive midline dissection. After the desired procedure is completed, the muscle, fascia, subcutaneous tissue, and skin are closed in individual layers.

Advantages and Limitations

Advantages of the posterior midline approach are surgeon familiarity, clear appreciation of the anatomy, and little or no risk of neurovascular injury. Limitations include possible excessive blood loss, extensive soft-tissue damage, and severe postoperative pain.

Lateral Lumbar Interbody Fusion

Lateral lumbar interbody fusion (LLIF) is a general term given to evolving methods of less invasive access to the lateral aspect of the spinal column via a retroperitoneal approach with the patient in the lateral decubitus position. Two types of LLIF have been described—direct (look) lateral interbody fusion (DLIF) and extreme lateral interbody fusion (XLIF).[31-36]

XLIF was originally described as a two-incision technique in which the first incision is made just lateral to the paraspinal muscles and a second incision is made in the midaxillary line.[31] The first incision allows the surgeon to mobilize the peritoneum away from the percutaneous application of tubular retractors that are inserted through the second incision.[31] As originally described, the tubular retractors are placed directly through the psoas muscle to dock onto the disk of interest.

In the DLIF technique, a single incision is made in the midaxillary line; often this incision is longer than that used in XLIF to allow the surgeon to directly look at the muscle layers and deep surgical anatomy.[33,34] The DLIF technique allows the surgeon to directly visualize the psoas muscle and place retractors anterior to rather than through the muscle. By directly visualizing the anatomy and approaching the spine anterior to the psoas, the DLIF technique may reduce injury to the lumbosacral plexus. This type of injury has been reported with the XLIF technique.[34]

Appropriate Levels

Lumbar levels from L2-L3 and L3-L4 can be accessed through LLIF, but L4-L5 and L5-S1 are difficult to approach secondary to the iliac crest. Some authors report that L4-L5 can be approached through increased lateral flexion of the patient, but the risk of L4 nerve injury should also be considered in preoperative planning and intraoperative execution.[32-34] The approach to levels above L2 is challenging because the ribs tend to deflect the retractors away from optimum disk access. In addition,

the diaphragmatic crus or diaphragm itself may inhibit access in this region. Transdiaphragmatic access is possible; however, the surgeon should be prepared to place a chest tube in this setting.

Positioning and Neuromonitoring

LLIF is performed with the patient in the lateral decubitus position to avoid injury to the inferior vena cava and allow the peritoneum to fall anterior and away from the surgical trajectory. The use of an adjustable table with a break placed at the disk space of interest (especially at lower lumbar levels and thoracolumbar levels) may facilitate safe access. Care should be taken to flex the ipsilateral hip, which may help in mobilization of the psoas without putting unnecessary pressure on the lumbar plexus during retractor placement. Intraoperative neuromonitoring and directional electromyography (EMG; free-run EMG through the dilators, which can be rotated) has been advocated to reduce plexus injury related to retractor placement.[35]

Surgical Steps

The correct level is identified through biplanar fluoroscopy or navigation, and a marking is placed on the flank corresponding to the center point of the targeted disk space. A 3-cm incision is placed on the left flank, and electrocautery is then used to cut through the external oblique fascia.[31,32] Depending on the number of affected levels, the skin incision can be extended. Blunt dissection with a finger or peanut is used to reach the retroperitoneum through the external oblique, internal oblique, and transverse abdominis muscles. Branches of the subcostal iliohypogastric and ilioinguinal nerves may be encountered either running freely in the retroperitoneum or, more commonly, between the internal oblique and transversus abdominus.[37] Abdominal wall denervation and dermatomal pain can occur if these branches are not protected. To reach the psoas, dorsal to ventral blunt dissection is used to move the peritoneum away from the surgical plane. Before passing through the psoas, the anterior vessels and posterior lumbar plexus are checked. To ensure their safety, the psoas should be separated between the middle and anterior third of the muscle, and the abdominal contents along with peritoneum are protected by placing handheld retractors. After the psoas muscle is visualized, sequential tubular dilators are passed through the muscle to reach the disk space. Dilators are rotated 360° while stimulating EMG leads to assess the proximity of the lumbar plexus.[35]

Complications

The most commonly observed complications of this approach (with a reported incidence of 0.7% to 19.7%

during long-term follow-up) are anterior thigh numbness and hip flexor weakness.[36] Vascular injury is uncommon, but it can be life-threatening because lateral positioning places barriers to and allows minimal access for timely vascular repair.[38]

Oblique Lumbar Interbody Fusion

Oblique lumbar interbody fusion (OLIF) is an alternative to LLIF. A retroperitoneal approach to the lumbar spine from L5-S1 to L1-L2 is achieved through a single skin incision. Advantages of OLIF over DLIF and XLIF are a decreased risk of neurologic injury and improved access to the L4-L5 and the L5-S1 levels.[39]

Positioning and Neuromonitoring

OLIF is performed with the patient in lateral decubitus position on a Jackson frame. Lumbosacral plexus injury risks are lower compared with XLIF, and the routine use of EMG neuromonitoring is less common.[39-41]

Surgical Exposure

The center point of the targeted disk space is marked under fluoroscopy. For a single level, OLIF uses an incision similar to that used in XLIF; however, it starts at the anterior edge of the disk (localized fluoroscopically) and extends 3 to 4 cm anteriorly in line with the disk. For multilevel procedures, an oblique skin incision of 5 to 10 cm is created in line with the fibers of the external oblique muscle along the lateral wall of the abdomen. The incision can be curved anteriorly along the anterior border of the anterior superior iliac spine (ASIS) and approximately 5 to 8 cm anterior to the anterior margin of the vertebral body[39] (**Figure 4**). Abdominal muscles can be bluntly separated with minimal cautery after dividing their fascia. The peritoneum is separated from underlying retroperitoneal structures by blunt finger dissection, and the abdominal contents are retracted anteriorly. The psoas muscle and the genitofemoral nerve are visualized, and the targeted disk space is then approached between the left psoas and the aorta. A spinal needle or Kirschner wire is placed in the disk space to confirm the surgical level fluoroscopically. The left-sided ureter and the sympathetic chain are mobilized anteriorly. In initial reports of this technique, the iliolumbar veins were not routinely ligated because the approach to the L4-L5 disk is lateral or anterolateral as opposed to directly anterior as performed in the anterior lumbar interbody fusion technique. This modification requires less retraction of the great vessels. Importantly, when approaching the L5-S1 level, the disk is removed lateral to the common

iliac vessels rather than in the bifurcation. Retraction of the peritoneum and vessels can be performed either with handheld retractors or using sequential dilators and self-retaining retractors as described previously in LLIF exposures.[39]

Complications

Complications of OLIF include ureteral injury, neurologic injury, and transient psoas weakness.[41]

Minimally Invasive Transforaminal Lumbar Interbody Fusion

The minimally invasive transforaminal lumbar interbody fusion (TLIF) technique has become increasingly popular because of the perceived advantages of preserving the posterior osteoligamentous (supraspinous and interspinous ligaments) tension band and the need for less retraction of lumbar multifidus muscles.[42-44] Disadvantages include a substantial learning curve, increased ionizing radiation exposure to the patient and staff, and reported increased risks of nerve root injury.[43]

Surgical Steps

The patient is placed prone on a Jackson frame and the affected spinal level is identified fluoroscopically. Guidewires are inserted into the pedicles via 1- to 2-cm paramedian incisions, and cannulated pedicle screws are placed over the guidewire. Performance of TLIF on the more symptomatic side is recommended. If substantial symptoms are present bilaterally, the contralateral side can be directly decompressed by depressing the thecal sac anteriorly and "crossing over" to the other side and performing the decompression. This decompression is technically demanding. If a durotomy occurs, it may not be repairable using this approach. Sequential soft-tissue dilators are then docked on the intervening facet and expanded to a desired working diameter of approximately 24 to 28 mm. Various additional retractors can be inserted over the tubular retractors to allow even greater visibility. The decompression of the lateral recess and foramen is performed through the ipsilateral facet and pars interarticularis. Contralateral decompression of the spinal canal can be performed by angling the retractor blades to the opposite side or by inserting the retractor on the contralateral side and repeating this step.[42] Bayoneted Kerrison and pituitary rongeurs can assist in decompressing the neural elements. Distraction of the pedicle screws allows for greater interpedicular access to the disk for TLIF. Pedicle screws are placed in a percutaneous fashion on the contralateral side to complete the construct.[42]

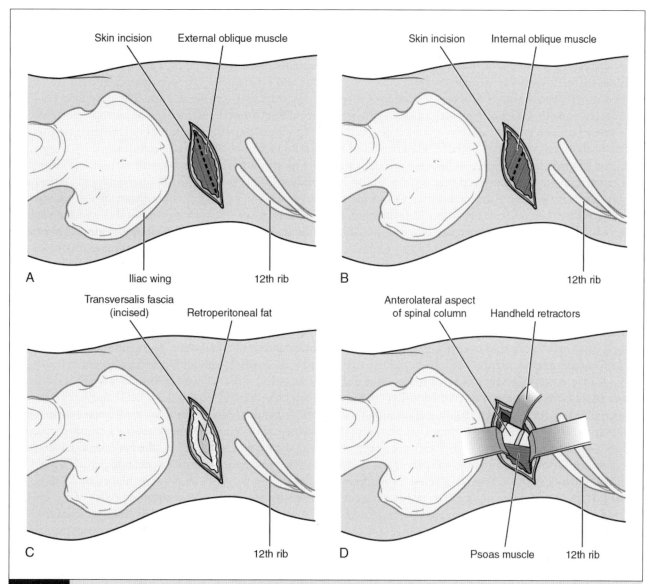

Figure 4 Schematic drawings depict the sequential layers of the surgical exposure for oblique lateral interbody fusion. **A,** With the patient in the lateral decubitus position, the skin is incised in diagonal fashion just proximal to the iliac crest. Below the subcutaneous fat, the external oblique muscle is encountered and can be divided parallel to the muscle fibers (dotted line). **B,** Below the external oblique muscle, the internal oblique muscle is encountered and can be divided parallel to the muscle fibers (dotted line). **C,** Below the internal oblique muscle, the transversalis fascia is encountered and can be divided in line with the skin incision. Below the transversalis fascia lies the retroperitoneal fat. **D,** The retroperitoneal contents are gently retracted anteriorly to expose the psoas muscle and anterolateral aspect of the lumbar spine.

Complications

Complications associated with minimally invasive TLIF are incidental durotomy, implant malposition, neural injury, and nonunion.

Anterior Lumbar Interbody Fusion

Anterior lumbar interbody fusion approaches the disk space from a nearly direct anterior retroperitoneal approach. Because this procedure provides wide access to the disk space, it can be used to treat a vast spectrum of conditions, including degenerative conditions, deformities, spondylolisthesis, and failed posterior surgery (such as pseudarthrosis).[45-48]

Surgical Exposure

Anterior lumbar interbody fusion is performed with the patient supine. To facilitate natural lumbar lordosis, a roll or a bump is placed under the lumbar spine. A vertical, paramedian skin incision may be needed for multiple levels; however, a low transverse Pfannenstiel incision can be used for exposure to L5-S1 and sometimes for L4-L5.[48] A left-sided retroperitoneal dissection allows easier dissection of the inferior vena cava. After the skin incision, further dissection through the fatty layer is performed using electrocautery to reach the anterior layer of the rectus sheath, which is then incised vertically. The peritoneum is separated using blunt finger dissection to create the retroperitoneal plane. The peritoneum is retracted from the left side toward the center using hand-held retractors to reach the anterior surface of the great vessels. Dissection is performed anterior to the psoas muscle; care must be taken to preserve the genitofemoral nerve, which lies on the anterior surface of the psoas. Each anatomic level has a different relationship to surrounding neurovascular structures.[48] At the L5-S1 disk level, the disk space is approached between bifurcation of the common iliac vessels, which are retracted laterally.[48] Care should be taken to ligate the middle sacral vein. Bipolar cautery is recommended to reduce the risk of presacral plexus injury, which can lead to sexual dysfunction, particularly retrograde ejaculation. At L4-L5, the left-sided common iliac vessels lie on the anterior surface of the disk. Typically, these vessels are retracted from left to right. When mobilizing the iliac veins, ligation of the iliolumbar vein may prevent traction to the right iliac vein during mobilization. Vertebral body osteophytes may obstruct vein mobilization. Obtaining a subperiosteal plane can facilitate vein mobilization around adherent osteophytes. At the L3-L4 disk level and higher, the inferior vena cava and the aorta are more easily mobilized to the patient's right side.

Complications

The most common specific complications of the anterior lumbar interbody fusion approach include bowel perforation, ureteral or bladder injury, vascular injury, retrograde ejaculation, deep vein thrombosis, and retroperitoneal hematoma resulting from failed hemostasis.[46]

Wiltse Approach

The Wiltse approach, also known as the paraspinal approach, is indicated for far lateral disk herniation, posterolateral bone grafting for fusion in situ, and pedicle screw placement.

Surgical Exposure

The Wiltse muscle-splitting approach involves the intermuscular plane between the multifidus and longissimus muscles.[49] The correct level is identified by placing a spinal needle in the paraspinal area corresponding to the intended disk level and confirming the position fluoroscopically. A vertical skin incision of 3 to 4 cm is made approximately 3 cm lateral from the midline. In thin patients, the intermuscular septum between the multifidus and longissimus can be palpated, and the incision is made directly over this septum. The deep fascia is identified and incised vertically. The septum between the longissimus and the multifidus is identified, and a second fascial incision is then made in the lateral most aspect of the multifidus. This allows gentle retraction of the multifidus toward the midline. Blunt, handheld appendiceal retractors can be helpful. Blunt finger dissection through the fatty plane between the multifidus and longissimus muscles is performed until the lateral aspect of the facets and the cephalad and caudal transverse processes can be palpated. After the lateral aspect of the facet joint is clearly visualized, a bipolar cautery facilitates release of the multifidus attachments from the facet. A Penfield No. 4 retractor is used to strip muscle from the cephalad and caudal transverse processes, thereby exposing the intertransverse membrane. The septum is then released from the medial superior border of the caudal transverse process and reflected proximally and laterally. Frequently, a facet bleeder will require coagulation during this maneuver. A Penfield No. 4 retractor also is used to mobilize perineural fat to expose the far lateral herniated fragment and the exiting nerve root. Most commonly, the nerve root is most easily mobilized cranially.

Advantages and Limitations

The Wiltse approach requires less bone removal than the conventional midline approach to treat lateral and far lateral disk herniations. The approach also allows clear visualization of the neuroforaminal and extraforaminal areas. Although the Wiltse approach is more appropriate for far lateral disk herniations, it becomes more challenging to use at the lower spinal levels, especially L5-S1, because of close approximation of the L5 transverse process and the sacral ala.[49] Other limitations include bleeding from surrounding muscles, injury to the nerve root, and difficulty in enucleating the disk.[50,51]

Bone Grafting

Autologous iliac bone graft is preferred for use in spine fusion. It is strongly recommended that spine surgeons have a working knowledge of the technique of obtaining graft from the anterior and posterior iliac crests. Both the anterior and posterior ilium are potential sources for cancellous, cortical, or combined bone graft; however, in terms of volume, bone graft of maximal quality can be obtained from the posterior iliac crest.

Posterior Iliac Bone Graft

Posterior iliac bone graft can be obtained through the same skin incision as used in the index spine procedure or through a separate skin incision. Using the same midline posterior incision to approach the posterior iliac crest is recommended if the index procedure included the lower lumbar spine. The posterior iliac crest is palpated, and a full-thickness flap is created over the dorsolumbar fascia. An assistant can use a Meyerding retractor on the flap as the surgeon uses a Cobb elevator and electrocautery to approach the iliac crest. A vertical incision is made along the middle of the iliac crest, and electrocautery facilitates subperiosteal release of the fascia and gluteal muscles laterally. If tricortical bone graft is needed, both the inner and outer tables of the ilium are exposed. An oscillating saw then can be used to harvest a tricortical graft. If only cancellous bone is needed, a cortical "cap" of the ilium can be removed with an osteotome, and bone gouges can then be used to scoop cancellous bone from between the inner and outer tables. It is recommended that the outer table be exposed to a depth of 3 inches. A Taylor retractor, which can retract the gluteus muscle as well as the entire superficial tissue flap, is inserted. A 0.5-inch osteotome is then used to remove a triangular piece of cortex from the external table. Large curets can then be used to harvest the graft to the depth of the inner table. After sufficient bone has been obtained, large pieces of thrombin-soaked cottonoid pledget can be packed against the exposed bone surface to achieve hemostasis. Alternatively, the posterior iliac bone graft can be obtained through a separate lateral skin incision placed along the border of the posterior iliac crest within 6 to 8 cm from the midline. Remaining steps are similar to those described previously. The complications associated with this technique are donor site pain, injury to cluneal nerves, and injury to the sciatic nerve or superior gluteal nerve or artery if dissection is too deep.

Anterior Iliac Bone Graft

The anterior iliac crest is a potential source of tricortical bone graft for anterior cervical fusions, and bone marrow aspirate from this region is a rich source of stem cells used for supplementing other bone graft material. An incision is made along the border of the iliac crest 4 cm posterior to the ASIS to avoid iatrogenic injury to the lateral femoral cutaneous nerve and avulsion of the ASIS. To obtain tricortical graft, the periosteum is elevated along with muscle attachments from inner and outer tables of the ilium. It is preferable to use an oscillating saw over the osteotome to avoid microfracture of the graft, and care should be taken to preserve the ASIS by ensuring that the graft harvest is at least 2 cm proximal to the ASIS. After tricortical bone graft is removed, more cancellous graft can be obtained, if needed, using a bone gouge. After removal of the bone graft, the fascial edges should be reapproximated with No. 1 synthetic absorbable sterile suture. to reduce the risk of hernia. The complications associated with this technique are donor site pain, meralgia paresthetica, avulsion fracture of the ASIS, hematoma formation, pelvic instability, and infection.

Summary

Each surgical approach to the spine has advantages and limitations. The use of minimally invasive approaches and muscle-sparing approaches is increasing rapidly. Minimally invasive surgical approaches facilitate earlier patient recovery and decrease the need for narcotics in the immediate postoperative period; however, long-term benefits have yet to be proved. Spine surgeons should monitor the literature for reports of complications associated with newer procedures and be mindful of the learning curve associated with incorporating new approaches and techniques into clinical practice.

Key Study Points

- The conventional anteromedial approach to the cervical spine is the preferred standard approach to manage disorders of the anterior subaxial spine (C3-C7).
- The surgical steps used for the posterior midline approach are similar when performing laminectomy or laminoplasty. Preservation of muscular attachments at C2 and C7 are of paramount importance in laminoplasty.
- The transpedicular approach is a circumferential approach to the thoracic spine. It has been effectively used in the treatment of thoracic vertebral body tumors and infection and may eliminate the need for aggressive thoracotomy.
- LLIF and OLIF are newer minimally invasive surgical approaches for performing lumbar interbody fusion anteriorly. Knowledge of the involved anatomy and careful evaluation of preoperative imaging studies are essential to avoid complications.
- Preserving the muscular attachments along the lateral facet joint is the key to keeping the midline approach minimally invasive when performing TLIF with a cortical bone trajectory.

1: Spine Anatomy and Biomechanics

Annotated References

1. Smith GW, Robinson RA: The treatment of certain cervical-spine disorders by anterior removal of the intervertebral disc and interbody fusion. *J Bone Joint Surg Am* 1958;40-A(3):607-624.

2. Beutler WJ, Sweeney CA, Connolly PJ: Recurrent laryngeal nerve injury with anterior cervical spine surgery risk with laterality of surgical approach. *Spine (Phila Pa 1976)* 2001;26(12):1337-1342.

3. Lu J, Ebraheim NA, Nadim Y, Huntoon M: Anterior approach to the cervical spine: Surgical anatomy. *Orthopedics* 2000;23(8):841-845.

4. Ebraheim NA, Lu J, Yang H, Heck BE, Yeasting RA: Vulnerability of the sympathetic trunk during the anterior approach to the lower cervical spine. *Spine (Phila Pa 1976)* 2000;25(13):1603-1606.

5. Fountas KN, Kapsalaki EZ, Nikolakakos LG, et al: Anterior cervical discectomy and fusion associated complications. *Spine (Phila Pa 1976)* 2007;32(21):2310-2317.

6. Lee MJ, Bazaz R, Furey CG, Yoo J: Risk factors for dysphagia after anterior cervical spine surgery: A two-year prospective cohort study. *Spine J* 2007;7(2):141-147.

7. Menezes AH, VanGilder JC: Transoral-transpharyngeal approach to the anterior craniocervical junction: Ten-year experience with 72 patients. *J Neurosurg* 1988;69(6):895-903.

8. McAfee PC, Bohlman HH, Yuan HA: Anterior decompression of traumatic thoracolumbar fractures with incomplete neurological deficit using a retroperitoneal approach. *J Bone Joint Surg Am* 1985;67(1):89-104.

9. Haller JM, Iwanik M, Shen FH: Clinically relevant anatomy of high anterior cervical approach. *Spine (Phila Pa 1976)* 2011;36(25):2116-2121.

    This anatomic study defines the relationship of various neurovascular structures encountered during anterior cervical dissection. The anatomic relationships of the hypoglossal nerve, internal and external superior laryngeal nerves, superior thyroid artery, and superior laryngeal artery to the cervical spine are defined. The authors concluded that these structures did not show any side-to-side variation.

10. Reindl R, Sen M, Aebi M: Anterior instrumentation for traumatic C1-C2 instability. *Spine (Phila Pa 1976)* 2003;28(17):E329-E333.

11. Vender JR, Harrison SJ, McDonnell DE: Fusion and instrumentation at C1-3 via the high anterior cervical approach. *J Neurosurg* 2000;92(suppl 1):24-29.

12. Vaccaro AR, Lim MR, Lee JY: Indications for surgery and stabilization techniques of the occipito-cervical junction. *Injury* 2005;36(suppl 2):B44-B53.

13. Goel A, Laheri V: Plate and screw fixation for atlanto-axial subluxation. *Acta Neurochir (Wien)* 1994;129(1-2):47-53.

14. Harms J, Melcher RP: Posterior C1-C2 fusion with polyaxial screw and rod fixation. *Spine (Phila Pa 1976)* 2001;26(22):2467-2471.

15. Takami T, Ichinose T, Ishibashi K, Goto T, Tsuyuguchi N, Ohata K: Importance of fixation angle in posterior instrumented occipitocervical fusion. *Neurol Med Chir (Tokyo)* 2008;48(6):279-282, discussion 282.

16. He H, Hu B, Wang L, Gao Y, Yan H, Wang J: The computed tomography angiography study of the spatial relationship between C1 transpedicular screw trajectory and V3 segment of vertebral artery. *Spine J* 2017;17(1):120-128.

    A close relationship was found between the C1 transpedicular screw trajectory and the V3 segment of the vertebral artery in a study of 62 patients using CT angiography. The authors recommended a medial inclination technique, especially for female patients. Level of evidence: IV.

17. Dewan MC, Godil SS, Mendenhall SK, Devin CJ, McGirt MJ: C2 nerve root transection during C1 lateral mass screw fixation: Does it affect functionality and quality of life? *Neurosurgery* 2014;74(5):475-480, discussion 480-481.

    Twenty-eight patients were included in a study performed to determine the consequences of C2 nerve root sectioning during placement of C1 lateral mass screws. C2 transection was performed in 8 patients and C2 was preserved in 20 patients. All patients were prospectively followed (mean follow-up, 27 months). It was concluded that even though C2 nerve root transection is associated with increased occipital numbness, clinical outcomes were not affected by C2 nerve root transection. Level of evidence: III.

18. Takeuchi K, Yokoyama T, Aburakawa S, et al: Axial symptoms after cervical laminoplasty with C3 laminectomy compared with conventional C3-C7 laminoplasty: A modified laminoplasty preserving the semispinalis cervicis inserted into axis. *Spine (Phila Pa 1976)* 2005;30(22):2544-2549.

19. Chiba K, Ogawa Y, Ishii K, et al: Long-term results of expansive open-door laminoplasty for cervical myelopathy: Average 14-year follow-up study. *Spine (Phila Pa 1976)* 2006;31(26):2998-3005.

20. Ruetten S, Komp M, Merk H, Godolias G: Full-endoscopic cervical posterior foraminotomy for the operation of lateral disc herniations using 5.9-mm endoscopes: A prospective, randomized, controlled study. *Spine (Phila Pa 1976)* 2008;33(9):940-948.

21. Gala VC, O'Toole JE, Voyadzis JM, Fessler RG: Posterior minimally invasive approaches for the cervical spine. *Orthop Clin North Am* 2007;38(3):339-349, abstract v.

22. Mikhael MM, Celestre PC, Wolf CF, Mroz TE, Wang JC: Minimally invasive cervical spine foraminotomy and lateral mass screw placement. *Spine (Phila Pa 1976)* 2012;37(5):E318-E322.

   This article describes posterior cervical decompression and lateral mass screw placement through a tubular retraction system. The posterior cervical spine was approached through the paramedian median muscle-splitting approach and lateral mass fixation was performed using tubular retractors.

23. Coric D, Adamson T: Minimally invasive cervical micro-endoscopic laminoforaminotomy. *Neurosurg Focus* 2008;25(2):E2.

24. Bilsky MH, Boland P, Lis E, Raizer JJ, Healey JH: Single-stage posterolateral transpedicle approach for spondylectomy, epidural decompression, and circumferential fusion of spinal metastases. *Spine (Phila Pa 1976)* 2000;25(17):2240-2249, discussion 250.

25. Wang JC, Boland P, Mitra N, et al: Single-stage posterolateral transpedicular approach for resection of epidural metastatic spine tumors involving the vertebral body with circumferential reconstruction: Results in 140 patients. Invited submission from the Joint Section Meeting on Disorders of the Spine and Peripheral Nerves, March 2004. *J Neurosurg Spine* 2004;1(3):287-298.

26. Cho DC, Sung JK: Palliative surgery for metastatic thoracic and lumbar tumors using posterolateral transpedicular approach with posterior instrumentation. *Surg Neurol* 2009;71(4):424-433.

27. Wong ML, Lau HC, Kaye AH: A modified posterolateral transpedicular approach to thoracolumbar corpectomy with nerve preservation and bilateral cage reconstruction. *J Clin Neurosci* 2014;21(6):988-992.

   Early results of single-stage posterolateral transpedicular corpectomy and fusion in the thoracolumbar spine are reported for five patients. At a mean follow-up of 3.3 months, patients with a preoperative neurologic deficit showed improvement in neurologic status.

28. Uribe JS, Smith WD, Pimenta L, et al: Minimally invasive lateral approach for symptomatic thoracic disc herniation: Initial multicenter clinical experience. *J Neurosurg Spine* 2012;16(3):264-279.

   This retrospective study highlights the safety and early results of a minimally invasive lateral approach for symptomatic thoracic herniated intervertebral disks. The authors evaluated 60 patients with symptomatic thoracic herniated disks treated using a mini open lateral approach and found a 6.7% overall complication rate. The results were comparable with open conventional modalities. It was concluded that minithoracotomy is a less invasive and viable option for the treatment of thoracic disk herniation.

29. Bartels RH, Peul WC: Mini-thoracotomy or thoracoscopic treatment for medially located thoracic herniated disc? *Spine (Phila Pa 1976)* 2007;32(20):E581-E584.

30. Mayer HM: Microsurgical anterior approach to T5–T10 (Mini-TTA), in Mayer HM, ed: *Minimally Invasive Spine Surgery*, ed 2. Berlin, Springer, 2006, pp 129-137.

31. Knight RQ, Schwaegler P, Hanscom D, Roh J: Direct lateral lumbar interbody fusion for degenerative conditions: Early complication profile. *J Spinal Disord Tech* 2009;22(1):34-37.

32. Ozgur BM, Aryan HE, Pimenta L, Taylor WR: Extreme lateral interbody fusion (XLIF): A novel surgical technique for anterior lumbar interbody fusion. *Spine J* 2006;6(4):435-443.

33. Berjano P, Balsano M, Buric J, Petruzzi M, Lamartina C: Direct lateral access lumbar and thoracolumbar fusion: Preliminary results. *Eur Spine J* 2012;21(suppl 1):S37-S42.

   This retrospective cohort review of 97 consecutive patients from three centers found that XLIF is a safe and effective technique for interbody fusion. No permanent neurologic impairment or vascular or visceral complications were reported. Transient neurologic complications were seen, but overall success was reported in 92% of cases.

34. Kwon B, Kim DH: Lateral lumbar interbody fusion: Indications, outcomes, and complications. *J Am Acad Orthop Surg* 2016;24(2):96-105.

   This review article focuses on various aspects of LLIF, including indications, relevant anatomy, surgical technique, complications, and outcomes. The authors suggest LLIF could provide safe and effective clinical outcomes with technical advancement and better understanding of the anatomy.

35. Tohmeh AG, Rodgers WB, Peterson MD: Dynamically evoked, discrete-threshold electromyography in the extreme lateral interbody fusion approach. *J Neurosurg Spine* 2011;14(1):31-37.

   This prospective multicenter study provides insight into the role of EMG in a surgical approach of LLIF. The authors strongly recommend using the real-time EMG threshold during the transpsoas approach to avoid lumbar plexus injury.

36. Cahill KS, Martinez JL, Wang MY, Vanni S, Levi AD: Motor nerve injuries following the minimally invasive lateral transpsoas approach. *J Neurosurg Spine* 2012;17(3):227-231.

   This retrospective chart review of 118 patients identified motor injuries in patients who had undergone LLIF. The study reported a 1.7% incidence of femoral nerve injury, with a level-specific incidence of 4.8% for procedures performed at the L4-L5 disk space, whereas other lumbar levels showed less risk. The authors recommended that care be taken to avoid injury to the T11 and T12 nerve roots during surgical closure. Proper closure of the abdominal

1: Spine Anatomy and Biomechanics

wall is needed to avoid abdominal muscle weakness and hernias.

37. Dakwar E, Le TV, Baaj AA, et al: Abdominal wall paresis as a complication of minimally invasive lateral transpsoas interbody fusion. *Neurosurg Focus* 2011;31(4):E18.

    This retrospective review reports on 568 patients who were treated with the minimally invasive lateral retroperitoneal transpsoas approach for interbody fusion. Abdominal wall paresis occurred in 10 patients as a complication of surgery. Abdominal wall paresis resolved in 8 of the 10 patients by the 6-month follow-up visit; the remaining 2 patients were lost to follow-up. It was concluded that abdominal wall paresis is a rare but known potential complication of lateral interbody fusion. Level of evidence: IV.

38. Aichmair A, Fantini GA, Garvin S, Beckman J, Girardi FP: Aortic perforation during lateral lumbar interbody fusion. *J Spinal Disord Tech* 2015;28(2):71-75.

    This case report concerns a rare intraoperative aortic injury that occurred during LLIF at level of L3-L4. While performing direct LLIF through a right-side mini transpsoas approach, the proximal aspect of the interbody implant broke. An attempt to impact the implant further resulted in violation of the L3 end plate and the anterior cortex, which subsequently injured the aorta.

39. Fujibayashi S, Hynes RA, Otsuki B, Kimura H, Takemoto M, Matsuda S: Effect of indirect neural decompression through oblique lateral interbody fusion for degenerative lumbar disease. *Spine (Phila Pa 1976)* 2015;40(3):E175-E182.

    In this prospective study of 28 patients with lumbar canal stenosis, OLIF was used to treat all the patients. Indirect decompression was performed by placing an interbody cage through an oblique lateral approach to the lumbar spine and then stabilizing the construct with posterior percutaneous pedicle screws.

40. Abe K, Orita S, Mannoji C, et al: Perioperative complications in 155 patients who underwent oblique lateral interbody fusion surgery: Perspectives and indications from a retrospective, multicenter survey. *Spine (Phila Pa 1976)* 2017;42(1):55-62.

    This retrospective multicenter review identified perioperative complications during OLIF. The study, which included 155 patients, reported 75 complications, including end plate fracture/subsidence (18.7%), transient psoas weakness and thigh numbness (13.5%), and segmental artery injury (2.6%). Most complications were transient, and only three patients had permanent damage, which included one uretal injury and two neurologic injuries. Level of evidence: III.

41. Silvestre C, Mac-Thiong JM, Hilmi R, Roussouly P: Complications and morbidities of mini-open anterior retroperitoneal lumbar interbody fusion: Oblique lumbar interbody fusion in 179 patients. *Asian Spine J* 2012;6(2):89-97.

    OLIF was used to treat 179 patients at a single institution. The authors found that minimally invasive OLIF was an easily performed and safe procedure for treating the lumbar spine from L2 to L5, and at L1-L2 in select patients.

42. Kim JS, Jung B, Lee SH: Instrumented minimally invasive spinal-transforaminal lumbar interbody fusion (MIS-TLIF); Minimum 5-years follow-up with clinical and radiologic outcomes. *J Spinal Disord Tech* 2012;Sept 28 [Epub ahead of print]

    This retrospective study evaluated clinical results of 44 patients who had undergone minimally invasive TLIF. The authors noted a significant decrease in visual analog scale pain scores and greater improvement in Oswestry Disability Index scores. Radiologic evidence of fusion was noted in nearly all patients with both isthmic and degenerative spondylolisthesis. Favorable clinical and radiologic results were achieved after single-level instrumented fusion.

43. Lau D, Lee JG, Han SJ, Lu DC, Chou D: Complications and perioperative factors associated with learning the technique of minimally invasive transforaminal lumbar interbody fusion (TLIF). *J Clin Neurosci* 2011;18(5):624-627.

    This retrospective comparison study of conventional TLIF and minimally invasive TLIF reported lower transfusion rates, a decreased need for postoperative surgical drains, and decreased time to mobility for patients who underwent minimally invasive TLIF. The authors noted that minimally invasive TLIF was associated with a higher rate of early complications.

44. Peng CW, Yue WM, Poh SY, Yeo W, Tan SB: Clinical and radiological outcomes of minimally invasive versus open transforaminal lumbar interbody fusion. *Spine (Phila Pa 1976)* 2009;34(13):1385-1389.

45. Rao PJ, Loganathan A, Yeung V, Mobbs RJ: Outcomes of anterior lumbar interbody fusion surgery based on indication: A prospective study. *Neurosurgery* 2015;76(1):7-23, discussion 23-24.

    This prospective clinical study of 125 patients who underwent anterior lumbar interbody fusion reported clinically successful outcomes in 86% of the patients. An overall 10% complication rate was reported. Complications included retroperitoneal hematoma, retrograde ejaculation, incisional hernia, and bowel obstruction.

46. Watkins R: Anterior lumbar interbody fusion surgical complications. *Clin Orthop Relat Res* 1992;284:47-53.

47. Gumbs AA, Bloom ND, Bitan FD, Hanan SH: Open anterior approaches for lumbar spine procedures. *Am J Surg* 2007;194(1):98-102.

48. Bianchi C, Ballard JL, Abou-Zamzam AM, Teruya TH, Abu-Assal ML: Anterior retroperitoneal lumbosacral spine exposure: Operative technique and results. *Ann Vasc Surg* 2003;17(2):137-142.

49. Wiltse LL, Bateman JG, Hutchinson RH, Nelson WE: The paraspinal sacrospinalis-splitting approach to the lumbar spine. *J Bone Joint Surg Am* 1968;50(5):919-926.

50. Pirris SM, Dhall S, Mummaneni PV, Kanter AS: Minimally invasive approach to extraforaminal disc herniations at the lumbosacral junction using an operating microscope: Case series and review of the literature. *Neurosurg Focus* 2008;25(2):E10.

51. Gioia G, Mandelli D, Capaccioni B, Randelli F, Tessari L: Surgical treatment of far lateral lumbar disc herniation: Identification of compressed root and discectomy by lateral approach. *Spine (Phila Pa 1976)* 1999;24(18):1952-1957.

1: Spine Anatomy and Biomechanics

Chapter 4

Spine Mechanics and Pathomechanics

John A. Hipp, PhD

Abstract

In routine clinical practice, it is challenging to objectively determine whether the load-bearing, motion-providing, and neurovascular protective capabilities of the spine have been compromised. An understanding of spine mechanics and pathomechanics can help identify functional abnormalities. This knowledge also is important in understanding how available surgical treatments for spine disorders alter the biomechanics of the spine, either as a consequence of decompression or in the process of providing stability. It is essential that clinicians be able to assess the biomechanical success of each spine surgery and understand the biomechanics of the spine and how implants can alter motion.

Keywords: cervical; kinematics; load-bearing capacity; lumbar; mechanics

Introduction

Healthcare providers appreciate that the spine provides structural support for the body and allows a wide range of movements while providing protection of the neurovascular elements within and about the spine. Collectively, load-bearing, motion-providing, and neurovascular protective capabilities are described as the biomechanical functions of the spine. In routine clinical practice, it is challenging to objectively determine compromise of these biomechanical functions. Because it is known that many radiographic and MRI abnormalities can be found in asymptomatic individuals, it can be difficult to determine whether imaging evidence of instability or degeneration

---

Dr. Hipp or an immediate family member serves as a paid consultant to or is an employee of and has stock or stock options held in Medical Metrics.

correlates with a patient's symptoms. These challenges must be addressed because most of the available surgical treatments for spinal disorders alter the biomechanics of the spine, either in the process of decompression or in the process of restoring stability. It is helpful for clinicians to understand the biomechanics of the spine and how implants can alter motion.

The basic biomechanics of the spine have been thoroughly reviewed in the previous literature.[1,2] In addition to those foundational texts, surgeons should keep current on recent findings regarding the spine's normal load-bearing capacity and arc of motion as well as the loading incurred through typical biomechanical alterations resulting from degenerative changes and pathologic processes.

Normal Spine Biomechanics

The spine usually supports loads that would cause a vertebral body to collapse if it did not have sufficient load-bearing capacity or would cause excessive displacement between vertebrae if the intervertebral motion restraints were incompetent. A healthy vertebra can support the load-bearing requirements needed to accomplish the normal and diverse activities of daily living (ADLs). A vertebral body will fail when the load-bearing capacity of the vertebra has been reduced (by age-related or pathologic bone loss) or when applied loads substantially exceed normal loads (as in trauma). Estimating the risk of fracture or when a previously injured or treated spine has regained sufficient load-bearing capacity to resume normal ADLs requires an understanding of both the spine's normal load-bearing requirements and its normal load-bearing capacity. The load-bearing capacity is partially determined by the material properties of the vertebral bone, but also by several other factors (**Figure 1**).

Spinal alignment can affect the loads applied to the spine and frequently has been described in relation to the overall biomechanics of the spine. Spinal alignment

---

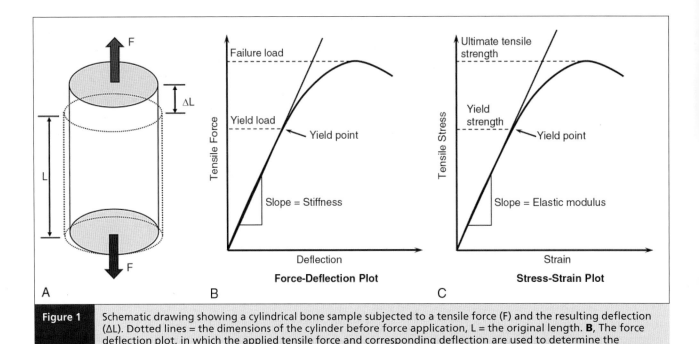

Figure 1 Schematic drawing showing a cylindrical bone sample subjected to a tensile force (F) and the resulting deflection (ΔL). Dotted lines = the dimensions of the cylinder before force application, L = the original length. **B,** The force deflection plot, in which the applied tensile force and corresponding deflection are used to determine the structural properties of the cylindrical bone. **C,** The stress-strain plot, in which the tensile force is normalized over the cross-sectional area of the bone sample and the deflection is normalized over the original length to determine the material properties of the bone. (Reproduced from Wang M, Rao RD: The biomechanics of the spinal column, in Rao RD, Smuck M, eds: *Orthopaedic Knowledge Update Spine 4.* Rosemont, IL, American Academy of Orthopaedic Surgeons, 2012, pp 19-31.)

is a complex topic that has been addressed in the recent scientific literature.[2]

Load-Bearing Requirements

Multiple techniques have been used to estimate the load-bearing requirements of the spine. These techniques range from simple free-body diagrams to sophisticated computer models. These techniques for estimating load-bearing requirements make use of data from load-measuring devices mounted to the spine, intervertebral disk pressure measurements, measurements of muscle activity, and measurements of the loads that an individual can apply with his or her body.

Measurements of the pressures within intervertebral disks are helpful in appreciating the relative load-bearing requirements of various ADLs because the forces that result in the measured pressures can be estimated. When a healthy individual with no degenerative changes or injuries to the spine is standing, the pressure within the L4-L5 disk is approximately 0.5 MPa.[3] That is nearly the pressure exerted on an object submerged to a depth of approximately 40 m. The compressive force required to create 0.5 MPa intradiscal pressure is approximately 530 N. Sitting can increase or decrease spinal loads by

up to 40% relative to those of standing, depending on whether the individual is supported or unsupported, the amount of thoracic kyphosis, and the position of the arms. Lying down can reduce pressure on the spine by 20% to 33% compared with standing. While supine, slight flexing of the legs can further reduce intradiscal pressure. Spikes and variations in pressure occur with changes in position. Intradiscal pressure measurements also help explain the gradual swelling of the disk that can occur after 7 hours of sleep, because pressures at the end of a sleep period are twice as high as at the start of a sleep period.

Activities that can substantially increase disk pressure include forward bending (pressure up to 3.6 times greater than that of standing, depending on how much the individual flexes forward), and lifting (as much as seven times greater pressure than standing, with stooped lifting creating pressure 35% greater than that of squat lifting). In a 2014 study, vertebral body replacements used in the management of L1-L3 trauma were modified to enable in vivo measurements of spinal loading.[4] Ten activities that resulted in particularly high spinal loads were identified (**Figure 2**). Maximum loads were found with lifting a weight from the ground and elevating a weight with arms extended straight out from the body. Simple activities such as tying a shoe can result in high

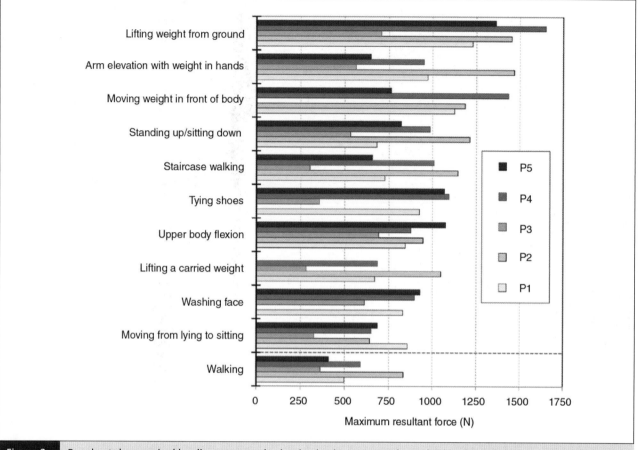

Figure 2 Bar chart shows spinal loading measured using in vivo instrumented vertebral body replacements in five patients (P1 to P5). The 10 activities with the highest measured loads are shown along with the variability in loading between patients and activities. These data can be used to educate patients on activities to avoid when greater spinal protection is needed (such as after spine surgery). (Adapted with permission from Rohlmann A, Pohl D, Bender A, et al: Activities of everyday life with high spinal loads. *PLoS ONE* 2014;9[5]:e98510.)

spinal loads. These data suggest that, in the setting of lumbar corpectomy with vertebral body replacement, the effect of bracing is unpredictable. Although only the portion of the load passing between the vertebral bodies was measured (some load was supported by the posterior elements), the load data are helpful in understanding differences in loading between activities in the setting of anterior column reconstruction.

Good data are available to support recommendations to patients for activities that can place the greatest mechanical stress on the lumbar spine.[3,4] In vivo measurements of lumbar spinal loads also may help in the decision to recommend an orthosis, because the data show that, although loads may be reduced in some patients, an orthosis can increase spinal loads in other patients.[5] Measurements of disk pressure in the cervical spine have been restricted to cadaver specimens and are not as helpful for understanding clinical load-bearing requirements.

Load-Bearing Capacity

The load-bearing capacity of vertebrae has been documented using ex vivo tests of isolated vertebrae subjected to controlled loading conditions. Whereas long bones have a safety factor because load-bearing capacity can substantially exceed load-bearing requirements,[6] documented failure loads for an intact vertebra have been in the range of the load-bearing requirements previously described.[7,8] This may partly be the result of the advanced age of the cadaver spines tested. A study on vertebral fracture risk reported that the estimated mean compression strength of vertebrae in postmenopausal women with no compressive fracture is $5,746 \pm 1,873$ N.[9] The factor of risk for a vertebral fracture has been defined as the load-bearing requirement divided by the load-bearing capacity.[10] The factor of risk for young spines varied between 0.07 for upright standing and 0.61 for lifting a 10-kg weight. For older spines, the factor of risk varied

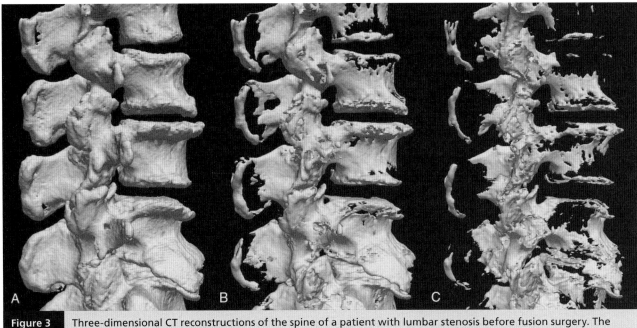

Figure 3 Three-dimensional CT reconstructions of the spine of a patient with lumbar stenosis before fusion surgery. The left half of the spine has been electronically removed to allow easier interpretation of the images. **A,** Image shows all tissue with a density of 180 Hounsfield units (HU) or higher. **B,** Image shows all tissue with a density of 480 HU and higher. **C,** Image obtained at a 780 HU threshold shows that the densest bone is found in the region of the pedicles, pars interarticularis, and lamina, and that posterior elements play an important role in spinal load bearing. If insertion of screws into the strongest bone is required, this imaging technique is helpful in locating the densest bone.

from 0.12 to 0.99, suggesting that in certain individuals with compromised vertebral bone quality, even loads encountered with normal ADLs could cause insufficiency failure.

It is important to appreciate that repetitive loading can increase the risk of fracture.[11] Because structural redundancy exists in normal vertebrae, failure can occur in a proportion of trabeculae within the vertebra without overall failure.[12] In osteoporotic vertebrae, however, structural redundancy is diminished because of the internal pattern of bone loss.[12] This is important because, unlike a long-bone fracture that can effectively prevent weight bearing, a compression fracture in the spine may result in some collapse of vertebral body height but does not prevent further weight bearing.

The posterior elements are important to the load-bearing capacity of the spine. The densest bone typically forms in regions where the highest loads are supported. For example, the densest bone is in the calcar region of the proximal femur, which is the location of convergence of trabeculae patterns that begin in the femoral head. The apparent brightness of bone on CT imaging is proportional to the density of the bone. Most software for viewing CT images allows tissue with low-signal intensity to be eliminated by adjusting how tissues of various densities appear on the display (**Figure 3**). Identifying the

bone with the highest density is helpful so that screws can be engaged in the densest bone when using the cortical bone trajectory technique for lumbar fusion[13,14]

Intervertebral Motion

In addition to maintaining the required load-bearing capacity of the vertebrae, the spine also must simultaneously facilitate a wide range of intervertebral motions while protecting the neurovascular elements passing through and near the spine. These difficult requirements are achieved in part by a complex system of soft-tissue structures, including the intervertebral disks and intervertebral ligaments, which control relative motion between vertebrae. The other essential elements in achieving diverse and controlled motions are the muscles and a nervous system that can sense the position of vertebrae and control the activity of the muscles. The intervertebral disk, intervertebral ligaments, and facet joints must work together to maintain intervertebral motion within normal limits.

The biomechanics of the intervertebral disk have been extensively studied, although much of this knowledge has yet to be effectively assimilated into validated diagnostic and treatment algorithms for routine clinical use. Resources are available that describe the fundamental structure of the normal intervertebral disk, including the anulus fibrosus and nucleus pulposus; the deformation of these structures during ADLs; and the role of soft-tissue structures in the diagnosis and treatment of spinal disorders.[15]

In clinical practice, overall motion through the spine can be measured using goniometers and electronic devices (including smart phones). Injuries or pathologic or degenerative changes to the disks or intervertebral ligaments may best be appreciated through precise measurements of the relative motion between vertebrae. In the sagittal plane, relative motion between vertebrae is commonly assessed from flexion-extension radiographs. The potential advantages of using upright flexion-extension MRI to assess abnormal intervertebral motion has been described but has not yet become a routine clinical tool.[16] Regardless of the imaging modality used, if the normal limits of translation are known, abnormal motion can be detected as translation outside of the normal limits.

Intervertebral motion in the sagittal plane has been extensively studied, although it is important to appreciate that the intervertebral motion that occurs in the coronal and axial planes during twisting or bending to the side may be important. Intervertebral motion also is coupled because, as the spine bends laterally, the vertebrae also will flex or extend and twist in the axial plane.[17] Coupled motion is less pronounced in sagittal plane flexion-extension because only small amounts of twisting or lateral bending occur between vertebrae with sagittal plane flexion-extension; therefore, intervertebral motion can be largely assessed in a single two-dimensional plane. One reason that sagittal plane flexion-extension radiography has been the primary clinical imaging modality for assessing instability is that only two-dimensional imaging is required. Axial rotation or lateral bending are best studied using three-dimensional imaging of the spine in multiple positions,[18] or using geometric detail from three-dimensional imaging combined with kinematic information from two-dimensional imaging;[19] however, these methods are not clinically practical in most situations. Even with two-dimensional imaging, variability in image acquisition protocols can confound diagnostic utility.

Substantial variability exists in the peer-reviewed literature for what is considered normal intervertebral motion.[20] Intervertebral motion classified as normal based on data from one study may be considered abnormal motion using similar data from a different study. This variability may be attributed in part to differences in the populations studied, but may largely result from variability in the instructions given to tested individuals as they are asked to perform spinal flexion and extension, or may

result from the specific methodology used to produce the motion measurements.

The effort that patients exert when asked to perform flexion and extension spinal movements also can result in large differences in apparent intervertebral motion.[21] A patient must apply enough stress to the spine during flexion and extension testing to allow a diagnosis of possible abnormal motion. An analogous situation involves the parameters that must be met when the anterior drawer test is used in the diagnosis of a torn anterior cruciate ligament (ACL). When the anterior drawer test is performed, it is appreciated that substantial force must be applied to the lower leg to assure that the examiner can detect that the ACL is being tensioned (if it is intact) and thereby confirm that the ACL can restrict translation of the tibia with respect to the femur. Similarly, if the goal is to determine if the disk and intervertebral ligaments can restrict intervertebral motion to within normal limits, then adequate force must be applied to the spine (by the patient during flexion and extension) to apply stress to the intervertebral motion restraints (if intact) and thereby assure a reliable diagnosis of any incompetent intervertebral motion restraints.[22] It is important for the clinician to assure that flexion-extension tests apply adequate stress to the spine to detect any incompetency of the intervertebral motion restraints. If insufficient stress is applied to the spine, the patient's radiation exposure during flexion-extension radiography is unjustified because spinal instability may not be detected. Criteria to determine whether flexion-extension spinal radiography is properly performed have been primarily based on studies of cadaver spines and the definitions of neutral and lax zones.

The concept of a neutral zone has been used to describe the small range of motion where vertebrae can move relatively freely with application of only small loads[23] (**Figure 4**). Within the neutral zone, the intervertebral motion restraints are not stressed to the point at which they substantially restrict intervertebral motion. Analogous to the previously mentioned anterior drawer test for an ACL injury in which a small amount of translation between the tibia and femur can occur before the ACL is tensioned, the healthy spine allows a small amount of intervertebral movement before the ligaments and disks begin to restrict motion (**Figure 5**). At the borders of the neutral zone in the spine, the disks, ligaments, and facet joints will begin to become mechanically stressed such that increasingly larger forces are required to achieve more intervertebral motion. The border of the neutral zone has been referred to as the lax zone.[24] Past the lax zone, there is a zone where the relationship between applied loads and displacements is approximately linear.

1: Spine Anatomy and Biomechanics

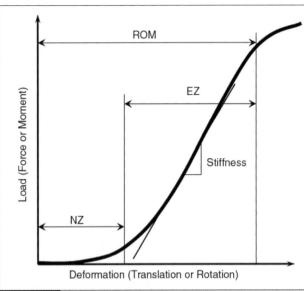

Figure 4	A typical load-displacement plot of a functional spinal unit when loaded along one of its six degrees of freedom. The neutral zone (NZ) represents the amount of displacement occurring near the neutral position of the spine, the elastic zone (EZ) represents the amount of displacement occurring in the physiologically loaded region, and the range of motion (ROM) represents the sum of the NZ and the EZ, as measured in millimeters (for translation) or degrees (for rotation). (Reproduced from Wang M, Rao RD: The biomechanics of the spinal column, in Rao RD, Smuck M, eds: *Orthopaedic Knowledge Update Spine 4.* Rosemont, IL, American Academy of Orthopaedic Surgeons, 2012, pp 19-31.)

A spine flexion-extension test should ideally load the spine sufficiently such that intervertebral motion is past the neutral and lax zones and into the linear elastic zone of the load versus deformation curve (**Figure 4**). The size of the combined neutral and lax zones can be measured in the laboratory by preparing the spine so that controlled loads can be applied while measuring resultant displacements.[24]

Although application of controlled loads to the spine is not practical in patients (so the size of the neutral zone cannot be directly measured and used diagnostically), laboratory measurements of the neutral zone can help determine how much intervertebral motion is needed to assure that the spine is stressed sufficiently to detect any incompetent intervertebral motion restraints. In the lumbar spine, laboratory data support that at least 5° of sagittal plane intervertebral rotation is required for the motion of the intervertebral level to be outside of the neutral and lax zones and into the linear elastic zone of the load-deformation curve[24] (**Figure 4**). In an asymptomatic population of volunteers who performed flexion and extension movements from a seated position, less than 5% of lumbar levels had less than 5° of intervertebral motion at any level of the spine, and the average intervertebral rotation was more than 11° at every level.[20] In the cervical spine, at least 4° of intervertebral rotation may be required to assure intervertebral motion occurs outside the neutral and lax zones.

The relative role of each individual intervertebral ligament and each component of an intervertebral disk in controlling intervertebral motion is complex. In the normal spine, the intervertebral disks, the intervertebral ligaments (anterior and posterior longitudinal ligaments, ligamentum flavum, interspinous ligaments, and supraspinous ligaments), and the facet joints (including the facet capsules) collectively contribute to the control of intervertebral motion.[25] Because this motion control system is complex, computer models are currently the most promising tool for understanding the role of each component.[26] These computer models may help in determining optimal diagnostic and treatment methods based on specific patterns of traumatic and degenerative compromises to the intervertebral motion restraints.

It is difficult to detect damage to intervertebral motion restraints by measuring the magnitude of rotation or translation between vertebrae. One explanation may be that the multiple intervertebral motion restraints provide redundancy in motion control; if one restraint is damaged, the others can maintain enough control that motion remains within limits. The quality of motion can be assessed based on the center of rotation and the translation per degree of rotation (TPDR). Objective measurement of TPDR may prove particularly valuable because the TPDR reduces dependency on patient effort.[20,27,28] The center of rotation is the point at which one vertebra appears to rotate with respect to an adjacent vertebra when comparing two or more positions of the spine. The center of rotation is dependent on the level analyzed, and it falls within a relatively narrow range in radiographically normal spines.[29]

Vertebral Morphology

Vertebrae have many morphologic features that help define how the spine moves and the loads that can be supported. Morphology can vary considerably between individuals. Characteristics such as the anterior-posterior width of the vertebra relative to the vertebral body height, the shape of the end plates, the size and orientation of the facet joints, the shape and spacing of the spinous processes, and variations in the uncovertebral joints of the cervical spine have been studied, and some evidence exists to support their clinical

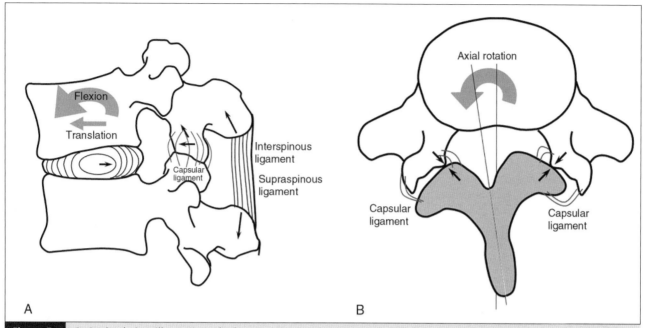

Figure 5 **A**, Sagittal-view illustration of a functional spinal unit demonstrates the resistance of posterior elements (facet joints, facet capsular ligaments, and interspinous and supraspinous ligaments [black arrows]) to displacement in flexion and anterior translation (gray arrows). **B**, Transverse-view illustration demonstrates the resistance of the facet joint and its capsular ligaments (black arrows) to axial rotation (gray arrow). (Reproduced from Wang M, Rao RD: The biomechanics of the spinal column, in Rao RD, Smuck M, eds: *Orthopaedic Knowledge Update Spine 4*. Rosemont, IL, American Academy of Orthopaedic Surgeons, 2012, pp 19-31.)

relevance. More research is needed to expand the number of validated clinical guidelines concerning the use of vertebral morphology in the diagnosis and treatment of spinal disorders.

Normal facet joints help guide motion between vertebrae and transmit loads between vertebrae, particularly in extension. The joint surfaces are covered with smooth cartilage and include a meniscus that helps provide smooth and cushioned motion between vertebrae, particularly during extension of the spine. A joint capsule surrounds each joint and helps control motion. The synovial lining inside the capsule keeps the joint lubricated.[30] A study of the effect of facet joint orientation on disk pressures found that, when facet joint orientation was closer to the sagittal plane, higher disk pressure resulted when the motion segment was exposed to a shear load.[31] Intuitively, facet joints that are more coronally oriented would resist anterior-posterior shear forces better than sagittally oriented facet joints (**Figure 6**). Transferring stress to the facet joints might protect the disk to an extent, but at the possible expense of greater propensity toward facet joint degeneration.

Vertebral end plate morphology also varies among individuals and may be an important factor in selecting the optimal treatment modality. A grading system for lumbar end plate morphology has been described, along

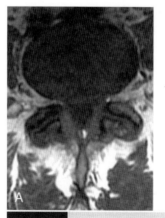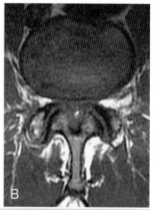

Figure 6 T1-weighted magnetic resonance images of sagittally (**A**) and coronally (**B**) oriented L4-L5 facet joints.

with its potential significance with respect to outcomes after lumbar disk arthroplasty.[32] A 2014 study reported better clinical outcomes at 2 years after disk arthroplasty in patients with flat or convex end plates versus hooked or concave end plates.[33] Although the findings may be specific to the design of the disk arthroplasty device used in the study, the need to consider the interaction between an implant and the shape of the end plate when planning surgery is indicated.

Pathomechanics

Trauma

Understanding and caring for patients with traumatic injury to the spine has been a primary motivation for much of the literature on spine biomechanics over the past seven to eight decades. Autopsy studies have shown that a wide range of injuries to spinal structures can occur from trauma. Soft-tissue injuries to the cervical spine are one of the most common patterns found in patients with severe blunt trauma.[34] Although clinically important, few diagnostic tests have been validated as sensitive and specific for the biomechanical consequences of soft-tissue injuries. Careful measurements obtained from thin-slice CT scans may allow a reliable diagnosis of some injuries by the documentation of abnormal separation between vertebrae or between the occiput and the upper cervical spine.[35,36] The frequency of use of these measurements in actual clinical practice is unknown.[37]

Presumably, abnormal separation would be associated with potentially harmful instability, although instability can be difficult to diagnose directly. The effect of soft-tissue injuries on the stability of the injured level(s) and on clinical outcomes is likely to depend on the severity of the injuries and the efficacy of attempts to stabilize the spine. Appreciating that patients can survive even severe dissociative injuries, it is important to understand best-available diagnostic approaches and stabilization practices.[38,39]

Whiplash

A subset of spine trauma is frequently grouped as whiplash injury. Whiplash injury is common, and the associated healthcare costs are high.[40] It is known from autopsy and laboratory studies that soft-tissue injuries can result from the accelerations and decelerations that can occur during rear-end vehicle collisions.[41] Injuries to the soft-tissue motion restraints may lead to abnormal intervertebral motion, and abnormal intervertebral motion can contribute to symptoms. Although damage to specific anatomic structures has not been reliably detected with currently available imaging studies in the setting of whiplash,[41,42] understanding the mechanisms of injury and the types of injuries that can occur may be helpful in making a diagnosis.

The mechanism of a common whiplash injury has been described.[41] Initially, a posterior translation of the head and neck is followed by extension of the cervical spine. Rapid forward acceleration of the head then brings the cervical spine into a flexed position. The actual movements of the head and neck relative to the body that occur during a motor vehicle collision or other blunt trauma can be highly variable, so it may be misleading in clinical practice to assume that a specific pattern of traumatic motion has occurred. Consistent with highly variable vehicle crash dynamics, a wide range of injuries has been documented, including damage to the facet joints, joint capsules, longitudinal ligaments, the intervertebral disk anulus fibrosus, and possibly, the muscle.[41] The relationship between the presence of the initial injuries and the subsequent development of clinical symptoms, particularly chronic symptoms, is poorly understood. Diagnostic tests that reliably detect specific soft-tissue injuries have yet to be fully validated.

A 2016 study identified radiographic disk metrics associated with whiplash-related symptoms.[43] The change in posterior disk height between flexion and extension divided by the amount of intervertebral rotation (reported as ± mean SD compared with radiographically normal symptomatic volunteers) was abnormally elevated in 19% of the patients who reported whiplash-related symptoms. This metric was found to be substantially higher when MRI revealed injury to the posterior intervertebral disk and/or posterior longitudinal ligament. Although this metric is not currently widely used in routine clinical practice and requires highly accurate measurements to detect the differences between normal and abnormal motion, it offers promise for the detection of the biomechanical consequences of soft-tissue injuries after blunt trauma. The posterior anulus fibrosus in the cervical spine can be thin compared with the anterior anulus fibrosus. This factor may substantially influence the propensity for damage to this region from a motor vehicle collision, and it is an important consideration when assessing magnetic resonance images for evidence of injuries. The best treatment approach for specific soft-tissue injuries remains to be determined.

Degeneration and Age-Related Changes

Degenerative changes in the spine are common.[44] It is well documented that degenerative changes can occur in asymptomatic individuals.[45] The development of symptomatic degenerative changes in the spine is determined by genetic and environmental factors, although the role of genetics is poorly understood.[46,47] Biomechanical changes associated with minor trauma from falls, overexertion during sporting and home activities, and repetitive job-related spinal loading likely contribute to degenerative changes. The degenerative changes resulting from the biomechanical effects of the loads supported by the spine can then alter intervertebral motion. Abnormal motion resulting from degenerative changes may contribute to the development of symptoms.

Limited understanding exists regarding how the myriad of observed degenerative changes affect the biomechanics of the spine and contribute to symptom development. Instability of the spine is the most commonly referenced potential biomechanical consequence of degenerative changes. A checklist for identifying clinical spinal instability has been described and provides a general framework for conceptually understanding the clinical use of the term instability, although it has a poorly defined role in routine patient care. [1,48,49] A well-validated objective diagnostic test for spinal instability is lacking.

The lack of objective metrics for defining spinal instability may help explain why a literature review of the effect of degeneration on spinal stability found only a trend toward increasing stiffness with degeneration.[44] A diagnostic test for instability can be used with confidence when documentation exists that the test detects true biomechanical abnormality and associations between clinical symptoms and abnormal test results and is useful in selecting the optimum treatment for the patient.

An association between spondylolisthesis and spinal instability is frequently inferred, although not all spondylolisthesis is unstable.[50] There are multiple confounding issues in determining the relationship of spinal instability and symptomatic spondylolisthesis.[51] During the natural history of spondylolisthesis, it is generally assumed that an unstable phase (defined as having abnormal intervertebral motion) will occur, but motion may return to normal or subnormal levels as the associated degeneration progresses.

Several phenomena associated with degeneration may help in the stabilization of a spinal level. Severe disk height loss, osteophyte formation, vertebral end plate sclerosis, and ligament ossification may offer evidence of restabilization.[51] However, instability cannot be definitively ruled out based only on radiographic signs of restabilization. Objective diagnostic metrics for instability may help resolve this dilemma. Instability has been defined as the presence of more than 3 mm of sagittal plane translation between flexion and extension.[50,52,53] Although this is a promising definition of instability, it is confounded by sensitivity to variable patient effort, variable radiographic magnification, and measurement error. A study of asymptomatic volunteers, which used a device to correct for differences in radiographic magnification, reported that the upper limit of normal translation was greater than 3 mm at most levels of the lumbar spine;[20] therefore, more than 16% of spinal levels in the asymptomatic volunteers would be classified as unstable. In clinical practice, a scaling device is not used to correct for radiographic magnification error, so the size of a vertebra measured from a radiograph can be 9% to 63% larger than the actual size of the vertebra.[54] In addition, if a patient exerts little effort when asked to flex and extend his or her spine

during radiography, the results may appear to indicate low translation when abnormally high translation is actually present (eg, when the patient bends to tie his or her shoe). For these reasons, the greater–than–3-mm criterion should be used with caution.

Another approach used to differentiate between static and dynamic spondylolisthesis is to compare the relative positions between vertebrae when the patient is supine (assessed with MRI or CT) with those of the patient when bearing weight (assessed using radiography).[55,56] A 2014 study reported that almost 40% of patients with spondylolisthesis as observed in upright standing radiographic examinations had reduction of the spondylolisthesis in supine imaging studies.[50]

Intervertebral Disk

Because intervertebral disks play a key role in controlling intervertebral motion, degeneration of a disk can alter intervertebral motion. Evidence indicates an increasing loss of intervertebral motion control during the early phases of disk degeneration; however, motion may return to normal levels or may remain at below-normal levels with severe degenerative changes. These changes were documented in a cadaver model;[57] however, in clinical practice, the changes in motion that occur with degeneration are subtle.[44] Using weight-bearing MRI, a study of 162 patients found an initial increase in translation in the early stages of intervertebral disk degeneration, followed by a decrease in translation with severe degeneration.[58] Using a cadaver model, no association was found between disk degeneration and the magnitude of sagittal plane translation when spines were subjected to shear loading;[59] however, it is unclear whether this was related to the stabilizing effect of the compressive load applied to the spine.

Compressive loading has been shown to have a stabilizing effect on the spine, which can be important when assessing instability.[60] If the vertebral end plates are nearly horizontal when imaging is obtained, gravitational forces may tend to force interlocking and stabilization of the vertebrae. If the end plates are substantially tilted with respect to a horizontal orientation, a large component of the gravitational forces will be exerted parallel to the disk space and can provoke translation between vertebrae that would increase the likelihood for detecting abnormal translation at an unstable level. A study of a large number of lumbar spines in patients with a wide range of ages showed that disk degeneration tended to occur after facet degeneration, and intervertebral translation initially increased with progressing degeneration and then decreased in those with advanced degeneration.[61] An association between facet and disk degeneration can be expected because

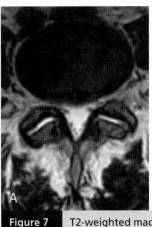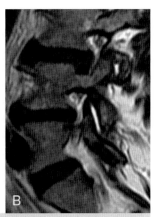

Figure 7   T2-weighted magnetic resonance images show fluid in a facet joint. If possible, it is helpful to confirm that the fluid is visible in both the sagittal (**A**) and axial (**B**) images.

incompetent motion control in one region will increase the burden on other elements of the intervertebral motion control system. Each pair of adjacent vertebrae and the intervertebral disk and ligaments forming the connection between the vertebrae form a functional spinal unit (FSU). Each FSU can be mechanically compromised in isolation, and this can in turn affect adjacent FSUs.

Facet Joints

The degenerative changes that can occur in the facet joints can be subjectively assessed using several grading systems.[62] It is unclear, however, how degenerative changes in facet joints affect spinal biomechanics and the relative contribution of degenerative changes in causing symptoms. Phenomenologically, it has been shown that patients with lumbar spondylolisthesis tend to have more sagittally oriented facet joints.[63] Spondylolisthesis is more likely in patients with L4-L5 facet joints oriented greater than 58° from the coronal plane.[64] This may be a consideration when assessing the potential value of a treatment such as uninstrumented decompression that requires inherent spinal stability. Recently, it has been reported that the orientation of the lumbar facet joints may depend, in part, on ethnicity.[65] This finding has not yet resulted in validated clinical guidelines for using facet joint orientation as a diagnostic tool or in treatment planning.

The presence of fluid in the facet joints observed with MRI is among the most accepted indicators of lumbar instability (**Figure 7**). Multiple studies have reported an association between the presence of fluid in the facet joints and dynamic spondylolisthesis.[55,66,67] In addition, it appears that the likelihood of dynamic instability correlates with the amount of fluid; however, it should be noted that gas can sometimes be seen on CT images of

the facet joints. Gas in the facet joints also is an accepted indicator of instability.[68] Gas appears black on a magnetic resonance image. The MRI fluid sign may be more sensitive (true in disease) than specific (false in health). Determining the actual sensitivity and specificity of any test for spinal instability is challenging because a true validated preferred test is required but has not yet been established. When assessing facet joints for a fluid sign, it is important to appreciate that lordosis is reduced in a supine patient, and the cranial-most aspect of the facet joints can open while the caudal-most aspect is closed. The accumulation of joint fluid may be seen in the resulting gap at the cranial-most aspect of the joint even at a stable level, so it is important to appreciate the amount of possible fluid at a stable level.

It has been shown that the amount of sagittal plane intervertebral translation that occurs (normalized to the amount of intervertebral rotation to control for variability in patient effort) is substantially higher when the facet fluid sign is present.[20] Because the TPDR is normally small,[20] TPDR may be a more reliable metric for determining instability, although only if sufficient patient effort has been exerted in flexion and extension to provoke an abnormal TPDR if present.

In the cervical spine, the morphology of the facet joints such as asymmetric hypertrophy is associated with pathomechanical changes such as degenerative spondylolisthesis.[69] Asymmetric hypertrophy is defined as a facet joint on one side having a much larger joint surface area than the facet joint on the opposite side. Spondylolisthesis in the cervical spine is more commonly observed in upright standing radiographs than in supine magnetic resonance images.[69] A large difference in the orientations of the left and right facet joints is associated with the presence of spondylolisthesis in the cervical spine.[70] Spondylolisthesis was found in 20% of symptomatic patients in one study.[71]

Vertebral Morphology

A study evaluating the relationship between MRI-based measurements of morphologic parameters for the lumbar spine reported little association with symptoms.[72] The thickness and cross-sectional area of the ligamentum flavum were among the few parameters that had significant association with clinical symptoms, but even those parameters explained less than 25% of the variability in Oswestry Disability Index scores. Imaging-based morphologic measurements have not been found to correlate with functional status.[73]

Iatrogenic Instability

Multiple studies have documented that resection of tissue to achieve a decompression objective can result in loss of stability or spondylolisthesis.[74-77] Increasing instability has been reported with increasingly greater resection of ligaments and resection of the lamina and facets.[78] Postoperative instability may be seen in 5.5% of patients following laminectomy or minimally invasive decompression without fusion.[75] In 40 patients with grade 1 spondylolisthesis who were treated with decompression using laminectomy only (no fusion), postoperative instability was more likely in patients with the following preoperative findings: intervertebral translation at the level of the spondylolisthesis greater than 1.25 mm, disk height greater than 6.5 mm, and facet joint angle greater than 50°.[74] Determining the true incidence of iatrogenic instability after uninstrumented decompression requires a validated test for instability, an evaluation of preoperative stability, and details of the decompressive procedure.

Repairing and Restoring Spine Biomechanics

All spine fusion, disk arthroplasty, and spine stabilization devices and related surgery are intended, at least in part, to influence spine biomechanics.

Fusion

Fusion is sometimes used to provide stability to a spinal level deemed unstable (unable to maintain normal alignment and intervertebral motion during ADLs). Fusion also may be used to provide stability to a level deemed likely to become unstable after decompression surgery. The goal of fusion is to create a mechanical environment conducive to the formation of bone that bridges between vertebrae. Because bridging bone only forms where motion is below a threshold, the primary technical goal is to reduce motion to below that maximum threshold. Many approaches to creating a fusion environment have been studied, from uninstrumented fusions to fusions with instrumentation in multiple regions, including anterior, lateral, posterior, and posterolateral regions. Pedicle screws are the preferred fixation method to enhance lumbar fusion and have been extensively studied in most clinically relevant scenarios.

Although the various approaches to achieving fusion can be modeled and compared using cadaver studies or computer models,[79] surgeons typically rely on experience and their perception of the need for using instrumentation to improve the stability of the treated level(s) in determining how much fixation is adequate for an individual patient. Although posterior lumbar systems can appear mechanically robust, these systems do not eliminate all motion between vertebrae. Most studies of fixation hardware in cadaver spines document some residual motion between vertebrae after instrumentation.[79] Because

mineralized bone can form only where there is minimal motion, the most likely locations for initial bone formation are areas with the lowest motion. After bone forms in a location, intervertebral motion is further reduced, thus providing a mechanical environment conducive to the formation of bridging bone at other locations. It is important that bridging bone forms a new path for transmission of forces between vertebrae before the hardware fails from the repetitive stress of providing the load transmission pathway.

Knowing the location of the densest bone in the spine may be beneficial when using instrumentation such as pedicle screws. Cortical screws recently have been clinically used for spinal fixation. These screws are placed in a pathway intended to mechanically engage with dense bone at multiple points along the inner pedicle and posterolateral aspects of the vertebral body[13] (**Figure 8**). Use of a cortical trajectory requires substantially higher torque for insertion.[80] Higher insertional torque is generally associated with a greater ability to transfer loads from the bone of one vertebra through the hardware and onto the bone of the adjacent vertebra. However, the shorter screw trajectory and the decreased length of cortical screws compared with pedicle screws require careful planning of the entire screw pathway to optimize biomechanical purchase and approximate or exceed the fixation strength of traditional trajectories that use larger screws.[81]

Optimal cortical screw size has been determined by measuring pullout strength. The most predictive factor of fixation strength is the percentage of screw length in the vertebral body. Higher percentages of screw length in the vertebral body correlate with stronger lumbar fixation. Screw diameter strongly correlates with pullout strength. It was determined that the ideal cortical screw has a diameter of 5.5 mm and a length of 35 mm. A major potential limitation is that most lumbar levels may not safely contain this size screw without surgical complication or an increased risk of pedicle or pars interarticularis fracture.

Because cortical screws do not generally traverse anterior and posterior to the center of rotation of a spinal segment, they have a mechanical disadvantage compared with longer screws that pass the center of rotation. For this reason, the use of cortical screws with interbody support is suggested. A 2013 study suggested that cortical screws without interbody support are less stiff than traditional pedicle screws only in axial rotation.[79] However, the biomechanical differences between cortical screws and traditional pedicle screws have yet to be fully evaluated, especially regarding clinical effect. One study reported higher failure rates of cortical screws in osteoporotic bone when tested under cyclical loading.[82]

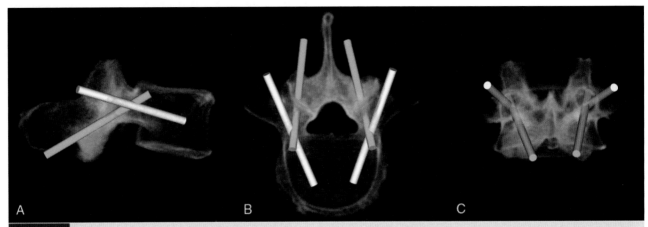

Figure 8 Illustrations compare the cortical screw trajectory (green) with the trajectory of traditional lumbar pedicle screws (white) for fixation of fusion hardware to the spine. Sagittal (**A**), axial (**B**), and coronal (**C**) views are shown.

Disk Arthroplasty

Preserving normal motion between vertebrae as opposed to stopping motion (as with fusion) is intuitively appealing. Substantial research has been undertaken on various motion-preserving strategies in the spine. The FDA approved several cervical and lumbar disk arthroplasty devices that are generally capable of providing motion between vertebrae, although the motion may not always fully reproduce the quantity and quality of normal motion. The quantity of motion is typically assessed in clinical trials of disk arthroplasty based on the magnitude of intervertebral rotation and translation. As previously discussed, these parameters can be difficult to interpret without understanding the protocol used to encourage patient effort in flexing and extending the spine. Analyzing motion at each individual level as a proportion of total motion (eg, rotation at C5-C6 as a percentage of C2 to C7 rotation) has been proposed as a better approach. It was found that disk arthroplasty tends to preserve the proportion of motion at each level, whereas fusion tends to distribute motion lost at the treated level to the other levels.[83,84] The long-term consequence of this finding is not yet fully understood.

The effect of disk arthroplasty on both the quantity and quality of intervertebral motion has been addressed using both data from clinical trials and computer models. Computer models are advantageous because important variables such as the effect of individual parameters can be precisely controlled. A limitation of computer models is the difficulty of representing the wide range of vertebral morphologies, soft-tissue properties, and patient activity levels that can occur. Despite the available knowledge base, the effect of most motion-preserving devices on the quality of spine motion and the effect of the quality of motion on long-term clinical outcomes remains poorly understood.

Using a retrospective analysis of data from an FDA-regulated study of a lumbar disk arthroplasty device, several variables significantly associated with clinical outcomes were identified.[33] Variables that proved important to good outcomes included disk height of less than 8 mm and a low level of lordosis at the treated level. A retrospective analysis of a cervical disk arthroplasty device reported that a preoperative short disk height or implanting a disk such that lordosis was increased by greater than 3° increased the risk of a poor outcome.[85] Finite element models showed that multilevel lumbar disk arthroplasties can substantially increase the motion occurring at the treated levels, and placing lumbar disks too far anterior or posterior can lead to abnormal motions and elevated forces across the facet joints.[86] Specific biomechanical consequences of disk arthroplasty can affect outcomes. Large studies that systematically assess the effects of biomechanical factors on outcomes are needed to create validated treatment guidelines.

Summary

Normal spine biomechanics enable a wide range of repetitive motions without structural failure while simultaneously protecting the neurovascular elements. Understanding the load-bearing requirements, load-bearing capacity, and normal motion of the spine can help in counselling patients about spinal disorders. A large body of peer-reviewed literature provides evidence for the many and varied injuries and degenerative changes that can occur in the spine. Nevertheless, validated diagnostic tests are not currently available that can identify specific causes for spine-related symptoms in many patients. It is likely that objective validated diagnostic tests could lead to substantial improvements in clinical outcomes for many patients with disorders of the spine. A large body of literature describing the biomechanical effects of many of the available surgical treatment modalities also is available; this information can aid surgeons in choosing the best treatment options for their patients. When available, the widespread use of validated spine biomechanical metrics in research studies will enable predictive analytics that can account for both clinical and biomechanical factors that predict the most effective treatment modalities.

Key Study Points

- Clinicians must understand the load-bearing requirements, the load-bearing capacity, and normal intervertebral motion to assess whether the biomechanics of the spine have been compromised.

- Assessment of intervertebral motion can be helpful in diagnosing incompetent intervertebral motion restraints, but only if the diagnostic test applied sufficient mechanic stress to the spine to allow a reliable diagnosis. The stability of the spine can be used to select the best treatment option.

- Clinical outcomes for multiple surgical treatment options depend in part on the interaction of the treatment with the morphology and mechanical properties of the spine.

Annotated References

1. White AA III, Panjabi MM: *Clinical Biomechanics of the Spine*, ed 2. Philadelphia, PA, JB Lippincott, 1990.

2. Oxland TR: Fundamental biomechanics of the spine: What we have learned in the past 25 years and future directions. *J Biomech* 2016;49(6):817-832.

   The understanding of spine biomechanics has advanced substantially since the publication of some of the original pioneering research. This review summarizes advancements in knowledge as well as gaps in knowledge that need to be addressed to better understand strategies for optimizing clinical outcomes.

3. Dreischarf M, Shirazi-Adl A, Arjmand N, Rohlmann A, Schmidt H: Estimation of loads on human lumbar spine: A review of in vivo and computational model studies. *J Biomech* 2016;49(6):833-845.

   This review paper provides a resource for information about the loads that must be supported by the spine during ADLs. This information may be helpful when counseling patients on recommended activity restrictions.

4. Rohlmann A, Pohl D, Bender A, et al: Activities of everyday life with high spinal loads. *PLoS One* 2014;9(5):e98510.

   This large database of loads measured by instrumented vertebral body replacements can serve as a reference when helping patients understand how to avoid activities with high spinal loads.

5. Rohlmann A, Zander T, Graichen F, Bergmann G: Effect of an orthosis on the loads acting on a vertebral body replacement. *Clin Biomech (Bristol, Avon)* 2013;28(5):490-494.

   Based on loads measured using an instrumented lumbar vertebral body replacement in patients, an orthosis was found to reduce loads in some patients and for some activities, whereas loads for other patients and other activities were increased. These results suggest caution when recommending use of an orthosis to restrict loading of the spine.

6. Biewener AA: Safety factors in bone strength. *Calcif Tissue Int* 1993;53(1 suppl 1):S68-S74.

7. Windhagen HJ, Hipp JA, Silva MJ, Lipson SJ, Hayes WC: Predicting failure of thoracic vertebrae with simulated and actual metastatic defects. *Clin Orthop Relat Res* 1997;344:313-319.

8. Zhao F-D, Pollintine P, Hole BD, Adams MA, Dolan P: Vertebral fractures usually affect the cranial endplate because it is thinner and supported by less-dense trabecular bone. *Bone* 2009;44(2):372-379.

9. Melton LJ III, Riggs BL, Keaveny TM, et al: Structural determinants of vertebral fracture risk. *J Bone Miner Res* 2007;22(12):1885-1892.

10. Bouxsein ML, Melton LJ III, Riggs BL, et al: Age- and sex-specific differences in the factor of risk for vertebral fracture: A population-based study using QCT. *J Bone Miner Res* 2006;21(9):1475-1482.

11. Gallagher S, Heberger JR: Examining the interaction of force and repetition on musculoskeletal disorder risk: A systematic literature review. *Hum Factors* 2013;55(1):108-124.

    This literature review aids in the appreciation of the magnitude of applied loads and the number of loading repetition interactions in determining the risk of musculoskeletal disorders.

12. Fields AJ, Nawathe S, Eswaran SK, et al: Vertebral fragility and structural redundancy. *J Bone Miner Res* 2012;27(10):2152-2158.

    Vertebrae can continue to provide load-bearing support after some trabeculae have failed because of structural redundancy. The combination of bone reduction within vertebrae and the loss of structural redundancy results in a much more serious vertebral fracture than can be explained by low bone volume fraction alone.

13. Su BW, Chaput CD: Treatment of spinal conditions in young adults: Cortical lumbar screw techniques. *Oper Tech Orthop* 2015;25(3):187-193.

Cortical screws used in fusion hardware fixation take advantage of the dense cortical bone in the region of the pars interarticularis. The surgical exposure can be less extensive than with traditional pedicle screws. Knowledge of the biomechanical and clinical support for fixation using cortical screws is presented.

14. Santoni BG, Hynes RA, McGilvray KC, et al: Cortical bone trajectory for lumbar pedicle screws. *Spine J* 2009;9(5):366-373.

15. Phillips FM, Lauryssen C: *The Lumbar Intervertebral Disc* .New York, NY, Thieme Medical Publishers, 2009.

16. Lao L, Daubs MD, Takahashi S, et al: Kinetic magnetic resonance imaging analysis of lumbar segmental motion at levels adjacent to disc herniation. *Eur Spine J* 2016;25(1):222-229.

    No effect of disk herniation on intervertebral motion at the adjacent levels was observed in a clinical study in which intervertebral motion was measured using magnetic resonance images obtained during the performance of lumbar flexion and extension.

17. Stokes IA, Gardner-Morse M: A database of lumbar spinal mechanical behavior for validation of spinal analytical models. *J Biomech* 2016;49(5):780-785.

    The authors of this study provide comprehensive reference data for intervertebral motion in the lumbar spine in a form usable for computer model validation.

18. Ishii T, Mukai Y, Hosono N, et al: Kinematics of the cervical spine in lateral bending: In vivo three-dimensional analysis. *Spine (Phila Pa 1976)* 2006;31(2):155-160.

19. Anderst WJ, Donaldson WF III, Lee JY, Kang JD: Three-dimensional intervertebral kinematics in the healthy young adult cervical spine during dynamic functional loading. *J Biomech* 2015;48(7):1286-1293.

    A sophisticated approach was used to measure three-dimensional intervertebral motion in young volunteers with no history of spine problems.

20. Staub BN, Holman PJ, Reitman CA, Hipp J: Sagittal plane lumbar intervertebral motion during seated flexion-extension radiographs of 658 asymptomatic nondegenerated levels. *J Neurosurg Spine* 2015;23(6):731-738.

    Reference data describing intervertebral motion in the lumbar spine of asymptomatic volunteers are presented. Data from prior publications are tabulated and support the need for standardization of lumbar flexion-extension studies.

21. Miyasaka K, Ohmori K, Suzuki K, Inoue H: Radiographic analysis of lumbar motion in relation to lumbosacral stability: Investigation of moderate and maximum motion. *Spine (Phila Pa 1976)* 2000;25(6):732-737.

22. Knutsson F: The instability associated with disc degeneration in the lumbar spine. *Acta Radiol* 1944;25:593-609.

23. Smit TH, van Tunen MS, van der Veen AJ, Kingma I, van Dieën JH: Quantifying intervertebral disc mechanics: A new definition of the neutral zone. *BMC Musculoskelet Disord* 2011;12(1):38.

    A mathematical definition is proposed for the neutral zone, which is a fundamental aspect of spine movement. Justification for the use of a flexion-extension study in the reliable diagnosis of instability is presented.

24. Crawford NR, Peles JD, Dickman CA: The spinal lax zone and neutral zone: Measurement techniques and parameter comparisons. *J Spinal Disord* 1998;11(5):416-429.

25. Yoganandan N, Kumaresan S, Pintar FA: Biomechanics of the cervical spine: Part 2. Cervical spine soft tissue responses and biomechanical modeling. *Clin Biomech (Bristol, Avon)* 2001;16(1):1-27.

26. Naserkhaki S, Jaremko JL, Adeeb S, El-Rich M: On the load-sharing along the ligamentous lumbosacral spine in flexed and extended postures: Finite element study. *J Biomech* 2016;49(6):974-982.

    Information is provided to aid in understanding the interaction of intervertebral disks, vertebral morphology, and intervertebral ligaments in the roles of simultaneously providing load-bearing capacity and stability.

27. Weiler PJ, King GJ, Gertzbein SD: Analysis of sagittal plane instability of the lumbar spine in vivo. *Spine (Phila Pa 1976)* 1990;15(12):1300-1306.

28. Kristjansson E, Leivseth G, Brinckmann P, Frobin W: Increased sagittal plane segmental motion in the lower cervical spine in women with chronic whiplash-associated disorders, grades I-II: A case-control study using a new measurement protocol. *Spine (Phila Pa 1976)* 2003;28(19):2215-2221.

29. Hipp JA, Wharton ND: Quantitative motion analysis (QMA) of the spine, in Yue JJ, Bertagnoli R, McAfee PC, An HS, eds: *Motion Preservation Surgery of the Spine.* New York, NY, Elsevier Health, 2008, pp 85-96.

30. Jaumard NV, Welch WC, Winkelstein BA: Spinal facet joint biomechanics and mechanotransduction in normal, injury and degenerative conditions. *J Biomech Eng* 2011;133(7):071010.

    Despite substantial research, a better understanding of the biomechanics of facet joints and their role in patient symptoms is needed. Existing knowledge of facet joint biomechanics and pathomechanics is presented.

31. Kim H-J, Chun H-J, Lee H-M, et al: The biomechanical influence of the facet joint orientation and the facet tropism in the lumbar spine. *Spine J* 2013;13(10):1301-1308.

    Using computer models, the authors documented little effect of lumbar facet orientation on intervertebral disk stresses resulting from bending moments; however, shear forces resulted in higher disk pressure with more sagittally oriented facet joints or facet tropism.

32. Oetgen ME, Yue JJ, la Torre JJ, Bertagnoli R: Does vertebral endplate morphology influence outcomes in lumbar total disc arthroplasty? Part II. Clinical and radiographic results as evaluated utilizing the Vertebral Endplate Yue-Bertagnoli (VEYBR) Classification. *SAS J* 2008;2(2):101-106.

33. Gornet MF, Schranck F, Wharton ND, et al: Optimizing success with lumbar disc arthroplasty. *Eur Spine J* 2014;23(10):2127-2135.

    Several variables can be measured from preoperative and postoperative radiographs and MRI studies that can explain variability in clinical outcomes. This variability may help in the formulation of strategies for optimizing clinical outcomes after lumbar disk arthroplasty.

34. Lador R, Ben-Galim PJ, Weiner BK, Hipp JA: The association of occipitocervical dissociation and death as a result of blunt trauma. *Spine J* 2010;10(12):1128-1132.

35. Radcliff KE, Ben-Galim P, Dreiangel N, et al: Comprehensive computed tomography assessment of the upper cervical anatomy: What is normal? *Spine J* 2010;10(3):219-229.

36. Chaput CD, Walgama J, Torres E, et al: Defining and detecting missed ligamentous injuries of the occipitocervical complex. *Spine (Phila Pa 1976)* 2011;36(9):709-714.

    Careful thin-slice CT examination measurements of the anatomic spacing between the occiput and the first and second cervical vertebrae are required to make a reliable diagnosis of injuries in this region. Reference data required for interpretation of measurements are presented.

37. Dreiangel N, Ben-Galim P, Lador R, Hipp JA: Occipitocervical dissociative injuries: Common in blunt trauma fatalities and better detected with objective computed tomography-based measurements. *Spine J* 2010;10(8):704-707.

38. Bellabarba C, Mirza SK, West GA, et al: Diagnosis and treatment of craniocervical dislocation in a series of 17 consecutive survivors during an 8-year period. *J Neurosurg Spine* 2006;4(6):429-440.

39. Mendenhall SK, Sivaganesan A, Mistry A, Sivasubramaniam P, McGirt MJ, Devin CJ: Traumatic atlantooccipital dislocation: Comprehensive assessment of mortality, neurologic improvement, and patient-reported outcomes at a Level 1 trauma center over 15 years. *Spine J* 2015;15(11):2385-2395.

    Failure to make a diagnosis of atlantooccipital dissociation is a predictor of mortality in patients with blunt trauma. Additional support for the need for careful CT-based measurements to reliably diagnose occipitocervical injuries is presented.

40. Hogg-Johnson S, van der Velde G, Carroll LJ, et al: The burden and determinants of neck pain in the general population: Results of the Bone and Joint Decade 2000-2010 Task Force on Neck Pain and Its Associated Disorders. *J Manipulative Physiol Ther* 2009;32(2 suppl):S46-S60.

41. Curatolo M, Bogduk N, Ivancic PC, McLean SA, Siegmund GP, Winkelstein BA: The role of tissue damage in whiplash-associated disorders: Discussion paper 1. *Spine (Phila Pa 1976)* 2011;36(25suppl):S309-S315.

    This review presents the most current knowledge regarding the biomechanics of whiplash injury.

42. Uhrenholt L, Grunnet-Nilsson N, Hartvigsen J: Cervical spine lesions after road traffic accidents: A systematic review. *Spine (Phila Pa 1976)* 2002;27(17):1934-1941, discussion 1940.

43. Gornet MF, Hipp JA, Copay AG, Schranck FW: Objective radiographic disc integrity metric identifies disc abnormalities in whiplash patients. *Spine J* 2016;16(10):S302.

    Using carefully assessed high-resolution MRI examinations as the preferred method, a simple metric that can be objectively measured from cervical flexion-extension radiographs was found to be substantially elevated in the presence of MRI abnormalities at the posterior anulus fibrosus and/or posterior longitudinal ligament.

44. Galbusera F, van Rijsbergen M, Ito K, Huyghe JM, Brayda-Bruno M, Wilke H-J: Ageing and degenerative changes of the intervertebral disc and their impact on spinal flexibility. *Eur Spine J* 2014;23(3 suppl 3):S324-S332.

    This literature review suggests that the mechanical behavior of the lumbar spine is altered by degenerative changes.

45. Brinjikji W, Luetmer PH, Comstock B, et al: Systematic literature review of imaging features of spinal degeneration in asymptomatic populations. *AJNR Am J Neuroradiol* 2015;36(4):811-816.

    The authors review the many publications documenting that degenerative changes in the spine are commonly seen in imaging studies of asymptomatic individuals.

46. Battié MC, Videman T, Kaprio J, et al: The Twin Spine Study: Contributions to a changing view of disc degeneration. *Spine J* 2009;9(1):47-59.

47. Rajasekaran S, Kanna RM, Reddy RR, et al: How reliable are the reported genetic associations in disc degeneration? The influence of phenotypes, age, population size, and inclusion sequence in 809 patients. *Spine (Phila Pa 1976)* 2016;41(21):1649-1660.

    The authors document how the apparent association between genetics and disk degeneration is influenced by many factors. Level of evidence: IV.

48. Panjabi MM: Clinical spinal instability and low back pain. *J Electromyogr Kinesiol* 2003;13(4):371-379.

49. Balderston RA, Auerbach JD: The definition of lumbar spinal instability and its clinical significance. *Seminars in Spine Surgery* 2005;17(4):240-242.

50. Even JL, Chen AF, Lee JY: Imaging characteristics of "dynamic" versus "static" spondylolisthesis: Analysis

using magnetic resonance imaging and flexion/extension films. *Spine J* 2014;14(9):1965-1969.

Instability is more likely when fluid is observed in the facet joint on MRI examination of the lumbar spine. Fluid in the space between spinous processes is also associated with instability.

51. Simmonds AM, Rampersaud YR, Dvorak MF, Dea N, Melnyk AD, Fisher CG: Defining the inherent stability of degenerative spondylolisthesis: A systematic review. *J Neurosurg Spine* 2015;23(2):178-189.

Multiple imaging-based observations can be identified that help predict stability at a lumbar intervertebral level with degenerative spondylolisthesis.

52. Boden SD, Wiesel SW: Lumbosacral segmental motion in normal individuals: Have we been measuring instability properly? *Spine (Phila Pa 1976)* 1990;15(6):571-576.

53. Snoddy MC, Sielatycki JA, Sivaganesan A, Engstrom SM, McGirt MJ, Devin CJ: Can facet joint fluid on MRI and dynamic instability be a predictor of improvement in back pain following lumbar fusion for degenerative spondylolisthesis? *Eur Spine J* 2016;25(8):2408-2415.

MRI showed that the probability of finding excessive intervertebral translation between flexion and extension increases with the thickness of fluid in the facet joint. Fluid in the facet joint may help predict the likelihood of achieving good outcomes after spinal fusion.

54. Ravi B, Rampersaud R: Clinical magnification error in lateral spinal digital radiographs. *Spine (Phila Pa 1976)* 2008;33(10):E311-E316.

55. Ben-Galim P, Reitman CA: The distended facet sign: An indicator of position-dependent spinal stenosis and degenerative spondylolisthesis. *Spine J* 2007;7(2):245-248.

56. Kuhns BD, Kouk S, Buchanan C, et al: Sensitivity of magnetic resonance imaging in the diagnosis of mobile and nonmobile L4–L5 degenerative spondylolisthesis. *Spine J* 2015;15(9):1956-1962.

The authors differentiate between static and dynamic spondylolisthesis. Spondylolisthesis is classified as dynamic when there is a substantial change in listhesis between supine and standing positions. Fluid in the facet joint is a clinical marker for dynamic spondylolisthesis.

57. Zirbel SA, Stolworthy DK, Howell LL, Bowden AE: Intervertebral disc degeneration alters lumbar spine segmental stiffness in all modes of loading under a compressive follower load. *Spine J* 2013;13(9):1134-1147.

The effect of degenerative changes on the biomechanics of an FSU are complicated but have been documented using laboratory testing of cadaver spines. The results of these laboratory studies can be helpful in further modeling and development of clinical diagnostics.

58. Lao L, Daubs MD, Scott TP, et al: Effect of disc degeneration on lumbar segmental mobility analyzed by kinetic magnetic resonance imaging. *Spine (Phila Pa 1976)* 2015;40(5):316-322.

MRI analyses of intervertebral motion of the lumbar spine in flexion and extension was used to document the development of instability in patients with mild to moderate disk degeneration and restabilization in those with severe degenerative disk changes. It should be appreciated that substantial variability exists—not all moderately degenerated disks are unstable and not all severely degenerated disks are stable.

59. Melnyk AD, Kelly A, Chak JD, et al: The effect of disc degeneration on anterior shear translation in the lumbar spine. *J Orthop Res* 2015;33(4):450-457.

Based on laboratory testing of cadaver spines, increasingly severe disk degeneration was not clearly associated with the amount of intervertebral shear translation when spines were tested with a superimposed compressive load.

60. Tawackoli W, Marco R, Liebschner MA: The effect of compressive axial preload on the flexibility of the thoracolumbar spine. *Spine (Phila Pa 1976)* 2004;29(9):988-993.

61. Kong MH, Morishita Y, He W, et al: Lumbar segmental mobility according to the grade of the disc, the facet joint, the muscle, and the ligament pathology by using kinetic magnetic resonance imaging. *Spine (Phila Pa 1976)* 2009;34(23):2537-2544.

62. Kettler A, Wilke HJ: Review of existing grading systems for cervical or lumbar disc and facet joint degeneration. *Eur Spine J* 2006;15(6):705-718.

63. Schuller S, Charles YP, Steib J-P: Sagittal spinopelvic alignment and body mass index in patients with degenerative spondylolisthesis. *Eur Spine J* 2011;20(5):713-719.

The authors of this study reported a significant association between the sagittal plan orientation of the pelvis, the body mass index of the patient, sagittally oriented facet joints, and the presence of spondylolisthesis.

64. Samartzis D, Cheung JP, Rajasekaran S, et al: Critical values of facet joint angulation and tropism in the development of lumbar degenerative spondylolisthesis: An international, large-scale multicenter study by the AOSpine Asia Pacific Research Collaboration Consortium. *Global Spine J* 2016;6(5):414-421.

Based on a large sample, good evidence was found that degenerative spondylolisthesis is more likely to occur in individuals with sagittally oriented facet joints. A threshold level of 58° was identified as predictive of degenerative spondylolisthesis.

65. Williams R, Cheung JP, Goss B, et al: An international multicenter study assessing the role of ethnicity on variation of lumbar facet joint orientation and the occurrence of degenerative spondylolisthesis in Asia Pacific: A study from the AOSpine Asia Pacific Research Collaboration Consortium. *Global Spine J* 2016;6(1):35-45.

This multinational, multiethnic study found that that ethnicity may not play a role in facet joint orientation in most patients with degenerative spondylolisthesis in the Asia-Pacific region.

66. Rihn JA, Lee JY, Khan M, et al: Does lumbar facet fluid detected on magnetic resonance imaging correlate with radiographic instability in patients with degenerative lumbar disease? *Spine (Phila Pa 1976)* 2007;32(14):1555-1560.

67. Chaput C, Padon D, Rush J, Lenehan E, Rahm M: The significance of increased fluid signal on magnetic resonance imaging in lumbar facets in relationship to degenerative spondylolisthesis. *Spine (Phila Pa 1976)* 2007;32(17):1883-1887.

68. Lefkowitz DM, Quencer RM: Vacuum facet phenomenon: A computed tomographic sign of degenerative spondylolisthesis. *Radiology* 1982;144(3):562.

69. Chaput CD, Allred JJ, Pandorf JJ, Song J, Rahm MD: The significance of facet joint cross-sectional area on magnetic resonance imaging in relationship to cervical degenerative spondylolisthesis. *Spine J* 2013;13(8):856-861.

Spondylolisthesis in the cervical spine was much more likely to be detected from a weight-bearing radiograph than a supine magnetic resonance image. The size of the facet joints and left-right asymmetry of the facet joints was more likely to be found when spondylolisthesis was observed.

70. Xu C, Lin B, Ding Z, Xu Y: Cervical degenerative spondylolisthesis: Analysis of facet orientation and the severity of cervical spondylolisthesis. *Spine J* 2016;16(1):10-15.

Asymmetry in the orientation of the left and right cervical facet joints is common. Although the magnitude of spondylolisthesis is not associated with this asymmetry, development of spondylolisthesis is more likely when asymmetry is present.

71. Suzuki A, Daubs MD, Inoue H, et al: Prevalence and motion characteristics of degenerative cervical spondylolisthesis in the symptomatic adult. *Spine (Phila Pa 1976)* 2013;38(17):E1115-E1120.

Spondylolisthesis of 2 mm or more was found in 20% of symptomatic patients, most commonly at C4-C5 and C5-C6. Translational motion was greater and spinal canal diameter smaller when spondylolisthesis was observed.

72. Kim YU, Kong YG, Lee J, et al: Clinical symptoms of lumbar spinal stenosis associated with morphological parameters on magnetic resonance images. *Eur Spine J* 2015;24(10):2236-2243.

This retrospective review of 117 patients with lumbar spinal stenosis reported that evaluation of integral morphologic parameters was more important than evaluation of individual morphologic parameters in these patients.

73. Alsaleh K, Ho D, Rosas-Arellano MP, Stewart TC, Gurr KR, Bailey CS: Radiographic assessment of degenerative lumbar spinal stenosis: Is MRI superior to CT? *Eur Spine J* 2017;26(2):362-367.

Based on imaging studies of 54 patients who underwent both a CT and an MRI examination, observer agreement in the assessment of lumbar stenosis was better using the MRI examination than the CT examination.

74. Blumenthal C, Curran J, Benzel EC, et al: Radiographic predictors of delayed instability following decompression without fusion for degenerative grade I lumbar spondylolisthesis. *J Neurosurg Spine* 2013;18(4):340-346.

Risk factors for instability after uninstrumented decompression included preexisting spondylolisthesis, preoperative intervertebral disk height greater than 6.5 mm, and sagittally oriented facet joints.

75. Guha D, Heary RF, Shamji MF: Iatrogenic spondylolisthesis following laminectomy for degenerative lumbar stenosis: Systematic review and current concepts. *Neurosurg Focus* 2015;39(4):E9.

Based on a systematic review of studies reporting data for a total of 2,496 patients, postoperative radiographic instability was reported in 5.5% of the patients. Instability was more common in patients with preexisting spondylolisthesis. Minimally invasive decompression may reduce postoperative instability.

76. Lee YP, Sclafani J: Lumbar iatrogenic spinal instability. *Seminars in Spine Surgery* 2013;25(2):131-137.

The authors provide a good overview of spinal instability and the potential for decompression surgery to create instability.

77. Hartmann F, Janssen C, Böhm S, Hely H, Rommens PM, Gercek E: Biomechanical effect of graded minimal-invasive decompression procedures on lumbar spinal stability. *Arch Orthop Trauma Surg* 2012;132(9):1233-1239.

Based on tests using cadaver spines, resection of regions of the cranial and caudal laminae (as might be performed during posterior decompression), and detachment of the supraspinous ligament resulted in substantial increases in intervertebral rotation between flexion and extension.

78. Delank K-S, Gercek E, Kuhn S, et al: How does spinal canal decompression and dorsal stabilization affect segmental mobility? A biomechanical study. *Arch Orthop Trauma Surg* 2010;130(2):285-292.

79. Perez-Orribo L, Kalb S, Reyes PM, Chang SW, Crawford NR: Biomechanics of lumbar cortical screw-rod fixation versus pedicle screw-rod fixation with and without interbody support. *Spine (Phila Pa 1976)* 2013;38(8):635-641.

Based on laboratory tests of cadaver spines, the reduction in intervertebral motion achieved using rods connected to cortical screws was no different than that of rods connected to conventional pedicles screws. This study also provides helpful data to document that substantial intervertebral motion can remain immediately after instrumented lumbar fusions.

1: Spine Anatomy and Biomechanics

80. Matsukawa K, Yato Y, Kato T, Imabayashi H, Asazuma T, Nemoto K: In vivo analysis of insertional torque during pedicle screwing using cortical bone trajectory technique. *Spine (Phila Pa 1976)* 2014;39(4):E240-E245.

    The torque required to implant a properly placed cortical screw was substantially higher than the torque required to implant a conventional pedicle screw. Level of evidence: II.

81. Matsukawa K, Yato Y, Imabayashi H, et al: Biomechanical evaluation of fixation strength among different sizes of pedicle screws using the cortical bone trajectory: What is the ideal screw size for optimal fixation? *Acta Neurochir (Wien)* 2016;158(3):465-471.

    Based on computer models, cortical screws with diameters larger than 5.5 mm, lengths greater than 35 mm, and a greater proportion of the length within the vertebral body have greater pull-out strength.

82. Akpolat YT, İnceoğlu S, Kinne N, Hunt D, Cheng WK: Fatigue performance of cortical bone trajectory screw compared with standard trajectory pedicle screw. *Spine (Phila Pa 1976)* 2016;41(6):E335-E341.

    The conventional pedicle insertion path was found to be more resistant to failure with repetitive loading compared with a path using cortical screws. In addition, some unique morphologies present challenges in using cortical bone screws.

83. Auerbach JD, Anakwenze OA, Milby AH, Lonner BS, Balderston RA: Segmental contribution toward total cervical range of motion: A comparison of cervical disc arthroplasty and fusion. *Spine (Phila Pa 1976)* 2011;36(25):E1593-E1599.

    The authors report that anterior cervical diskectomy and fusion resulted in increased segmental motion adjacent to the fusion level, whereas no change in adjacent level motion occurred after cervical disk arthroplasty. The clinical importance is not documented in this study, but concern exists that the increased motion adjacent to fusion levels may accelerate adjacent level degeneration.

84. Auerbach JD, Jones KJ, Milby AH, Anakwenze OA, Balderston RA: Segmental contribution toward total lumbar range of motion in disc replacement and fusions: A comparison of operative and adjacent levels. *Spine (Phila Pa 1976)* 2009;34(23):2510-2517.

85. Rihn JA, Radcliff K, Hipp J, et al: Radiographic variables that may predict clinical outcomes in cervical disk replacement surgery. *J Spinal Disord Tech* 2015;28(3):106-113.

    Multiple factors explaining variability in clinical outcomes can be measured from preoperative and postoperative radiographs of the cervical disk of patients treated with disk arthroplasty. Clinical outcomes of cervical disk arthroplasty may be optimized by careful attention to the preoperative condition of the disk space and careful sizing and placement of the arthroplasty device.

86. Schmidt H, Galbusera F, Rohlmann A, Zander T, Wilke H-J: Effect of multilevel lumbar disc arthroplasty on spine kinematics and facet joint loads in flexion and extension: A finite element analysis. *Eur Spine J* 2012;21(5suppl 5):S663-S674.

    Computer models were used to help understand how the placement of a lumbar disk arthroplasty device can affect intervertebral motion and resultant forces on the facet joints. Some implant positions can result in separation of the device from the vertebral end plates during flexion or extension. The importance of correct placement of disk arthroplasty devices is emphasized.

Diagnostics in Spine Care

SECTION EDITOR:

Charles H. Cho, MD, MBA

Chapter 5

Physical Examination in Spine Care

John P. Metzler, MD

Abstract

An appropriate physical examination preceded by a patient history should lead to a differential diagnosis in patients with spinal pain or neurologic symptoms. The physical examination is needed to determine the presence and severity of neurologic impairment. Every initial examination should establish the presence or absence of an upper or lower motor neuron lesion by assessing gait, balance, strength, sensation, and reflexes. For the patient with spinal pain, provocative testing of joints, neural tissue, and soft tissue can aid in the localization of a pain generator.

Keywords: diagnostic subgroup; neural tension test; neurologic symptoms; pain provocation; physical examination

Introduction

After taking an appropriate history, the physician should have a differential diagnosis and a firm grasp of the concerns, beliefs, and motives that led the patient to seek consultation from a spine specialist. The physical examination can help determine the presence of spinal and nonspinal structural pathology, identify and localize neurologic impairment, and determine the source(s) of pain. Imaging studies, laboratory tests, and other diagnostic studies may or may not be indicated based on the examination findings. Patients may bring imaging studies and/or reports requested by other physicians to the examination and be primarily concerned with addressing the listed findings. Degenerative changes, disk protrusions, and spinal stenosis can be present in asymptomatic individuals.[1-3] An appropriately detailed history and physical

examination is an important tool for sorting out the clinical significance of imaging findings. A patient's history and physical examination findings, along with imaging when appropriate, are necessary to guide the selection of medications, therapy, injections, and surgery.

Every physical examination of a new patient should include some components of inspection, palpation, range of motion, and neurologic evaluation. Depending on the presenting symptoms, the differential diagnosis, and the prior imaging findings and administered treatments, the level of detail in various parts of the examination may vary. The nature of the patient's symptoms can give the examiner an idea of which parts of the examination may require more emphasis. **Table 1** outlines diagnostic subgroups based on presenting symptoms that may be useful to consider when performing a spinal physical examination.

Neurologic Symptoms

Bilateral Symptoms

In the patient with neurologic symptoms in the bilateral upper or lower extremities, the examination should include tests for signs of myelopathy or cauda equina compression. Patients with myelopathy may report numbness or weakness in the bilateral upper and/or lower extremities and may have impaired balance, gait, or coordination. Patients with further progression of myelopathy may have symptoms of urinary urgency or incontinence. Extradural compression of the spinal cord often produces concomitant reports of pain in the distribution of a specific nerve root or roots. Pain is less common in patients with intradural lesions. In those presenting with painless weakness, intradural compression and other neurologic conditions that can damage the spinal cord should be considered before ascribing degenerative changes seen on imaging studies as the definitive cause of weakness. Retrospective reviews of patients with amyotrophic lateral sclerosis have shown a high incidence of spinal decompressive surgery performed for neurologic symptoms that were later determined to be early symptoms of amyotrophic lateral sclerosis.[4,5]

Table 1

Diagnostic Subgrouping of Spinal Symptoms

Neurologic Symptoms

Bilateral extremity

  Myelopathy concern

  Cauda equina concern

  Other neurologic disease

Unilateral extremity

  Radiculopathy concern

  Peripheral nerve

Pain Symptoms

Radiating limb pain

  Radicular

  Referred

Axial Pain

  Flexion based

  Extension based

  Other

Spinal masqueraders (pain from a nonspinal etiology)

  Musculoskeletal

   Shoulder

   Hip

   Posterior pelvis/sacroiliac

  Visceral

If a patient is suspected of having myelopathy, he or she may be initially evaluated from behind, with the examiner looking for a wide-based gait (the feet farther apart than a normal distance of 2 to 4 inches) and the trunk showing excessive lateral sway. Formal gait analysis has shown that patients with more advanced disease will have increased stance width, decreased stride length, and increased time spent in the stance phase.[6]

In a patient with myelopathy, the upper extremities may demonstrate normal, diminished, or brisk reflexes depending on the level of spinal cord compression. If the exiting nerve root at the stenotic level also is compressed, the corresponding reflex may be diminished (for example, C6-7 stenosis may compress the exiting C7 nerve root and cause an absent or diminished triceps reflex). Spinal levels below the compression will be disinhibited and, thus, patellar and Achilles reflexes are typically hyperreflexic and symmetric. Sharply dorsiflexing the foot with continued pressure will place a stretch on the gastrocnemius muscle-tendon unit and may elicit ankle clonus, which further confirms an upper motor neuron pathology.

The examiner also should test for the presence of pathologic reflexes. Withdrawal of the lower extremity from a painful stimulus is a primitive reflex present at birth. Between 12 and 24 months of age, the motor cortex develops and maintains suppression of this flexion reflex. The reappearance of the reflex typically signifies organic interference in one of the upper motor neuron pathways.[7] Several different methods, including the Babinski, Chaddock, and Oppenheim methods, can be used to test for a pathologic flexion reflex.[7] The Hoffmann reflex is flexion of the thumb that is elicited by flicking the distal phalanx of the long or middle finger; this reflex may be seen in patients with myelopathy. The Hoffmann reflex is thought to be caused by hyperreflexia of the finger flexors, not by the presence of a pathologic reflex.[7]

Impaired hand coordination is a common symptom of myelopathy. Hand dexterity can be tested by asking the patient to grip and release his or her hand as many times as possible in 15 seconds. In an individual without myelopathy, this task normally can be performed 25 to 30 times in 15 seconds; however, a patient with myelopathy will exhibit substantial impairment in the ability to perform the test. After surgical decompression, substantial improvement can be seen.[8]

If a patient reports bowel or bladder dysfunction or reduced sensation in the saddle area, an assessment of rectal tone and perianal and saddle sensation should be performed. Urgent care is needed if there is suspicion of cauda equina syndrome.[9] Substantial sphincter dysfunction has been described as a predictor of a poor clinical outcome.[10]

Unilateral Symptoms

Symptoms of weakness, numbness, or pain in a single extremity should lead the examiner to consider the possibility of nerve root impairment. Included in this differential diagnosis are traumatic and entrapment injuries of the brachial or lumbosacral plexus and their associated peripheral nerves. In the cervical spine, the strength examination should include the C5 to T1 myotomes. In the lumbar spine, the L2 to S1 myotomes should be examined. If a specific muscle demonstrates focal weakness, further manual muscle testing may elucidate whether the entrapment site is at the nerve root level or more peripheral. Weakness with abduction of the fingers can be seen in both C8 radiculopathy and peripheral ulnar nerve entrapment. With further examination of index finger extension and thumb abduction, the examiner can determine whether the entrapment most likely lies at the C8 level or is more distally located in the ulnar nerve. The extensor indices

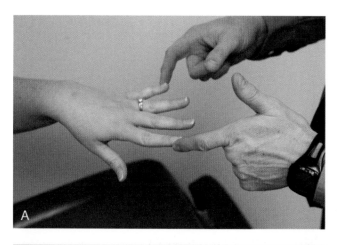

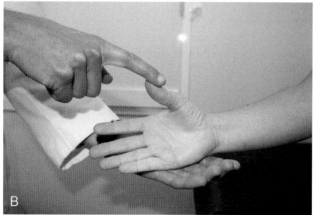

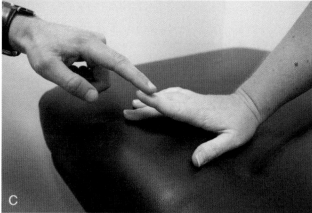

Figure 1 Clinical photographs showing C8 distribution manual muscle testing. With C8 motor involvement, all three muscles are weak. Weakness isolated to only one test suggests a more peripheral nerve entrapment site. **A,** Ulnar nerve–finger abduction. **B,** Median nerve–thumb abduction. **C,** Radial nerve–index finger extension.

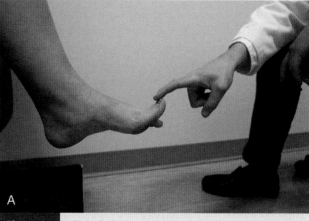

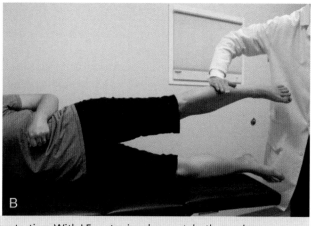

Figure 2 Clinical photographs showing L5 distribution weakness testing. With L5 motor involvement, both muscles are weak. Weakness isolated to only one test suggests a more peripheral nerve entrapment site. **A,** Peroneal nerve–great toe extension. Weakness can be seen with L5 radiculopathy or peroneal nerve entrapment **B,** Superior gluteal nerve–hip abduction. Weakness with hip abduction and great toe extension is consistent with L5 radiculopathy.

and abductor pollicis brevis both have C8 contributions, but they are supplied by the radial and median nerves, respectively (**Figure 1**). Similarly, if findings of weakness with ankle dorsiflexion and/or great toe extension are present, weakness with hip abduction can be expected if the entrapment is at the L5 nerve root level (**Figure 2**).

The sensory examination should look for sensory abnormalities in the distribution of a particular dermatome or the peripheral nerves. Many dermatomal maps exist with variations among them, which may make it difficult to determine sensory impairment at a specific nerve root level. Several factors can contribute to

2: Diagnostics in Spine Care

Table 2

Muscle Stretch Reflexes and Corresponding Nerve Innervations

Reflex	Nerve Roots
Biceps	C5, C6
Brachioradialis	C5, C6
Pronator teres	C6, C7
Triceps	C6, C7, C8
Quadriceps	L2, L3, L4
Medial hamstring	L4, L5, S1, S2
Gastrocnemius	L5, S1, S2

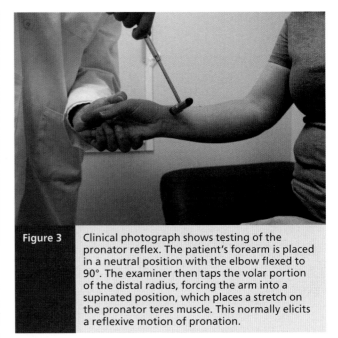

Figure 3 Clinical photograph shows testing of the pronator reflex. The patient's forearm is placed in a neutral position with the elbow flexed to 90°. The examiner then taps the volar portion of the distal radius, forcing the arm into a supinated position, which places a stretch on the pronator teres muscle. This normally elicits a reflexive motion of pronation.

difficulty in identifying the nerve root level of the impairment, including the connections between nerve roots, the transmission of sensory modalities to the same area of skin by different nerve roots, and the substantial overlap between dermatomes.[11] Because of the substantial overlap of corresponding dermatomes, it is rare for entrapment of a single nerve root to cause dense numbness. Rather, the numbness is usually vague and poorly defined. An area of dense numbness should lead to a more rigorous examination for peripheral nerve entrapment or more widespread peripheral neuropathy.

Muscle stretch reflexes of the upper and lower extremities should be assessed for an asymmetric diminished or an absent reflex, which would suggest nerve root impingement. **Table 2** lists specific reflexes and their corresponding innervations. The pronator teres reflex and medial hamstring reflex are less commonly evaluated but can be clinically useful. To elicit the pronator reflex, the forearm is held in a neutral position with the elbow flexed to 90° and resting in the patient's lap. The examiner then taps the volar portion of the distal radius; this forces the arm into a supinated position and places a stretch on the pronator teres muscle and normally elicits a reflexive motion of pronation[12] (**Figure 3**). The medial hamstring reflex is most easily elicited with the patient prone, with the ankle of the leg being tested crossed over the opposite ankle (**Figure 4**). The reflex is typically more difficult to elicit than the patellar and Achilles reflexes; however, the presence of asymmetry can provide useful diagnostic information.

Pain Symptoms

Important clues that aid in the diagnosis of a disorder and the determination of appropriate treatment can be gained by observing the patient's gait and posture. If the patient lurches off to the side during ambulation, it is necessary to determine if the gait is antalgic or has a Trendelenburg pattern. A patient with an antalgic gait will lurch toward the painful side during weight bearing on the affected limb to decrease the pull of painful hip abductors. A patient with a Trendelenburg (or gluteus medius) gait has weak hip abductors. When the affected side is in stance phase, the contralateral hip will drop (sound-side sag). With a compensated Trendelenburg gait, the patient will list the trunk over the weak side to maintain his or her center of gravity.

Observation of the patient in the examination room can yield information about postures or habits that may be contributing to tissue overload. In the patient with a head-forward posture and rounded shoulders, tissue overload can be expected in the upper trapezius or rhomboids, with associated pain and tenderness in this region. After assessing posture, the examiner can select a few muscles for palpation to look for confirmatory tenderness and tautness. When palpating selected muscles, it is helpful to ask the patient if there is any radiating pain and if his or her typical pain is being reproduced. Positive findings are suggestive of myofascial pain.

In acute conditions, the patient may adopt positions that help offload painful structures. In the presence of cervical radiculopathy or brachial plexopathy, the patient may rest the hand of the affected upper extremity on top of his or her head to alleviate tension on the affected nerves. The examiner may notice the patient in this position (Bakody sign) or may request that the patient adopt this position and then ask if there is pain relief

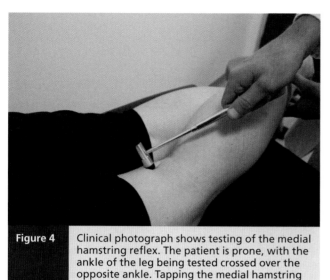

Figure 4 Clinical photograph shows testing of the medial hamstring reflex. The patient is prone, with the ankle of the leg being tested crossed over the opposite ankle. Tapping the medial hamstring tendon normally elicits a palpable or visible contraction of the medial hamstring.

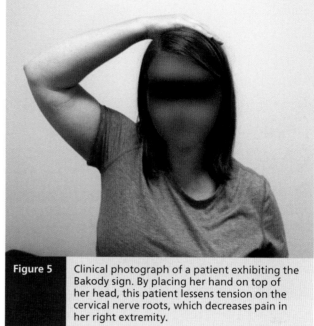

Figure 5 Clinical photograph of a patient exhibiting the Bakody sign. By placing her hand on top of her head, this patient lessens tension on the cervical nerve roots, which decreases pain in her right extremity.

(shoulder abduction test)[13,14] (**Figure 5**). A lateral shift of the lumbar spine correlates highly with the presence of an acute disk herniation. Most commonly, the patient's body will be shifted to the side that is contralateral from the herniation.[15]

Standing behind the patient, the examiner can look for and palpate asymmetries of the paraspinal muscles, scapula, rib cage, iliac crest, and greater trochanters that may signify a scoliotic deformity. Lack of alignment of the cervicothoracic junction to the gluteal cleft suggests coronal plane decompensation.[16]

During the thoracic and lumbar examination, forward bending should be assessed by observing the patient from the side. Forward bending is a combination of thoracic, lumbar, and hip flexion. In assessing movement impairments that may be contributing to a painful condition, it is important to note the relative contribution of each of these areas. Normally, the forward bending motion is initiated with a posterior sway of the hips. The lumbar spine then reverses its normal curvature and ends in a flattened position.[17]

In patients with low back pain, repetitive end-range flexion and extension and side-gliding/rotation can be performed to determine if the pain has a directional preference (ie, whether the pain lessens with repetitive end-range movements in a particular direction). In patients demonstrating a directional preference, matching the patient's directional preference to a physical therapy program that uses the favored direction has been shown to provide a better outcome than therapy programs that do not use a directional preference.[18,19]

In the patient with radiating pain, a provocative test may be used to help determine if the pain is caused by radiculopathy. The Spurling test is performed by tilting the patient's head toward the painful side to see if this elicits reproduction of the patient's typical cervical radicular symptoms. If needed, pressure then can be placed on top of the patient's head in a further attempt to elicit symptoms. The test has a higher level of specificity (92% to 100%) than sensitivity (40% to 60%).[20]

Pain radiating into the extremity is an indication for performing a dural stretch test. Reproduction of radiating extremity pain is considered a sign of possible radiculopathy. Classically, this test is performed in the lower extremity by putting tension on the L5 and S1 nerve roots via a straight leg raise test with the patient supine. The test also can be performed in the seated position, with increased tension on the dura obtained by having the patient flex the neck and thoracolumbar spine (ie, slumped position)[21] (**Figure 6**). Tension can be placed on the upper lumbar nerve roots (L2 through L4) via the femoral nerve stretch test (**Figure 7**). With the patient prone, the examiner flexes the patient's knee as far as possible and then adds hip extension, looking for reproduction of the patient's typical radiating symptoms of pain or paresthesias. If the patient is unable to lie prone, side lying can be used as an alternative option.

The cervical nerve roots can be similarly tested with upper limb tension tests[21] (**Figure 8**). The C5 through C8 nerve roots can be strained and displaced inferolaterally. To perform the test, the patient is supine and the

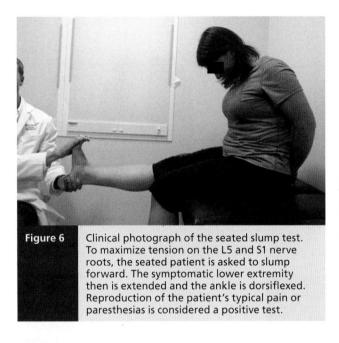

Figure 6 Clinical photograph of the seated slump test. To maximize tension on the L5 and S1 nerve roots, the seated patient is asked to slump forward. The symptomatic lower extremity then is extended and the ankle is dorsiflexed. Reproduction of the patient's typical pain or paresthesias is considered a positive test.

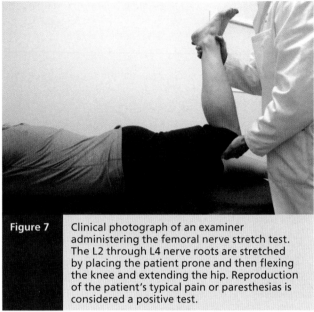

Figure 7 Clinical photograph of an examiner administering the femoral nerve stretch test. The L2 through L4 nerve roots are stretched by placing the patient prone and then flexing the knee and extending the hip. Reproduction of the patient's typical pain or paresthesias is considered a positive test.

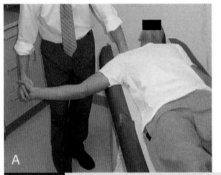 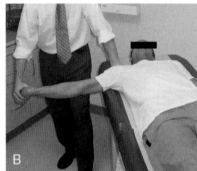 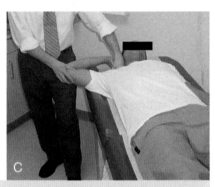

Figure 8 Clinical photographs of upper limb tension tests. Upper extremity nerves are placed under tension and the patient is asked if typical pain or paresthesias is reproduced. **A,** To create median nerve bias, the patient is placed supine and the shoulder is depressed, abducted, and externally rotated; the elbow, wrist, and fingers are extended. **B,** Radial nerve bias is created by placing increased tension on the radial nerve. The patient's shoulder is abducted and internally rotated, the elbow is extended, the forearm is pronated, and the wrist and fingers are flexed. **C,** Ulnar nerve bias is created to place increased tension on the ulnar nerve. The shoulder is abducted to 90° and the patient's hand is brought to his ear, thereby flexing the elbow, supinating the forearm, and extending the wrist and fingers.

shoulder is depressed, abducted, and externally rotated; the elbow, wrist, and fingers are extended.[22] If the examiner wants to more selectively stress the C7 nerve root or radial nerve, the patient's shoulder is abducted and internally rotated, the elbow is extended, the forearm is pronated, and the wrist and fingers are flexed. Selective bias of the C8 root and ulnar nerve can be achieved by abducting the shoulder to 90° and then bringing the patient's hand to his or her ear, thereby flexing the elbow, supinating the forearm, and extending the wrist and fingers.[21] Upper limb tension has been demonstrated to have a high sensitivity but low specificity in making a diagnosis of cervical radiculopathy.[23,24]

Pain in the posterior pelvic girdle (defined as the area between the posterior iliac crest and the gluteal fold or area around the sacroiliac [SI] joint) can originate from outside the spine. Physical examination of this region relies on using a constellation of findings to determine if the SI joint and surrounding soft tissues are potential pain generators. Palpation just inferior to the posterior superior iliac spine over the long dorsal ligament frequently reveals tenderness. Tenderness to palpation may also be found at the symphysis pubis. Difficulty in performing the active straight leg raise is a common finding, and its presence suggests a lack of motor control that may help perpetuate a chronic painful condition caused

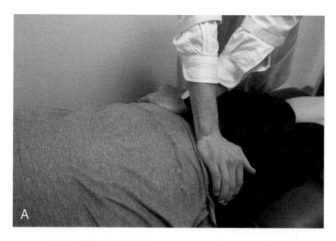
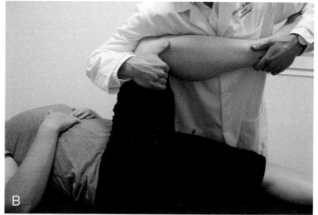
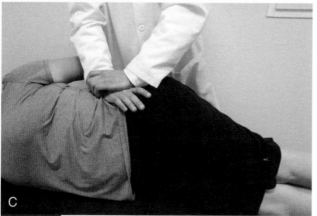
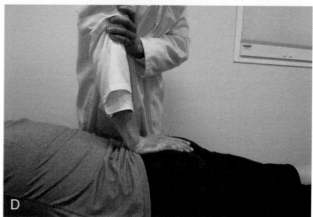

Figure 9 Clinical photographs of a patient undergoing sacroiliac joint provocation tests. Tests are consider positive if there is reproduction of the patient's typical pain. **A,** The distraction test. With the patient supine, the examiner's hands are placed on the anterior superior iliac spine of each ilia and a lateral and posterior force is applied. **B,** The thigh thrust test. With the patient supine and the hip flexed to 90°, a posteriorly directed force is applied to the femur, placing a shearing stress on the sacroiliac joint. **C,** The compression test. The patient lies on the asymptomatic side and the examiner places pressure on the superior iliac crest, directing it toward the opposite iliac crest. **D,** The sacral thrust test. With the patient prone and the ilia fixed against the examination table, the examiner's hand is placed in the center of the sacrum. An anteriorly directed force is then applied.

by repetitive mechanical irritation of pain-sensitized structures.[25-27]

No single isolated provocation test of the SI joint correlates well with a diagnostic intra-articular or lateral branch block. All SI joint provocation tests stress additional tissues outside the SI joint, which makes interpretation of a single test difficult. However, when four provocative tests are applied (distraction, thigh thrust, compression, and sacral thrust) and two or more tests are positive for reproducing the patient's typical symptoms, there is a strong correlation with relief from a diagnostic SI joint block.[4,28] In addition, when all four tests are negative, the SI joint can effectively be ruled out as the source of the patient's typical pain.[4,28] **Figure 9** demonstrates the provocation tests. The distraction test is performed with the patient supine. With the examiner's hands on the anterior superior iliac spine of each ilia, a lateral and

posterior force is applied. The thigh thrust or posterior shear test is performed with the patient supine and the hip flexed to 90°. A posteriorly directed force is then applied to the femur, placing a shearing stress on the SI joint. To perform the compression test, the patient lies on the asymptomatic side and the examiner places pressure on the superior iliac crest, directing it toward the opposite iliac crest. The sacral thrust test is performed with the patient prone and the ilia fixed against the examination table. The clinician's hands are placed one on top of the other in the center of the sacrum. An anteriorly direct force is then applied, and the presence or absence of pain provocation is noted.[29,30]

The differential diagnosis for spinal pain and radiating pain is extensive and extends to systems outside the spine. Initial suspicion of a nonspinal etiology may occur when the patient's history is being taken. Pain that is modified by the state of the viscera (eg, pain after eating, with urination, with exertion) should heighten awareness of a possible nonspinal pain generator. In addition, associated systemic symptoms such as fever, nausea, or shortness of breath should lead to examination of associated systems.

Summary

A multitude of techniques exist for spinal examination. By paying close attention to a patient's history, the clinician can select an appropriate examination that will detect and localize neurologic impairment and determine pain generators. By spending an appropriate amount of time and thoughtfully performing the physical examination, an appropriate diagnostic modality or treatment can be determined.

Key Study Points

- Depending on the patient's symptoms, the physical examination may be varied to help further differentiate a diagnosis and determine specific treatments.
- An appropriately detailed neurologic examination is necessary to diagnose urgent and emergent spinal conditions, localize spinal pathology, and detect other neurologic disorders.
- Observation, palpation, and provocative testing can assist in the detection of spinal pain generators and nonspinal pain generators that mimic spinal conditions.
- The physical examination can help guide the selection of appropriate imaging and treatment options.

Annotated References

1. Boden SD, Davis DO, Dina TS, Patronas NJ, Wiesel SW: Abnormal magnetic-resonance scans of the lumbar spine in asymptomatic subjects: A prospective investigation. *J Bone Joint Surg Am* 1990;72(3):403-408.

2. Boden SD, McCowin PR, Davis DO, Dina TS, Mark AS, Wiesel S: Abnormal magnetic-resonance scans of the cervical spine in asymptomatic subjects: A prospective investigation. *J Bone Joint Surg Am* 1990;72(8):1178-1184.

3. Wood KB, Garvey TA, Gundry C, Heithoff KB: Magnetic resonance imaging of the thoracic spine: Evaluation of asymptomatic individuals. *J Bone Joint Surg Am* 1995;77(11):1631-1638.

4. Kraemer M, Buerger M, Berlit P: Diagnostic problems and delay of diagnosis in amyotrophic lateral sclerosis. *Clin Neurol Neurosurg* 2010;112(2):103-105.

5. Srinivasan J, Scala S, Jones HR, Saleh F, Russell JA: Inappropriate surgeries resulting from misdiagnosis of early amyotrophic lateral sclerosis. *Muscle Nerve* 2006;34(3):359-360.

6. Nishimura H, Endo K, Suzuki H, Tanaka H, Shishido T, Yamamoto K: Gait analysis in cervical spondylotic myelopathy. *Asian Spine J* 2015;9(3):321-326.

   The authors of this study report on 98 patients with cervical spondylotic myelopathy and 34 normal control patients who underwent gait analysis. The severity of the gait abnormalities corresponded with the severity of Nurick grade.

7. Ahlskog JE; Mayo Foundation for Medical Education and Research: *Clinical Examinations in Neurology* ,ed 6. St. Louis, MO, Mosby, 1991, pp 247-248.

8. Hosono N, Sakaura H, Mukai Y, Kaito T, Makino T, Yoshikawa H: A simple performance test for quantifying the severity of cervical myelopathy. *J Bone Joint Surg Br* 2008;90(9):1210-1213.

9. Fraser S, Roberts L, Murphy E: Cauda equina syndrome: A literature review of its definition and clinical presentation. *Arch Phys Med Rehabil* 2009;90(11):1964-1968.

10. Kennedy JG, Soffe KE, McGrath A, Stephens MM, Walsh MG, McManus F: Predictors of outcome in cauda equina syndrome. *Eur Spine J* 1999;8(4):317-322.

11. De Luigi AJ, Fitzpatrick KF: Physical examination in radiculopathy. *Phys Med Rehabil Clin N Am* 2011;22(1):7-40.

    Part of this review concerns lumbar and cervical radiculopathy. Extensive citations are provided regarding the sensitivity and specificity of various physical examination maneuvers used for patients with radiculopathy symptoms.

12. Malanga GA, Campagnolo DI: Clarification of the pronator reflex. *Am J Phys Med Rehabil* 1994;73(5):338-340.

13. Davidson RI, Dunn EJ, Metzmaker JN: The shoulder abduction test in the diagnosis of radicular pain in cervical extradural compressive monoradiculopathies. *Spine (Phila Pa 1976)* 1981;6(5):441-446.

14. Johnson I: Bakody sign. *Surg Neurol* 1977;7(6):370.

15. Zhu Z, Zhao Q, Wang B, et al: Scoliotic posture as the initial symptom in adolescents with lumbar disc herniation: Its curve pattern and natural history after lumbar discectomy. *BMC Musculoskelet Disord* 2011;12:216.

    The authors report on 26 adolescents who presented with a lumbar disk herniation and scoliosis. Most of the patients had a short lumbosacral curve and a long thoracic curve and their bodies were shifted to the contralateral side of the disk herniation. All patients showed improvement in their scoliosis after diskectomy.

16. Newton PO, ed: *Adolescent Idiopathic Scoliosis*. Rosemont, IL, American Academy of Orthopaedic Surgeons, 2004, pp 11-21.

17. Sahrmann S: *Diagnosis and Treatment of Movement Impairment Syndromes*. London, England, Mosby, 2002.

18. Long A, Donelson R, Fung T: Does it matter which exercise? A randomized control trial of exercise for low back pain. *Spine (Phila Pa 1976)* 2004;29(23):2593-2602.

19. Donelson R, Long A, Spratt K, Fung T: Influence of directional preference on two clinical dichotomies: Acute versus chronic pain and axial low back pain versus sciatica. *PMR* 2012;4(9):667-681.

    Data show that patients with low back pain and a directional preference respond well to treatment that uses directional preference. The location and duration of pain and the presence of neurologic impairment are not predictive of response.

20. Viikari-Juntura E, Porras M, Laasonen EM: Validity of clinical tests in the diagnosis of root compression in cervical disc disease. *Spine (Phila Pa 1976)* 1989;14(3):253-257.

21. Butler D: *Mobilisation of the Nervous System*. Edinburgh, Scotland, Churchill Livingstone, 1991.

22. Lohman CM, Gilbert KK, Sobczak S, et al: Cervical nerve root displacement and strain during upper limb neural tension testing: Part 1. A minimally invasive assessment in unembalmed cadavers. *Spine (Phila Pa 1976)* 2015;40(11):793-800.

    The cervical nerve roots in 11 cadavers were examined using radiolucent markers under fluoroscopy. This is the first study to measure displacement and strain of the cervical roots during the median biased upper limb neural tension test. Level of evidence: II.

23. Rubinstein SM, Pool JJ, van Tulder MW, Riphagen II, de Vet HC: A systematic review of the diagnostic accuracy of provocative tests of the neck for diagnosing cervical radiculopathy. *Eur Spine J* 2007;16(3):307-319.

24. Rubinstein SM, van Tulder M: A best-evidence review of diagnostic procedures for neck and low-back pain. *Best Pract Res Clin Rheumatol* 2008;22(3):471-482.

25. Beales DJ, O'Sullivan PB, Briffa NK: Motor control patterns during an active straight leg raise in chronic pelvic girdle pain subjects. *Spine (Phila Pa 1976)* 2009;34(9):861-870.

26. Vleeming A, Albert HB, Ostgaard HC, Sturesson B, Stuge B: European guidelines for the diagnosis and treatment of pelvic girdle pain. *Eur Spine J* 2008;17(6):794-819.

27. Hu H, Meijer OG, Hodges PW, et al: Understanding the active straight leg raise (ASLR): An electromyographic study in healthy subjects. *Man Ther* 2012;17(6):531-537.

    The authors describe normal muscle activation patterns in healthy individuals performing the active straight leg raise test with and without an SI belt. A lack of force closure is proposed as a cause of an impaired active straight leg raise test.

28. Laslett M, Aprill CN, McDonald B, Young SB: Diagnosis of sacroiliac joint pain: Validity of individual provocation tests and composites of tests. *Man Ther* 2005;10(3):207-218.

29. Laslett M, Williams M: The reliability of selected pain provocation tests for sacroiliac joint pathology. *Spine (Phila Pa 1976)* 1994;19(11):1243-1249.

30. Ombregt L, Bisschop P, ter Veer H: *A System of Orthopaedic Medicine*. London, England, Elsevier Health Sciences, 2003, pp 950-951.

2: Diagnostics in Spine Care

Chapter 6

Spine Imaging

Charles H. Cho, MD, MBA   Robert M. Kurtz, MD

Abstract

The primary modalities for imaging of the spine are standard radiography followed by advanced imaging with CT, myelography, MRI, bone scanning, and positron emission tomography. Intraoperative fluoroscopy and CT are becoming common for image-guided procedures. The requesting clinical team and the equipment user should understand the risks and benefits involved for any imaging delivery, including the energy used (radiation, magnetic force) and the introduced medication (iodinated contrast, gadolinium contrast, radioactive isotope). Throughout this process, familiarization with the national guidelines for the specific imaging study is important for optimal patient care with value in care delivery.

Keywords: guidelines in spine imaging; risks of spine imaging; spine imaging modalities

Introduction

Of the five major imaging modalities (radiography, CT, MRI, nuclear scintigraphy, and positron emission tomography [PET]), lumbar radiography remains the starting point for imaging evaluation of individuals with spine pain. Understanding spine imaging involves awareness of a few key components, including familiarity with the basic strengths and weaknesses of the individual imaging modality, the risks and contraindications of the imaging source, and understanding the evolving clinical guidelines in the appropriate use of imaging.

Dr. Cho or an immediate family member serves as a board member, owner, officer, or committee member of the North American Spine Society. Neither Dr. Kurtz nor any immediate family member has received anything of value from or has stock or stock options held in a commercial company or institution related directly or indirectly to the subject of this chapter.

Radiography

Although there are fewer indications than before for the use of spine radiography because of the widespread availability and excellent capability of CT to depict osseous structures, existing indications include neck or back pain without or with trauma, need for preoperative planning, postoperative assessment, and evaluation of scoliosis.

The typical radiographic views of the spine are AP and lateral. Additional oblique views are used to evaluate the degree of neural foraminal narrowing in the cervical spine or to evaluate the pars interarticularis in the lumbar spine. A cone-down lateral view of the lumbosacral junction is also often obtained. In the cervical spine, an odontoid view is added because the skull base obscures the odontoid on standard AP views, and a swimmer's view can be added because the shoulder often overlaps the C7-T1 junction. Flexion/extension views are used to evaluate subluxation from injury to the cervical ligamentous structures, although this is not recommended in individuals with acute trauma because of muscle spasms. These views are usually obtained with maximum passive flexion and extension. Significant observations are most frequently considered to be changes greater than 2 mm in the amount of spondylolisthesis or an 11° change in angulation.

When evaluating the thoracic spine, labeling the correct thoracic level is imperative before any surgical treatment because transitional anatomy often exists at the L5 or S1 level. Counting the upper thoracic vertebrae is often difficult on the lateral view because the shoulders obscure details. Therefore, obtaining AP views to localize the first and last ribs often is the best method to determine the correct level for surgical treatment.

Many national medical societies publish guidelines for spine imaging. The American College of Radiology (ACR) publishes Appropriate Use Criteria (AUC) for multiple clinical variations in the use of imaging.[1] In trauma, radiographs are considered appropriate with a strong clinical indication but not appropriate without it. For chronic back pain, radiographs are appropriate and often the initial imaging study of choice. In patients with uncomplicated low back pain, radiographs of the lumbar spine are usually not appropriate and imaging is often not warranted. However, if low back pain is complicated by conditions such as low-velocity trauma, advanced age, osteoporosis, or chronic steroid use, the recommendation to obtain radiographs of the spine becomes appropriate.

For evaluating the degenerative lumbar spine, the North American Spine Society suggests lateral radiographs as the most appropriate noninvasive test, and when possible, the lateral radiograph should be obtained while the patient is bearing weight.[2] For patients with isthmic spondylolisthesis, weight-bearing radiographs with or without oblique views or dynamic view radiographs are recommended as the most appropriate imaging test. For situations in which the radiographic results are indeterminate, CT is suggested as the next appropriate imaging study.[3]

Computed Tomography

CT uses the same principles as radiography, but with the addition of multiple projections to create cross-sectional images of the body. Photons generated by an x-ray tube are sent through the body. The photons are absorbed (attenuated) more by dense structures (such as metal, bone, and calcium). Detectors measure the remaining photons after they pass through the body and the information is used to re-create images from many different rotational angles. The CT number (Hounsfield unit [HU]) is calculated by normalizing the attenuation of each voxel to that of water (water measures at 0 HU). The Hounsfield unit values range from –1,000 to 3,000. The images can be "windowed" to emphasize different features by altering the center of the values and the range of values being displayed. The typical bone window has a center of 300 HU and a range of 2,000 HU. A soft-tissue window has a center of 40 HU and a range of 400 HU. CT can now be performed quickly using multidetector CT scanners. Multiplanar (sagittal and coronal) and three-dimensional reconstructions are created easily and quickly.

CT is ideal for evaluation of the bones, in particular for fractures, degenerative arthropathy, postoperative osseous fusion, and destructive osseous lesions. Fractures are well characterized with excellent detail regarding the number of fracture fragments and the presence of fragment displacement, angulation, distraction, and rotation. Degenerative arthropathy is demonstrated with osseous sclerosis, osteophytosis, loss of joint space, and subchondral cystic change (**Figure 1**). The degree of osseous narrowing of the neural foramina and the spinal canal also can be evaluated, noting that the soft-tissue (disk or ligamentous) contribution to narrowing is not as

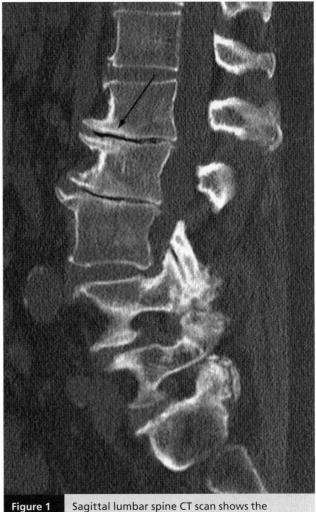

Figure 1 Sagittal lumbar spine CT scan shows the narrowed disk space and end plate sclerosis (arrow) resulting from degenerative disease.

clearly defined as with MRI, particularly in the cervical spine. Bone union following fusion is shown by solid bone mass bridging the disk space, facet joints, or other sites of osseous fusion. As tumors replace bone marrow, either sclerotic expansion or soft-tissue replacement of the normal bony trabeculae or cortical bone occurs and is shown better on CT (**Figure 2**). Radiographs may not show lytic lesions until 30% of the trabeculae are eroded and/or replaced. CT also is a good modality for preoperative planning. The size of pedicles is well demonstrated to help plan for screw placement. Three-dimensional reconstructions can help visualize complex anatomy.

A disadvantage of CT regarding evaluation of the spine is that demonstration of soft-tissue edema and/or infection and inflammation of soft tissue is limited. Although inflammation or edema can be seen as fluid density and stranding within the paraspinal fat, these

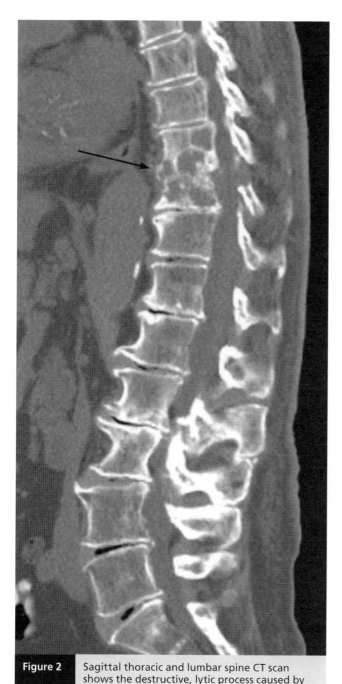

Figure 2 — Sagittal thoracic and lumbar spine CT scan shows the destructive, lytic process caused by the tumor at T9 and T10 (arrow).

viscous contents that show density similar to soft tissue on CT images and often can be missed, particularly in the psoas muscle, which is a common location for edema and abscess with spinal column infection. The spinal cord and nerve roots are not well seen because of their relatively small sizes, attenuations similar to cerebrospinal fluid (CSF), and poor penetration of the spinal canal by x-ray photons, which is attributable to the dense surrounding bone of the spinal column (resulting in poor definition of the contents of the canal).

Iodinated Contrast Material: Use and Risks

The use of iodinated contrast material often is not necessary for indications for which CT is requested, especially in the spine. The most common setting for which contrast material is used is if concern exists for an infectious process or tumor and MRI is contraindicated in the patient. Contrast material also can help evaluate for abscess by showing a distinct rim of enhancement around a fluid density collection (**Figure 3**). Soft-tissue tumors can show solid, heterogeneous, or peripheral enhancement.

Allergic-like reactions can occur when iodinated contrast material is administered. The mechanism of the reaction is not clearly understood, but an antigen-antibody response is not always found. The reactions are considered idiosyncratic. An individual who already has experienced an allergic-like reaction to contrast material is at higher risk of having another reaction (10% to 35% risk in the future if not premedicated), usually to a similar degree as any prior reaction. Occasionally, a more severe reaction will occur. Irrespective of this, the reactions are treated similarly to true allergic reactions and the patient should be premedicated before future studies with steroids and with or without an antihistamine. Using a different contrast agent for future injections also can be considered. Prior allergic-like reactions to iodinated contrast material should not preclude injections with gadolinium-based contrast agents for MRI because no cross-reactivity has been shown to occur, but patients with a history of atopy or reactions to other agents may have a greater tendency to have reactions to either.[4]

Patients with acute or chronic renal failure also may be at risk for the development of worsening renal function following the administration of iodinated contrast agents. This theory has been questioned because many patients whose creatinine levels increase after contrast administration have other comorbidities, and many previous studies involved patients who received intra-arterial contrast material for cardiac angiography (which administers a more concentrated dose of contrast material to the kidneys than intravenous administration).[5] Therefore, a distinction is now made between contrast material–induced

processes are shown much better on MRI, particularly when the muscles, spinal canal, or bone marrow is involved. For example, discitis and osteomyelitis can be seen on CT as narrowing of the disk space with end plate irregularity and potential loss of vertebral body height, possibly with edema in the surrounding paraspinal soft tissues. The additional findings of bone marrow edema, epidural abscess, and soft-tissue abscess are seen much better on magnetic resonance images. Abscesses can have

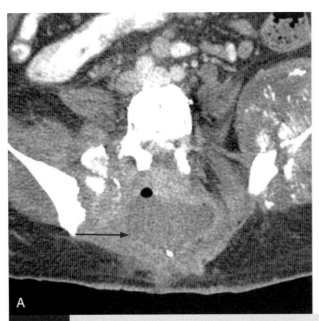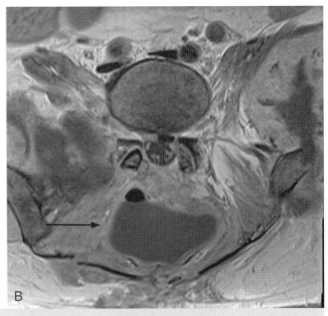

Figure 3 **A,** Contrast material–enhanced axial CT scan of spinal level L5 shows abscess fluid with trapped air (arrow). Note signal enhancement and edema in adjacent muscle. **B,** Axial postcontrast T1-weighted magnetic resonance image at the same level as panel **A** shows enhancement around the abscess (arrow).

nephropathy and postcontrast acute kidney injury, which avoids faulting the contrast material. No cutoff value of creatinine or estimated glomerular filtration rate (eGFR) has been agreed on for which iodinated contrast media is contraindicated. A risk-benefit analysis must be performed before administering contrast agents to any patient, accounting for all risks, benefits, and alternatives. A cutoff eGFR value of 30 mL/min/1.73 m² can be used in patients with chronic renal insufficiency and alternatives considered in the setting of acute kidney injury.[6] Patients with end-stage renal disease who are anuric and undergoing routine hemodialysis are not at risk for postcontrast kidney injury because their kidneys are nonfunctioning.

If iodinated contrast material is administered in the setting of renal insufficiency, hydration is the only prophylactic therapy consistently shown to be effective. Isotonic solutions are preferred, with a protocol example of 0.9% saline at 100 mL/h administered for 6 to 12 hours before contrast material administration and continuing for 4 to 12 hours after. Decreasing the dose of contrast material at lower eGFR levels (theoretically decreasing the risk to the kidneys because of reduced contrast material load) can be considered as long as diagnostic information can be obtained with the smaller dose.[4]

CT Radiation Dose

With CT, radiation doses are calculated based on the imaging parameters used, including the length of the scan, and are normalized to the expected dose based on measurements using a phantom. Actual patient doses can vary from the calculated dose for given imaging parameters, depending on patient cross-sectional diameter and attenuation, with smaller patients receiving a higher actual dose and larger patients receiving a smaller dose than estimated. Radiation dose is measured in millisieverts (mSv). The average dose for a spine CT scan is 5 to 6 mSv, which corresponds to an individual's amount of natural radiation exposure over approximately 2 years.

Adverse events associated with radiation exposure are stratified into those that have threshold radiation exposures and those that result from cumulative exposure without a set threshold level. One type of event that occurs with a set threshold level is skin damage from direct radiation exposure. This occurrence is uncommon at levels of radiation used for CT scanning, but is more common with long interventional fluoroscopic studies. The primary concern of cumulative radiation exposure over time is the induction of cancer. This risk is greater in those who undergo multiple imaging studies and in children, who are more radiosensitive than adults. In these settings, it may be prudent to perform MRI rather than CT.[7] In all cases, a common principle in radiology is to keep doses "as low as reasonably achievable" by optimizing each scan to obtain diagnostic information while keeping the radiation dose at a reasonably low level and considering acceptable alternatives that do not use ionizing radiation (such as ultrasonography or MRI).

CT Guidelines and Recommendations

The most important recent change in imaging recommendations for trauma to the spine is the replacement of radiography with CT. Radiography is reserved for patients in whom suspicion for spine injury is low. The ACR's AUC recommend non–contrast-enhanced CT for the evaluation of patients with trauma to the cervical, thoracic, and lumbar spine regions, as indicated by clinical criteria.[1] Using CT data, sagittal and coronal reconstruction images should be obtained to improve the evaluation of fractures and subluxations. Arterial injury including dissection is a concern in patients with cervical spine injury. The evidence for obtaining a CT angiogram to evaluate for dissection is minimal. Given the low concern for arterial injury in blunt trauma, disagreement exists on the use of CT angiography for this group of patients. For lumbar degenerative spondylolisthesis, the North American Spine Society guidelines suggest CT myelography as the most appropriate study for those patients in whom MRI is contraindicated.[2]

CT Myelography

CT myelography is performed following injection of iodinated contrast material into the thecal sac, usually by means of lumbar puncture. The use of CT myelography has declined sharply over the past few decades as a result of the widespread use and availability of MRI in the evaluation of the spinal canal, cord, and nerve roots. CT myelography can be used when MRI is contraindicated, such as in the setting of an implanted device for which MRI would be unsafe, when the patient is too claustrophobic to withstand MRI, with image degradation because of metallic implants, or if symptoms are not explained by MRI findings. More implanted devices are being manufactured with an "MRI-conditional" designation; patients with these devices can undergo MRI under appropriate imaging conditions.[8] Before determining a patient cannot undergo MRI, the safety of a device must be verified by using the device card or by the performing surgeon. Myelography also can be useful in addition to MRI when a cystic collection/arachnoid cyst in the spinal canal is suspected, to assess for continuity with the subarachnoid CSF space and to delineate the margins of the cyst; to evaluate for a CSF leak; or to define anatomy in the setting of suspected spinal cord herniation.

Fluoroscopic guidance usually is used for the procedural portion of the examination. If lumbar puncture is difficult because of anatomy or extensive osseous fusion, CT guidance or cervical puncture may be necessary. Cervical puncture also can be used in the setting of active infection in the lumbar soft tissues, which increases the risk of seeding the infection along the needle tract, or

in the setting of obstruction of cranial flow of contrast material because of severe spinal canal stenosis in the thoracic or lumbar region during evaluation of the cervical or thoracic canal.

The presence of contrast material in the thecal sac allows for evaluation of the spinal cord and nerve roots on their course through the spinal canal and into the neural foramina because the dural sheath follows the nerves for a short distance into the foramen. The spinal cord can be assessed for focal or diffuse thickening of caliber if concern exists for active myelitis or cord tumor or for cord thinning in the setting of myelomalacia. The degree of narrowing of the thecal sac and spinal canal, deformity of the cord, and the presence of obstruction of CSF flow are well shown. However, the internal architecture of the cord is not well assessed using myelography. Nerve roots can be evaluated for thickening and/or compression with myelography. MRI findings may underestimate the degree of nerve root compression in the lateral recess compared with CT myelograms and may underestimate the width of the spinal canal and neural foramina. Myelography and CT myelography also allow dynamic imaging, both temporally for the evaluation of thecal sac filling and to assess for site of leakage in patients with intracranial hypotension.

Relative contraindications to myelography include the presence of a coagulopathy or anticoagulation medicine. Use of the anticoagulant usually needs to be withheld for a variable length of time before the procedure. The presence of iodinated contrast material in the subarachnoid spaces also can reduce the threshold for seizure, especially in the presence of certain medications. These medications (mostly antidepressant and antipsychotic medications) are often withheld for 48 hours before and 24 hours following the procedure.[9] It is important to consult with the performing radiologist and/or the prescribing clinician to answer any questions about whether a medication needs to be or can safely be withheld for the procedure.

The same precautions used with CT also need to be used with myelography, including the risks of radiation to pregnant and pediatric patients or in patients who may have an allergy to iodinated contrast.[10]

Magnetic Resonance Imaging

MRI uses a strong magnetic field along with a series of radiofrequency waves to render representations of the contents of the body. The magnetic field strength of the current units most commonly used are 1.5 Tesla (15,000 gauss) and 3.0 Tesla (30,000 gauss), with lesser strengths available for open and office-based MRI systems. Because of the high magnetic field strength, the

2: Diagnostics in Spine Care

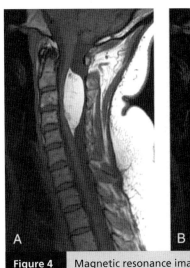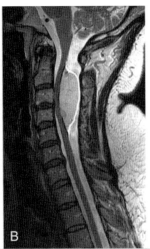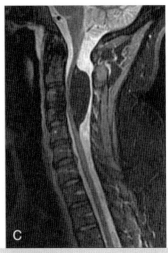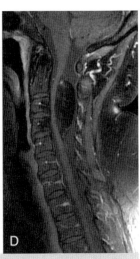

Figure 4 Magnetic resonance images of the cervical spine demonstrate a spinal canal dermoid. T1-weighted (**A**) and fast T2-weighted (**B**) images show fat with bright signal intensity in the dermoid. **C,** Short tau inversion recovery sequence nulls the fat signal in the dermoid. **D,** Contrast material–enhanced T1-weighted image with fat saturation nulls the fat content signal in the dermoid and subcutaneous tissues.

installation and use of the machines is highly regulated because patients or staff with implanted ferromagnetic materials and certain devices cannot be near the unit.

A major benefit of MRI over CT and radiography is that no ionizing radiation is used. Therefore, MRI is an excellent modality for imaging in patients who will need to undergo multiple follow-up examinations; for imaging in children, who are more sensitive to the effects of ionizing radiation; and for imaging in pregnant patients. MRI is ideal for imaging the paraspinal soft tissues, disks, epidural space, neural foramina, and contents of the thecal sac, including the spinal cord and nerve roots.

MRI Sequences

When imaging the spine, several different sequences are commonly used. The two most well known and used are T1- and T2-weighted sequences (most clinical protocols use fast T2-weighted sequences). The T1-weighted sequences show fat as appearing bright (hyperintense) and water as dark (hypointense); T2-weighted sequences (fast spin-echo) show fat as bright and water also as being bright. A fat saturation method can be used to null the fat signal intensity (or turn it hypointense) on the T1-weighted and (fast) T2-weighted sequences. Alternatively, a short tau inversion recovery (STIR) sequence can be used to obtain similar results by changing the bright T2 fat signal intensity to a dark signal. Using either T2-weighting with fat saturation or a STIR sequence, the bright fat is removed to accentuate the edema/fluid in the T2-weighted images. This helps identify pathologic processes in the bone marrow, spinal canal, and paraspinal soft tissues (**Figure 4**).

In the spine, T1-weighted sequences are primarily used to evaluate the signal intensity of bone marrow. Bone marrow is typically hyperintense on T1-weighted sequences because of the high fat content within the marrow in adults (children with a greater concentration of cellular hematopoietically active marrow would show relatively dark signal intensity on a T1-weighted sequence because of the reduced composition of fat). The fatty content of the marrow can be assessed by comparing it with the intervertebral disks and paraspinal muscles. If marrow appears darker than the paraspinal muscles in adults, then a pathologic process should be considered. This is true for both diffuse (lymphoma, leukemia) and focal (myeloma, metastasis, edema) processes. Benign processes that cause diffuse low signal intensity in the marrow are a result of the conversion to red marrow, such as in the setting of anemia or rebound activation of the marrow following chemotherapy. Focal marrow lesions that are bright on T1-weighted sequences are almost always benign and usually represent hemangiomas (which have a high fat content), with exceptions including hemorrhagic blood products (**Figure 5**). Fractures are often seen well on T1-weighted sequences, showing up as a hypointense signal line through the fatty marrow, with varying degrees of confluent surrounding hypointense signal intensity representing edema.

T1-weighted sequences are also well suited for the evaluation of the epidural space and of the contents of the neural foramina because both have high adipose content. Any pathologic process that results in filling in or replacement of the normal fat in these locations should result in close attention given to these regions on the other sequences.

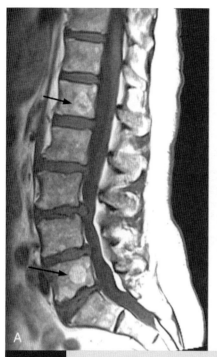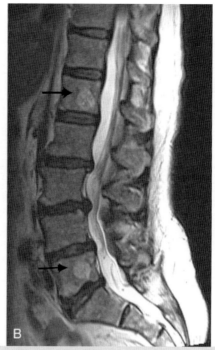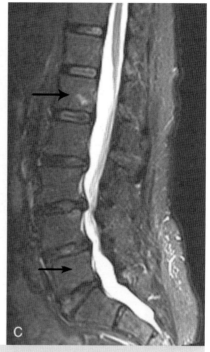

Figure 5 Sagittal spine magnetic resonance images show hemangiomas at L1 and L5 (arrows). **A,** T1-weighted image shows the bright signal intensity of the fat content in the lesion. **B,** T2-weighted image also shows the bright fat in the hemangioma. **C,** Short tau inversion recovery sequence shows the fat signal nulled, with a small amount of fluid of the hemangioma in L1.

The disks and paraspinal muscles show up as intermediate to dark signal intensity on T1-weighted sequences, with ligaments appearing dark on all sequences because of their relative lack of fluid. T1-weighted sequences are good for the evaluation of ligaments in the setting of trauma to assess for discontinuity. Most other pathologies, including infectious and inflammatory processes, are better evaluated on the T2-weighted and STIR sequences.

On T2-weighted sequences, marrow also shows up as bright, although slightly less so than on T1 sequences. The cartilaginous end plates show up as dark signal. The disks are hyperintense centrally in the nucleus pulposus, with a thin peripheral rim of hypointense signal intensity arising from the anulus fibrosus. Most pathology will show up as bright signal intensity on T2-weighted images, including edema related to fracture as well as infectious and inflammatory processes. CSF appears bright on T2-weighted images, resulting in excellent contrast with the spinal cord and nerve roots, which show up as dark. T2-weighted sequences are well suited for the evaluation of spinal cord signal and to evaluate for nerve root compression of the intrathecal portions of the nerves. T2-weighted images also show good delineation of the nerve roots in the neural foramina because they are surrounded by hyperintense fat.

Disk pathology is well seen on T2-weighted sequences, including loss of disk height and disk desiccation (appearing as darkening of the disk on T2-weighted images because of fluid loss). Annular tears (linear or irregular bright signal), disk protrusions, disk extrusions, and resultant thecal sac and neural foraminal encroachment are well evaluated on T2-weighted sequences.

Gadolinium contrast agent administration may help when concern exists for neoplasm (**Figure 6**) or infection (**Figure 7**) or for the evaluation of the postoperative lumbar spine. Gadolinium results in shortening of the T1 signal because of paramagnetic effects of the heavy metal, resulting in increased signal intensity. In the postoperative lumbar spine, recurrent or residual disk protrusions/extrusions and granulation tissue have similar signal intensity on the non–contrast enhanced sequences, and differentiation between the two is difficult. With the administration of gadolinium agents, granulation tissue should be enhanced, whereas the disk will remain dark (but often with a thin rim of surrounding enhancement).

MRI and Spinal Fixation Hardware

Although MRI is generally considered to be safe in the presence of spinal fixation hardware, the makeup of the material (iron, cobalt, nickel, stainless steel) can affect the images by substantial artifact degradation

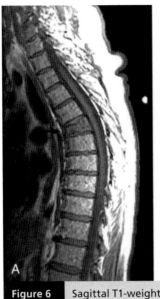
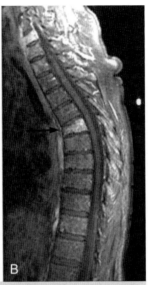

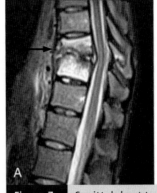
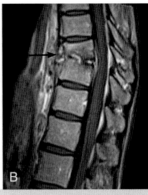

Figure 7 Sagittal short tau inversion recovery sequence magnetic resonance images obtained from a patient with discitis show edema in the disk space and adjacent bone marrow and diffuse enhancement (arrow) before (**A**) and after (**B**) contrast material administration.

Figure 6 Sagittal T1-weighted spine magnetic resonance images obtained before (**A**) and after (**B**) contrast material administration show diffuse enhancement of the vertebral body infiltrated by a tumor (arrow).

attributable to susceptibility effects of ferromagnetic materials, which could render the images nondiagnostic. Some techniques can be used with MRI to reduce the effects of metal artifact degradation. This degradation is becoming less of an issue as titanium implants are more commonly used.[11]

In general, magnetic susceptibility effects are less at lower field strengths, so 1.5 Tesla is preferred to 3.0 Tesla or higher field strength. Most imaging centers have set sequences available called metal artifact reduction sequences. Adjusting technical imaging parameters of voxels, matrix size, and bandwidth can minimize the artifact.[11]

MRI Safety

MRI can result in a safety hazard to a subset of patients and staff. Therefore, an extensive screening process needs to be implemented before allowing anyone to enter the environment of the magnetic field. For patients who will be in the imager, the screening process involves filling out a form about history of surgery, implanted devices, and the possibility of foreign metallic bodies, including any history of working with metal, for which concern exists for the presence of metal fragments within the orbit. Any patient who answers positively to any question will require further evaluation to assess the exact nature of the foreign device or material to determine if MRI is safe to perform. The materials that can cause a safety hazard are composed of ferromagnetic material, which can result in

heating/burning or dislodgement/torque that can injure the surrounding tissues.

Implanted devices are designated as MRI safe, MRI conditional, or MRI unsafe. MRI-safe devices should not cause any adverse effects when exposed to the magnetic field or the radiofrequency pulses within the unit. MRI-conditional devices have several requirements as designated by the manufacturer that need to be followed to safely perform imaging. As long as these recommendations are adhered to, MRI poses no known hazards for patients with MRI-conditional devices.[8,12] It is important to keep in mind that some devices are only suitable for imaging certain parts of the body (such as only the brain or extremities), and torso or spine imaging may be excluded. Clear identification of the manufacturer and device model number is mandatory before permitting the patient to undergo MRI.

All facilities that contain an MRI unit are required to have zones set up that are clearly demarcated and allow safe movement of people within and around the MRI environment. Zone 1 includes all areas that are freely accessible by the public. Zone 2 is still a public area but serves as an interface between public zone 1 and strictly controlled zone 3. Patient screening often occurs in zone 2. Zone 3, which usually consists of the control room where the technologist works, needs to be separated by a locked door that allows ready access only by prescreened staff. Zone 4 is the imaging room. Any time zone 3 or 4 is entered, it is important to adhere to the technologist's requests to ensure everyone's safety. This adherence is critical especially in urgent situations of patient decompensation or cardiopulmonary arrest, which requires multiple members of the code team who may be unfamiliar with the risks of the magnetic field.

Gadolinium agents also can result in a safety hazard to patients. The major concerns associated with gadolinium are the possibility of an allergic-type reaction and of nephrogenic systemic fibrosis, a disease that can result in fibrosis of the skin and internal organs related to the administration of gadolinium-containing agents in patients with renal insufficiency. Gadolinium-based contrast agents are not considered nephrotoxic at the routinely administered doses.

Allergic-type reactions to gadolinium agents, although less frequent and often less severe than the reactions that patients have to iodinated CT contrast agents, are serious and treated with the same intensity. These are not true allergic reactions because patients can have a reaction without ever having been exposed to the agent before and often will not consistently have the reaction with every subsequent exposure. An antigen-antibody response is not always identified. Therefore, the responses are currently considered an idiosyncratic reaction, and can consist of rash, hives, throat swelling, difficulty breathing, or anaphylactoid reactions resulting in hypotension, cardiorespiratory failure, and death. As with iodinated contrast reactions, patients should be premedicated with a regimen of corticosteroids with or without an antihistamine before injection to attempt to decrease the risk of injection and a different contrast agent may be used. For more severe reactions, consideration should be given to performing a noncontrast study. If contrast is absolutely necessary, the study should be performed in the hospital setting with trained staff and appropriate anesthesia support available.[4]

Nephrogenic systemic fibrosis can result in fibrosis of the skin and internal organs, similar to systemic scleroderma. Gadolinium has been found in the affected tissues. The group most commonly affected is patients with stage IV renal failure who are undergoing routine hemodialysis, but it has also been seen, albeit less frequently, in patients with acute renal failure or lesser degrees of chronic renal insufficiency. Gadolinium-based agents are usually considered safe in patients with chronic renal failure who have an eGFR greater than 30 mL/min/1.73 m^2, but the agents should be used cautiously in patients with acute renal failure or with an eGFR less than 30 mL/min/1.73 m^2.[4,13] If contrast is deemed necessary, a risk-benefit assessment should be performed and there should be direct discussion between the referring clinician and approving radiologist. The patient also should be made aware of the risks associated with the gadolinium-based agent and informed consent should be obtained.

MRI Guidelines and Recommendations

For cervical trauma, the AUC of the ACR consider MRI an appropriate and complementary imaging modality to CT.[1] MRI also is the study of choice for patients with neurologic symptoms concerning for spinal cord injury, hematoma, or disk herniation, as well as ligamentous injury. Some controversy exists regarding the use of MRI in patients with normal CT examination findings. The ACR suggests using MRI in patients whose neurologic status cannot be fully evaluated after 48 hours, even with normal CT examination results.[1]

For lumbar degenerative spondylolisthesis, MRI is suggested as the most appropriate noninvasive test for imaging spinal stenosis by North American Spine Society guidelines.[2] In patients with clinical concern for disk herniation, MRI is the recommended study of choice, but CT myelography should be performed in patients for whom MRI is contraindicated. For lumbar spinal stenosis, MRI is recommended as the most appropriate imaging study, with CT myelography performed for patients in whom MRI is contraindicated. In addition, workgroup consensus suggests MRI as the first-line diagnostic study for patients with spinal stenosis.[14]

Imaging recommendations for low back pain are evolving. For uncomplicated acute low back pain, the ACR suggests no imaging studies because the pain is a benign self-limiting process. However, in patients with red flags for serious injury or with prolonged pain after medical management, MRI is recommended, although many payers will require radiographic evaluation prior to approving MRI.[1] Many patients have no correlative abnormal imaging findings. Also, imaging abnormalities can exist in people without back pain. As summarized by the AUC of the ACR, the challenge for practicing physicians is to identify the small subgroup of patients within the large population that requires spinal imaging in whom serious disease should be suspected.[1]

Nuclear Scintigraphy and PET

Bone scintigraphy and PET are the modalities most often used in the diagnosis of spine disease. Bone scintigraphy (also called bone scanning) is useful for bone lesions, including the spine, and used less for soft tissues. The isotope technetium Tc-99 methylene diphosphonate (^{99}Tc MDP) and planar or multiplanar single-photon emission computed tomography images are obtained a few hours after injection. ^{99}Tc MDP binds to hydroxyapatite crystals in proportion to local blood flow and osteoblastic activity, making the agent a good marker for bone turnover and bone perfusion.

Fractures, osteomyelitis, and osteolytic metastatic tumors (**Figure 8**) all show increased "hot" activity in the bone scan. Occasionally, areas that show a lack of activity ("cold") may exist in aggressive metastatic lesions,

2: Diagnostics in Spine Care

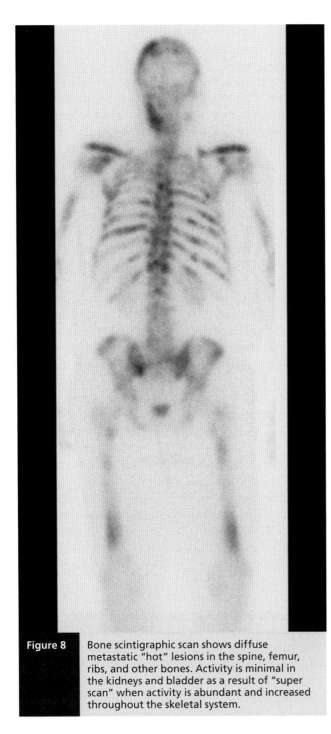

Figure 8 Bone scintigraphic scan shows diffuse metastatic "hot" lesions in the spine, femur, ribs, and other bones. Activity is minimal in the kidneys and bladder as a result of "super scan" when activity is abundant and increased throughout the skeletal system.

The amount of radiation from bone scanning is low compared with that from CT. Although the isotope adheres to the bone, it is excreted through the kidneys. Therefore, the largest pool of radioactive activity is in the bladder and urine, lasting approximately 24 hours. Patients should be instructed in proper voiding and hand hygiene after the procedure by the nuclear medicine personnel.

PET is used for the detection of metastatic disease in the spine and soft tissues of the body. Although the literature reports conflicting sensitivities for PET compared with bone scanning, many medical practices use PET because it can help identify both bone and soft-tissue tumors.[15]

The ^{18}F fluorodeoxyglucose (FDG) produced from a cyclotron is administered via venous injection. After a short period, CT images are obtained followed by multiple sections of the body obtained with PET. Both PET and CT are performed with the same scanner, with registration of both sets of images.

The isotope ^{18}F FDG shows increased activity in tissues with elevated glycolytic activity. Ceroplastic cells have increased glycolysis; therefore, the cells show abnormally elevated activity with PET. False-positive FDG uptake can occur in infection, inflammation, and sarcoidosis (**Figure 9**).

MRI of the spine is often performed to complement PET findings for defining tumor involvement. Although PET/CT has a CT component, the images are of lesser quality and used mostly for localization purposes. Additional high-quality CT often is needed for surgical planning.

Administrative logistics are involved in obtaining reimbursement for PET scans from the Centers for Medicare and Medicaid Services. A requirement is data entry into the National Oncologic PET Registry,[16] with a limited number of allowable PET scans for the patient incident creating some delay for emergent PET scans for patients with Medicare as the primary insurance.

Intraoperative Fluoroscopy

Fluoroscopy is frequently used in the operating suite to localize the surgical level and to guide the placement of radiopaque implants. Understanding the basic radiation exposure precautions is important for both the patient and the equipment user and surgical team when performing image-guided spine procedures.

The ACR presented a white paper on radiation doses in medicine.[17] High-dose radiation has increased the risk of stochastic effects of carcinogenesis. However, the more immediate concern is the deterministic effect of

indolent healing abscesses, plasmacytomas, or disruption of blood flow such as with bone infarcts or prostheses.

A three-phase bone scan is available to examine for blood flow, blood pool, and delayed images for infection. However, in spine imaging, MRI with contrast is more frequently the imaging modality of choice to detect infection. The predominant use of ^{99}Tc MDP bone scanning is to image areas of fractures or metastatic bone lesions in the spine.

The equipment user and the team should follow a few guidelines when using intraoperative fluoroscopy. For the equipment user, the main concern relates to scatter radiation. Because radiation decreases with distance, the equipment user should stay away from the patient as much as possible when using C-arm fluoroscopy. A lead apron is mandatory when close to the intraoperative C-arm for all personnel. Wearing a thyroid shield is strongly recommended because the shield substantially decreases radiation to the thyroid gland. Protective goggles are recommended as often as possible. Avoiding placement of the equipment user's hands in direct exposure of the radiation beam is important. If possible, collimation (narrowing aperture at the source) should be used to deliver radiation only to the essential part of the imaging target to minimize overall radiation exposure.[19]

Intraoperative CT

Intraoperative CT is being used more often because of its increased accuracy in the placement of spine hardware. The surgeon and other personnel should be outside the operating room or behind sufficient lead shielding during intraoperative CT to minimize scatter radiation. The two settings selected are peak kilovoltage and milliamperes. Most CT scanning programs automate the peak kilovoltage and milliampere variables to produce best-quality images, often at a high radiation dose. Manual minimization of the two variables will result in poor image quality, but at a low radiation dose to the patient. Increasing the two variables will produce better image quality, but at a high radiation dose to the patient. Larger body size also requires a higher radiation dose to visualize the spine structures. Therefore, close interaction with the technologist in determining the optimal setting becomes an important component to understand when using intraoperative CT. Otherwise, the radiation delivered to the patient will increase. In addition, decreasing the total number of scans decreases overall radiation to the patient, which is preferred.

After the images are acquired, the data can be formatted to accentuate the tissue of interest. Another component of the CT image focuses on software processing of the acquired data, described as a CT algorithm. After obtaining the CT scan, the data can be formatted into different algorithms. If soft tissue is of interest, a lower kernel algorithm (approximately 30 HU) is used. For bone or hardware, a higher kernel algorithm (approximately 60 HU) creates sharp bone margins. Repeat scanning is not necessary to obtain images with these different algorithms because the technologist can reformat the data into the preferred algorithm. After the data are formatted,

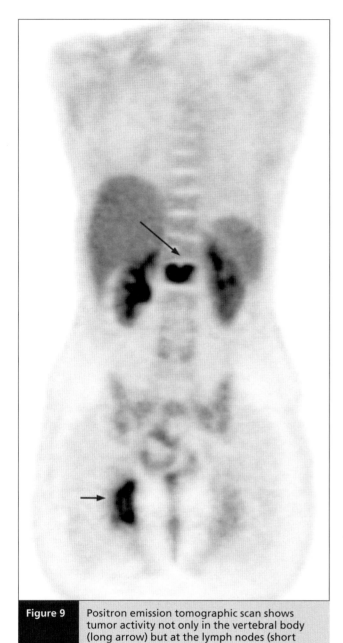

Figure 9 Positron emission tomographic scan shows tumor activity not only in the vertebral body (long arrow) but at the lymph nodes (short arrow).

radiation dose to the body surface, including erythema, skin damage, hair loss, cataracts, and radiation sickness. Therefore, the FDA mandates the display of cumulative radiation delivered from new fluoroscopic equipment, which requires close monitoring by the equipment user and the technologist.[18]

It is essential that the user of the fluoroscopic unit in the operating suite understand the basic risks and the use of the equipment, including the measurement units of Grays for radiation dose and sieverts for the equivalent dose based on the type of radiation (x-ray, α, β radiation, and so forth).

2: Diagnostics in Spine Care

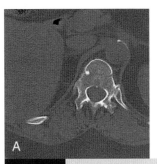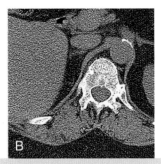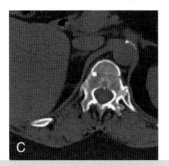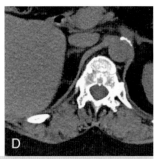

| Figure 10 | Axial CT scans of the spine show a bone algorithm and bone window (**A**), a bone algorithm and soft-tissue window (**B**), a soft-tissue algorithm and bone window (**C**), and a soft-tissue algorithm and soft-tissue window (**D**). |

the window setting (Hounsfield levels) can be changed so that the tissue of interest can be seen. This concept is best understood as a 2 × 2 matrix (**Figure 10**). When examining soft tissue, a lower kernel algorithm and soft-tissue window is optimal. When looking for a bone fracture, a higher kernel algorithm with bone window is preferred. A soft-tissue algorithm with bone window will still show bone margins of acceptable quality, but with less sharpness. A bone algorithm with soft-tissue window often is not of nondiagnostic use.

A recent meta-analysis compared a less invasive surgical approach with open spine surgery and showed an increase in radiation exposure to the surgeon and the team.[20] Many variables affect the magnitude of increase in the delivered radiation and scattered radiation. Many imaging specialists think that the amount of radiation increase may not be significant, although the overall effect of the increase in radiation is not known. Therefore, it becomes prudent to decrease radiation whenever possible by understanding the basics of radiation delivery and by determining ways to minimize radiation to the equipment user and the patient. Concepts in radiation-based image guidance are an important educational component in the use of image-guided intraoperative procedures.

Summary

Imaging of the spine entails understanding of the various imaging modalities available that will provide the best imaging information for subsequent patient treatment. The provider or the referring clinical team also must understand the limitations of imaging and the risks associated with the delivery of energy for image acquisition. Also, understanding the available national guidelines for the appropriate use of imaging is important for the safety of the patient and the quality of clinical treatment.

Key Study Points

- Understanding the basic concepts of radiation dose is important in requesting imaging studies and in the use of intraoperative imaging equipment.
- Myelography, MRI, and PET have detailed assessments performed before and after imaging that are required for patient safety.
- Guidelines and appropriate use for imaging of the spine continue to be developed among multiple national societies and should be referenced whenever possible to plan directed, value-based treatment.

Annotated References

1. American College of Radiology: ACR Appropriateness Criteria. Update 2016. Available at: http://www.acr.org/Quality-Safety/Appropriateness-Criteria. Accessed January 30, 2017.

   The ACR AUC are evidence-based guidelines designed to assist referring clinicians in ordering the most appropriate study based on clinical presentation. Expert panels including radiologists and other specialists developed the guidelines.

2. North American Spine Society: Evidence-based clinical guidelines for multidisciplinary spine care: Diagnosis and treatment of degenerative lumbar spondylolisthesis. Revised 2014. Available at: https://www.spine.org/Portals/0/Documents/ResearchClinicalCare/Guidelines/Spondylolisthesis.pdf. Accessed January 30, 2017.

   Evidence-based guidelines for the treatment of lumbar spondylolisthesis and recommendation grades based on high-level evidence are presented.

3. North American Spine Society: Evidence-based clinical guidelines for multidisciplinary spine care: Diagnosis and treatment of adult isthmic spondylolisthesis. 2014. Available at: https://www.spine.org/Portals/0/Documents/

ResearchClinicalCare/Guidelines/AdultIsthmicSpondylolisthesis.pdf. Accessed January 30, 2017.

Evidence-based guidelines for the treatment of lumbar isthmic spondylolisthesis and recommendation grades based on high-level evidence are presented.

4. American College of Radiology: Manual on contrast media v10.2. 2016. Available at: http://www.acr.org/quality-safety/resources/contrast-manual. Accessed January 30, 2017.

This manual produced by the ACR Committee on Drugs and Contrast Media presents up-to-date information and an evidence-based discussion of the use of contrast media in radiology, with a focus on enhancing safe and effective use.

5. Davenport MS, Cohan RH, Khalatbari S, Ellis JH: The challenges in assessing contrast-induced nephropathy: Where are we now? *AJR Am J Roentgenol* 2014;202(4):784-789.

The authors review the history of contrast-induced nephropathy and discuss difficulties in establishing a causative relationship between currently used low-osmolar contrast media and contrast-induced nephropathy in the clinical setting. They suggest that contrast-induced nephropathy is real, but it is rare. Level of evidence: IV.

6. Davenport MS, Khalatbari S, Cohan RH, Dillman JR, Myles JD, Ellis JH: Contrast material-induced nephrotoxicity and intravenous low-osmolality iodinated contrast material: Risk stratification by using estimated glomerular filtration rate. *Radiology* 2013;268(3):719-728.

The authors report on a retrospective study of 20,242 patients who underwent CT either without or with intravenous contrast. It was concluded that intravenous low-osmolar iodinated contrast is a risk factor for acute kidney injury, but not in patients with a stable serum creatinine level less than 1.5 mg/dL. Level of evidence: III.

7. Lin EC: Radiation risk from medical imaging. *Mayo Clin Proc* 2010;85(12):1142-1146, quiz 1146.

8. Nazarian S, Beinart R, Halperin HR: Magnetic resonance imaging and implantable devices. *Circ Arrhythm Electrophysiol* 2013;6(2):419-428.

The authors discuss MRI in patients with implanted defibrillators, focusing on physics, nonclinical testing, prior clinical studies, safety protocols, and MRI quality.

9. Fedutes BA, Ansani NT: Seizure potential of concomitant medications and radiographic contrast media agents. *Ann Pharmacother* 2003;37(10):1506-1510.

10. Harreld JH, McMenamy JM, Toomay SM, Chason DP: Myelography: A primer. *Curr Probl Diagn Radiol* 2011;40(4):149-157.

The authors discuss the use of myelography in patients with spinal pathology and neck or back pain, including indications, patient workup and planning, procedure technique, and postmyelographic care. Level of evidence: IV.

11. Hargreaves BA, Worters PW, Pauly KB, Pauly JM, Koch KM, Gold GE: Metal-induced artifacts in MRI. *AJR Am J Roentgenol* 2011;197(3):547-555.

This article reviews the source of imaging artifacts arising from metallic hardware and includes a discussion on how to reduce artifacts by adjusting imaging parameters to produce more clinically useful images. Level of evidence: IV.

12. Shellock FG, Woods TO, Crues JV III: MR labeling information for implants and devices: Explanation of terminology. *Radiology* 2009;253(1):26-30.

13. Kaewlai R, Abujudeh H: Nephrogenic systemic fibrosis. *AJR Am J Roentgenol* 2012;199(1):W17-W23.

A detailed discussion of nephrogenic systemic fibrosis, including history, possible pathophysiology, and presentation/diagnosis, is presented. The authors provide recommendations for safe use of gadolinium-based contrast agents in the setting of known or possible renal dysfunction. Level of evidence: IV.

14. North American Spine Society: Evidence-based clinical guidelines for multidisciplinary spine care: Diagnosis and treatment of degenerative lumbar spinal stenosis. Revised 2011. Available at: https://www.spine.org/Portals/0/Documents/ResearchClinicalCare/Guidelines/LumbarStenosis.pdf. Accessed on January 30, 2017.

Evidence-based guidelines for lumbar spinal stenosis and recommendation grades based on high-level evidence are presented.

15. Fogelman I, Cook G, Israel O, Van der Wall H: Positron emission tomography and bone metastases. *Semin Nucl Med* 2005;35(2):135-142.

16. National Oncologic PET Registry. Available at: https://www.cancerpetregistry.org/clinicians.htm. Accessed March 13, 2017.

The purpose of this registry is to safeguard access to Medicare reimbursement for certain types of PET scans.

17. Amis ES Jr, Butler PF, Applegate KE, et al; American College of Radiology: American College of Radiology white paper on radiation dose in medicine. *J Am Coll Radiol* 2007;4(5):272-284.

18. US Food and Drug Administration: CFR—Code of Federal Regulations Title 21. Revised April 1, 2016. Available at: http://www.accessdata.fda.gov/scripts/cdrh/cfdocs/cfcfr/CFRSearch.cfm?FR=1020.32. Accessed January 30, 2017.

This FDA report provides guidelines for monitoring the performance of ionizing radiation–emitting products.

19. Kaplan DJ, Patel JN, Liporace FA, Yoon RS: Intraoperative radiation safety in orthopaedics: A review of the ALARA (As low as reasonably achievable) principle. *Patient Saf Surg* 2016;10:27.

This review article discusses the basics of fluoroscopy and methods to decrease the dose of radiation to the patient,

2: Diagnostics in Spine Care

operator, and other staff in an orthopaedic operating room.

20. Yu E, Khan SN: Does less invasive spine surgery result in increased radiation exposure? A systematic review. *Clin Orthop Relat Res* 2014;472(6):1738-1748.

This systemic review of radiation exposure in spine surgery was performed to determine the difference in radiation exposure in open versus less invasive spine procedures, radiation exposure based on the position of the surgeon, and radiation exposure using C-arm fluoroscopy compared with fluoroscopy with computer-assisted navigation.

Chapter 7

Electrodiagnostic Testing and Intraoperative Neurophysiologic Monitoring

Berdale Colorado, DO, MPH   James O. Sanders, MD   Kenneth Foxx, MD

Abstract

Electrodiagnostic studies play an important role in the assessment of patients with neuromuscular disorders. Office-based testing consists primarily of nerve conduction studies and needle electromyography, whereas intraoperative testing and monitoring consists of somatosensory-evoked potentials, motor-evoked potentials, and spontaneous and triggered electromyography. It is helpful to be familiar with all forms of testing, including the indications and limitations of nerve conduction studies and needle electromyography for suspected spine disorders, as well as the clinical practice guidelines for intraoperative neurophysiologic monitoring.

Keywords: intraoperative neurophysiologic monitoring; needle electromyography; motor-evoked potential; motor unit action potential; nerve conduction study, somatosensory-evoked potential

Electrodiagnostic Testing

Berdale Colorado, DO, MPH

Introduction

Electrodiagnostic testing is first and foremost an extension of the clinical examination. A focused history and physical examination is essential for guiding electrodiagnostic testing.

Electrodiagnostic studies provide a measure of the electrical activity of muscles and nerves and can serve as a valuable tool in treating patients with suspected spine disorders. Although neuroimaging detects structural abnormalities, only electrodiagnostic testing can assess functional or physiologic abnormalities. Multiple electrodiagnostic tests exist; however, nerve conduction studies and needle electromyography (EMG) are the most commonly performed office-based tests. Information regarding localization, severity, duration, and prognosis of a nerve disorder often can be obtained through electrodiagnostic testing. An overview of nerve conduction and needle EMG studies is presented along with a discussion of the indications for electrodiagnostic testing for suspected spine disorders, the limitations of electrodiagnostic testing, and a framework for confirming that appropriate electrodiagnostic testing has been completed for commonly encountered diagnoses.

Overview of Testing
Nerve Conduction Studies
Nerve conduction studies measure the ability of peripheral nerves to conduct electrical impulses. These studies are typically performed before needle EMG because the results of the nerve conduction studies may influence which muscles are tested with needle EMG and the interpretation of the needle EMG findings. Nerve conduction studies can be generally divided into motor nerve conduction studies, sensory nerve conduction studies, and

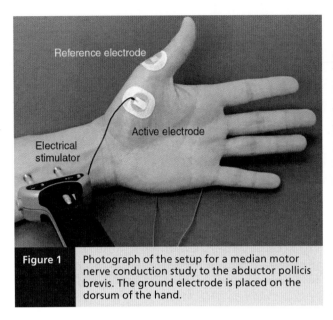

Figure 1 Photograph of the setup for a median motor nerve conduction study to the abductor pollicis brevis. The ground electrode is placed on the dorsum of the hand.

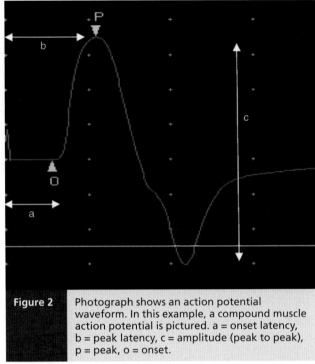

Figure 2 Photograph shows an action potential waveform. In this example, a compound muscle action potential is pictured. a = onset latency, b = peak latency, c = amplitude (peak to peak), p = peak, o = onset.

Table 1

Selected Nerve Conduction Study Waveform Parameters

Waveform Parameter	Unit of Measurement	Description
Onset latency	Milliseconds	Interval between delivery of an electrical stimulus and the onset of an evoked waveform
Peak latency	Milliseconds	Interval between delivery of an electrical stimulus and the peak of an evoked waveform
Amplitude	Microvolts (sensory) Millivolts (motor)	The maximum voltage difference between two points, usually peak-to-peak or baseline-to-peak
Conduction velocity	Meters per second	Speed of propagation of an action potential along a nerve or muscle fiber

mixed nerve conduction studies. The basic setup for nerve conduction studies involves a ground electrode and two recording electrodes (an active and a reference electrode). The active electrode is placed over the muscle of interest in motor nerve conduction studies and over the nerve of interest in sensory nerve conduction studies. An electrical stimulator is positioned at a specific distance from the active electrode along the course of the nerve (**Figure 1**). When an electrical impulse is applied by the stimulator, an action potential is recorded at the active electrode and is displayed on the EMG machine as a waveform (**Figure 2**). Various waveform parameters, including onset latency, peak latency, amplitude, and conduction velocity, are measured and interpreted by an electrodiagnostician (**Table 1**).

The recorded potential in a motor nerve conduction study is known as a compound muscle action potential (CMAP), which represents the summation of all underlying individual muscle fiber action potentials. Onset latency (the time required for an electrical stimulus to initiate an evoked potential) and amplitude (reflecting the number of muscle fibers activated) of the CMAP are measured. After a distal and a proximal site have been stimulated, a conduction velocity can be calculated, which is the speed an impulse travels along a nerve.

Latency and conduction velocities reflect the fastest conducting fibers and are primarily dependent on the integrity of the myelin sheath.

The recorded potential in a sensory nerve conduction study is known as a sensory nerve action potential

(SNAP), which represents the summation of all the individual sensory fiber action potentials. Because nerve conduction occurs in both directions following nerve depolarization, sensory nerve conduction studies can be performed using either orthodromic (in the direction of physiologic conduction) or antidromic (opposite of physiologic conduction) techniques. Although the antidromic technique is often preferred, particularly because of the higher amplitude compared with the orthodromic technique, both techniques have advantages and disadvantages. Peak latency (reflecting the latency along most of the sensory fibers) and amplitude (reflecting the number of sensory fibers activated) of the SNAP are measured.

Late response studies such as the F-wave and H-reflex studies are sometimes used to assess more proximal nerve segments. These studies can provide additional information in the evaluation of radiculopathies, plexopathies, polyneuropathies, and proximal peripheral neuropathies.

Taken altogether, the numeric values of the latency, amplitude, and conduction velocity of the various nerve conduction studies can point to a focal nerve lesion such as an entrapment or a diffuse neurogenic process such as a peripheral polyneuropathy.

Needle Electromyography

Needle EMG is typically performed after completion of the nerve conduction studies. The basic setup for needle EMG involves a needle electrode (either monopolar or concentric), a reference electrode (if using a monopolar needle), and a ground electrode (**Figure 3**). Monopolar and concentric needles each have advantages and disadvantages, but both are widely used.

The needle is inserted into each muscle of interest, and several additional small, brief insertions are made to adequately sample each muscle. Insertional activity and spontaneous activity are assessed while the muscle is at rest. In a normal muscle, there should be electrical silence shortly after needle movement. Increased insertional activity is defined as any electrical activity that lasts longer than 300 ms after brief needle movement, with the exception of end plate potentials, which can be seen if a needle is placed near the motor end plate. Increased insertional activity is seen with denervation. Spontaneous activity is defined as any electrical activity at rest that lasts longer than 3 seconds. Two types of spontaneous activity commonly seen with denervation are fibrillations and positive sharp waves. These represent abnormal electrical activity generated from denervated single muscle fibers. Fibrillations and positive sharp waves are graded based on their distribution and intensity, ranging from 1+ (persistent single runs in two areas) up to 4+ (continuous discharges in all areas of the muscle).

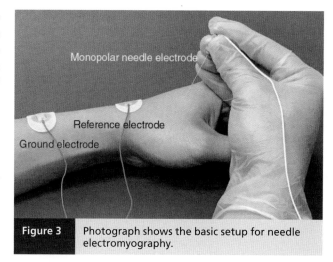

Figure 3 Photograph shows the basic setup for needle electromyography.

After assessment of insertional and spontaneous activity, analysis of motor unit action potentials (MUAPs) is performed. This assessment involves voluntary contraction of the muscles of interest. MUAPs are analyzed for amplitude, duration, number of phases, and recruitment (**Table 2**).

Amplitude is measured from the most positive to the most negative peak, and the normal value is typically 1-2 mV. Amplitude can be increased in the setting of reinnervation, often indicating a chronic neurogenic disorder. Duration is measured from the initial baseline departure to the final return to baseline, and the normal value is typically 5-15 ms. Duration can be increased in the setting of reinnervation, often indicating a subacute neurogenic disorder.

Phases of the MUAP refer to the number of times the MUAP crosses the baseline; the normal value is typically two to four phases. Increased phases, or polyphasicity, can be seen in the setting of reinnervation, often indicating a subacute neurogenic disorder. With increasing muscle contraction force, additional MUAPs can be activated, and the MUAP recruitment pattern can be analyzed. In normal recruitment, when the first MUAP fires at a rate of approximately 10 Hz, a second MUAP is recruited and begins to fire at a rate of approximately 5 Hz. As the firing frequency increases by approximately 5 Hz, an additional MUAP is recruited. With maximal contraction, a complete interference pattern may be seen in which the screen of the EMG machine is filled with four or more overlapping MUAPs and no individual MUAP can be distinguished. With denervation, recruitment is often reduced and only one or a few MUAPs are seen, even with maximal contraction. In this case, the interference pattern would be reduced.

2: Diagnostics in Spine Care

Table 2			
Selected Motor Unit Action Potential Analysis Parameters			
Parameter	Unit of Measurement	Description	Representation
Amplitude	Millivolts	Interval between most positive peak to most negative peak of waveform	Represents the muscle fibers recorded near the needle electrode
Duration	Milliseconds	Interval between waveform's initial deflection from baseline to its final return	Represents the number of muscle fibers within the motor unit
Phases	Number of phases	Number of times the waveform crosses the baseline	Represents the synchronicity of muscle fiber action potentials firing
Recruitment	Hertz (for recruitment frequency)	The successive activation of the same and additional units with increasing strength of voluntary muscle contraction	Represents the pattern of motor unit action potential recruitment

Electrodiagnostic Testing for Spine Disorders

The timing of performance of electrodiagnostic testing is dependent on the clinical differential diagnosis. Electrodiagnostic testing may be indicated in the assessment of any suspected nerve disorder. Patients with symptoms such as arm or leg pain, weakness, or numbness or tingling are commonly referred for electrodiagnostic testing. Testing can confirm the presence of a radiculopathy; rule out peripheral nerve disorders, which can affect similar anatomic distributions; and identify the presence of multiple coexistent nerve disorders. For example, a patient may simultaneously have a cervical radiculopathy, carpal tunnel syndrome, and a peripheral polyneuropathy. Identifying these disorders may have a substantial effect on the treatment plan. Electrodiagnostic testing also can be helpful in patients with a physical examination that does not clearly localize the etiology of their symptoms or with imaging findings that do not correlate with their symptoms. The needle EMG and nerve conduction studies may be abnormal when all other test findings, including neuroimaging, are unremarkable.

The timing or performance of electrodiagnostic testing also depends to some extent on the type of information desired. A common misconception is that it is necessary to wait 2 to 3 weeks after a nerve injury before obtaining needle EMG or nerve conduction studies. This misconception is based on the idea that wallerian degeneration, which may take several days to weeks, must first occur before meaningful information can be obtained. However, a substantial axonal injury can be seen immediately, and this information may aid in early localization of the injury. The primary limitation to early performance of electrodiagnostic testing is the difficulty in differentiating a conduction block from an axonal injury immediately after a nerve injury. In a patient with a cervical or lumbosacral radiculopathy, it is a commonly held belief that changes of denervation on needle EMG are seen first in the paraspinal muscles at approximately 2 weeks. This is followed by changes of denervation in the peripheral muscles (proximal to distal) at approximately 3 weeks. This belief is not supported in the literature; several studies have concluded that radiculopathies do not follow a predictable time course of denervation.[1-4]

Pitfalls and Limitations of Electrodiagnostic Testing
Nerve Conduction Studies

Nerve conduction studies can be affected by numerous factors that must be taken into account when interpreting data. These can be subdivided into physiologic and nonphysiologic factors. Temperature is the most important physiologic factor affecting nerve conduction studies. A decrease in temperature can cause prolonged latency, increased amplitude, increased duration, and decreased conduction velocity. Conduction velocity decreases approximately 2.4 m/s per 1°C decrease, and distal latency can be prolonged by 0.2 ms per 1°C decrease. Normal temperature is approximately 32°C for the upper extremity and 30°C for the lower extremity. Other physiologic factors that can influence nerve conduction studies include age, height, sex, edema, obesity, and anomalous innervation.[5] Therefore, these factors must be taken into consideration when determining what is "normal."

Nonphysiologic factors affecting nerve conduction studies refer to technical considerations that can influence the recorded data. These include improper electrode placement, suboptimal stimulation, inaccurate measurements, and failure to recognize artifacts. These factors can create inaccurate latency, amplitude, and conduction velocity measurements, which can result in incorrect conclusions. Recognition of potential technical factors is imperative when conducting nerve conduction studies.

Needle Electromyography

In the electrodiagnostic evaluation of a cervical or a lumbosacral radiculopathy, nerve conduction studies are typically normal, and the diagnosis is made primarily on the results of needle EMG. Needle EMG is the best electrodiagnostic procedure for detecting radiculopathies. However, the primary limitation of needle EMG is that it does not detect all compressive radiculopathies. A "negative needle EMG" cannot be used to exclude a radiculopathy. Sensitivities of needle EMG for cervical radiculopathy range from 50% to 71%, and sensitivities for lumbosacral radiculopathy range from 49% to 86%.[1] Specificity of needle EMG for radiculopathy is high. A 2011 study reported that when only positive sharp waves or fibrillations were considered abnormal, specificity ranged from 92% to 97% in lumbosacral radiculopathy.[6] Low sensitivity can result from an inadequate number of affected motor nerve root fibers, inadequate sampling of fibers during needle EMG, or because the needle EMG was performed after reinnervation had occurred. A pure sensory radiculopathy would result in a normal needle EMG because of sparing of the dorsal root ganglion. These are important considerations when electrodiagnostic testing is negative for needle EMG abnormalities.

Needle EMG has limited effectiveness for identifying the cause or etiology of a nerve lesion. Also, the specific nerve root involved may not be accurately identified by the needle EMG because of myotome overlap or anomalous root innervation. These are important considerations when electrodiagnostic testing is positive for needle EMG abnormalities.

Interpretation of Electrodiagnostic Testing

Although detailed interpretation of electrodiagnostic data can be challenging to a clinician who does not perform such testing, a general understanding can help clinicians identify a high-quality EMG report.

The electrodiagnostic testing for radiculopathy should include both nerve conduction studies and needle EMG. Although the nerve conduction studies are typically normal, they are necessary to exclude a peripheral neuropathy. Low CMAP amplitudes may occur, however, in the setting of a radiculopathy with substantial axonal degeneration. At least one motor nerve conduction study and one sensory nerve conduction study should be performed in the involved limb. The sensory nerve conduction study

ideally should be in the distribution of the suspected radiculopathy. The screening for a suspected radiculopathy should examine at least five to seven muscles, including the paraspinal muscles.[7] The screening should include muscles that represent all relevant myotomes of the involved limb, with emphasis on the myotome in question.

No consensus exists regarding which muscles should be included in the initial screening. If one muscle is abnormal, the screening is expanded. The optimal number of muscles tested for both cervical and lumbosacral radiculopathy screenings has been proposed to be six muscles and should include the paraspinal muscles.[8,9] A needle EMG study is considered "positive" for a radiculopathy if EMG abnormalities are present in two or more muscles that receive innervation from the same root (preferably by different peripheral nerves), but muscles innervated by adjacent nerve roots are normal. The EMG report should include the nerve conduction studies performed as well as the muscles tested on needle EMG. These findings are typically presented in a table format. A diagnosis of a radiculopathy based on findings of fibrillations and positive sharp waves is considered highly convincing. A diagnosis of a radiculopathy based on findings of decreased recruitment or increased polyphasicity is considered less strong.

Diagnostic Ultrasonography as an Adjunct to Electrodiagnostic Testing

The use of neuromuscular ultrasonography has rapidly increased over the past decade and is a valuable adjunct to electrodiagnostic testing. Ultrasonography may be considered in situations in which peripheral nerve entrapment is part of the differential diagnosis, but electrodiagnostic test findings are negative for evidence of any entrapment neuropathy. Nerve enlargement in the region of the entrapment site is commonly seen with ultrasonography; however, the cause of this enlargement is not completely understood.[10] Although the current application of neuromuscular ultrasonography has focused more on distal peripheral nerve assessment, recent research has explored the use of ultrasonography in the assessment of spinal nerve roots.[11]

Intraoperative Neurophysiologic Monitoring

James Sanders, MD
Kenneth Foxx, MD

Introduction

Intraoperative neurophysiologic monitoring (IONM) consists of several modalities combined to provide continuous assessment of neurologic structures at risk of injury during spine surgery, including the spinal cord, nerve roots, and

2: Diagnostics in Spine Care

peripheral nerves. Iatrogenic injury to these structures can occur from contusion, mechanical compression, vascular compromise, or a combination of these factors. IONM can potentially identify evolving insults, which allows the surgical team to pursue corrective action and prevent permanent injury.[12] The most commonly used modalities in spine surgery include somatosensory-evoked potentials (SSEPs), motor-evoked potentials (MEPs), free-running or spontaneous electromyography (sEMG), and stimulus or triggered electromyography (tEMG). Multimodality IONM is often used in complex spine procedures, and the selection of the appropriate modality depends on the anatomic surgical location and associated risks.

The first widely used technique for intraoperative assessment of neurologic structures was the Stagnara wake-up test.[13-15] Because this clinically based test involves the patient's emergence from general anesthesia and neurologic examination in the operating room, it only provides an approximate assessment of motor tracts, but no information regarding the integrity of sensory tracts, specific nerve roots, or specific peripheral nerve structures. Because feedback is not continuous, it may not allow for timely corrective action. The Stagnara wake-up test also is associated with risks such as recalling intraoperative events, extubation, and difficulty performing the test in certain patient populations such as those with cognitive deficits.

SSEP monitoring was the first type of IONM reported and remains its cornerstone. MEPs were first described as high-voltage, single-pulse, transcranial stimulation of the cerebral cortex with induction of contralateral motor activity, but single-pulse stimulation was highly susceptible to the effects of anesthesia. The development of multipulse stimulation and refinement of anesthetic techniques led to the widespread use of MEPs in spine surgery. tEMG has become popular for assessing pedicle screw placement, and sEMG is used for the continual evaluation of nerve roots. The current aggregate of IONM modalities has become a critical tool in spine surgery.

Neuromonitoring Modalities
Somatosensory-Evoked Potentials
SSEPs are used to monitor the dorsal column-medial lemniscus pathway, which carries tactile discrimination, vibratory sensation, proprioception, and stereognosis from the periphery to the postcentral gyrus. The posterior spinal artery supplies the vascular territory of the dorsal columns. Information from receptors in skin, tendons, and muscles is relayed via heavily myelinated fibers from first-order neurons whose soma is in the dorsal root ganglion. These fibers travel in peripheral nerves, which combine in plexuses of their extremity, and are distributed to several nerve roots, leading to dermatomal overlap. Axons from first-order neurons travel in the ipsilateral fasciculi gracilis and cuneatus and are somatotopically organized with sacral fibers located medially in the fasciculus gracilis and cervical fibers located laterally in the fasciculus cuneatus. These axons synapse with second-order neurons in the nucleus gracilis and nucleus cuneatus, and decussate in the medulla to travel in the medial lemniscus to the ventral posterolateral nucleus of the thalamus. Information is then ultimately relayed to the primary somatosensory cortex in the postcentral gyrus and distributed in the somatotopically organized sensory cortical homunculus.[13-15]

Typical upper extremity SSEP stimulation sites are the median nerve (C6, C7, C8, and T1 nerve roots) and ulnar nerve (C8 and T1 nerve roots).[13-15] Use of the ulnar nerve in the upper extremity is preferred by some clinicians because its lower nerve root entry affords a more complete assessment of the cervical spinal cord. In the lower extremity, the posterior tibial nerve (L4, L5, S1, and S2 nerve roots) and peroneal nerve (L4, L5, and S1 nerve roots) are used. The electrical stimulation applied to a peripheral nerve creates an afferent signal that is ultimately measured by electrodes on the scalp. On scalp recordings, a negative potential is seen approximately 20 ms after upper extremity stimulation and is referred to as the N20 potential. A positive potential is seen approximately 37 ms after lower extremity stimulation and is termed the P37 potential.[15] Potentials are assessed for both amplitude and latency (**Figure 4**). Amplitude is measured in microvolts and defined as the distance from baseline to peak or from peak to trough. Latency is measured in milliseconds and refers to the period of time from peripheral stimulation to the recording of a potential.

A single cortical compound action potential cannot be detected because of background electroencephalography-related noise captured on scalp recordings. The signals generated by multiple stimulation sweeps must be averaged to obtain meaningful results.[15] With scalp recordings, the signal-to-noise ratio varies depending on the location of the electrodes relative to the corresponding cortical region. Recordings with higher signal-to-noise ratios require fewer sweeps to obtain and produce more reliable results. Scalp electrodes are generally placed using a standard montage, but fine adjustments are recommended to optimize the signal-to-noise ratio, which allows for more rapid and accurate signal change detection.[15,16]

Electrodes also are placed to obtain recordings along the dorsal column-medial lemniscus pathway at the level of the brainstem and select peripheral nerve structures such as the brachial plexus, popliteal fossa, and lumbar

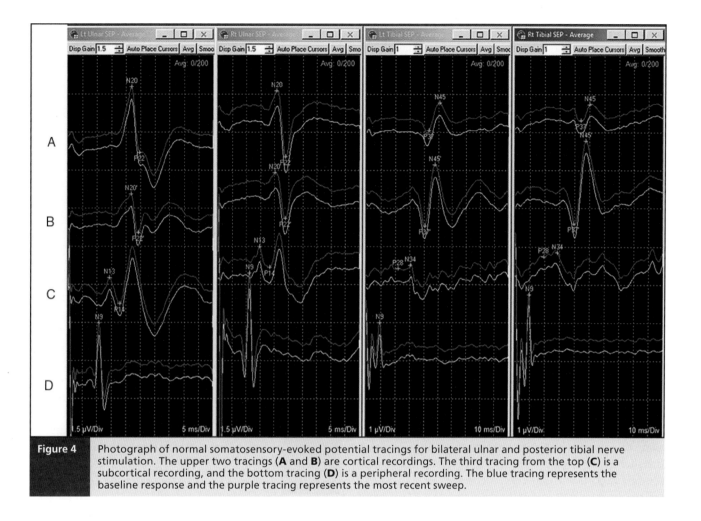

Figure 4 Photograph of normal somatosensory-evoked potential tracings for bilateral ulnar and posterior tibial nerve stimulation. The upper two tracings (**A** and **B**) are cortical recordings. The third tracing from the top (**C**) is a subcortical recording, and the bottom tracing (**D**) is a peripheral recording. The blue tracing represents the baseline response and the purple tracing represents the most recent sweep.

plexus.[14] The signal generated by the medulla and midbrain is referred to as the subcortical response. A P31/N34 (positive potential 31 ms and negative potential 34 ms after stimulation) complex subcortical response is seen with posterior tibial nerve stimulation, and a P14/N18 (positive potential 14 ms and negative potential 18 ms after stimulation) complex subcortical response is recorded with median nerve stimulation. Subcortical recordings are less susceptible to the effects of anesthesia than cortical recordings, and they are useful in determining whether a change in cortical monitoring is the result of anesthesia or neurologic insult. However, subcortical recordings are technically more difficult to obtain and are prone to muscle-related noise.[17] Recordings at peripheral nerve sites are used to determine whether the peripheral stimulus is adequate, and they are useful in the detection of peripheral nerve compression and limb ischemia.[14]

A 50% reduction in signal amplitude or a 10% increase in latency are considered important and require surgeon notification. Even in ideal situations, SSEPs can take up to 5 minutes to detect a significant change.[13,15,17] Amplitude changes are more sensitive to the onset of injury when compared with latency changes.[13] In a large multicenter survey, a 92% sensitivity and 98.9% specificity were reported for the detection of new postoperative deficits with SSEP monitoring.[18] SSEPs can be profoundly affected by hypotension, hypothermia, halogenated inhalational anesthetics, and intravenous sedation. The surgical and intraoperative monitoring teams must work together to recognize and minimize the effects of these confounders. Anesthetic effects are dose related and can be controlled with nitrous oxide supplementation.[17] SSEPs are used to assess spinal cord sensory tracts and are good basic indicators of spinal cord function. However, baseline SSEPs may be diminished in patients with severe myelopathy, spinal cord tumor, obesity, or peripheral neuropathy.[13] The role of SSEPs in the assessment of the motor tracts is limited. SSEPs are more sensitive to motor changes secondary to mechanical injury than changes resulting from vascular insult such as anterior spinal artery occlusion.[17] The corticospinal tracts and the anterior horn cells are perfused by the anterior spinal artery. During corrective spinal

2: Diagnostics in Spine Care

surgery, small radiomedullary arteries may be stretched or compressed, causing ischemia or infarction. In addition, SSEPs cannot reliably monitor the integrity of individual nerve roots.[14]

Motor-Evoked Potentials

MEPs monitor the corticospinal tract, which originates in the neurons of the primary motor cortex of the precentral gyrus. The upper motor neuron axons converge in the internal capsule and continue to the medulla before reaching the spinal canal. Seventy-five percent to 90% of the axons cross in the pyramidal decussation and continue in the contralateral lateral corticospinal tract. The ventral corticospinal tract contains the remaining ipsilateral axons, which cross over at their dedicated spinal level. A small number of upper motor neurons synapse directly with alpha motor neurons in the anterior gray matter, and the remainder act through intermediate neurons. Each alpha motor neuron innervates a single motor unit.[15]

MEPs are produced by transcranial anodal stimulation with subdermal scalp electrodes placed over the primary motor cortex.[14,15] A low-output impedance electrical stimulator generates a high-volume, short-duration pulse train via the subdermal electrodes.[13] With application of a short train of 5 to 7 electrical pulses, the alpha motor neurons receive enough stimulation to reach their firing thresholds. MEPs can be recorded either as D-waves over the spinal cord with epidural electrodes or as CMAPs via recording needles placed in the muscles of interest.[19]

D-waves do not require activation of lower motor neurons, which renders the technique more robust and less variable, with proven utility in intramedullary spinal cord tumor resection. Complete loss of MEPs with at least 50% preservation of D-wave amplitude is usually associated with transient motor deficit, whereas a complete loss of D-wave amplitude is predictive of permanent paralysis.[14] However, the D-wave recording has been shown to have a high rate of false-positive results during scoliosis surgery, and it is unable to detect a unilateral spinal cord injury. The recording electrode must be placed in the epidural space, either percutaneously or through a laminotomy distal to the surgical level. D-wave recordings can be made only at spinal levels where the corticospinal tract is large enough to generate a recordable signal, which restricts its use to above the T11 level.[15]

CMAP recordings are used much more frequently than D-wave recordings because of their relative ease of use, ability for use distal to T11, and ability to detect unilateral injury. CMAPs are more easily monitored from more distal muscles because of their richer corticospinal tract innervation compared with proximal muscles. Commonly used muscles include the abductor pollicis

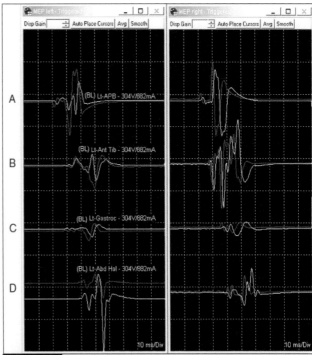

Figure 5 Photograph of transcranial motor-evoked potential tracings recorded from the following bilateral muscles: abductor pollicis brevis (**A**), tibialis anterior (**B**), gastrocnemius (**C**), and abductor hallucis brevis (**D**). The blue tracing represents the baseline recording and the purple tracing represents the most recent response. A possible change in the left abductor hallucis brevis is indicated.

brevis, abductor hallucis brevis, gastrocnemius, and tibialis anterior (**Figure 5**), although the biceps, deltoid, and quadriceps also can be monitored.[19]

Prior to initiation of a surgical procedure, baseline MEP threshold voltages and CMAP baseline amplitudes are obtained for each side of the body. The starting stimulus voltage is typically 100V and is increased in 50V increments until a CMAP response can be recorded in each of the monitored muscles. The stimulation voltage required to produce a CMAP response in each of the monitored muscles is termed the threshold voltage. CMAPs are polyphasic waveforms that are variable in morphology.[15] CMAP amplitude is typically calculated as the area under the curve of the recorded potential. Latency time is usually 20 ms in the hand and 45 ms in the foot, although these values are dependent on a variety of factors, including body temperature, patient height, and preexisting neuromuscular pathology.[13,14]

As a result of the variability of MEP responses, four methods of interpretation have been developed. (1) The all-or-nothing criterion requires a complete loss of the baseline MEP signal. It is indicative of a clinically important event and warrants an immediate corrective action per recommendations of the American Society of Neuromonitoring (ASNM).[15,20] This method of interpretation may not be appropriate for degenerative and spine deformity surgery in which a temporary postoperative motor deficit is unacceptable. It may be more suitable for intradural surgery. (2) The amplitude criterion requires an 80% decrease in signal amplitude in at least one of the six recording sites for a change to be considered clinically important.[15] This technique has shown 100% sensitivity and 91% specificity for the detection of a postoperative motor deficit.[14] (3) The threshold criterion involves analysis of increases in the stimulation threshold required to maintain CMAP responses.[14] If an increase of greater than 100V is required for at least 1 hour to maintain CMAP responses, a neurologic insult is presumed to have occurred.[14] The amplitude and threshold criteria are considered moderate criteria by the ASNM because of their tendency to generate false-positive results.[15,20] (4) The morphology criterion focuses on changes in the pattern and duration of MEP waveforms. A transition from a polyphasic to a biphasic waveform is indicative of a motor deficit. A complete loss of waveform is associated with a higher risk of permanent injury. Morphologic changes also can occur because of anesthetic agents, hypothermia, hypotension, patient positioning, or technical issues.[14] The ASNM has not made recommendations for using this criterion in spine surgery.[15,20]

Although MEPs can effectively monitor the corticospinal tracts, they are subject to several limitations and confounding factors. As with SSEPs, it may be impossible to obtain MEP signals in patients with preoperative neurologic deficits. CMAPs are dependent on transsynaptic activation of spinal motor neurons, and paralytic agents need to be avoided entirely or maintained at a subparalytic level.[19] Because halogenated agents can depress synaptic transmission and spinal motor neuron function, total intravenous anesthesia is strongly preferred.[19] CMAP interpretation also may be confounded by substantial variability in waveform amplitude and morphology secondary to activation of a small number of different low-threshold spinal motor neurons by each descending corticospinal volley.[19] MEP monitoring may be difficult in some children younger than 6 years because of incomplete electrophysiologic maturation of the corticospinal tract, which finalizes by age 13 years. However, it often can be used effectively in young children. Because MEPs only monitor 4% to 5% of the corticospinal tract neuron pool, a complex motor deficit may rarely occur without any monitoring abnormalities.[21] In addition, as a result of radicular overlap and limited

sampling, a single nerve root injury will frequently be missed with MEP monitoring.[17]

Although MEP monitoring is generally considered quite safe, the possibility of injury exists.[17] Thermal injuries, which are estimated to occur in 0.01% of cases, can result from improper technique. Bite injuries, which occur in approximately 0.2% of cases, are the result of contraction of the mastication muscles, which is likely mediated by corticobulbar pathway activation, trigeminal nerve stimulation, or direct muscle stimulation. A soft bite-block is a standard precaution. Seizures from transcranial stimulation are rare, with an estimated incidence of 0.03%, and are usually self-limited. Cardiac arrhythmia also is possible, but its occurrence has been rarely reported. The ASNM guidelines do not include any absolute contraindications to MEP monitoring, but epilepsy, cortical lesions, skull defects, intracranial vascular clips, shunts, cranial electrodes, pacemakers, and other implanted bioelectric devices are listed as relative contraindications. However, the ASNM guidelines also note that no proof exists that any of these conditions increase complication rates, and many patients with one or more of these conditions have undergone uneventful MEP monitoring.[20]

Electromyography
Neither SSEP nor MEP monitoring provide reliable monitoring of single nerve root function during spine surgery. Electromyographic techniques can detect excessive nerve root retraction, mechanical injury, thermal injury, or medial cortical breach of a pedicle screw.

Segmental nerve root monitoring can be used to assess the function of motor unit axons via sEMG and tEMG. CMAPs are recorded from needle electrodes placed in muscles innervated by the cervical, thoracic, lumbar, and sacral nerve roots. The typically monitored muscles innervated by cervical nerve roots include the following: (1) trapezius and sternocleidomastoid (C2, C3, C4), (2) biceps and deltoid (C5, C6), (3) flexor carpi radialis (C6, C7), and (4) abductor pollicis brevis and abductor digiti minimi (C8, T1). Commonly used muscles innervated by thoracic nerve roots include the following: (1) upper rectus abdominis (T5, T6), (2) middle rectus abdominis (T7, T8), (3) lower rectus abdominis (T9, T10, T11), and (4) interior rectus abdominis (T12). Typically monitored muscles innervated by lumbar and sacral nerve roots include the following: (1) vastus medialis (L2, L3, L4), (2) tibialis anterior (L4, L5, S1), (3) peroneus longus (L5, S1), (4) gastrocnemius (S1, S2), and (5) the external anal sphincter (S2, S3, S4).[22]

Spontaneous Electromyography
Surgical manipulation such as traction or compression of a nerve root produces neurotonic discharges, which

2: Diagnostics in Spine Care

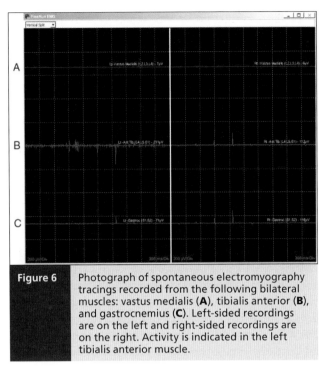

Figure 6 Photograph of spontaneous electromyography tracings recorded from the following bilateral muscles: vastus medialis (**A**), tibialis anterior (**B**), and gastrocnemius (**C**). Left-sided recordings are on the left and right-sided recordings are on the right. Activity is indicated in the left tibialis anterior muscle.

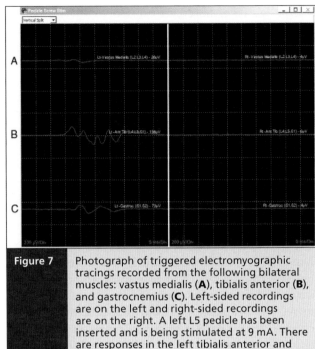

Figure 7 Photograph of triggered electromyographic tracings recorded from the following bilateral muscles: vastus medialis (**A**), tibialis anterior (**B**), and gastrocnemius (**C**). Left-sided recordings are on the left and right-sided recordings are on the right. A left L5 pedicle has been inserted and is being stimulated at 9 mA. There are responses in the left tibialis anterior and gastrocnemius.

results in the production of CMAPs that can be recorded from the muscles innervated by the nerve root. Because there is a certain degree of redundancy in muscle innervation, monitoring one muscle group per nerve root is usually considered adequate.[14,23] The only exception is the C5 nerve root, which is at high risk of injury during cervical procedures, and concurrent monitoring of the deltoid and biceps is recommended. sEMG is continuously recorded and may be sent to a speaker to provide auditory feedback. Paralytic agents should not be used, and train-of-four testing should indicate that at least three of four twitches are present.[14]

A normal resting nerve root in the anesthetized patient does not significantly activate the muscles that it innervates, which translates to a flat line and silence on sEMG recordings.[23] Abnormal recordings can be described as spikes, bursts, or trains. Spikes and bursts are the result of nerve root irritation from traction, compression, or thermal injury and can inform the surgeon of proximity to a nerve root[14] (**Figure 6**). With an increasing degree of trauma to the nerve, the amplitude and frequency of these discharges increases and trains of activity are observed. Trains of activity represent extensive nerve fiber recruitment and indicate impending nerve injury with sustained manipulation.[14]

sEMG provides continuous feedback throughout the surgical procedure and has a high sensitivity for the detection of nerve root injury. A review of 213 patients who underwent thoracolumbar spine surgery with sEMG

recordings found a 100% sensitivity but only a 23.7% specificity for the detection of new postoperative neurologic deficits.[24] sEMG recordings are sensitive to temperature changes such as irrigation with cold water or the use of cautery devices. Electrocardiography leads and use of a high-speed drill can produce artifact. The presence of preoperative neurologic deficits or underlying neuromuscular disorders may make sEMG recordings unreliable.[14]

Triggered Electromyography

A major risk of pedicle screw placement is a medial or an inferior breach resulting in injury to the dura, nerve roots, or spinal cord.[14,15] The tEMG technique relies on the principle that the electrical resistance of bone is higher than that of surrounding tissues. With accurate placement of the screw, the surrounding cortical bone acts as an insulator to electrical conduction. If a medial breach occurs, a low resistance pathway is formed between the screw and the adjacent tissues, allowing for nerve root stimulation and generation of a CMAP in the muscles innervated by that nerve root.[23]

tEMG is performed by directly stimulating a pedicle screw with monopolar, cathodal, and constant current via an insulated ball-tip probe, with an anodal reference needle electrode placed in the paraspinal muscle. The current is gradually increased until CMAPs are elicited. It is important to place the stimulation probe directly on top of the screw, not on the tulip, to optimize the current flow from the screw to the reference electrode.[14] A close correlation exists between the intensity of stimulation required to elicit CMAPs and the risk of neurologic injury.[23] Stimulation thresholds differ among cervical, thoracic, and lumbar pedicles because of the variations in thickness and shape of the bone.[14] A stimulation threshold more than 15 mA indicates safe placement of the pedicle screw regardless of the level. Lumbar and thoracic pedicle screws thresholds of less than 7 mA and 6 mA, respectively, are suggestive of a medial wall breach.[14,25-27] Although tEMG is rarely used in posterior cervical fusion surgery, it has been reported that a stimulation threshold of less than 10 mA warrants further investigation.[28] Although stimulation threshold values can be predictive of screw misplacement, their false-positive rate is quite high, with more than 75% of the threshold values below 6 mA representing appropriately placed screws.[23,26] A 6 mA threshold value in conjunction with a 60% to 65% decrease from the average of the threshold values obtained from all other pedicle screws may be a more reliable warning sign of a medial pedicle breach.[26] An example of tEMG tracing is shown in **Figure 7**.

tEMG also is prone to false-negative findings resulting from anesthesia, technical difficulties, or preexisting nerve injury. Paralytic agents should be avoided, and four of four twitches should be present on train-of-four testing.[14] Current shunting can occur because of the presence of soft tissues, blood, or other fluid around the screw head.[14,15] The use of pedicle screws coated with hydroxyapatite, which reduces the conductive capacity of the screws, may produce false-negative results.[14] Chronically irritated nerve roots typically have higher direct triggering thresholds ranging from 6 mA to more than 10 mA, compared with 2 mA in a normal nerve root.[15] Performing a direct stimulation test is recommended to establish a baseline stimulation threshold when a nerve root is known to be chronically irritated.[14]

Multimodal Techniques and Guidelines

IONM should be tailored to the location and type of surgical procedure because each modality has limitations, and none can sufficiently monitor all neural structures at risk of injury.[14] Several groups have published position statements on IONM use.[29-34] A joint position statement by the American Association of Neurological Surgeons and the Congress of Neurological Surgeons Joint Section on Disorders of the Spine and Peripheral Nerves states that IONM may assist in diagnosing neurologic injury, but notes that "there currently exists no evidence such monitoring either reduces the incidence of neurological injury or mitigates the severity of it."[33] A recommendation is made that IONM "should be performed in procedures

when the operating surgeon feels that the diagnostic information is of value, such as deformity correction, spinal instability, spinal cord compression, intradural spinal cord lesions, and when in proximity to peripheral nerves or roots."[33] The statement also makes specific recommendations regarding the use of sEMG and tEMG.

Cervical and Thoracic Spine Surgery

Preservation of spinal cord integrity is of prime importance during cervical and thoracic spine surgery. Combined SSEP and MEP monitoring provides an excellent assessment of the entire spinal cord, and their combined use increases the sensitivity and specificity of detecting an injury. Some authors recommend the use of sEMG during surgical procedures performed in proximity to the C5 nerve root, which is at particular risk of injury. The reliability and use of electrophysiologic monitoring during surgery for cervical myelopathy or radiculopathy is not clear.[30] Because the thoracic cord is at risk of ischemia during anterior procedures involving segmental artery ligation, some authors recommend temporary occlusion of segmental arteries under MEPs before ligation to identify critical vessels and avoid spinal cord infarction.[13]

Lumbosacral Spine Surgery

In the lumbosacral spine, the focus of IONM shifts from the spinal cord to the nerve roots. The use of SSEPs in combination with sEMG, as the optimal multimodal technique for continuously monitoring nerve root integrity, has been recommended by some authors.[14] tEMG can be used during pedicle screw placement as a method for detecting medial pedicle screw breach, although this technique has a high false-positive rate.[23,26]

Minimally Invasive Spine Surgery

The limited exposure and confined work space afforded by minimally invasive surgery can place neurologic structures at risk. These conditions make IONM particularly attractive, and the modalities used depend on the location of the procedure, with sEMG and tEMG potentially helpful for monitoring at-risk nerve roots or peripheral nerves.

Spine Deformity Surgery

Neurologic impairment is a rare but potentially devastating complication of modern surgery for spine deformity. The probability of hardware misdirection is probably higher in surgery to correct a deformity because of the abnormal curvature and rotation of the vertebrae, and the risk of spinal cord injury is likely higher because the spinal cord tends to be positioned along the medial wall of the concave pedicles. However, the greatest risk of spinal cord injury occurs during distraction of the spine.

2: Diagnostics in Spine Care

Checklist for the Response to Intraoperative Neuromonitoring Changes in Patients with a Stable Spine

GAIN CONTROL OF ROOM	ANESTHETIC/SYSTEMIC	TECHNICAL/NEUROPHYSIOLOGIC	SURGICAL
❑ Intraoperative pause: stop case and announce to the room	❑ Optimize mean arterial pressure (MAP)	❑ Discuss status of anesthetic agents	❑ Discuss events and actions just prior to signal loss and consider reversing actions:
❑ Eliminate extraneous stimuli (e.g. music, conversations, etc.)	❑ Optimize hematocrit	❑ Check extent of neuromuscular blockade and degree of paralysis	❑ Remove traction (if applicable)
❑ Summon ATTENDING anesthesiologist, SENIOR neurologist or neurophysiologist, and EXPERIENCED nurse	❑ Optimize blood pH and pCO_2	❑ Check electrodes and connections	❑ Decrease/remove distraction or other corrective forces
		❑ Determine pattern and timing of signal changes	❑ Remove rods
	❑ Seek normothermia		❑ Remove screws and probe for breach
❑ Anticipate need for intraoperative and/or perioperative imaging if not readily available	❑ Discuss POTENTIAL need for wake-up test with ATTENDING anesthesiologist	❑ Check neck and limb positioning; check limb position on table especially if unilateral loss	❑ Evaluate for spinal cord compression, examine osteotomy and laminotomy sites

ONGOING CONSIDERATIONS
❑ REVISIT anesthetic/systemic considerations and confirm that they are optimized
❑ Wake-up test
❑ Consultation with a colleague
❑ Continue surgical procedure versus staging procedure
❑ IV steroid protocol: Methylprednisolone 30 mg/kg in first hr, then 5.4 mg/kg/hr for next 23 hrs

❑ Intraoperative and/or perioperative imaging (e.g. O-arm, fluoroscopy, x-ray) to evaluate implant placement

Date of Revision: 2/26/2014

Figure 8 Example of a checklist for use in spinal deformity surgery for patients with a stable spine. This checklist would not be applicable for vertebral column resections or a patient with an unstable spine. (Reproduced with permission from Vitale MG, Skaggs DL, Pace GI, et al: Best practices in intraoperative neuromonitoring in spine deformity surgery: Development of an intraoperative checklist to optimize response. *Spine Deform* 2014;2[5]:333-339.)

In an information statement, the Scoliosis Research Society (SRS) states that IONM "can assist in the early detection of complications and possibly prevent postoperative morbidity."[34] The SRS also notes that the use of IONM in deformity surgery is not investigational and is used routinely by most SRS members. The SRS considers IONM the "preferred method for the early detection of an evolving or impending spinal cord deficit during surgical manipulation." The SRS also notes that the wake-up test is a useful adjunct to IONM.[34]

The value of using surgical checklists, particularly during high-stress situations such as IONM alerts, has been demonstrated. Some institutions also incorporate discussion of the specific IONM modalities to be used, anesthetic issues, and a review of alarm criteria in the initial surgical timeout.[23] A consensus clinical practice guideline established an intraoperative checklist to optimize responses to IONM changes in deformity surgery[29] (**Figure 8**). A systematic process for the team to follow is divided into the following five main categories: (1) gain control of the room, (2) anesthetic/systemic, (3) technical/neurophysiologic, (4) surgical, and (5) ongoing considerations (**Table 3**).

Summary

Electrodiagnostic testing is valuable in identifying or excluding peripheral nerve disorders that may mimic radicular symptoms. In addition to localizing a nerve disorder, electrodiagnostic testing can provide information regarding the severity, duration, and prognosis for the spinal disorder.

Table 3

Consensus-based Best Practice Guidelines for IONM Practices in the United States

Intraoperative neuromonitoring is best performed with a team approach. The surgeon, anesthesiologist, and qualified neuromonitoring personnel all should be involved in the identification and communication of neuromonitoring changes.

SSEPs should be used in all spine deformity cases.

TcMEPs and/or descending neurogenic-evoked potentials should be used in all spine deformity cases.

A 50% degradation in SSEP signal amplitude from baseline and/or a sustained decrease in TcMEP signal amplitude and/or a decrease in descending neurogenic-evoked potential signal of 60% constitute "significant warning criteria" in spine deformity surgery.

A wake-up test should always be considered in spine deformity cases with persistent signal degradation or in patients who cannot be monitored.

IONM = intraoperative neurophysiologic monitoring, SSEPs = somatosensory-evoked potentials, TcMEP = transcranial motor-evoked potential.

Reproduced with permission from Vitale MG, Skaggs DL, Pace GI, et al: Best practices in intraoperative neuromonitoring in spine deformity surgery: Development of an intraoperative checklist to optimize response. *Spine Deform* 2014;2[5]:333-339.

The most commonly used IONM modalities are SSEPs, MEPs, sEMG, and tEMG. The dorsal column-medial lemniscus pathway, which carries tactile discrimination, vibratory sensation, proprioception, and stereognosis from the periphery to the postcentral gyrus are monitored with SSEPs. MEPs are used to monitor the corticospinal tract, which originates in the upper motor neurons of the primary cortex and extends to their connections with alpha motor neurons. sEMG continuously monitors the integrity of individual nerve roots. tEMG is used to detect a medial breach of pedicle screws. Multimodality IONM is often used in complex spinal procedures, and appropriate selection depends on the anatomic location and associated risks. Guidelines and consensus statements have been published regarding use of IONM.

Key Study Points

- Electrodiagnostic testing is valuable in identifying or excluding peripheral nerve disorders that may mimic radicular symptoms.
- Electrodiagnostic testing has moderate sensitivity but high specificity for radiculopathy.
- SSEPs and MEPs primarily monitor the integrity of the spinal cord.
- sEMG is used to continuously monitor the integrity of individual nerve roots.
- tEMG is used to detect medial breach of pedicle screws.

Acknowledgment

Dr. Sanders and Dr. Foxx would like to acknowledge Sarah Gannon, R. EEG/EP T./CNIM for her help obtaining and preparing some of the figures used in this chapter.

Annotated References

1. Dillingham TR: Evaluating the patient with suspected radiculopathy. *PM R* 2013;5(5suppl):S41-S49.

   An overview of the electrodiagnostic evaluation of patients with suspected radiculopathy is presented.

2. Dillingham TR, Pezzin LE, Lauder TD: Cervical paraspinal muscle abnormalities and symptom duration: A multivariate analysis. *Muscle Nerve* 1998;21(5):640-642.

3. Pezzin LE, Dillingham TR, Lauder TD, et al: Cervical radiculopathies: Relationship between symptom duration and spontaneous EMG activity. *Muscle Nerve* 1999;22(10):1412-1418.

4. Dillingham TR, Pezzin LE, Lauder TD, et al: Symptom duration and spontaneous activity in lumbosacral radiculopathy. *Am J Phys Med Rehabil* 2000;79(2):124-132.

5. Buschbacher RM, Prahlow ND: *Manual of Nerve Conduction Studies*, ed 2. New York, NY, Demos Medical, 2006.

6. Tong HC: Specificity of needle electromyography for lumbar radiculopathy in 55- to 79-yr-old subjects with low back pain and sciatica without stenosis. *Am J Phys Med Rehabil* 2011;90(3):233-238, quiz 239-242.

   An assessment of the specificity of needle EMG for lumbar radiculopathy in patients with low back pain and sciatica without stenosis is presented.

2: Diagnostics in Spine Care

7. Wilbourn AJ, Aminoff MJ; American Association of Electrodiagnostic Medicine: AAEM minimonograph 32: The electrodiagnostic examination in patients with radiculopathies. *Muscle Nerve* 1998;21(12):1612-1631.

8. Dillingham TR, Lauder TD, Andary M, et al: Identifying lumbosacral radiculopathies: An optimal electromyographic screen. *Am J Phys Med Rehabil* 2000;79(6):496-503.

9. Dillingham TR, Lauder TD, Andary M, et al: Identification of cervical radiculopathies: Optimizing the electromyographic screen. *Am J Phys Med Rehabil* 2001;80(2):84-91.

10. Cartwright MS, Walker FO: Neuromuscular ultrasound in common entrapment neuropathies. *Muscle Nerve* 2013;48(5):696-704.

    This study reviews common ultrasound findings in entrapment neuropathies and focuses on the use of ultrasonography in four common entrapment neuropathies: carpal tunnel syndrome, ulnar neuropathy at the elbow and wrist, and fibular neuropathy at the knee.

11. Kim E, Yoon JS, Kang HJ: Ultrasonographic cross-sectional area of spinal nerve roots in cervical radiculopathy: A pilot study. *Am J Phys Med Rehabil* 2015;94(2):159-164.

    The use of high-resolution ultrasonography in patients with cervical radiculopathy is explored. The cross-sectional areas of the nerve roots between the affected and unaffected sides are compared.

12. Samdani AF, Belin EJ, Bennett JT, et al: Major perioperative complications after spine surgery in patients with cerebral palsy: Assessment of risk factors. *Eur Spine J* 2016;25(3):795-800.

    This prospective case-control study of patients undergoing spine surgery for idiopathic scoliosis reported that identification and correction of offending factors after an intraoperative alert resulted in normal neurologic function equivalent to that of patients who had no alerts during surgery. These results stress the importance of acting properly when IONM alerts occur. Level of evidence: II.

13. Devlin VJ, Schwartz DM: Intraoperative neurophysiologic monitoring during spinal surgery. *J Am Acad Orthop Surg* 2007;15(9):549-560.

14. Gonzalez AA, Jeyanandarajan D, Hansen C, Zada G, Hsieh PC: Intraoperative neurophysiological monitoring during spine surgery: A review. *Neurosurg Focus* 2009;27(4):E6.

15. Rabai F, Sessions R, Seubert CN: Neurophysiological monitoring and spinal cord integrity. *Best Pract Res Clin Anaesthesiol* 2016;30(1):53-68.

    This is a comprehensive review article of intraoperative neurophysiologic monitoring. Level of evidence: V.

16. MacDonald DB, Al Zayed Z, Stigsby B: Tibial somatosensory evoked potential intraoperative monitoring: Recommendations based on signal to noise ratio analysis of popliteal fossa, optimized P37, standard P37, and P31 potentials. *Clin Neurophysiol* 2005;116(8):1858-1869.

17. Malhotra NR, Shaffrey CI: Intraoperative electrophysiological monitoring in spine surgery. *Spine (Phila Pa 1976)* 2010;35(25):2167-2179.

18. Nuwer MR, Dawson EG, Carlson LG, Kanim LE, Sherman JE: Somatosensory evoked potential spinal cord monitoring reduces neurologic deficits after scoliosis surgery: Results of a large multicenter survey. *Electroencephalogr Clin Neurophysiol* 1995;96(1):6-11.

19. Mendiratta A, Emerson RG: Neurophysiologic intraoperative monitoring of scoliosis surgery. *J Clin Neurophysiol* 2009;26(2):62-69.

20. Macdonald DB, Skinner S, Shils J, Yingling C; American Society of Neurophysiological Monitoring: Intraoperative motor evoked potential monitoring: A position statement by the American Society of Neurophysiological Monitoring. *Clin Neurophysiol* 2013;124(12):2291-2316.

    The authors present a comprehensive review of MEP monitoring technique and a position statement of the American Society of Neurophysiological Monitoring. Level of evidence: V.

21. Sloan TB, Janik D, Jameson L: Multimodality monitoring of the central nervous system using motor-evoked potentials. *Curr Opin Anaesthesiol* 2008;21(5):560-564.

22. Leppanen RE: Intraoperative monitoring of segmental spinal nerve root function with free-run and electrically-triggered electromyography and spinal cord function with reflexes and F-responses. A position statement by the American Society of Neurophysiological Monitoring. *J Clin Monit Comput* 2005;19(6):437-461.

23. Lall RR, Lall RR, Hauptman JS, et al: Intraoperative neurophysiological monitoring in spine surgery: Indications, efficacy, and role of the preoperative checklist. *Neurosurg Focus* 2012;33(5):E10.

    This study documents the inclusion of IONM in the surgical pause and its ability to make the surgical team aware of issues that may need to be addressed.

24. Gunnarsson T, Krassioukov AV, Sarjeant R, Fehlings MG: Real-time continuous intraoperative electromyographic and somatosensory evoked potential recordings in spinal surgery: Correlation of clinical and electrophysiologic findings in a prospective, consecutive series of 213 cases. *Spine (Phila Pa 1976)* 2004;29(6):677-684.

25. Calancie B, Madsen P, Lebwohl N: Stimulus-evoked EMG monitoring during transpedicular lumbosacral spine instrumentation: Initial clinical results. *Spine (Phila Pa 1976)* 1994;19(24):2780-2786.

26. Raynor BL, Lenke LG, Kim Y, et al: Can triggered electromyograph thresholds predict safe thoracic pedicle screw placement? *Spine (Phila Pa 1976)* 2002;27(18):2030-2035.

27. Glassman SD, Dimar JR, Puno RM, Johnson JR, Shields CB, Linden RD: A prospective analysis of intraoperative electromyographic monitoring of pedicle screw placement with computed tomographic scan confirmation. *Spine (Phila Pa 1976)* 1995;20(12):1375-1379.

28. Djurasovic M, Dimar JR II, Glassman SD, Edmonds HL, Carreon LY: A prospective analysis of intraoperative electromyographic monitoring of posterior cervical screw fixation. *J Spinal Disord Tech* 2005;18(6):515-518.

29. Vitale MG, Skaggs DL, Pace GI, et al: Best practices in intraoperative neuromonitoring in spine deformity surgery: Development of an intraoperative checklist to optimize response. *Spine Deform* 2014;2(5):333-339.

    This study used the Delphi method to establish best practices concerning IONM in patients with stable spines undergoing deformity correction surgery. A checklist was developed to assist surgical and IONM team members during stressful situations.

30. Resnick DK, Anderson PA, Kaiser MG, et al; Joint Section on Disorders of the Spine and Peripheral Nerves of the American Association of Neurological Surgeons and Congress of Neurological Surgeons: Electrophysiological monitoring during surgery for cervical degenerative myelopathy and radiculopathy. *J Neurosurg Spine* 2009;11(2):245-252.

31. Resnick DK, Choudhri TF, Dailey AT, et al; American Association of Neurological Surgeons/Congress of Neurological Surgeons: Guidelines for the performance of fusion procedures for degenerative disease of the lumbar spine: Part 15. Electrophysiological monitoring and lumbar fusion. *J Neurosurg Spine* 2005;2(6):725-732.

32. Sharan A, Groff MW, Dailey AT, et al: Guideline update for the performance of fusion procedures for degenerative disease of the lumbar spine: Part 15. Electrophysiological monitoring and lumbar fusion. *J Neurosurg Spine* 2014;21(1):102-105.

    This guideline, based on expert opinion, specifically focuses on the use of IONM during surgery for lumbar degenerative disease.

33. AANS/CNS: Updated Position Statement: Intraoperative Electrophysiological Monitoring, 2014. Available at: http://www.spinesection.org/files/pdfs/IOM Position Statement 04.24.2014.pdf. Accessed March 30, 2017.

    This position statement identifies specific issues found in the IONM literature and quotes the original articles. It makes no attempt to present either a literature consolidation or systematic review.

34. Scoliosis Research Society: Neuromonitoring Information Statement. SRS Information Statement, 2009. Available at: http://www.srs.org/about-srs/quality-and-safety/position-statements/neuromonitoring-information-statement. Accessed March 30, 2017.

2: Diagnostics in Spine Care

Chapter 8

Diagnostic Procedures in Spine Care

D. Scott Kreiner, MD   Timothy Sanford, MD

Abstract

Proper diagnosis regarding the etiology of low back pain is important to guide appropriate management, improve outcomes, optimize resources, and reduce medical costs. Several diagnostic procedures are associated with each source of low back pain. These include diskography for intervertebral disk pain, medial branch blocks for zygapophyseal joint–mediated pain, intra-articular sacroiliac joint blocks for sacroiliac joint pain, and selective nerve root blocks for radiculopathy and/or radicular pain.

Keywords: diagnostic; diskography; medial branch blocks; sacroiliac joint; selective nerve root blocks, SI joint

Introduction

Back pain and its subsequent management is often generalized. To properly manage back pain, accurate assessment and diagnosis are crucial. Accurate diagnosis of back pain will help guide management, improve outcomes, optimize resources, and reduce medical costs. Several structures, including muscles, tendons, ligaments, bones, nerves, joints (zygapophyseal and sacroiliac), and intervertebral disks, can cause back pain. To define a structural basis for the pain, back pain is commonly categorized as axial or radicular. Chronic axial pain most commonly occurs in three main structures, which forms a basis for categorical division: disk-mediated, zygapophyseal joint (Z joint)–mediated, and sacroiliac (SI) joint–mediated pain. Several

Dr. Kreiner or an immediate family member serves as a board member, owner, officer, or committee member of the North American Spine Society. Neither Dr. Sanford nor any immediate family member has received anything of value from or has stock or stock options held in a commercial company or institution related directly or indirectly to the subject of this chapter.

diagnostic procedures can be used to help determine the etiology of low back pain.

Axial Back Pain

Pain located in the intervertebral disk, Z joint, and SI joint comprises 90% of chronic axial back pain. Pain resulting from vertebral fractures, pelvic fractures, Baastrup syndrome, and fusion hardware accounts for the remaining 10%. In a study of 170 patients, intervertebral disk–mediated pain accounted for 41.8% of low back pain, Z joint–mediated pain for 30.6% of low back pain, and SI joint–mediated pain for 18.2% of low back pain[1] (**Table 1**).

Discogenic Back Pain

Disk-mediated pain is the most common etiology of back pain.[1] Imaging can depict disk abnormalities at multiple levels, and determining the concordant pain level can be challenging. One study reported that MRI findings of a disk protrusion with a high-intensity zone (HIZ) correlated with pain provocation; however, a bulging disk with an HIZ, disk degeneration without HIZ, and disk protrusion without HIZ did not correlate with pain provocation.[2] Therefore, it is difficult to determine whether the disk is the pain generator and at which level, especially if MRI findings demonstrate multilevel disk abnormalities. Other studies have demonstrated abnormal disk findings in asymptomatic patients,[3,4] including disk degeneration, herniation, or bulge seen on MRI. One study found that 61% of study subjects (mean age, 42 years) had disk abnormalities.[4]

An algorithmic approach should be followed in the diagnostic workup of axial low back pain. In addition to a detailed history, examination, and imaging studies, initial diagnostic procedures should include medial branch blocks for Z joint–mediated pain and SI joint diagnostic injections followed by diskography, a diagnostic procedure used to help determine whether the intervertebral disk is the pain generator of axial low back pain. One of the main reasons that initial diagnostic procedures should include the Z joint and SI joint is that good evidence

Table 1

Etiology and Prevalence of Low Back Pain

Etiology	Prevalence (170 Patients)	Mean Age (±SD)
Intervertebral disk	41.8%	43.7 (10.3)
Lumbar zygapophyseal joint	30.6%	59.6 (13.1)
Sacroiliac joint	18.2%	61.4 (17.7)
Other (fracture, hardware, and others)	9.4%	NA

NA = not available.
Data from Depalma MJ, Ketchum JM, Saullo T: What is the source of chronic low back pain and does age play a role? *Pain Med* 2011;12(2):224-233.

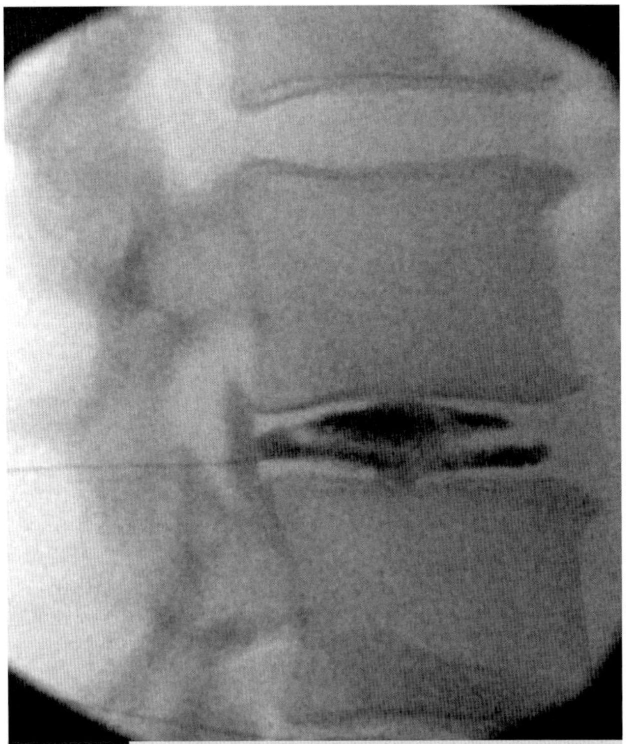

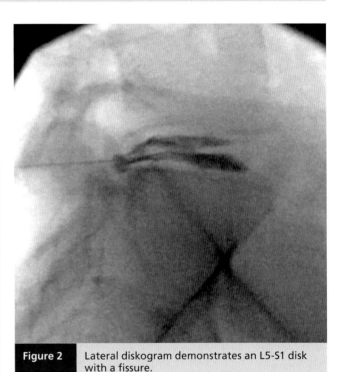

Figure 1 Lateral diskogram demonstrates an L3-L4 disk with a tear.

Figure 2 Lateral diskogram demonstrates an L5-S1 disk with a fissure.

supports these procedures in the diagnosis of their respective pain generator, and currently, the evidence to support diskography is controversial.

Diskography has been a topic of debate because the literature both supports and questions its diagnostic and prognostic value, as well as its risk profile. In addition, treatments of discogenic pain such as intradiscal electrothermal therapy, lumbar disk arthroplasty, and spinal fusion have become less common, questioning the need to perform diskography. Diskography comprises two separate yet complementary procedures: provocation lumbar diskography (PLD) and analgesic diskography.

Provocation Lumbar Diskography

PLD is used to determine the presence of an annular fissure and to confirm the disk as a source of pain if the injection of contrast material into the disk reproduces the patient's pain. Image guidance (fluoroscopy or CT) is used to direct a needle into the disk, and contrast material is injected to pressurize the disk. In addition, the contrast media can confirm the presence of a fissure (**Figures 1, 2, and 3**), which also can be confirmed using CT after diskography. Optimal diagnostic results require adherence to strict criteria. The 2013 International Spine Intervention Society's (ISIS) guidelines for a definitively positive diskogram result include concordant pain of 6 or greater on a scale of 1 to 10, pain reproduced with pressure less than 50 psi greater than opening pressure, and stimulation of two adjacent disks that reproduces no pain.[5] It is important that strict diagnostic criteria be followed. The inconsistency in diagnostic criteria has resulted in the variable outcomes seen in the literature, mainly with high rates of false-positive results. One review concluded that if strict operational criteria are used during diskography, the rate of false-positive results improves substantially.[6]

Analgesic Diskography

Analgesic diskography is the process of injecting a local anesthetic into a disk that has been confirmed to be the source of the patient's pain using PLD. One study demonstrated at least a 50% reduction in low back pain in 80% of disks that were considered the source of pain by PLD after injection of 4% lidocaine.[7] Another study compared the outcomes of interbody fusion based on positive results of analgesic diskography compared with PLD and demonstrated significant improvement in low back pain and disability at 1-, 2-, and 3-year follow-up in the analgesic diskography group.[8] Congruence has been reported between the analgesic diskography and PLD.[7]

Diagnostic Value of Diskography

Controversial discussions regarding the diagnostic and prognostic value and the risk of diskography are referencing PLD and not analgesic diskography. There was no consensus in the early literature as to whether diskography provided high diagnostic value. However, a recent systematic review and meta-analysis demonstrated that following ISIS guidelines strictly can result in a clinically acceptable cumulative low false-positive rate of 9.3% per patient.[9] In previous studies in which the diagnostic criteria varied, higher false-positive rates were demonstrated.[6,9-24]

Prognostic Value of Diskography

In determining whether positive discographic results lead to better surgical outcomes, a review of the literature suggests variable outcomes regarding the prognostic outcomes of lumbar fusion in those in whom the diagnosis was made via diskography versus clinical and imaging assessment alone.[25,26] However, the studies that demonstrated no improved outcomes after lumbar fusion did not follow the strict ISIS guidelines. One prospective study demonstrated that with adherence to the strict ISIS guidelines, those who underwent lumbar fusion in the setting of positive PLD results experienced improvement in function (specifically with daily activities) and were three times more likely to have less back pain than those who had positive discographic results but did not undergo surgery.[26]

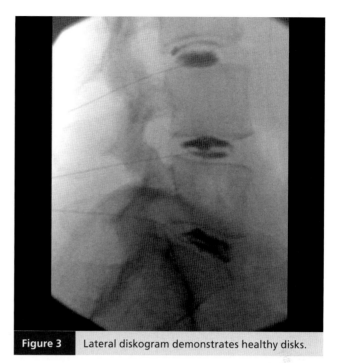

Figure 3 Lateral diskogram demonstrates healthy disks.

Complications Related to Diskography

Acute complications are rare and are mostly limited to case reports; they include acute disk herniation, discitis, vascular insult, meningitis, abscess, nerve/cord injury, and hemorrhage. Chronic complications can include future disk degeneration; whether diskography predisposes to future disk degeneration or injury is a current topic of debate. A recent 10-year matched cohort study reported that diskography results in an increased risk of clinical disk injury.[21] In contrast, a 2013 study reported no acceleration of disk degeneration at 5-year follow-up.[27] Other human and animal studies have also demonstrated mixed results and interpretation as to whether diskography results in future disk injury.[20,28,29]

Z Joint–Mediated Back Pain

Z joint–mediated back pain is the second most common etiology of low back pain.[1] The medial branches of the dorsal rami innervate the posterior elements of the vertebrae and the corresponding segment of the multifidus muscle. Pain arising from the Z joint can be diagnosed by injecting local anesthetic into the Z joint directly, or by nerve block at the medial dorsal rami branches with local anesthetic (**Figure 4**). Nerve block at the medial branches supplying a Z joint is the preferred method of diagnosing Z joint pain because this method has been validated;[30,31] intra-articular injections have not been validated as a diagnostic method. This procedure is used as a potential precursor to radiofrequency ablation of these nerves.

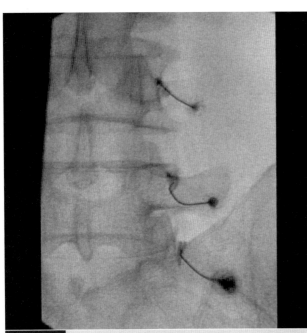

Figure 4 AP spinal radiograph demonstrates nerve blocks of the medial branches of the dorsal rami at levels L3 and L4, and of the L5 dorsal ramus.

To make an accurate diagnosis of Z joint pain, dual blocks should be performed on the same nerves on two separate occasions because of the unacceptably high rate of false-positive results. The second injection should be performed only if the first injection provided at least an 80% reduction in pain for a time frame commensurate with the local anesthetic used. If the second injection produces at least an 80% reduction in pain commensurate with the duration of a local anesthetic, the Z joint can be attributed as the cause of the patient's pain. A positive response to dual diagnostic nerve blocks predicts a positive response to radiofrequency neurotomy of these nerves.

Complications associated with a medial branch block are minimal. These include the general risks associated with any procedure that involves puncture of the skin such as infection, bleeding, bruising, and pain. This procedure is performed on the posterior spine and is thus distal to the neuroaxis (that is, the spinal cord). This dramatically reduces the risk of injury to the spinal cord directly by the needle or indirectly by injury to a spinal cord radicular feeder vessel. Additional risks are associated with therapeutic radiofrequency ablation because the goal is to create permanent tissue damage; however, a detailed discussion is beyond the scope of this chapter.

Sacroiliac Joint–Mediated Pain

SI joint pain as the etiology of axial low back pain is often overdiagnosed. SI joint–mediated pain is not the most common cause of chronic low back pain.

One retrospective review of 358 patients demonstrated an approximate 18% prevalence rate of SI joint–mediated pain.[1] The prevalence of pain increased with age and prior lumbosacral fusion. However, accurate diagnosis of SI joint–mediated pain can be difficult, and if dual nerve blocks are used to confirm the diagnosis of low back pain, only 20% to 30% of patients with expected SI joint pain will meet the diagnostic criteria based on physical examination and imaging or with a history of lumbar fusion.[32,33] Diagnosing intra-articular SI joint pain as the etiology of low back pain via history and physical examination is unreliable. Intra-articular SI joint blockade is the most widely accepted procedure for the diagnosis of SI joint pain.

Dual diagnostic blocks promote stricter criteria regarding the diagnosis of SI joint–mediated low back pain by lowering the rate of false-positive results. ISIS Guidelines[5] state that at least 75% relief is needed to be considered a positive response. Studies that used 50% to 74% relief as the cutoff had higher rates of false-positive results.[34,35]

Intra-articular blockade must be performed under image guidance (fluoroscopy or CT) to ensure proper delivery of the anesthetic by means of contrast administration through the spinal needle directly into the SI joint. The use of ultrasonography to guide needle placement has been studied.[36] Only a small amount of anesthetic should be used to avoid aberrant flow and false-positive findings.

The prognostic value of this procedure regarding outcomes with SI joint fusion is not currently known. Favorable outcomes have been noted with intra-articular corticosteroid injections after an appropriate response to dual diagnostic nerve blockade.[37]

Complications associated with intra-articular SI joint blockade are limited to those associated with any intra-articular injection. Complications include infection, bleeding, bruising, and additional pain.

Radiculopathy

The terms radiculopathy and radiculitis are often used interchangeably; however, they should be properly and carefully differentiated. Radiculopathy refers to pathology affecting a nerve root that may result in weakness, decreased tone, diminished reflexes, and/or bodily dysfunction (such as bladder incontinence). Radiculitis or radicular pain refers to irritation of the nerve root but does not necessarily reflect a neurologic deficit. Irritation

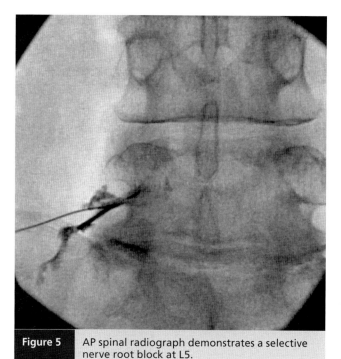

Figure 5   AP spinal radiograph demonstrates a selective nerve root block at L5.

of the nerve root is often what results in pain and abnormal sensation in a dermatomal pattern. Radiculopathy and radiculitis can coexist, resulting in a constellation of symptoms such as radicular pain in a dermatomal distribution, with weakness affecting the musculature supplied by the affected nerve root.

Radiculopathy and radiculitis are most commonly the sequelae of disk herniation. Other causes of radiculopathy and radiculitis include canal and foraminal stenosis and mass effect (such as Z joint cysts or tumors). Advanced imaging, such as MRI, often helps determine the root cause of the radiculopathy and/or radiculitis. When imaging demonstrates multilevel spinal pathology or is inconclusive, additional diagnostic procedures including electrodiagnostic studies and/or selective nerve root blocks (SNRBs) may be needed to help determine the appropriate nerve root level (**Figure 5**).

Electrodiagnostic studies such as electromyography and nerve conduction velocity studies are used to determine nerve pathology, and can help distinguish the location (for example, nerve root, plexopathy, distal mononeuropathy, and peripheral neuropathy), chronicity, and severity of nerve pathology. Electrodiagnostic studies will only demonstrate abnormalities if a radiculopathy (physiologic change in nerve function) is present, but results will be normal if only nerve irritation, or radiculitis, is present.

Regarding radiculopathy, electrodiagnostic studies can be used to help determine the specific nerve root level affected, especially when imaging demonstrates multilevel pathology or is inconclusive. A drawback to electromyography in the diagnosis of radiculopathy is that although highly specific, sensitivity can be as low as 34%.[38] In these situations, an SNRB can help determine the nerve level involved.

SNRB is an anesthetic block performed at a specific nerve root level. A needle is advanced to the neural foramen under fluoroscopic guidance, contrast through the needle confirms placement, and an anesthetic is injected to provide a temporary block to the specific nerve root level. Although technically similar to transforaminal epidural steroid injections, the goal of a SNRB is to block the nerve root only and minimize both injection into the epidural space and spread of the anesthetic to other levels. Dissimilar to electrodiagnostic studies, SNRB also can help in the diagnosis of radiculitis, even when radiculopathy is not present. Multiple studies have determined the specificity of SNRB to be 90% or higher,[39-41] and the sensitivity to be 85% or higher.[39,41,42] One study reported a positive predictive value of 70% to 95% for good surgical outcomes in patients who underwent surgery following positive results for SNRB.[41] The range in the positive predictive value is a result of inclusion criteria; the positive predictive value decreases to 70% if those who declined surgery are categorized as having had unsuccessful surgery. One study reported that spinal nerve blockade did not predict improved outcomes of surgery compared with MRI.[43] However, negative nerve blocks were predictors of poor outcome. Often, a corticosteroid is injected after the anesthetic for therapeutic purposes.

Complications with SNRBs are rare, but they can be serious and include infection, bleeding, bruising, increased pain, headache, dural puncture, and permanent nerve lesion and/or paralysis. The neurologic risks increase the more cephalad the procedure is performed (the risk increases as the procedure level progresses from the lumbosacral nerve roots to levels at which the spinal cord is present).

Summary

In addition to the history, physical examination, and imaging, the specific diagnosis regarding the etiology of low back pain often can be facilitated by diagnostic procedures. Diskography remains a controversial procedure in the diagnosis of discogenic back pain and should be used only after other diagnostic procedures, imaging, history, and physical examination have rendered inconclusive results. Adherence to strict discographic guidelines can result in favorable surgical outcomes.

Medial branch blocks for Z joint–mediated pain, intra-articular SI joint blockade for SI joint pain and SNRB for radiculopathy and/or radicular pain are procedures with high diagnostic and prognostic value and should be used in the workup of low back pain when appropriate.

Key Study Points

- Diskography, although controversial, can be a useful diagnostic procedure with low false-positive rates, when performed using the strict criteria set forth by the ISIS guidelines committee.
- Evidence is mixed regarding whether diskography results in future disk degeneration.
- Anesthetic block of the medial branch of the dorsal ramus is the preferred procedure for the diagnosis of Z joint–mediated pain.
- Intra-articular anesthetic blockade with dual diagnostic blocks provides the strictest criteria in the diagnosis of SI joint pain; injection must be performed under fluoroscopic or CT guidance to ensure proper delivery of anesthetic.
- Studies have demonstrated that SNRB has high sensitivity and specificity and can be used to help determine the level of nerve root pathology or irritation if findings from the history, physical examination, imaging, and electrodiagnostic studies are inconclusive.

Annotated References

1. DePalma MJ, Ketchum JM, Saullo T: What is the source of chronic low back pain and does age play a role? *Pain Med* 2011;12(2):224-233.

   The intervertebral disks are the most common source of chronic low back pain in adults. The younger the patient, the more likely it is that the disk is the pain generator. Facet joint and SI joint–mediated pain is more prevalent in older patients.

2. Kang CH, Kim YH, Lee SH, et al: Can magnetic resonance imaging accurately predict concordant pain provocation during provocative disc injection? *Skeletal Radiol* 2009;38(9):877-885.

3. Boden SD, Davis DO, Dina TS, Patronas NJ, Wiesel SW: Abnormal magnetic-resonance scans of the lumbar spine in asymptomatic subjects: A prospective investigation. *J Bone Joint Surg Am* 1990;72(3):403-408.

4. Jensen MC, Brant-Zawadzki MN, Obuchowski N, Modic MT, Malkasian D, Ross JS: Magnetic resonance imaging of the lumbar spine in people without back pain. *N Engl J Med* 1994;331(2):69-73.

5. Bogduk N, ed: *Practice Guidelines for Spinal Diagnostic and Treatment Procedures*, ed 2. San Francisco, CA, International Spine Intervention Society, 2013.

   The most current evidence regarding spinal procedures is summarized, and descriptions are provided on how to perform the procedures.

6. Bogduk N, Aprill C, Derby R: Lumbar discogenic pain: State-of-the-art review. *Pain Med* 2013;14(6):813-836.

   Discogenic pain can be diagnosed using strict operational criteria to reduce the likelihood of false-positive results.

7. DePalma MJ, Lee JE, Peterson L, Wolfer L, Ketchum JM, Derby R: Are outer annular fissures stimulated during diskography the source of diskogenic low-back pain? An analysis of analgesic diskography data. *Pain Med* 2009;10(3):488-494.

8. Ohtori S, Kinoshita T, Yamashita M, et al: Results of surgery for discogenic low back pain: A randomized study using discography versus discoblock for diagnosis. *Spine (Phila Pa 1976)* 2009;34(13):1345-1348.

9. Wolfer LR, Derby R, Lee JE, Lee SH: Systematic review of lumbar provocation discography in asymptomatic subjects with a meta-analysis of false-positive rates. *Pain Physician* 2008;11(4):513-538.

10. Carragee EJ, Tanner CM, Yang B, Brito JL, Truong T: False-positive findings on lumbar discography: Reliability of subjective concordance assessment during provocative disc injection. *Spine (Phila Pa 1976)* 1999;24(23):2542-2547.

11. Carragee EJ: Is lumbar discography a determinate of discogenic low back pain: Provocative discography reconsidered. *Curr Rev Pain* 2000;4(4):301-308.

12. Carragee EJ, Chen Y, Tanner CM, Hayward C, Rossi M, Hagle C: Can discography cause long-term back symptoms in previously asymptomatic subjects? *Spine (Phila Pa 1976)* 2000;25(14):1803-1808.

13. Carragee EJ, Chen Y, Tanner CM, Truong T, Lau E, Brito JL: Provocative discography in patients after limited lumbar discectomy: A controlled, randomized study of pain response in symptomatic and asymptomatic subjects. *Spine (Phila Pa 1976)* 2000;25(23):3065-3071.

14. Carragee EJ, Paragioudakis SJ, Khurana S: Lumbar high-intensity zone and discography in subjects without low back problems. *Spine (Phila Pa 1976)* 2000;25(23):2987-2992.

15. Carragee EJ, Tanner CM, Khurana S, et al: The rates of false-positive lumbar discography in select patients

2: Diagnostics in Spine Care

without low back symptoms. *Spine (Phila Pa 1976)* 2000;25(11):1373-1380, discussion 1381.

16. Carragee EJ, Alamin TF, Miller J, Grafe M: Provocative discography in volunteer subjects with mild persistent low back pain. *Spine J* 2002;2(1):25-34.

17. Carragee EJ, Barcohana B, Alamin T, van den Haak E: Prospective controlled study of the development of lower back pain in previously asymptomatic subjects undergoing experimental discography. *Spine (Phila Pa 1976)* 2004;29(10):1112-1117.

18. Carragee EJ, Alamin TF, Carragee JM: Low-pressure positive discography in subjects asymptomatic of significant low back pain illness. *Spine (Phila Pa 1976)* 2006;31(5):505-509.

19. Carragee EJ, Lincoln T, Parmar VS, Alamin T: A gold standard evaluation of the "discogenic pain" diagnosis as determined by provocative discography. *Spine (Phila Pa 1976)* 2006;31(18):2115-2123.

20. Carragee EJ, Don AS, Hurwitz EL, Cuellar JM, Carrino JA, Herzog R: Does discography cause accelerated progression of degeneration changes in the lumbar disc: A ten-year matched cohort study. *Spine (Phila Pa 1976)* 2009;34(21):2338-2345.

21. Cuellar JM, Stauff MP, Herzog RJ, Carrino JA, Baker GA, Carragee EJ: Does provocative discography cause clinically important injury to the lumbar intervertebral disc? A 10-year matched cohort study. *Spine J* 2016;16(3):273-280.

    The disk puncture and pressurized injection performed during PLD can increase the risk of clinical disk problems in patients.

22. Derby R, Lee SH, Kim BJ, Chen Y, Aprill C, Bogduk N: Pressure-controlled lumbar discography in volunteers without low back symptoms. *Pain Med* 2005;6(3):213-221, discussion 222-224.

23. Derby R, Kim BJ, Lee SH, Chen Y, Seo KS, Aprill C: Comparison of discographic findings in asymptomatic subject discs and the negative discs of chronic LBP patients: Can discography distinguish asymptomatic discs among morphologically abnormal discs? *Spine J* 2005;5(4):389-394.

24. Shin DA, Kim HI, Jung JH, Shin DG, Lee JO: Diagnostic relevance of pressure-controlled discography. *J Korean Med Sci* 2006;21(5):911-916.

25. Madan S, Gundanna M, Harley JM, Boeree NR, Sampson M: Does provocative discography screening of discogenic back pain improve surgical outcome? *J Spinal Disord Tech* 2002;15(3):245-251.

26. Cooper G, Kahn S, Lutz GE: Predictive value of provocative lumbar disc stimulation: International Spine Intervention Society Annual Meeting Abstracts. *Pain Med* 2008;9:968.

27. Ohtori S, Inoue G, Orita S, et al: No acceleration of intervertebral disc degeneration after a single injection of bupivacaine in young age group with follow-up of 5 years. *Asian Spine J* 2013;7(3):212-217.

    Imaging did not demonstrate acceleration of disk degeneration at 5 years after a single injection of bupivacaine into the intervertebral disks.

28. Flanagan MN, Chung BU: Roentgenographic changes in 188 patients 10-20 years after discography and chemonucleolysis. *Spine (Phila Pa 1976)* 1986;11(5):444-448.

29. Kahanovitz N, Arnoczky SP, Sissons HA, Steiner GC, Schwarez P: The effect of discography on the canine intervertebral disc. *Spine (Phila Pa 1976)* 1986;11(1):26-27.

30. Bogduk N: Diagnostic nerve blocks in chronic pain, in Breivik HS, ed: *Pain Best Practice & Research Compendium*. Edinburgh, Elsevier, 2007, pp 47-55.

31. Curatolo MB: Diagnostic and therapeutic nerve blocks, in Fishman SM, Ballantyne JC, Rathmell JP, eds: *Bonica's Management of Pain*. Philadelphia, PA, Wolters Kluwer, 2010, pp 1401-23.

32. Liliang PC, Lu K, Liang CL, Tsai YD, Wang KW, Chen HJ: Sacroiliac joint pain after lumbar and lumbosacral fusion: Findings using dual sacroiliac joint blocks. *Pain Med* 2011;12(4):565-570.

    The SI joint can be a potential source of pain after lumbar and lumbosacral fusions. The clinical presentation of postoperative SI joint pain differs from that of preoperative SI joint pain.

33. Maigne JY, Aivaliklis A, Pfefer F: Results of sacroiliac joint double block and value of sacroiliac pain provocation tests in 54 patients with low back pain. *Spine (Phila Pa 1976)* 1996;21(16):1889-1892.

34. van der Wurff P, Buijs EJ, Groen GJ: A multitest regimen of pain provocation tests as an aid to reduce unnecessary minimally invasive sacroiliac joint procedures. *Arch Phys Med Rehabil* 2006;87(1):10-14.

35. Irwin RW, Watson T, Minick RP, Ambrosius WT: Age, body mass index, and gender differences in sacroiliac joint pathology. *Am J Phys Med Rehabil* 2007;86(1):37-44.

36. Soneji N, Bhatia A, Seib R, Tumber P, Dissanayake M, Peng PW: Comparison of fluoroscopy and ultrasound guidance for sacroiliac joint injection in patients with chronic low back pain. *Pain Pract* 2016;16(5):537-544.

    The authors report on 40 patients with chronic low back who were randomly assigned to receive ultrasound-guided or fluoroscopy-guided SI joint injections. Ultrasound-guided SI joint injections with confirmation via fluoroscopy had similar accuracy to injections guided by fluoroscopy alone.

37. Liliang PC, Lu K, Weng HC, Liang CL, Tsai YD, Chen HJ: The therapeutic efficacy of sacroiliac joint blocks with triamcinolone acetonide in the treatment of sacroiliac joint

dysfunction without spondyloarthropathy. *Spine (Phila Pa 1976)* 2009;34(9):896-900.

38. Haueisen DC, Smith BS, Myers SR, Pryce ML: The diagnostic accuracy of spinal nerve injection studies: Their role in the evaluation of recurrent sciatica. *Clin Orthop Relat Res* 1985;198:179-183.

39. Dooley JF, McBroom RJ, Taguchi T, Macnab I: Nerve root infiltration in the diagnosis of radicular pain. *Spine (Phila Pa 1976)* 1988;13(1):79-83.

40. Stanley D, McLaren MI, Euinton HA, Getty CJ: A prospective study of nerve root infiltration in the diagnosis of sciatica: A comparison with radiculography, computed tomography, and operative findings. *Spine (Phila Pa 1976)* 1990;15(6):540-543.

41. van Akkerveeken PF: The diagnostic value of nerve root sheath infiltration. *Acta Orthop Scand Suppl* 1993;64(suppl 251):61-63.

42. Anderberg L, Annertz M, Brandt L, Säveland H: Selective diagnostic cervical nerve root block: Correlation with clinical symptoms and MRI-pathology. *Acta Neurochir (Wien)* 2004;146(6):559-565, discussion 565.

43. Sasso RC, Macadaeg K, Nordmann D, Smith M: Selective nerve root injections can predict surgical outcome for lumbar and cervical radiculopathy: Comparison to magnetic resonance imaging. *J Spinal Disord Tech* 2005;18(6):471-478.

Medical Management of Spine Disorders

SECTION EDITOR:

Scott R. Laker, MD

Chapter 9

Transdisciplinary Care for Cervical Spine Disorders

Gregory Whitcomb, DC

Abstract

The neck comprises a system of highly integrated biomechanical, neurophysiologic, and vascular functions that cannot be considered in isolation. Overlapping cervical spine pathologies exist, and a variety of interventions have evolved for each. In contrast, the clinical care systems developed for patients with neck disorders have resulted in a relatively segregated approach, which has been influenced by the training and biases of the healthcare providers. In addition to physical factors, psychosocial influences are equally critical to achieve effective care and outcomes. Healthcare providers disregard the sum of these variables at potentially great cost to patients and society. In the context of cervical spine disorders, it is increasingly important to address the mounting evidence for the broader and more dynamic framework of transdisciplinary care.

Keywords: care models; cervical spine; transdisciplinary care

Introduction

Transdisciplinary care is not purely situational. Rather, it is dynamic and additive, resulting in collective problem solving in the milieu of evidence-based care. Transdisciplinarity is a process that extends beyond simple provider juxtaposition or the latest biotechnologic advances; it is based on the recognition that no single best approach exists to treat neck pain,[1] and that fundamental change is needed in the care delivery process to improve access, augment evaluation and diagnosis, and coordinate treatment in ways that can effectively and affordably meet the myriad needs of patients with cervical spine disorders and the communities in which they live and work.

Epidemiologic Considerations

The reach of cervical spine disorders is substantial and extends beyond affected individuals to families, communities, healthcare organizations, employers, governmental agencies, and health insurance systems.

Neck pain ranks as the fourth leading cause of disability globally,[2] following low back pain, depression, and arthralgias; notably, these conditions often overlap. Up to one-half of adults will experience a clinically meaningful episode of neck pain during their lifetime.[3] Data show similarly high rates of neck pain in the adolescent population.[4] Study design variables have resulted in wide variability in population–based prevalence rates, ranging from 12% to as high as 70% and affecting up to 48% of workers, 11% to 14% of whom report related functional limitation. Neck pain and headaches are strongly correlated.[5] Disability from neck pain is present in up to 12% of adults, and a progressive increase in emergency department visits for neck pain has occurred over the past 3 decades.[6]

Presenteeism, or working while sick, can cause productivity loss, poor health, exhaustion, and workplace epidemics. Absenteeism has historically received extensive attention in the human resource sciences; however, presenteeism only recently has received scientific attention.[7] Presenteeism rates are among the highest for individuals with neck and upper back pain, and psychosocial factors have a substantial relationship to reporting, recovery,[8] and disability.[9]

Although disability caused by neck pain has a greater effect in the industrialized world, data now show that it is a global problem, with a greater effect on women

3: Medical Management of Spine Disorders

than men. Neck problems are expected to compound substantially in the future because of increasing child survival and aging rates.[2]

The costs related to treatment of neck pain are substantial, with precipitous increases in surgical and nonsurgical treatment over the past 2 decades. Moreover, disparity in access to services[10] as well as looming changes related to reimbursement and medical malpractice[11] reflect the cost ineffectiveness of the current spine care system.[12] Compounded by a crisis in opioid use,[13] this perceived lack of value has resulted in governmental, institutional, and even public criticism of spine care providers, particularly spine surgeons.[14*]

At the same time, the overall well-being of physicians in the United States is in decline, with high rates of stress, impaired work-life balance, and burnout. Burnout in physicians is twice as high as in the general working population.[15] Although the dynamics associated with this trend are complex, an increasingly corporatized[16] and productivity-driven healthcare delivery system is clearly associated with physical and psychologic stress,[17] and spine surgeons are among those most directly affected.[18]

Traditionally, decision making for spine surgery is an individualized process, with many options resulting in essentially equivalent outcomes.[19] When serious structural neck pathology may cause irreversible impairment, surgery may ultimately be the most conservative approach.

Given the comparatively small percentage of patients likely to benefit from surgery, optimal patient selection has resulted in strained access to surgeons who spend substantial time treating distinctly nonsurgical spine issues in high-volume outpatient clinics. Given the increasing emphasis on optimizing patient-provider alignment and value, a spine surgeon's time and skills are clearly most effective when providing truly tertiary care. Intuitively, data confirm that the time spent performing surgery is associated with higher work satisfaction for surgeons.[15]

Given the prevalence and personal and societal costs of cervical spine conditions, as well as the associated stresses on those who care for patients with these conditions, current patient care models clearly are not sustainable. New thinking and broad systemic changes are needed to optimize outcomes and reduce costs for patients with neck disorders.

Spine Care in a World of Global Transformation

The ability of emerging technologies to quickly disseminate information is accelerating profound change at every level of human interaction, including healthcare delivery and patient expectations. Internet access has resulted in a fundamental transition from the patient as a passive recipient to an active consumer of health care.[20] Patients can be overwhelmed by the volume of information (often of variable quality) and multiple treatment options.[21]

Compounding work stress for healthcare providers,[22] electronic medical record (EMR) technologies now allow almost immediate contact between providers and their patients, who are demanding faster access to clinical care. Accordingly, spine clinicians are often tasked with rapid decision making that can extend beyond the scope of their training and have potential medicolegal ramifications.

Although marketed as a public benefit, information technologies are progressively being used to monitor provider financial performance against patient satisfaction, with powerful ramifications for healthcare systems. This data management will likely result in new reimbursement strategies with direct effects on providers and healthcare institutions.[23] In addition, an increasingly diverse patient population is demanding new competencies to resolve disparities in health care.[24]

Viewed collectively, these broad and compounding systemic effects require integrated problem-solving across the disciplinary spectrum, and new healthcare management strategies must play a central role in meeting the needs of patients and those who bear the costs of their care.[25] This will require a shift from historically silo-oriented biomedical neck care to vastly different strategies. For example, a recent study showed the relative superiority of mindfulness-based stress reduction and cognitive behavioral therapy compared with usual spine care,[26] which led to the observation that "there is an urgent need to rethink and reorganize care (for axial pain) at all levels, so that the safest and most effective treatments are the most readily accessible."[27]

Achieving Transdisciplinarity: The Chaordic Management Model

The following three questions were central to the foundation of Visa International, which has risen to become the largest single block of consumer purchasing power in the global economy.[28] (1) Why are institutions everywhere, whether political, commercial, or social, increasingly unable to manage their affairs? (2) Why are individuals, everywhere, increasingly in conflict with, and alienated from the institutions of which they are part? (3) Why are the society and the biosphere in disarray? The essence of transdisciplinarity systems resides in a narrow overlap between chaos and order, termed chaordic, and is generally defined as any self-organizing, self-governing organization, community, or system with behavior that harmoniously blends characteristics of both chaos and order.[28]

Proponents of chaordic management propose that the newtonian hierarchical command and control strategies of the Industrial Age have resulted in most of the larger problems currently confronting society, and integrated heterarchical solutions achieved through a constitution and defining mission of a variety of invested stakeholders are necessary to meet these problems. This thinking has direct relevance to the complexities of spine care in a rapidly evolving and global healthcare system.

A Historical Perspective on Care Models

The Biomedical Model and the Importance of the Intervertebral Disk

The Greco-Roman tradition of medicine was grounded in holism, which is the concept of treating the whole person by considering spiritual, mental, and sociocultural factors, rather than just the physical symptoms of a disease. This view of patient care was lost in the orthodoxy of the Middle Ages. By the 17th century, Vesalius and Descartes had laid the foundations for modern anatomic study and mind-body dualism. With the rapid advancement in the natural and biologic sciences in the 1800s, Koch, Pasteur, and Virchow effectively codified the biomedical model as the centerpiece of 20th-century Western health care.[29]

Arguably, the single largest step toward the pathology model of spine pain was Mixter and Barr's 1934 publication, *Herniation or Rupture of the Intervertebral Disk with Involvement of the Spinal Canal*.[30] In a profoundly biomedical fashion, their work made structural pathology the basis for axial disorders and ultimately paved the way for the use of arthrodesis in treating neck and back pain.

Given the advancements in instrumented and genetically enhanced fusion, infection control, and anesthesia, and compounded by the infusion of corporate capital and aggressive hospital marketing, the rate of spine surgery in the United States (as opposed to much of the world) increased at a greater rate than even that of total hip arthroplasty between 1998 and 2008. Costs also soared.[31] Despite evidence showing good outcomes for select candidates, the massive increase in surgery has not yielded proportional benefits.[12] Payer and public repercussions have been strident. Criteria and consensus for optimal surgical candidate selection remain priorities for the spine surgical research community.

A Return to Holism, Complementary Alternative Medicine, and Physical Therapy

Holism and vitalism (the doctrine that living organisms possess a nonphysical inner force or energy that gives them the property of life) was popular during the 18th and 19th centuries, and evidence confirms the use of manual treatment of spinal disorders throughout history and across widely disparate cultures. Counter to biomedical sensibilities, osteopathic and chiropractic practitioners were soon attributing spine pain and systemic disease to such entities as somatic dysfunction and vertebral subluxation, without an objective basis for these conditions, let alone the wide-ranging effects attributed to them. Legislation quickly became an agent to define and regulate the practice of medicine, and such practices were effectively outlawed as ineffective quackery. However, in contrast to biomedical models, perhaps the most important contribution of these professions was the philosophy that health is a part of the natural expression of the vitality innate in life. Wellness through lifestyle is increasingly supported by science, and since 1948, the World Health Organization's constitution has defined health as "a state of complete physical, mental, and social well-being and not merely the absence of disease or infirmity."[32]

By the 1990s, increasing numbers of patients were seeking care for axial pain outside standard medical practice. In addition, patients were willing to obtain this care at substantial out-of-pocket expense.[33] This exodus powerfully demonstrated patient dissatisfaction with the limitations of biomedical spine care.

Accompanying the expansion of care in other nonmedical spine specialties has been the rapid growth of physical therapy. After World War II, physical therapists assumed a critical role in the rehabilitation of thousands of US soldiers, which resulted in the increasing awareness of the functional aspects of musculoskeletal disorders. Particularly in countries other than the United States, physical therapists also expanded the use of manual treatment. For decades, the physical therapy profession functioned largely in the shadow of medical physicians; however, physical therapists are now contributing to musculoskeletal research, and the profession has become integral with spine care in most healthcare systems.

This constellation of nonmedical healthcare providers has contributed to the scientific understanding of neck pain and options for its treatment. However, the competition for cultural authority among these professions often has proved confusing for both patients and medical physicians. Systems are needed to identify and align the benefits of each.

The Biopsychosocial Model

With advancement in the mental health sciences, the concept of biomedicine was critically challenged at another level. In the late 1970s, a more comprehensive approach to patient care was proposed[34] and the biopsychosocial model has since been validated and widely embraced in spine care.

3: Medical Management of Spine Disorders

Subsequent work expanded on the concept of "illness behavior," and extensive research by spine-oriented psychologists has validated that nonphysical factors are equally if not more influential on recovery and progression from acute to chronic axial pain and related disability than is physical pathology.[35] Despite recognition of the importance of psychosocial factors in best-evidence clinical guidelines, incorporation of the biopsychosocial model has lagged.[36]

In addition, advances in pain research have confirmed that nociception is centrally processed and interpreted in complex ways, and chronic pain results in functional changes in the brain.[37] These discoveries are blurring the margins of psychology and neuroscience, and reinforce the importance of a better understanding of disability attributed to spinal pain. Evidence supports the importance of mind-body approaches such as cognitive-based therapy as critical to effective spine care.[38] Strategies to address central pain processing are gaining validity in biopsychosocial neck and back pain management.[39]

From Monodisciplinary to Transdisciplinary Care

As a consequence of a long-standing silo-orientated approach to axial pain, patients have been confronted by a daunting array of treatments and confusion about selecting the best care.[21] Multidisciplinary spine programs became increasingly prevalent in the 1990s, partly as a result of the disproportionate costs associated with the care of a small subset of spine patients. These programs were often lengthy, intensive, and focused on the small percentage of patients with the most chronic and debilitating back and neck pain. Although outcomes were generally favorable, the expense and duration of these programs compromised their value, necessitating alternative strategies.[40]

Subsequently, an interdisciplinary approach to spine care has gained momentum. Intrinsic to both multidisciplinary and interdisciplinary program approaches are structured multiprovider team evaluations and prescriptive clinical pathways that can create bottlenecks to access and duplicative or overlap services. Efforts to improve effectiveness have resulted in other strategies. Optimal provider-patient alignment through subgrouping has shown some promise, but more work is needed.[41,42]

Large healthcare systems have promoted management of axial pain at the primary care level; however, family and primary medical practitioners are in short supply and musculoskeletal skills sets are lacking at this level.[43] Direct access to subspecialty spine care should not be limited to patients with complex conditions, and evidence suggests that early care for patients with comparatively straightforward neck problems may limit the progression to chronicity.[44]

Globalization and integration have resulted in an increasing recognition of the importance of transdisciplinary research and organizational management. Paralleling nature, transdisciplinary systems spontaneously self-organize in response to both external and internal challenges. In the clinical setting, transdisciplinarity offers flexibility and expediency in both access and patient care.

Transdisciplinary Care for Cervical Spine Disorders

Implicit in transdisciplinary care is an understanding that the needs of patients exceed the knowledge, training, and skills of any single provider. The transdisciplinary approach is responsive on its margins, allowing dynamic patient-provider interaction through the unique blending of multiple disciplines (**Figure 1**). Committing to this process can be uncomfortable to those cultured in the biomedical hierarchy of command and control biomedical management.

The transdisciplinary care model requires dynamic interaction among a variety of disciplines, thus enabling the exchange of information, knowledge, expertise, and clinical skills necessary to team-based problem solving. This approach is gaining traction in other healthcare milieus such as oncology and nursing. Although more studies regarding its implementation are needed, transdisciplinary care has been shown to contribute to both clinician satisfaction and a favorable patient experience in a biopsychosocial functional restoration program.[45]

Structurally, a transdisciplinary model is inherently patient-centric, heterarchical, and integrated. Through direct connection with any one provider, the patient has connectivity to the entire system, as does each provider (**Figure 2**). Although sensitive to best-evidence practice guidelines, it allows clinicians to adapt to a patient's needs. At the same time, however, a transdisciplinary milieu is self-policing through interprovider accountability. Importantly, this requires clear prospective group agreement regarding the sometimes difficult process of conflict resolution.

Transdisciplinarity need not apply only to patient care; it can potentially enhance clinical administration with positive effects for patients and providers from initial contact to discharge and subsequent care. For example, patients may freely make comments to nonprovider staff members that could prove critical in ways that exceed the classic boundaries of patient-provider interaction. A systemic approach recognizes the perceptions and input of all individuals involved in the process of clinical care, including administrative personnel such as receptionists and schedulers.

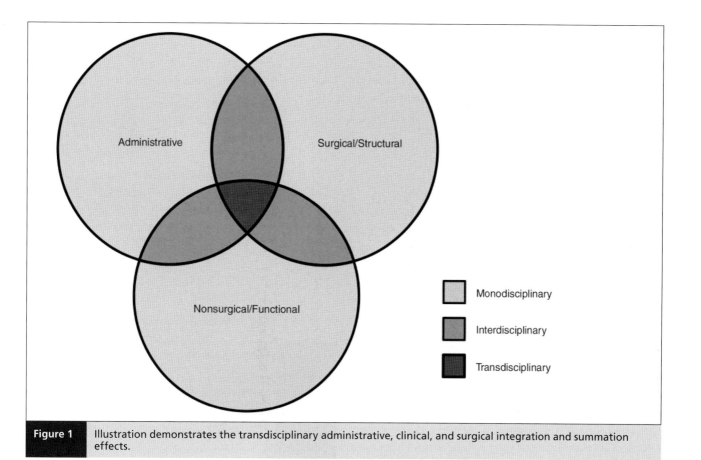

Figure 1 Illustration demonstrates the transdisciplinary administrative, clinical, and surgical integration and summation effects.

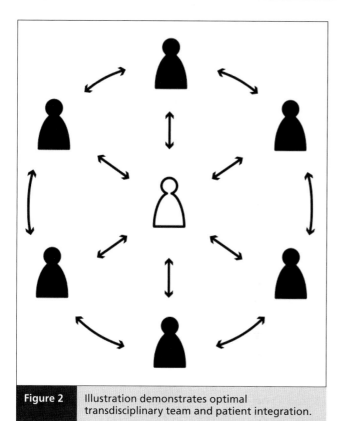

Figure 2 Illustration demonstrates optimal transdisciplinary team and patient integration.

Foundations of a Transdisciplinary Team

The concept of transdisciplinarity has received considerable attention outside the realm of spine care. One study stresses the Institute of Medicine's recommendation for healthcare teams as a key step toward improving the quality of care and cogently characterizes the process and structural differences between multidisciplinary, interdisciplinary, and transdisciplinary functions. It is noted that "the multidisciplinary model involves vertical communication from supervisor to subordinates, with each member contributing an assessment after applying a discipline-specific skillset (with) little discussion between team members (that) the interdisciplinary model acknowledges the overlap in knowledge of (team) members and facilitates horizontal communication at many points in the (evaluation and care process) and that the transdisciplinary model of care takes collaboration to a still higher level, incorporating ongoing cross-disciplinary education (and) regulated overlapping roles."[46]

Best-evidence practice guidelines help to define key players in a transdisciplinary approach to cervical spine disorders. Spine-specialized neurologic and orthopaedic surgeons, physiatrists, physical and occupational

3: Medical Management of Spine Disorders

therapists, chiropractors, interventional pain specialists, psychologists, nurse practitioners, physician's assistants, and registered nurses contribute the most fundamental elements of a clinical team; however, vocational rehabilitation, social, and even lay community members can enhance care strategies in the broader context of biopsychosocial spine care and disability management.

Viable transdisciplinary teams require healthcare providers to work across historic boundaries and processes; without doing so, care coordination will ultimately degrade. The chaordic approach to business management[28] is based on foundational principles that have been characterized as the Six Lenses on Organization[47] (**Figure 3**). Effective transdisciplinary teams are created and sustained using these concepts. Without leadership dedicated to these concepts, individual or discipline-specific agendas will invariably undermine an integrated care milieu.

Transdisciplinarity in Biopsychosocial Care

The education of medical students in the biopsychosocial care model has lagged substantially behind that of biomedical interventions.[48] Given their broad reach, effective transdisciplinary programs also require a commitment to biopsychosocial patient care. Psychosocial factors are critical to the patient experience and can be addressed at virtually every level of patient interaction. Best-evidence advice that most imaging findings are benign and reassurance that normal activity is not injurious will improve outcomes. When repeated across multiple patient-provider interactions through transdisciplinary team care, the effect of such advice is compounded and powerfully supports active care strategies.

Depression, anxiety, catastrophizing, fear-avoidance behaviors, and other psychosocial stressors have a well-established correlation with axial pain and the progression to chronic pain and disability. Early risk recognition and psychosocial interventions are facilitated in an environment of cross-trained providers. Routine clinical interventions such as addressing fear-avoidance behaviors during exercise and stability training, discussing emotional distress at medical reassessments, or talking about passive treatment dependency during chiropractic follow-ups can supplement structured mental health care.

The Benefits of Transdisciplinary Triage and Care Access

Accreditation and reimbursement are increasingly tied to access and patient satisfaction. Balanced against value propositions, it is critically important to optimize patient access to the providers or groups of providers who can

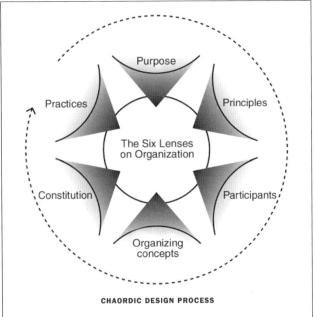

CHAORDIC DESIGN PROCESS

| Figure 3 | Illustration of the Six Lenses on Organization Chaordic Design Process. Purpose is a clear statement that defines and binds the community in worthy pursuit. Principles are clear, commonly understood statements reflecting how participants conduct themselves in pursuit of purpose. Participants are the group that defines just, equitable, and effective relationships that all can trust to achieve purpose in accordance with principles. Organizing concepts are activities and process trusted as equitable, effective, and in accordance with organizational purpose and principles. The constitution is the codification of participant rights, obligations, and relationships that forms an organizational entity. Practices are activities, products, or services through which participants pursue the organization's purpose and create value. |

most effectively initiate and coordinate evidence-based spine care. Patient preference also has been shown to affect satisfaction and outcome. More than any single discipline, transdisciplinary care teams have greater flexibility to meet the preferences and clinical needs of patients with neck disorders.

A small percentage of patients with acute or first-episode cervical spine disorders are likely to experience chronicity; therefore, early identification of risk factors is critical. In a transdisciplinary model, screening for prospective disability risks facilitates broader care coordination with employers and other stakeholders.[49]

Information technology can facilitate patient triage. Potentially serious pathology, including red flags, psychosocial yellow flags, and patient preferences, usually can be identified initially via a skilled telephone interview (conducted by a registered nurse or equivalent professional) and/or other preclinical mechanism. For patients with complex issues (for example, serious comorbid health status, third-party liability claims, debilitating pain with current work absence), preappointment telephone triage performed by a nurse can inform clinical assessment while reducing both the amount of waiting time before coming to the clinic and the length of the consultation session.

Initial clinical evaluation by well-trained nonmedical spine specialists is acceptable to patients.[50] Evidence shows that most patients with acute neck pain will respond favorably to basic care such as NSAIDs, muscle relaxant medications, manual therapy, and postural and relaxation training. Early access to providers of nonmedical spine care can reduce time to evaluation and provide timely care. Nurse practitioners, physician assistants, chiropractors, and physical therapists can hasten the identification of patients with red flags that warrant early evaluation by a spine surgeon.

Transdisciplinary Clinical Assessment
The flexibility of the transdisciplinary model allows a range of clinical assessments from targeted to comprehensive. Most patients present with axial neck pain and stiffness in combination with dysfunctional stabilization mechanics, postural faults, and lifestyle factors warranting functional treatment and rehabilitation.

In the absence of red flag indicators or recent trauma, routine imaging studies are not likely to inform treatment. Both standard and advanced radiographs show a high prevalence of age-consistent degenerative findings, which are poorly correlated with axial neck pain.[51] However, treatment risk and benefit considerations vary by discipline, and transdisciplinary consideration should be given to imaging studies to address indications or contraindications (for example, the appropriate level for an injection or osteoporosis for spinal manipulation) or in the absence of projected improvement after an initial course of care.

Best available scientific evidence generally does not support more than a temporary effect with any stand-alone treatment, although treatment of pain and stiffness can ease early rehabilitation and reactivation. Although medication, interventional procedures, and manual therapy have specific uses, unattended functional deficits such as motor control and stability dysfunction or work exposures likely will result in recurrent or progressive neck problems. In a transdisciplinary care setting, functionally oriented physical and occupational therapy evaluations are critical to rehabilitation, and include behavioral modification, targeted exercise (for motor control, flexibility, and strength training), and positive lifestyle changes.

Standardized screening tools can inform clinical care.[52] For example, expert reassurance and guidance help modify behavioral barriers such as fear avoidance or active endurance during routine follow-up care. However, in more difficult cases, psychologic assessment should be considered based on the input of a team member at any time during the patient's clinical course.

Transdisciplinary Care Planning and Coordination
Synthesizing a treatment plan requires communication. In the transdisciplinary setting, EMR systems afford virtual interprovider communication, although real-time staff consultation should occur at the discretion of any provider during the patient's clinical course.

Based on discipline-specific training or experience, factors such as new symptoms, findings, or patient noncompliance may become apparent to certain clinicians before others, and the ability to confer and respond can be critical. Variation between team members' recommendations for treatment and care must be addressed and resolved early and continuously. Because of a lack of superiority of any single treatment approach, the transdisciplinary model is well suited to communication and timing, and treatments can be uniquely tailored to meet the evolving needs or preferences of patients.

Although further research is needed, concurrent treatments may be complementary in the continuum of care. For example, neuromotor and stabilization training can be limited by pain and stiffness, which can be reduced through manual treatment and/or interventional pain procedures. With transdisciplinary care emphasizing clinical interventions to support functional rehabilitation, patients and providers must remain open to alternative options in the absence of improvement, including cessation or alteration of treatment.

In cases refractory to active care, referral to a chronic medical and psychologic pain specialist may be necessary; however, evidence suggests that integrated care in a biopsychosocial model shows promise in reducing the incidence of disability from chronic pain and related work absence.[53]

Transdisciplinary Clinical Care: Case Examples
These case examples are vignettes based on actual cases presenting to an integrated academic spine center.

Case Example One
A 39-year-old woman employed as an oncology nurse reported a history of neck pain and stiffness dating back to childhood. Team evaluation was initiated at the recommendation of her primary care physician. Her work had

3: Medical Management of Spine Disorders

not required stressful lifting or patient transfer, and she had no history of recent or remote neck or shoulder injury. Within 2 weeks preceding her baseline visit to a primary care physician, radiating right arm pain suddenly developed with distributed numbness from the right shoulder to the right dorsal midline forearm and hand. The primary care physician prescribed opioid analgesics and oral corticosteroids, without recommendation for follow-up.

Within 1 week of the evaluation by her primary care physician, she presented with improved symptoms, including decreased axial pain and arm/hand numbness and tingling. Physiatric evaluation confirmed positional aggravation of neck pain and right arm paresthesias without evidence of ipsilateral peripheral neuropathy or neurologic deficit. Imaging was deferred, and the patient was advised to continue taking the prescribed medications and follow up with a physician assistant in 2 weeks. The patient was encouraged to continue with her usual work and basic daily activities.

Within the next week, she presented for same-day physical therapy and chiropractic evaluation after completing her course of oral steroids. In addition to painful neck stiffness and poor deep neck flexor recruitment, the physical therapy evaluation demonstrated dysfunctional axial, glenohumeral, and scapulothoracic motor control, with grade 4/5 right elbow flexor and 3/5 serratus anterior weakness.

Chiropractic consultation confirmed the patient's history of first-time arm symptoms and an absence of any recent severe or atypical headache, vision change, facial numbness, contralateral upper or lower extremity pain/paresthesia or weakness, or incipient bowel or bladder dysfunction. Obstetric history was para 3, gravida 3 with a history of antepartum low back pain without symphalgia. The patient acknowledged a long-standing history of nonlimiting, intermittent, and consistently mild episodes of low back pain. Although able to continue basic daily activity and work (10-hour work days), the patient reported worsening pain and a sense of global right arm heaviness.

Examination confirmed an otherwise healthy-appearing, alert, oriented, and articulate middle-aged woman in modest distress. Sitting and standing postures were slumped with the head/neck in anterior and slightly left lateral weight bearing. Lumbar lordosis was exaggerated with poor lower abdominal tone and dysfunctional axial stabilization mechanics. A costal breathing pattern was present with asymmetric right scalene group and multilevel segmental cervical/thoracic tenderness and low-grade cervical extensor spasm.

Neck motions were limited to greater than 50% in extension and right lateral bending because of immediate provocation of radiating arm pain and paresthesias extending to the right dorsal forearm and hand, which was consistent with a positive Spurling test result. Flexion was comparatively well tolerated with adequate lordotic reversal. The Lhermitte sign was absent.

Anterior neck examination was remarkable for right supraclavicular fossa tenderness and increased right arm pain and paresthesia on plexus compression. No palpable cervical adenopathy was noted. Examination of the right shoulder showed asymmetric shoulder internal rotation and extension motion deficit without evidence of cuff impingement or labral compromise. Right scapular dyskinesis was evident without gross scapular winging.

Comparative neurologic evaluation showed interim onset 3-4/5 right biceps, triceps, and wrist flexor muscle weakness, decreased sensitivity to pinprick in a right C6-C7 distribution, bilateral lower extremity hyperreflexia, and bilateral Hoffman responses. Muscle bulk and tone of the arm and hands was grossly normal. The Tinel sign was absent at the right elbow and wrist. Finger escape, crossed adductor response, and clonus were negative, and gait was smooth.

Given the clear evidence of sudden deterioration in neurologic status, cervical MRI was performed before any further care (particularly, regional manual treatment) was considered. MRI demonstrated a large left parasagittal and lateral C6-C7 disk herniation with extension into the neural foramen, and cervical cord compression and displacement without signal intensity change or substantial bony neuroforaminal or central canal narrowing. A spine surgical consultation was accommodated almost immediately. The patient was treated with a single-level anterior cervical decompression and fusion.

Surgical considerations notwithstanding, this patient's best outcome clearly extends beyond root decompression and segmental fusion; her history and clinical findings were demonstrative of a long-standing movement disorder and postural stress relative to more chronic axial neck and back pain and shoulder stiffness. Transdisciplinarity afforded a seamless transition to postoperative management of pain and stiffness and care of her preexisting dysfunctional axial and shoulder girdle stabilization mechanics. Treatment of all conditions was equally critical to an optimal outcome.

Case Example Two

A 29-year-old woman employed as a professional singer and administrative assistant requested a chiropractic evaluation. She reported more than 10 years of neck and upper back pain and generalized (symmetric suboccipital to bitemporal distribution) headaches. She denied other symptoms, and a review of systems and medical history were reportedly otherwise unremarkable. She did not exercise and maintained a multiyear smoking habit of one pack of cigarettes per day.

Although the patient had undergone monthly full spine chiropractic manipulations for several years, she acknowledged no more than temporary benefit from these treatments. She had not been examined by a physician or physical therapist for her current symptoms. She admitted to depression regarding her persistent symptoms and anxiety about degenerative changes noted on her cervical radiographs.

She had a dysphoric, asthenic, and fatigued appearance with slouched posture. The patient was intermittently tearful during her appointment. Widespread tenderness was reported with even superficial palpation, which resulted in a withdrawal response. No focal midline or anterior neck tenderness was elicited.

Passive neck motions were grossly physiologic, with pain in all planes but primarily in extension, with associated upper thoracic stiffness and discomfort. The Spurling test result was negative for radicular-type symptoms; however, neck pain was elicited with even light vertex pressure, indicating a positive axial loading test result. Deep neck flexor recruitment was suboptimal with anterior head carriage. Bilateral shoulder ranges of motion were full and locally painless, and clinical examination showed no finding suspicious for rotator cuff, bicipital tendon, or glenoid labral compromise. Scapulothoracic motions were grossly normal. Upper extremity neuromotor, reflex, and sensory examinations were normal without neural tension or long tract signs. After the examination, the patient's relatively benign findings were explained and she was reassured that further diagnostic testing was unnecessary. She was distressed, expressing that she hoped to undergo MRI to determine the cause of her symptoms.

A transdisciplinary approach was recommended, including physical therapy, physiatric evaluations, and brief but time-limited regional manual treatment. The behavioral findings were addressed with careful inquiry into any unreported prior injury. The patient volunteered a history of sustained sexual, physical, and emotional abuse during late childhood, for which she had never received counseling. Her pain was explained in the context of chronicity, central processing, and a lack of supportive mental health care. Additional physical treatments were contingent on coordinated psychologic assessment, to which the patient agreed.

The patient reported substantial improvement in all symptoms in a matter of weeks. Manual therapy was withdrawn and further gains were reported at follow-ups over 6 months, during which psychologic counseling continued. She reported increasing optimism regarding her ability to effectively self-manage symptoms by means of spine stabilization exercises, relaxation techniques, and walking. Her sleep had improved, and she was willing to transition to self-directed care. Two years later, she returned with a flare-up in symptoms after experiencing strain while lifting during a household move and confirmed general successful independent management of her symptoms with a continuing exercise program. Tobacco use had continued, but at decreased levels, and she reported improvement in anxiety and depression while continuing mental health care at an outside facility.

What Can We Learn?

These two case examples represent relative extremes on the spectrum of neck pain disorders. The first case is a well-defined instance of acute-onset neurologic compromise, and the second case involved nonspecific physical finding in a patient with prevalent long-standing psychosocial distress, unnecessary treatment dependency, and a history of abuse that strongly correlated with progression to chronic pain. Neither patient had previously received evidence-oriented clinical care. From a strictly biomedical perspective, both patients were ostensibly candidates for physically oriented treatment (stand-alone surgery in the first case and extensively repetitive chiropractic treatments in the second case) without prior consideration of the broader clinical pictures. Critical to care optimization was transdisciplinary recognition of a combination of physical and psychosocial factors that if unaddressed may have resulted in unnecessary physical treatments, poor outcomes, and significant patient ramifications.

These examples demonstrate the broad changes that confront the future of orthopaedic practice and "significant cooperation on behalf of all involved healthcare providers will be necessary to ensure that quality of care does not suffer while efforts for cost containment continue"[54] and the emerging realization that transdisciplinarity will be critical to patients and providers negotiating a new era in health care.

Summary

The current approach to cervical spine care is unsustainable. Cervical spine disorders are endemic, highly recurrent, and commonly involve psychosocial and other complexities that exceed the management capacity of any single spine specialist. Compounded by the extraordinary internal and external stresses of a rapidly changing healthcare environment, transdisciplinarity is urgently needed in patient care. Although efforts to refine physical treatment

3: Medical Management of Spine Disorders

should continue, transdisciplinarity in health care has the potential to improve outcomes, patient satisfaction, and treatment value and enhance the work experience of providers.

Embracing and implementing a transdisciplinary biopsychosocial care model requires a willingness to think and work in new ways. A chaordic model of management may hold the key to this evolution in health care.

Key Study Points

- Cervical spine disorders are highly prevalent, with substantial personal and societal costs.

- Extant management models have resulted in neck care that is largely biomedical, expensive, poorly coordinated, and ineffective.

- Psychosocial factors are equally, if not more, influential on treatment outcomes and the progression to neck pain disability. Broad access to biopsychosocial neck care is needed.

- Despite some single-treatment effectiveness, the scope of cervical disorders exceeds that of any single discipline.

- Transdisciplinary health care has the potential to expedite access while improving outcomes, value, and patient satisfaction.

Annotated References

1. Verhagen AP, van Middelkoop M, Rubinstein SM, et al: Effect of various kinds of cervical spinal surgery on clinical outcomes: A systematic review and meta-analysis. *Pain* 2013;154(11):2388-2396.

   The differences in benefits and harms between the various surgical techniques are small. The surgeon, patient, and healthcare provider can therefore decide to implement any surgical technique based on experience, preferences, or costs.

2. Hoy D, March L, Woolf A, et al: The global burden of neck pain: Estimates from the global burden of disease 2010 study. *Ann Rheum Dis* 2014;73(7):1309-1315.

   This study reported that the global prevalence of neck pain was 4.9% (95% confidence interval [CI]: 4.6–5.3). Disability-adjusted life-years increased from 23.9 million (95% CI: 16.5–33.1) in 1990 to 33.6 million (95% CI: 23.5–46.5) in 2010. Additional research is needed to better understand the predictors and clinical course of neck pain, as well as methods to prevent and better manage neck pain.

3. Hogg-Johnson S, van der Velde G, Carroll LJ, et al; Bone and Joint Decade 2000-2010 Task Force on Neck Pain and Its Associated Disorders: The burden and determinants of neck pain in the general population: Results of the Bone and Joint Decade 2000-2010 Task Force on Neck Pain and Its Associated Disorders. *Spine (Phila Pa 1976)* 2008;33 (4 suppl):S39-S51.

4. Ehrmann Feldman D, Shrier I, Rossignol M, Abenhaim L: Risk factors for the development of neck and upper limb pain in adolescents. *Spine (Phila Pa 1976)* 2002;27(5):523-528.

5. Ashina S, Bendtsen L, Lyngberg AC, Lipton RB, Hajiyeva N, Jensen R: Prevalence of neck pain in migraine and tension-type headache: A population study. *Cephalalgia* 2015;35(3):211-219.

   It was reported that neck pain is highly prevalent in the general population, even more prevalent in individuals with primary headaches, and most prevalent in those with coexistent migraine plus tension-type headaches, followed by those with pure tension-type headache and migraine alone. Myofascial tenderness is substantially increased in individuals with neck pain.

6. Martin BI, Turner JA, Mirza SK, Lee MJ, Comstock BA, Deyo RA: Trends in health care expenditures, utilization, and health status among US adults with spine problems, 1997-2006. *Spine (Phila Pa 1976)* 2009;34(19):2077-2084.

7. Aronsson G, Gustafsson K, Dallner M: Sick but yet at work. An empirical study of sickness presenteeism. *J Epidemiol Community Health* 2000;54(7):502-509.

8. Yang H, Hitchcock E, Haldeman S, et al: Workplace psychosocial and organizational factors for neck pain in workers in the United States. *Am J Ind Med* 2016;59(7):549-560.

   Intervention programs that address issues related to workplace risk factors may be beneficial for workers with neck pain. Future studies should examine psychosocial risk factors and physical risk factors.

9. Lee H, Hübscher M, Moseley GL, et al: How does pain lead to disability? A systematic review and meta-analysis of mediation studies in people with back and neck pain. *Pain* 2015;156(6):988-997.

   This systematic review and meta-analysis was designed to identify and examine the extent to which putative mediators explain the effect of pain on disability in people with low back pain or neck pain. The methodologic quality of these studies was low; however, the results suggest substantial mediating effects of self-efficacy, psychologic distress, and fear, which underpin the direct targeting of these constructs in treatment.

10. Weiner BK, Black KP, Gish J: Access to spine care for the poor and near poor. *Spine J* 2009;9(3):221-224.

11. Epstein NE: It is easier to confuse a jury than convince a judge: The crisis in medical malpractice. *Spine (Phila Pa 1976)* 2002;27(22):2425-2430.

12. Martin BI, Deyo RA, Mirza SK, et al: Expenditures and health status among adults with back and neck problems. *JAMA* 2008;299(6):656-664.

13. Manchikanti L, Helm S II, Fellows B, et al: Opioid epidemic in the United States. *Pain Physician* 2012;15 (3 suppl):ES9-ES38.

   The use of therapeutic opioids is escalating. Narcotic analgesic prescriptions now exceed 238 million prescriptions. Opioid analgesics are now responsible for more deaths than the number of deaths from both suicide and motor vehicle crashes, or deaths from cocaine and heroin combined.

14. Langreth R: Why you should never get fusion surgery for plain back pain. (2011). Available at: https://www. forbes.com/sites/robertlangreth/2011/01/10/why-you-should-never-get-fusion-surgery-for-plain-back-pain/#559714bb519d. Accessed February 27, 2017.

15. Shanafelt TD, Balch CM, Bechamps GJ, et al: Burnout and career satisfaction among American surgeons. *Ann Surg* 2009;250(3):463-471.

16. Peterson LE, Baxley E, Jaén CR, Phillips RL: Fewer family physicians are in solo practices. *J Am Board Fam Med* 2015;28(1):11-12.

   During the past 20 years, there has been a trend toward fewer family physicians identifying as being in solo practice. The reasons for this decline and its effect on access to care should be studied because rural areas are more dependent on solo practitioners.

17. Ariely D, Lanier WL: Disturbing trends in physician burnout and satisfaction with work-life balance: Dealing with malady among the nation's healers. *Mayo Clin Proc* 2015;90(12):1593-1596.

   A main reason for burnout and dissatisfaction with the current health management system among physicians arises from the view of the practice of medicine as a production function as opposed to as a research and development activity.

18. McAbee JH, Ragel BT, McCartney S, et al: Factors associated with career satisfaction and burnout among US neurosurgeons: Results of a nationwide survey. *J Neurosurg* 2015;123(1):161-173.

   The rate of burnout was high in this survey study of US neurosurgeons. The negative effects of burnout on the lives of surgeons, patients, and their families require further study and will probably necessitate the development of interventional programs at local, regional, and even national levels.

19. Lubelski D, Williams SK, O'Rourke C, et al: Differences in the surgical treatment of lower back pain among spine surgeons in the United States. *Spine (Phila Pa 1976)* 2016;41(11):978-986.

   Substantial differences exist among US spine surgeons in the treatment of LBP. These differences are associated with the geographic location of the practice, the specialty, the practice type, and fellowship training.

20. Diaz JA, Griffith RA, Ng JJ, Reinert SE, Friedmann PD, Moulton AW: Patients' use of the Internet for medical information. *J Gen Intern Med* 2002;17(3):180-185.

21. Haldeman S, Dagenais S: A supermarket approach to the evidence-informed management of chronic low back pain. *Spine J* 2008;8(1):1-7.

22. Shanafelt TD, Dyrbye LN, Sinsky C, et al: Relationship between clerical burden and characteristics of the electronic environment with physician burnout and professional satisfaction. *Mayo Clin Proc* 2016;91(7):836-848.

   In this large national study, physician satisfaction with EMRs and computerized physician order entry was generally low. Physicians who used EMRs and computerized physician order entry were less satisfied with the amount of time spent on clerical tasks and were more likely to experience professional burnout.

23. Greenwald AS, Bassano A, Wiggins S, Froimson MI: Alternative reimbursement models: bundled payment and beyond: AOA critical issues. *J Bone Joint Surg Am* 2016;98(11):e45.

   Healthcare providers, including orthopaedic surgeons, healthcare professionals at postacute care institutions, and product suppliers, all must help determine strategies for success of reimbursement models included under The Bundled Payments for Care Improvement initiative.

24. Tait RC, Chibnall JT: Racial/ethnic disparities in the assessment and treatment of pain: Psychosocial perspectives. *Am Psychol* 2014;69(2):131-141.

   Racial and ethnic disparities are prevalent throughout the US healthcare system and have proven refractory to change. Such disparities are present in the treatment of patients with chronic pain conditions, which exacts high personal and societal costs.

25. Weeks WB, Ventura J, Justice B, Hsu E, Milstein A: Multistakeholder recommendations for improving value of spine care: Key themes from a roundtable discussion at the 2015 NASS Annual Meeting. *Spine J* 2016;16(7):801-804.

   At the 2015 North American Spine Society Annual Meeting a group of providers, insurers, employers, advocates, and researchers convened to explore methods for improving value of healthcare services for patients with spine-related disorders. Guided by the Institute of Medicine's six aims of care (safe, effective, patient-centered, timely, efficient, and equitable care) the group defined multiple evidence-based approaches to improving value.

26. Cherkin DC, Sherman KJ, Balderson BH, et al: Effect of mindfulness-based stress reduction vs cognitive-behavioral therapy or usual care on back pain and functional

3: Medical Management of Spine Disorders

limitations in adults with chronic low back pain: A randomized clinical trial. *JAMA* 2016;315(12):1240-1249.

Without statistical difference, mindfulness-based stress reduction and cognitive-behavioral therapy resulted in greater improvement at 26 weeks than usual care. Mindfulness-based stress reduction may be an effective care for chronic low back pain.

27. Should mindfulness meditation be a standard treatment for chronic low back pain? The Back Letter. 2016;31(6):61-69. Available at: http://journals.lww.com/backletter/ Citation/2016/06000/Should_Mindfulness_Meditation_ Be_a_Standard.1.aspx. Accessed February 27, 2017.

28. Hock D: *One From Many: VISA and the Rise of the Chaordic Organizations* .San Francisco, CA, Berret-Koehler Publishers, 2005.

29. Waddel G: *The Back Pain Revolution* ,ed 2. Edinburgh, Churchill-Livingstone Publishers, 2004.

30. Mixter WJ, Barr JS: Herniation or rupture of the intervertebral disk with involvement of the spinal canal. *N Engl J Med* 1934;211:210-215.

31. Rajaee SS, Bae HW, Kanim LE, Delamarter RB: Spinal fusion in the United States: Analysis of trends from 1998 to 2008. *Spine (Phila Pa 1976)* 2012;37(1):67-76.

The frequency, utilization, and hospital charges for spinal fusion have increased at a higher rate than other notable inpatient procedures from 1998 to 2008.

32. Constitution of the World Health Organization: Principles. World Health Organization website. Available at: http:// www.who.int/about/mission/en/. Accessed February 14, 2017.

33. Eisenberg DM, Kessler RC, Foster C, Norlock FE, Calkins DR, Delbanco TL: Unconventional medicine in the United States. Prevalence, costs, and patterns of use. *N Engl J Med* 1993;328(4):246-252.

34. Engel GL: The need for a new medical model: A challenge for biomedicine. *Science* 1977;196(4286):129-136.

35. Waddell G, Bircher M, Finlayson D, Main CJ: Symptoms and signs: Physical disease or illness behaviour? *Br Med J (Clin Res Ed)* 1984;289(6447):739-741.

36. Zusman M: Belief reinforcement: One reason why costs for low back pain have not decreased. *J Multidiscip Healthc* 2013;6:197-204.

Several large-scale education programs were recently developed in different countries to align knowledge of the public (including general practitioners) with evidence-based best practice. The aim was to change beliefs (such as dysfunctional patient behavior and biomedical practice on the part of clinicians); however, these programs had no influence on behavior or costs in three of the four countries in which they were implemented. One suggested reason for the overall lack of success is that altering the potentially disabling belief among the lay public that low back pain has a structural mechanical cause is extremely difficult.

37. Wager TD, Atlas LY, Lindquist MA, Roy M, Woo CW, Kross E: An fMRI-based neurologic signature of physical pain. *N Engl J Med* 2013;368(15):1388-1397.

The authors describe a functional MRI neurologic signature that discriminates between the sensations of painful heat and nonpainful heat and is specific for physical pain.

38. Chou R, Loeser JD, Owens DK, et al; American Pain Society Low Back Pain Guideline Panel: Interventional therapies, surgery, and interdisciplinary rehabilitation for low back pain: An evidence-based clinical practice guideline from the American Pain Society. *Spine (Phila Pa 1976)* 2009;34(10):1066-1077.

39. Nijs J, Paul van Wilgen C, Van Oosterwijck J, van Ittersum M, Meeus M: How to explain central sensitization to patients with 'unexplained' chronic musculoskeletal pain: Practice guidelines. *Man Ther* 2011;16(5):413-418.

Prior to commencing rehabilitation in cases of unexplained chronic musculoskeletal pain, maladaptive illness perceptions must be changed to alter maladaptive pain cognitions and reconceptualize pain. This can be accomplished by patient education about pain physiology, a continuous process initiated during the educational sessions and continued within both the active treatment and during longer term rehabilitation.

40. Petit A, Roche-Leboucher G, Bontoux L, et al: Effectiveness of three treatment strategies on occupational limitations and quality of life for patients with non-specific chronic low back pain: Is a multidisciplinary approach the key feature to success. Study protocol for a randomized controlled trial. *BMC Musculoskelet Disord* 2014;15:131.

In this report, a multidisciplinary approach is hypothesized as the key feature to success in reducing social and occupational impairment in patients with chronic low back pain. It is possible to achieve the same results with less intensive strategies if a multidisciplinary approach is maintained.

41. Fritz JM, Delitto A, Erhard RE: Comparison of classification-based physical therapy with therapy based on clinical practice guidelines for patients with acute low back pain: A randomized clinical trial. *Spine (Phila Pa 1976)* 2003;28(13):1363-1371, discussion 1372.

42. Main CJ, Sowden G, Hill JC, Watson PJ, Hay EM: Integrating physical and psychological approaches to treatment in low back pain: The development and content of the STarT Back trial's 'high-risk' intervention (StarT Back; ISRCTN 37113406). *Physiotherapy* 2012;98(2):110-116.

A screening and targeted approach was found to be more effective and cost-effective in treating low back pain than current best practice. Three different interventions targeted patients identified at low, medium, or high risk depending on the presence of psychosocial risk factors. The authors describe the development and content of the STarT Back trial's high-risk intervention in the context of a systematic approach, termed psychologically informed practice.

43. Schmale GA: More evidence of educational inadequacies in musculoskeletal medicine. *Clin Orthop Relat Res* 2005;437:251-259.

44. Horn ME, Brennan GP, George SZ, Harman JS, Bishop MD: A value proposition for early physical therapist management of neck pain: A retrospective cohort analysis. *BMC Health Serv Res* 2016;16:253.

    This study found that healthcare systems that provide pathways for patients to receive early physical therapy for neck pain may realize improved patient outcomes, greater value, and higher efficiency in decreasing disability and pain compared with delayed management. Additional studies are needed.

45. Cartmill C, Soklaridis S, David Cassidy J: Transdisciplinary teamwork: The experience of clinicians at a functional restoration program. *J Occup Rehabil* 2011;21(1):1-8.

    This study reported that transdisciplinary teams with multiple healthcare providers are suitable for treating patients with complex needs and with chronic injuries. Input from organizational and communication levels is required to effectively contribute to both clinician satisfaction and to improved coordination in patient care.

46. Ruddy G, Rhee K: Transdisciplinary teams in primary care for the underserved: A literature review. *J Health Care Poor Underserved* 2005;16(2):248-256.

47. Chaordic Commons: Six Lenses on Organization. Available at: http://www.chaordic.org. Accessed January 23, 2017.

48. Waldstein SR, Neumann SA, Drossman DA, Novack DH: Teaching psychosomatic (biopsychosocial) medicine in United States medical schools: Survey findings. *Psychosom Med* 2001;63(3):335-343.

49. Linton SJ, Boersma K, Traczyk M, Shaw W, Nicholas M: Early workplace communication and problem solving to prevent back disability: Results of a randomized controlled trial among high-risk workers and their supervisors. *J Occup Rehabil* 2016;26(2):150-159.

    Interventions aimed at both the worker and the workplace achieved substantially larger improvements in work absence caused by pain, health perception, and healthcare use than usual treatment in workers at high risk for disability from back pain.

50. Rempel J, Busse JW, Drew B, et al: Patients' attitudes toward nonphysician screening of low back and low back related leg pain complaints referred for surgical assessment. *Spine (Phila Pa 1976)* 2017;42(5):E288-E293.

    Patients referred for surgical consultation for low back pain or low back–related leg pain are largely willing to accept screening by nonphysician healthcare providers.

51. Nakashima H, Yukawa Y, Suda K, Yamagata M, Ueta T, Kato F: Abnormal findings on magnetic resonance images of the cervical spines in 1211 asymptomatic subjects. *Spine (Phila Pa 1976)* 2015;40(6):392-398.

    Cervical disk bulging, spinal cord compression, and increased signal intensity changes were evaluated with cervical MRI for 1,211 healthy volunteers. Disk bulging, spinal cord compression, and increased signal intensity were found in 87.6%, 5.3%, and 2.3% subjects, respectively. The frequency of spinal cord compression and increased signal intensity increased after age 50 years.

52. Karlen E, McCathie B: Implementation of a quality improvement process aimed to deliver higher-value physical therapy for patients with low back pain: case report. *Phys Ther* 2015;95(12):1712-1721.

    Implementation of a quality improvement process was measured by year-over-year improved clinical outcomes, decreased utilization, and increased adherence to evidence-based physical therapy, which was associated with higher-value care.

53. Dunstan DA, Covic T: Compensable work disability management: A literature review of biopsychosocial perspectives. *Aust Occup Ther J* 2006;53(2):67-77.

54. Rossi VJ, Ahn J, Bohl DD, Tabaraee E, Singh K: Economic factors in the future delivery of spinal healthcare. *World J Orthop* 2015;6(5):409-412.

    The bundled episode reimbursement has gained popularity as a potential alternative to the current fee-for-service system. In the newer model, the spine surgeon will become increasingly responsible for controlling costs. The evolving interests of hospital systems could result in the devaluation of the surgeons' services. Buy-in by all involved healthcare providers will be necessary to ensure that quality of care does not suffer while efforts for cost containment continue.

3: Medical Management of Spine Disorders

Chapter 10

Interdisciplinary Care for Lumbar Spine Disorders

Michael L. Reed, DPT, OCS   S. Raymond Golish, MD, PhD, MBA   Jerome Schofferman, MD

Abstract

Spinal impairment is the leading cause of disability worldwide, with lumbar spine–related problems the most common cause of disability among all the axial skeletal disorders. The medical and socioeconomic burdens of spinal disorders have outpaced those related to depressive disorders, cardiac syndromes, chronic obstructive pulmonary disease, migraines, diabetes, and falls. Although specialties in other fields such as cardiology have successfully reduced disease-related disability rates, spine specialists have not achieved the same success. The incidence of spinal disability has continued to escalate despite advances in diagnostics and nonsurgical and surgical care.

It is helpful to be familiar with the potential stakeholders involved in an episode of spine-related dysfunction and to explore the needs and expectations of the stakeholder groups and the value proposition for each in a coordinated system of care. Understanding the interdisciplinary model of care for patients with spinal disorders, evidence for and against an interdisciplinary care system, established guidelines that support the concept of an integrated model, along with an examination of organizations that have achieved extraordinary success by establishing their own versions of an interdisciplinary process of spine care will benefit those who care for patients with lumbar spine disorders. Physicians also should be familiar with the role of medication in the care of patients with acute and chronic low back pain.

Keywords: antidepressant; anti-inflammatory drug; interdisciplinary; lumbar spine; medication; multidisciplinary; NSAID; patient navigator; patient triage; performance improvement; opioid; stakeholder; value equation; value proposition

Dr. Reed or an immediate family member serves as a board member, owner, officer, or committee member of the North American Spine Society. Dr. Golish or an immediate family member serves as a paid consultant to the FDA, Icotec AG, Intrinsic Therapeutics, Medacta, and Simplify Medical; serves as an unpaid consultant to and has stock or stock options held in Cytonics; and serves as a board member, owner, officer, or committee member of the American Academy of Orthopaedic Surgeons, ASTM International, and the North American Spine Foundation. Dr. Schofferman or an immediate family member serves as a board member, owner, officer, or committee member of the North American Spine Society.

Introduction

In the United States, 51 million individuals report having a disability, of which 14 million (27.5%) report spine impairment as the primary cause.[1] Disabled individuals are 71% more likely to experience an economic decline to the poverty level compared with their healthy peers.[2] Spine-related impairment is the most common cause of disability in the United States.[3,4]

In the United States, $357 billion of public funds is spent annually supporting those who are disabled.[5] Total costs associated with spine-related impairment in the United States have been estimated at between $253 billion and $600 billion, which represents a cost increase of at least 91% in just over a decade.[6] Over the past 20 years, the cost of spine-related impairment and associated musculoskeletal disorders has escalated by nearly four times the rate of increase in the gross domestic product.[6] Sixty-six percent of the total cost associated with spine-related impairment in the United States is attributed to productivity loss and absenteeism, which accounts for annual losses for US employers of $28 billion.[5,7]

3: Medical Management of Spine Disorders

The Social Security Disability Insurance Program pays out $144 billion per year, with approximately $40 billion paid to beneficiaries with spine-related impairments.[1,8] The total number of these beneficiaries increased by 43% between 2003 and 2013.[9] Approximately 40% of work absence is caused by back pain, and 20% of those with spine pain report they cannot continue working.[10] Back pain caused 671 million bed days and 385 million lost work days in 2008.[11] Spine-related impairment affects women more frequently than men.[6]

Spine impairment is currently the leading cause of disability of veterans of the US Army.[12] During deployment, 7% of noncombat-related medical evacuations are for episodes of spinal pain, which is the most common cause.[13] Among Iraq and Afghanistan veterans, 10 times as many discharges from the military occurred because of long-term spine pain that was unrelated to a combat injury compared with discharges that were attributed to blast injuries.[14]

Millions of children have spine deformities and conditions that reduce their quality of life and longevity, with 94% of children with spine-related impairment reporting some level of associated disability.[15,16] The relative risk of becoming disabled for a young individual of working age in the United States is 25%.[17] It is estimated that 30.7% of occupational disability claims are related to musculoskeletal disorders, and most can be attributed to spine-related complaints.[18]

The evolving value-based medical system is encouraging spine specialists and spine care delivery systems to become better integrated, coordinated, efficient, and cost-effective. Along with patients and their families, many other stakeholders are now demanding meaningful, measurable, and rapid improvement in spine care outcomes and associated costs. An aging population, the increase in the number of beneficiaries covered under the Patient Protection and Affordable Care Act, and a contracting physician workforce have resulted in an urgent need for effective and less expensive interdisciplinary spine care.

Having a comprehensive platform of primary care support in a medical system is the most critical step to ensuring appropriate and efficient management of community health and wellness.[19] Leveraging the support of ancillary providers within a primary care hub in coordination with primary physicians and information systems can secure adequate access and coordinated care resulting in optimal care quality, reduced utilization, and improved cost control. Access, reassurance, education, alignment of expectations, care coordination, intraprofessional and extraprofessional communication, outcomes tracking, and feedback for systematic learning and refinement are all lacking in the current spine management model, except for some notably successful examples.

A "second curve" of change in the delivery of US health care has been described.[20] Silos of traditional specialty departments that grow and contract based on patient demand are antiquated. It is predicted that medical systems will evolve to function as integrated units that collectively and cooperatively manage medical conditions with shared accountability. Value will be derived by ensuring optimal outcomes, efficiently using resources, and coordinating care across various disciplines in a manner that engages patients and their families to be active participants.

Definitions and Distinctions

In any system of shared communication, an established understanding of terminology, meanings, and context is of critical importance. For the purpose of ensuring clarity and preventing misunderstandings, the definitions and distinctions presented in **Table 1** will apply in this chapter.

The differences between the terms "multidisciplinary" and "interdisciplinary" have been described in the literature.[21] Multidisciplinary systems often reference fragmented and uncoordinated patient care through cross referrals between multiple specialties. As a result, the clinical pathways become redundant and costly. More importantly, without adequate care management and communication between and among specialists, patients are ushered down a corridor of care that becomes increasingly more complex, invasive, and expensive. Omissions related to the psychosocial contributing factors may be missed or ignored if they do not fit within a specialty area, leading to unnecessary treatments and chronicity.

Interdisciplinary care now represents the preferred integrated system and has won acclaim from prestigious organizations. In an interdisciplinary care model, despite professional heterogeneity, team members coordinate and communicate the care process through a collaborative and purposeful process. Patients often enter the system early after the onset of spine-related symptoms by interfacing with a spine navigator. This affords the patient an opportunity to receive rapid attention and consideration, regardless of the urgency of the case. Early counsel can mitigate the risk for the development of a chronic issue or disability.[22] The navigator also assumes the responsibility of triage, ensuring that the patient-care pathway is most efficient and follow-through is achieved.

In addition to the navigator role, an interdisciplinary team approach includes a physician team leader who further stratifies a case based on risk (medical comorbidities and psychosocial factors) and assists in team coordination.

Table 1

Definitions of Important Terms/Concepts Related to Interdisciplinary Care

Term or Concept	Working Definition
Extraprofessional team	A team of professionals who are not from the same profession, such as a surgeon, radiologist, neurologist, and nurse collaborating on the same case.
Integrated	To make into a whole by bringing all parts together; unify.
Interdisciplinary team	A group of healthcare professionals from diverse fields who work in a coordinated fashion toward a common goal for the patient.
Intraprofessional team	A team of professionals who are all from the same profession, such as three physical therapists collaborating on the same case.
Multidisciplinary team	A team of professionals including representatives of different disciplines who coordinate the contributions of each profession, which are not considered to overlap, to improve patient care.
Performance improvement	Evaluating organizational processes as a means of identifying opportunities for systematic refinement to enhance efficiency, quality, and cost savings.
Patient navigator	A designated healthcare professional who manages the deliberate organization of patient care activities between two or more participants (including the patient) involved in a patient's care to facilitate the appropriate delivery of healthcare services.
Stakeholder	Any person or party with an interest in the financing, implementation, or outcome of a service, practice, process, or decision related to managing a patient's care.
Value proposition	The promise of the overall experience and resulting benefits that a specific stakeholder can realize from the use or consumption of a product, service, or solution.

By evaluating a patient in a holistic manner—considering all potential contributing domains such as his or her medical, physical, biomechanical, psychosocial, economic, occupational, ergonomic, and goal-related expectations—a targeted and properly planned management program can be developed with all disciplines included, considered, and leveraged, as needed. Using this approach, gaps can be filled before they degrade the care process and the potential outcome.[21]

Stakeholders and Associated Needs

Historically, the primary stakeholders afforded the greatest consideration in the US medical system have included the patients, clinicians, hospitals, medical companies (pharmaceutical and devices), and third-party payers. Given the preponderance of reimbursement arrangements between clinicians and health insurance companies, many business-minded healthcare economists have likened the patient to a "consumer," the third-party payer to a "customer," the clinician to a "service provider," and hospital/medical company to "supplier." These relationships and assumed roles have caused incentives to become misaligned and asynchrony has ensued.

The playing field in medicine has expanded dramatically as patient care has become more holistic. Greater consideration is now given to nontraditional stakeholders, including the patient's family, the primary care physicians, ancillary clinicians, employers, disability insurers, and taxpayers. A closer perspective on the various stakeholders, their potential challenges as they relate to an episode of spine care, and their anticipated needs in an interdisciplinary system is presented in **Table 2**.

Value Proposition

Two important articles published in 2010 described the concept of the value equation, which is some quantifiable measure of outcome quality divided by associated cost (value = outcomes/cost).[23,24] In this formula, an increase in outcome quality and a correlative decrease in cost will increase value. At face value, if the denominator is driven down to just $1 and the numerator is raised as high as possible, then value optimization would be achieved. Unfortunately, depending on who the individual is and the factors that affect his or her perception of value, the metrics input into this equation may not accurately measure applicable value for that individual. In fact, the equation may not reach an equitable level across all potential stakeholder groups. Without a clear understanding of the needs and expectations of all stakeholders considered in balance, an interdisciplinary system might meet the

Table 2

Stakeholder Profiles

Stakeholder	Role	Potential Challenges Related to a Lumbar Spine Episode of Care	Anticipated Needs and Expectations
Patient	Consumer	Prolonged pain and suffering; barriers to access and delayed care; fear, anxiety, and helplessness; confusion and frustration caused by discontinuity of information and messaging; unreasonable recovery expectations; unnecessary occupational absenteeism and presenteeism; functional decline and deconditioning; fragmented care coordination; loss of wages and income; social isolation and dysfunction; unnecessary disability	Ameliorate symptoms and suffering; cure quickly; if condition cannot be cured, help manage the condition; be available when needed; help patient understand the condition and expected course; rapid return to work; ease of communication and care coordination; consistent messaging across clinicians; reasonable cost
Patient's family member	Consumer	Fear, anxiety, and helplessness; confusion and frustration due to discontinuity of information and messaging; unreasonable recovery expectations; loss of family income and financial distress; social isolation and dysfunction	Ameliorate family member's anxiety; be available when needed; help family understand the condition and expected course; rapid return to work; ease of communication and care coordination; consistent messaging across clinicians; reasonable cost
Primary care physician	Provider	Having to properly stratify cases with lumbar-related symptoms; identify relevant red flags; identify factors that might predispose the patient to a prolonged recovery and unnecessary disability; access specialist support, if needed; satisfying the expectations of a patient who is in pain; demand for opiate medication; access to opiate alternatives; time and stress of care coordination; poor patient cooperation and compliance; meeting reporting requirements relative to access to care and associated outcomes; cost overruns and unnecessary staff time; inadequate reimbursement for effort and time expended	A process of stratification and triage; guidance with respect to the identification of red flags; uniform guidelines on cost-efficient pathways; access to reliable specialist's support when needed; access to nonopioid pain management alternatives; ease of communication and care coordination; patient cooperation and compliance; feedback with respect to the outcome of an episode of care; reasonable remuneration for services provided
Spine specialist physician	Provider	Having to properly evaluate patients who may not be candidates for discipline-specific services; unavailable or irrelevant case-related data; nonexistent or inadequate communication between co-treating clinicians; time and stress of care coordination; lack of uniform care management algorithms; difficulty accessing reliable providers that offer best practice approaches; patient cooperation and compliance; meeting reporting requirements relative to access to care and associated outcomes; cost overruns and unnecessary staff time; inadequate reimbursement for effort and time expended	Discipline appropriate referrals; access to relevant data and information on case; ease of communication and care coordination; uniform guidelines on cost-efficient pathways; ensure access to reliable specialist support when needed; patient cooperation and compliance; feedback with respect to the outcome of an episode of care; reasonable remuneration for services provided

Table 2

Stakeholder Profiles (continued)

Stakeholder	Role	Potential Challenges Related to a Lumbar Spine Episode of Care	Anticipated Needs and Expectations
Ancillary clinician	Provider	Having to properly evaluate patients who may not be candidates for discipline-specific services; unavailable or irrelevant case-related data; nonexistent or inadequate communication between co-treating clinicians; time and stress of care coordination; lack of uniform care management algorithms; patient cooperation and compliance; meeting reporting requirements relative to access to care and associated outcomes; cost overruns and unnecessary staff time; inadequate reimbursement for effort and time expended	Discipline appropriate referrals; access to relevant data and information on case; ease of communication and care coordination; uniform guidelines on cost-efficient pathways; ensure access to reliable specialist support when needed; patient cooperation and compliance; feedback with respect to the outcome of an episode of care; reasonable remuneration for services provided
Hospital administrator	Supplier	Inadequate or irrelevant data from referring clinicians; asynchronous diagnostic and treatment algorithms; inadequate or inefficient communication and care coordination; lack of reliable specialist support; poor patient cooperation and compliance; risk of complications and subsequent readmissions; inadequate or incomplete follow-up with respect to outcome; inadequate reimbursement for the provision of services	Access to relevant data and information on case; uniform guidelines on cost-efficient pathways; ease of communication and care coordination; ensure access to reliable specialist support when needed; patient cooperation and compliance; minimize risk of complications and readmissions; feedback with respect to the outcome of an episode of care; reasonable remuneration for resources provided
Medical company	Supplier	Same as that of hospital administrator	Same as that of hospital administrator
Patient's employer	Customer	Fear, anxiety, and helplessness; confusion and frustration caused by discontinuity of information and messaging; unreasonable recovery expectations; unnecessary occupational absenteeism and presenteeism; loss of productivity and income; cost of rehiring and retraining; potential for reduced staff morale	Ameliorate employee's symptoms and suffering so that he or she can return to work; cure employee, quickly; if condition cannot be cured, help employee manage the condition so that he or she can continue to work; be available when needed; help employer understand the condition and expected course; ease of communication and care coordination; consistent messaging across clinicians; reasonable cost, especially for self-insured employers

expectations of some stakeholders and underperform for others within a single episode of care.

By identifying and developing shared goals, all stakeholders can, collectively, properly align efforts that will improve system-wide performance and properly assign accountability.[24] Value in health care cannot be measured only by assessing the patient outcome divided by the monetary expense of care. A medical system devoted to achieving value in this manner will ultimately degrade benefits for the providers, suppliers, payers, and society.

Often, the patient does not play the role of a customer. Rather, through a third-party payer arrangement, the customer role is subordinated to a health insurance company that, in turn, negotiates reimbursement with the providers and suppliers on behalf of their patients and their own third-party payer organizations. Patients simply become

Table 2

Stakeholder Profiles (continued)

Stakeholder	Role	Potential Challenges Related to a Lumbar Spine Episode of Care	Anticipated Needs and Expectations
Third-party payer	Customer	Confusion and frustration caused by discontinuity of information and messaging; unreasonable recovery expectations; fragmented care coordination; unnecessary diagnostic and treatment utilization; unnecessary costs; suboptimal outcomes leading to continued healthcare utilization	Ameliorate beneficiary symptoms and suffering quickly; if condition cannot be cured, help beneficiary manage the condition in a self-sufficient manner; be available when needed by the beneficiary; ease of communication and care coordination; consistent messaging across clinicians; reasonable and predictable cost, using the minimal amount of resources to secure an optimal outcome
Disability insurer	Customer	Confusion and frustration caused by discontinuity of information and messaging; unreasonable recovery expectations; unnecessary occupational absenteeism; functional decline and deconditioning; fragmented care coordination; loss of wages and income; unnecessary disability	Ameliorate beneficiary's symptoms and suffering so that return to work can be achieved; if condition cannot be cured, help the beneficiary manage the condition so that he or she can continue to work; be available when needed by beneficiary; ease of communication and care coordination; consistent messaging across clinicians
Taxpayer	Customer	Inefficient and ineffective care delivery system; overutilization of declining resources; unnecessary cost caused by delayed care; inadequate management; prolonged treatment, work loss, reduced productivity, and disability	Ameliorate the patient's symptoms and suffering; quickly cure the patient; if the patient cannot be cured, help the patient manage the condition in a self-sufficient manner; help the patient return to work and avoid disability; be available when the patient needs help; ease of communication and care coordination; consistent messaging across clinicians; reasonable and predictable cost, using the minimal amount of resources to secure an optimal outcome

the consumers of healthcare services and products and relinquish their authority to control the cost of their care; in addition, they are not incentivized to critically evaluate the need for services. Often, patients attempt to access the maximum amount of available resources permitted by the third-party payer; this strategy potentially increases associated costs and negatively affects the value equation. Until the consumer and customer are synchronized and aligned, providers and suppliers will struggle to enhance the value equation. Clearly, optimizing care quality and cost-efficiency will enhance value; however, the formula for value determination must consider the proposition of a favorable return on investment for all stakeholders, including the US taxpayer.

With respect to multidisciplinary integration, the derived value of care should be referenced against the collective effort rather than one particular service provider or intervention.[24] The team should get the credit, not just one player. The need for focused factories is disputed, and integrated systems where accountability can only be attributed to the whole process is championed. Although this perspective has been widely praised and supported, the prospect of creating an interdisciplinary system must deliver more than just the best care at the lowest cost. Rather, the needs and expectations of providers and suppliers also must be considered. In doing so, all stakeholders will be incentivized to create interdisciplinary systems of care integration that are balanced with respect to shared value.

A 2014 article offers an important perspective regarding value and cost-effectiveness.[25] Most healthcare institutions and providers consider individual patient preferences and available resources as the guiding factors in determining the appropriateness of medical interventions.

However, societal preferences supported by the general public are more suitable. If the taxpayer is considered a customer stakeholder, the value proposition of an interdisciplinary model should favor the needs and expectations of those who are making provisions to fund health care. From this standpoint, the value proposition would best be calculated in a manner that considers the needs and contributions attributable to all stakeholders, not just individual patients, providers, or payers.

Assuming successful implementation of an interdisciplinary system of care for lumbar disorders, **Table 3** outlines the expected value proposition for each stakeholder previously identified in this chapter. This list and the associated deliverables may not be exhaustive. Many factors, including unique geographic, occupational, economic, social, and cultural idiosyncrasies, will influence the particular characteristics of each group. The diversity and variability among stakeholders necessitates special interdisciplinary consideration and attention.

Evidence for Interdisciplinary Care for Spine Disorders

Ascertaining the presence of red flags such as severe or rapidly progressing neurologic compromise, a history of major trauma, or atypical symptoms has been one of the primary justifications for early intervention. On the one hand, these red flag issues are relatively rare and, in most instances, patients seek urgent care when these problems occur. On the other hand, patients who are at a high risk for the development of a chronic or disabling disorder because of poor coping strategies, unreasonable recovery expectations, anxiety, depression, occupational stress, or social factors may require early intervention. Patients in whom chronic low back pain (LBP) develops have a greater frequency of comorbid psychological conditions such as depression and anxiety.[26] The cost burden for these patients also is much higher because resource utilization is much greater than that of control patients. Given the fact that 7.6 million adults in the United States report having a chronic and disabling low back issue, the influence and management of nonmedical factors make early access to care a priority for this patient population. Early intervention can mitigate the effect of psychosocial factors, prevent inappropriate coping strategies caused by hopelessness and fear, and expedite return to work.[27]

Early intervention combined with risk stratification implemented by either primary care physicians or a frontline patient navigator is an expanding model throughout the United States.[28] A risk stratified tool called the Keele STarT Back Screening Tool is a simple prognostic questionnaire that helps clinicians identify modifiable risk factors (biomedical, psychological, and social) for back pain disability. This tool was used in a multipractice study. The resulting questionnaire score was used to stratify patients into low-, medium-, or high-risk categories. A 2014 study compared usual medical management to stratified care of patients with LBP.[29] A total of 1,647 adults with LBP participated in the study. Results showed that, compared with traditional care, patients who received stratified care had substantially less disability, 50% less time off from work, and used fewer healthcare services. Other studies on stratified primary care management support these findings.[30,31]

If initial single provider care is unsuccessful in patients with nonradicular low back symptoms, consensus exists that these patients can benefit considerably from an interdisciplinary approach.[32,33] Patients who might traditionally be considered surgical candidates because of the failure of typical single-provider care often decline surgery when provided functionally based interdisciplinary rehabilitation.[34] Stronger support of risk stratification, triage, and early interdisciplinary care has been reported in studies that have shown that a structured clinical pathway can lead to a reduction in inappropriate referrals to spine surgeons while maintaining surgical candidate volume.[35,36] Proper vetting of a patient before consultation with a surgeon is a meaningful and valuable process outcome because the surgeon's time is better spent with a patient who is an appropriate surgical candidate.

In a 2015 study, 41 trials consisting of 6,858 subjects were analyzed to determine the efficacy of an integrated biopsychosocial rehabilitation program for patients with chronic LBP.[37] Participants had a mean duration of LBP of more than 1 year, and nonsurgical treatment had been unsuccessful. The authors found moderate-quality evidence in support of an integrated model of care with respect to improvements in pain and daily function when compared with usual care. In addition, moderate evidence showed that the collaborative approach doubled the likelihood that a patient would return to work within 6 to 12 months compared with the comparison group.

Evidence Against Interdisciplinary Care for Spine Disorders

Despite the various advantages and benefits previously described in this chapter, some notable caveats exist. When evaluating the value proposition for all stakeholders as opposed to the patient only, the return on an investment may not be as favorable for all the stakeholders. For example, in medical surgical progressive care units, patient navigators have contributed to improvements in patient safety, fewer complications, and reduced readmission

Table 3

Value Propositions

Stakeholder	Value Proposition
Patient	Early intervention and counsel
	Reassurance and support
	Opportunity to properly align expectations before irrational overlay
	Identification of urgent care needs
	Strategies to manage symptoms in a proactive manner
	Prevention of chronicity and/or disability through identification of high-risk patients
	Early identification and management of patients that may need long-term monitoring
	Enhanced education with consistent messaging through continuum of care
	Ease of communication and care coordination
	Expedited return to work
	Prevention of functional decline and deconditioning
	Preservation of income and socioeconomic viability
	Uniform and cost-efficient management
Patient's family member	Early intervention and counsel
	Enhanced education with consistent messaging through continuum of care
	Ease of communication and care coordination
	Expedited return to work
	Prevention of functional decline and deconditioning
	Preservation of income and socioeconomic viability
	Uniform and cost-efficient management
Primary care physician	Team-established process of stratification and triage
	Clear understanding of red flags and identification strategies
	Team-established guidelines for cost-efficient pathways
	Access to reliable specialist support, when needed
	Access to nonopioid pain management alternatives
	Ease of communication and care coordination
	Enhanced patient cooperation and compliance
	Feedback with respect to the outcome of an episode of care
	Enhanced remuneration for services provided
Spine specialist physician	Discipline appropriate referrals, optimizing time and effort
	Access to relevant data and information on case
	Ease of communication and care coordination
	Team-established guidelines for cost-efficient pathways
	Access to reliable specialist support, when needed
	Enhanced patient cooperation and compliance
	Feedback with respect to the outcome of an episode of care
	Optimized remuneration for services provided
Ancillary clinician	Same as that of spine specialist physician

rates; however, patient satisfaction ratings were shown to be reduced in programs that leverage midlevel support as first responders.[28]

In a 2016 study, 58 patients were randomly assigned to two groups. One group was examined within 2 weeks of the onset of LBP and were deemed to have received early intervention.[38] The comparison group remained on a waiting list for 12 weeks before consultation. Both groups received the same intervention, which consisted of an outpatient, intensive back school. Although the study authors acknowledged that this preliminary study was underpowered, they reported that both groups had an equitable amount of lost work days. Despite this finding, study limitations include the small number of patients,

Table 3

Value Propositions (continued)

Stakeholder	Value Proposition
Hospital administrator	Access to relevant data and information on case
	Team-established guidelines for cost-efficient pathways
	Ease of communication and care coordination
	Ensure access to reliable specialist support when needed
	Enhanced patient cooperation and compliance
	Mitigated risk of complications and readmissions
	Feedback with respect to the outcome of an episode of care
	Optimized remuneration for resources provided
Medical company	Same as that of hospital administrator
Patient's employer	Early intervention, enhancing patient understanding of condition and appropriateness of return to work strategies
	Enhanced understanding of the condition and expected course
	Decreased absenteeism and enhanced productivity
	Ease of communication and care coordination
	Consistent messaging
	Reasonable cost, especially for self-insured employers
Third-party payer	Early intervention and counsel
	Timely attention to benefactor's symptoms and suffering
	Enhanced management of the condition in a self-sufficient manner
	Ease of communication and care coordination
	Consistent messaging across clinicians
	Reasonable and predictable cost, using the minimal amount of resources to secure an optimal outcome
Disability insurer	Early intervention and counsel
	Timely attention to benefactor's symptoms and suffering
	Enhanced management of the condition in a self-sufficient manner
	Expedited return to work
	Reduced absenteeism
	Increased productivity
	Ease of communication and care coordination
	Consistent messaging across clinicians
Taxpayer	Early intervention and counsel
	Timely attention to patient symptoms and suffering
	Improved care management and service delivery
	Enhanced management of the condition in a self-sufficient manner
	Expedited return to work
	Prevention of work loss and disability
	Reasonable and predictable cost, using the minimal amount of resources to secure an optimal outcome

the author's definition of "early" with respect to waiting time, and the homogenous method of intervention.

In a study of 351 employees that were listed as sick because of LBP, a brief intervention with reassuring advice was compared with a multidisciplinary intervention involving a team of spine specialists and a case manager.[39] The treatment costs, volume of healthcare utilization, and amount of sick leave were calculated to determine the cost-effectiveness of the two approaches. Results showed that the brief intervention with reassurance led to fewer sick leave weeks and considerably less cost. The only subgroup that seemed to benefit from the multidisciplinary approach were sick-listed employees who had a self-perceived risk of job loss and feelings of little influence over their work situation. It is possible that this program may have had greater success with an upfront triage and stratification process, or it may show that many patients do well with reassurance and self-care.

Despite the general acceptance and support among spine specialists for incorporating a biopsychosocial approach, there remains a paucity of integrated programs throughout the United States. Barriers to incorporation may include fear of autonomy loss by providers, lack of understanding with respect to interdisciplinary roles, limited professional resources, inadequate leadership, difficulty staying up-to-date on the latest advances, implementing electronic medical record solutions, and capitalizing anticipated upfront costs. In a constantly changing and complex medical system with evolving regulations, the need to care for an increasing number of patients, and the increasing documentation required for each patient, the prospect of adopting a new, integrated system may be too daunting for many practitioners to consider.[40]

Discussion: Evidence for and Against Interdisciplinary Care

Considering the evidence both for and against interdisciplinary care for lumbar disorders, the preponderance of data suggests that an integrated model can better meet the needs of all stakeholders in several expectation domains. Extra effort is required to ensure that patients are fully satisfied with the level of attention they are receiving in an early interventional triaged process. Some reported deficiencies might reflect unsettled emotional attachment to the traditional model of seeing a doctor as the frontline care provider versus being treated using a nontraditional triage process in which a midlevel clinician or ancillary specialist serves as the first point of contact.

Using the literature, the status of achieving the previously proposed value proposition for each stakeholder can be evaluated. Clearly, more research is required to examine the expectations of each stakeholder in an integrated model and to verify that all aspects of the value proposition are being achieved.

Consensus Guidelines

It is interesting to consider the needs of all stakeholder groups as those needs pertain to clinical guidelines. If providers and suppliers are aware of their consumer and customer assumptions, the clinical guidelines used to meet those needs will be more meaningful, relevant, and impactful. One study examined the understanding of patients and the public regarding clinical guidelines, what patients and the public expected to be included in a clinical guideline to help support the health care they receive, and the decisions they make about diagnostic and treatment choices.[41] The awareness of clinical guidelines was found to be low. Participants expected clinical guidelines to include the presentation and clarification of treatment options, with a provision for some level of expected outcome for each option. In addition, the study participants expressed the need for provider guidance, especially from general practitioners.

In 2007, the American College of Physicians (ACP) collaborated with the American Pain Society (APS) to publish clinical guidelines for the diagnosis and treatment of LBP. Interestingly, these guidelines recommended a triage process, stratification, and identification of symptom severity and neurologic compromise as a means of establishing thresholds to trigger various treatment pathways, along with patient education, evidence-informed decision making, and interdisciplinary care for conditions that are recalcitrant to early nonsurgical treatment.[42]

In 2009, the National Institute for Health and Care Excellence published a guideline on LBP in adults.[43] This guideline references nonspecific LBP of no less than 6 weeks' duration and no more than 12 months' duration. An intent of this guideline is to effectively reduce the effect of nonspecific LBP as it relates to disability and the socioeconomic status of affected individuals. Self-management and education are key recommendations. Having uniform educational messages across the continuum of care is of critical importance. Particular mention is made of an interdisciplinary process whereby communication between the clinicians and patients is uniform, robust, and relevant. Detailed attention to tailoring an approach to the needs of multiple stakeholders, including those of the patient's family, are encouraged. The patient's family is invited to participate in the shared decision-making process.

A systematic review performed to identify international guidelines on the management of nonspecific LBP found that 15 such guidelines were published between 2000 and 2008.[44] The content of those guidelines was noted to be very similar with respect to the use of diagnostic and therapeutic procedures. A common theme of early intervention, optimistic assurance, discouragement of bed rest, consideration of psychosocial factors, multidisciplinary care, and gradual reactivation was reported.

A literature search of articles from 2002 to 2010 identified 13 relevant clinical guidelines on the management of LBP.[45] A universal consensus regarding the use of a triage and stratification process was noted. Generally accepted recommendations were noted for patient education, consideration of psychosocial factors, exercise, and multidisciplinary care management.

In 2016, the Agency for Healthcare Research and Quality published a guideline regarding the medical treatment of LBP.[46] A strong emphasis was placed on early return to work, cessation of ineffective treatments, and provision and documentation of education so that a patient can be an active participant in the decision to pursue a treatment pathway and articulate the purpose of diagnostic and treatment procedures. Most importantly, this guideline encourages an interdisciplinary approach, including psychological or psychosocial evaluations and treatments in patients meeting specific criteria. The guideline specifically states that care management should be driven by interdisciplinary programs that emphasize collective and coordinated evaluations, goal setting, planning, and execution. These programs are designed for patients with complex multifactorial disorders.

Practical Clinical Applications

The goals of any spine care management paradigm are coordination, efficiency, and adequate quality that ensures the most optimal outcome in a cost-effective manner. Some patients need only simple reassurance and encouragement during the natural recovery process and require the attention of a single provider. Others, although more rarely, demand a complex array of medical, pain management, rehabilitation, and psychosocial support services to secure the most desirable outcome. The challenge is determining the proper level of care for each patient, the timing of care, the extent of care, and how to pay for the associated expenses.

Observations and recommendations from a 2008 article about interdisciplinary care at an academic spine center can be adopted by private and group practices, nonacademic hospitals, and within medical communities where providers conduct their business independently but have the resources to collaborate via any number of communication strategies.[47] The keys to success include having a common mission that resonates with the entire interdisciplinary team; integrated scheduling and triage; and leveraging spine specialist physiatrists to screen, classify, and manage a coordinated process of care. In addition, the need to attend to patient expectations and care pathway preferences tempered by evidence-based guidance and cost-effective resources is emphasized. At the spine center described in the study, the members of the interdisciplinary team worked in close proximity to each other and weekly group meetings were held.

A 2013 study used a systematic review of the literature on interdisciplinary teamwork and the perceptions of

253 staff members working in interdisciplinary systems within 11 rehabilitation systems to determine the 10 key factors that characterize a good interdisciplinary system[48] (**Table 4**).

Three well-known organizations, the Texas Back Institute (TBI), the Virginia Mason Medical Center (VMMC), and Dartmouth-Hitchcock Medical Center (DHMC) have successfully implemented integrated interdisciplinary models for the management of lumbar spine disorders.

The TBI model was inspired by a specialty program at Rancho Los Amigos Hospital in California. The founders of the TBI program envisioned an integrated multidisciplinary team in which patients with spine disorders benefit from systematic care coordination and an institutional focus on combining high-quality care with research and public education. By 1982, TBI was garnering national attention that, with time, vaulted the organization to international acclaim. Commonly referred to as the world's best and most impactful "pracademic" (referencing the combination of active clinical practice with research and scientific inquiry) spine center of excellence, the founders created a strong interdisciplinary team, a robust process of coordinated communication and care, and outcomes-driven research. TBI is currently considered one of the most comprehensive interdisciplinary spine specialty institutions in the world.

In 2000, VMMC in Seattle, Washington, developed an innovative performance improvement initiative after recognizing that its traditional fragmented system of care was inefficient and financially not sustainable. This institution created an integrated, interdisciplinary, and value-driven model that achieved extraordinary success and now serves as a model for other US institutions.[49] VMMC made a commitment to ensuring that the organization operated from the top down, with a common vision and mission among local and national leadership to deliver quality health care and service. VMMC performed a comprehensive analysis of its processes and resources to develop a model of "lean" methodology similar to that used by the Toyota Production System, with a determined focus on eliminating waste and inefficiency. The model was called the Virginia Mason Production System; implementation began in 2004. The stated vision and mission and the new process of efficiency achieved enhanced patient outcomes, higher performance ratings, greater employee satisfaction, and fiscal growth. In addition, the system of interdisciplinary care inspired external collaborations with nontraditional stakeholders such as employers, third-party payers, community leaders, and political representatives. This marketplace collaborative led to better aligned expectations and attention to favorable

Table 4

Key Factors That Characterize a Good Interdisciplinary System

Themes	Description
Leadership and management	Having a clear leader of the team, with clear direction and management; democratic; shared power; support/supervision; personal development aligned with line management; leader who acts and listens
Communication	Individuals with communication skills; ensuring that there are appropriate systems to promote communication within the team
Personal rewards, training, and development	Learning; training and development; training and career development opportunities; incorporates individual rewards and opportunity, morale, and motivation
Appropriate resources and procedures	Structures (eg, team meetings, organizational factors, team members working from the same location); ensuring that appropriate procedures are in place to uphold the vision of the service (eg, communication systems, appropriate referral criteria, etc)
Appropriate skill mix	Sufficient/appropriate skills, competencies, practitioner mix, balance of personalities; ability to make the most of other team members' backgrounds; having a full complement of staff, timely replacement/cover for empty or absent posts
Climate	Team culture of trust, valuing contributions, nurturing consensus; need to create an interprofessional atmosphere
Individual characteristics	Knowledge, experience, initiative, knowing strengths and weaknesses, listening skills, reflexive practice; desire to work on the same goals
Clarity of vision	Having a clear set of values that drive the direction of the service and the care provided; portraying a uniform and consistent external image
Quality and outcomes of care	Patient-centered focus; outcomes and satisfaction; encouraging feedback; capturing and recording evidence of the effectiveness of care and using that as part of a feedback cycle to improve care
Respecting and understanding roles	Sharing power; joint working; autonomy

Reproduced with permission from Nancarrow SA, Booth A, Ariss S, Smith T, Enderby P, Roots A: Ten principles of good interdisciplinary team work. *Human Resources for Health* 2013;11:19.

mutual returns on investments, with an enhanced value proposition for all stakeholders.

The marketplace collaborative led to multiple plenary sessions that resulted in the development of "clinical value streams" for various medical conditions that represented high volume, high cost, and inadequate outcomes.[49] These clinical value streams represented optimal care plans and were developed with consideration of the needs of all stakeholders (**Figure 1**). These shared needs formed the definition of quality within the VMMC community collaborative. The five key domains included patient satisfaction, evidence-based care, rapid access to care, rapid return to function, and cost.

Specific to the VMMC value stream for back care, the measurable outputs include more efficient use of physician time, accommodation of a 64% increase in patient volume without the need for extra space, and more efficient billing (an uptick to 58.3 relative value units on an average per day basis compared with 28.1 under the old system).[49] Costs to self-insured employers also decreased. Rapid access to care

resulted in a 50% decrease in lost work days by patients and less use of healthcare resources. For patients requiring spine surgery, the new approach resulted in lower complication rates and enhanced patient safety[50] (**Figure 2**).

The DHMC developed its integrated spine center in collaboration with the Dartmouth Institute and launched the specialized facility in 1997. The mission of the Spine Center is to provide a comprehensive program of interdisciplinary care that is both high quality and cost-efficient.[51] The DHMC Spine Center publicly presents itself as a "one-stop shop" that provides an interdisciplinary experience that is stratified and triaged from the outset. Through this care continuum, 90% of patients complete the care process without needing surgery. The DHMC Spine Center uses a collaborative and cooperative approach that places a high value on team member input and, in turn, leverages the skill sets and knowledge of each team member to the highest level of his or her licensure. The result is an inspired employee and patient experience that is supported by written care

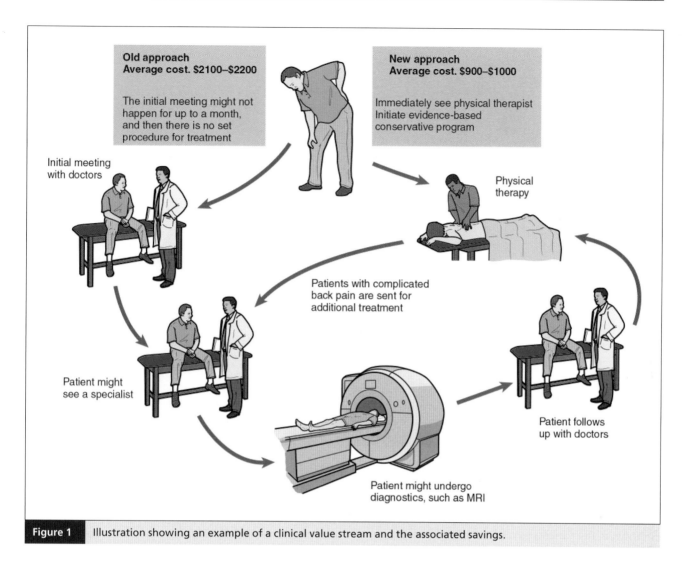

Old approach
Average cost. $2100–$2200

The initial meeting might not happen for up to a month, and then there is no set procedure for treatment

New approach
Average cost. $900–$1000

Immediately see physical therapist
Initiate evidence-based conservative program

Initial meeting with doctors

Physical therapy

Patients with complicated back pain are sent for additional treatment

Patient might see a specialist

Patient follows up with doctors

Patient might undergo diagnostics, such as MRI

Figure 1 Illustration showing an example of a clinical value stream and the associated savings.

pathways, data collection, outcomes analysis, and continuous refinement for performance improvement and enhanced multi-stakeholder value attainment.

The organizational vision of the DHMC Spine Center, the inclusive and collaborative interdisciplinary environment, the recognition of unique and important value propositions specific to all stakeholders, and a culture of objective data collection and analytics have elevated the program to national acclaim and serve as an excellent interdisciplinary model for other US spine programs.

The Role of Medication in Managing Low Back Pain

Medications play a small but often important role in managing both acute and chronic LBP. Some medications are used for both acute and chronic LBP, whereas other medications are used for only acute or only chronic LBP.

Acute Low Back Pain

In patients with acute LBP, medication is used to decrease pain, maintain or improve function, and lessen the chance of progression to a chronic state. To date, most medications have not been shown to improve on the natural history of LBP. Most patients with acute LBP recover fully, but one-third do not recover.[52] Patients with higher levels of initial pain, poorer function, and only minimal pain improvement after 1 week seem to have the worst long-term outcomes.[52] Patients should be reevaluated approximately 1 week after their initial presentation for reassessment of pain, disability, and medication use. If no improvement is seen, a different management approach should be considered.

Acetaminophen

Acetaminophen had been recommended by multiple systematic reviews and guidelines,[42,53] but a recent study showed acetaminophen to be no better than placebo.[54] In

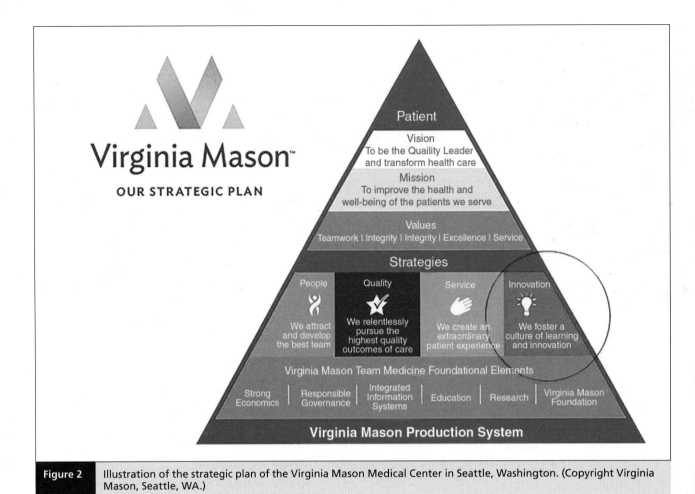

Figure 2 Illustration of the strategic plan of the Virginia Mason Medical Center in Seattle, Washington. (Copyright Virginia Mason, Seattle, WA.)

addition, many patients have already tried acetaminophen and might be skeptical of a physician who recommends this over-the-counter drug.

Nonsteroidal Anti-inflammatory Drugs

NSAIDs are also often recommended, but these drugs cannot be relied on. Some studies and systematic reviews have suggested efficacy (although often without a clinically meaningful improvement) in patients with acute LBP, but others have not.[46,55,56] However, NSAIDs are used frequently to manage LBP and appear to help some patients. No criteria are available that can help in the selection of patients who might have a positive response to NSAIDs.[42,46,53,55,56] It is clear that no one NSAID is better than any other. Side effects of NSAIDs are more common than those of a placebo, but with short-term use, adverse effects are rarely serious. No additional relief is gained by using a skeletal muscle relaxant or low-dose opioid in addition to an NSAID.[57] A reasonable clinical strategy may be to try using an NSAID in low-risk patients. If there is no benefit in approximately 7 days, NSAID use should be discontinued in favor of other medication or nonpharmacologic treatments. For radicular pain, NSAIDs do not appear to be helpful.[58]

Skeletal Muscle Relaxants

Skeletal muscle relaxants are beneficial to some patients with acute LBP and may be appropriate for initial treatment.[59,60] Even with short-term use, adverse side effects, including dyspepsia, sedation, and dizziness are common but usually not serious with short-term use. Elderly patients are quite susceptible to the relaxants' anticholinergic effects, and there is potential for abuse and dependence on these medications. There is no benefit to combining a skeletal muscle relaxant with an NSAID.[57] No single skeletal muscle relaxant is better than another. The use of skeletal muscle relaxants should be limited to 10 to 14 days.

Corticosteroids

Corticosteroids are generally ineffective for acute LBP. A single dose of intravenous dexamethasone can reduce pain for at least 24 hours and reduce the length of stay in the emergency department, but benefits are neither substantial nor sustained.[61] The use of prednisone in the emergency department has not proven helpful.[62]

Opioid Analgesics

Opioid analgesics for acute LBP have not been specifically studied, but opioids have been found to be effective in other acute musculoskeletal conditions.[63] Short-term use of opioids might reduce pain and help maintain function.[64] In a study of early users of opioids, 5% become long-term users, although it is not known whether this resulted from the severity of injury, opioid misuse, addictive disease, or other causes.[65]

After weighing the benefits and risks, it seems reasonable to consider an opioid trial if a patient continues to have moderate to severe pain at approximately 1 week after initial presentation. Prior to initiating opioid treatment, it is appropriate to obtain a history of any opioid, alcohol, or chemical dependence; learn the psychosocial situation of the patient; and consult a state prescription drug-monitoring database. For acute pain, only a short-acting opioid should be used, preferably a drug without acetaminophen. The dose should be sufficient to provide meaningful relief. Low-dose opioids do not add analgesic benefits to naproxen.[57] It is strongly recommended that the initial prescription of opioids be for a maximum of 7 days and only enough to last until a scheduled follow-up visit. The prescription should not be automatically refilled without a patient visit. It is reasonable to assume that it is not the first prescription of the opioid that creates the highest potential for subsequent opioid misuse. Problems are more likely associated with an unwarranted refill, too high a dose, allowing refill without a patient visit, or oversupply without proper disposal.[65]

Other Medications

Other medications such as antidepressants and anticonvulsants do not have a role in managing acute LBP.

Chronic Low Back Pain

Most patients with acute LBP recover in approximately 3 months, although recovery may take up to 6 months in some patients. After 3 months, however, recovery is much less likely. Chronic LBP can be defined as LBP that is present after 3 to 6 months. The pain can be primarily axial, primarily in an extremity, or a combination of both. Causes can be nociceptive, neuropathic, or mixed.[66,67] These distinctions affect the choice of medication.

Acetaminophen

Acetaminophen is not very helpful for chronic LBP, but many patients use it. Because of potential liver toxicity,

patients should be counselled against using more than 2 g of over-the-counter acetaminophen per day. It is especially important to determine if the patient is taking any prescription drugs that also contain acetaminophen.

Nonsteroidal Anti-inflammatory Drugs

It is worthwhile for patients with chronic LBP to try NSAIDs, but benefits and the degree of relief (if any) are unpredictable.[46,68] A small number of patients respond well enough to consider long-term use. However, long-term use has a high potential for adverse effects, some of which can be serious, especially in elderly patients and those with medical comorbidities. After an explanation of risks versus benefits, it seems reasonable to offer a low-risk patient a therapeutic trial of NSAIDs. If a good response occurs, NSAID use can be continued with frequent monitoring of the clinical response along with renal, hepatic, and hematologic laboratory studies.

Skeletal Muscle Relaxants

Because the effectiveness of skeletal muscle relaxants usually wanes after approximately 10 to 14 days, there is limited or no role for this type of medication in chronic LBP, except perhaps for acute flares.

Corticosteroids

No studies are available evaluating corticosteroid use managing chronic LBP. Anecdotally, there are some patients who benefit from oral prednisone for severe flares.

Antidepressants

As opposed to earlier teachings, neither tricyclic antidepressants nor selective serotonergic antidepressants improve pain or function in patients with chronic LBP.[46] However, duloxetine has been shown to lower the intensity of pain and improve function in some patients with unspecified chronic LBP and those with axial and extremity neuropathic pain.[69] It appears that in some patients with chronic axial LBP, the underlying mechanism is neuropathic rather than nociceptive.[68,69] The prevalence of neuropathic pain in chronic axial LBP is reported to be as high as 12% to 37%,[67,70] thus making it an important problem to recognize and treat.

Anticonvulsants

In patients with a neuropathic component to their LBP, anticonvulsants such as pregabalin can be helpful, especially for extremity pain. Pregabalin also can be effective for managing LBP in patients with spinal stenosis by reducing pain and improving walking distance, sleep quality, and gait.[71] However, pregabalin does not appear

Table 5

Relative Indications for Long-Term Opioid Analgesic Therapy

Physician is experienced with long-term opioid analgesic therapy

Patient and physician should have reasonable expectations of ≥ 50% improvement

Chronic pain lasting at least 3 to 6 months

Moderate to severe pain

Low risk of addiction; no prior history of substance abuse

No severe psychological disorder

Identifiable structure or neuropathic disorder, which is not amenable to surgical correction

Refractory to good rehabilitation

Good response to opioid trial

to be effective in patients with sciatica.[72] Topiramate has been useful for some patients with nonspecific chronic LBP as well as patients with neuropathic leg pain.[73]

Opioid Analgesics

Long-term opioid analgesic therapy is fiercely debated. The serious increase in opioid-related deaths, overdoses, and other adverse events has been well publicized in professional journals and the lay press. Few discussions have been published about patients taking opioids who have good pain control, better quality of life, and few adverse events. The lack of evidence regarding the efficacy and safety of long-term opioid analgesic therapy for chronic LBP is well known, but is due in part to the paucity of studies on this subject. A few observational and retrospective studies have suggested longer-term efficacy and safety.[74,75] In well-selected patients, approximately one-third will discontinue opioid use because of side effects, one-third will have limited relief that may not justify continuing opioid therapy, and the remainder will have meaningful improvement.[75] A Cochrane review reiterated that high-quality long-term studies are lacking, but in shorter-term studies of patients with chronic LBP, opioids were better than placebo for pain control and probably for function.[46,76]

Based on the best available evidence, there is a role for long-term opioid analgesic therapy in a small number of well-selected patients with chronic, severe, and refractory spine pain[77-79] (Table 5). After selection, patients should have a trial of opioid use, and only those with meaningful improvement should continue long-term therapy.

It is essential to consider each patient individually and balance potential risks and benefits. Risks to individual patients include death, overdose, addiction, disability, and a path to illegal opioid use. Risks to public health include diversion (purposeful misuse or theft), other adverse events, and increased healthcare and disability costs.[77-79]

Chronic severe intractable pain also has risks, including pain-related disability, decreased quality of life, deteriorating family interactions, psychological disorders, and even suicide.[77] Risks to the public good include lost work along with its sequelae and increased healthcare utilization. It is probably best that patients requiring long-term opioid use be treated by a physician who is experienced in medical pain management.

Summary

A systematic and consistent interdisciplinary process for lumbar spine care that includes objective metrics, meaningful data collection, and actionable analytics can optimize efficiencies, enhance patient outcomes, and decrease costs. Strong and committed leadership is required because a paradigm shift in providing spine care can be unsettling to those accustomed to the fragmented, fee-for-service model. Considering the needs and expectations of all stakeholders and communicating those requirements openly and honestly can overcome many of the barriers to successful implementation.

Efficient and cost-effective interdisciplinary lumbar spine care models incorporate a navigator and uniform thresholds at which spine specialist providers become engaged within the coordinated team. By providing early access to care, patients at risk for the development of chronic and disabling syndromes can be identified early and given appropriate support. Rational self-management can be encouraged, rapid return to function can be achieved, overutilization of healthcare services can be prevented, and optimal outcomes at the lowest expense can be realized.

Customization of an interdisciplinary lumbar spine care model is required for different practice settings, geographic nuances, and cultural distinctions. Proven models of success can serve as a road map in all types of settings, including academic, pracademic, and private practice.

The role of medication in managing both acute and chronic LBP should be considered and used in the proper circumstances and in appropriately selected patients. Medication can aid in reducing pain and restoring function.

With proper leadership, all spine service lines can take part in a system that delivers the highest quality care at the most reasonable costs, with enhanced efficiency and expediency to adequately meet the needs of all stakeholders.

Key Study Points

- A systematic and consistent interdisciplinary process for lumbar spine care that is laden with objective metrics, meaningful data collection, and actionable analytics can optimize efficiencies, enhance patient outcomes, and save money.

- Efficient and cost-effective interdisciplinary lumbar spine care models incorporate a navigator and uniform thresholds at which spine specialist providers become engaged within the coordinated team.

- Staying up to date on the latest advances, caring for an increasing volume of patients, documenting each case, implementing electronic medical record solutions, and maintaining compliance with the ever-changing regulatory mandates make it difficult for spine specialists to effectively participate in an interdisciplinary lumbar spine care model.

- Customization of an interdisciplinary lumbar spine care model is required for different practice settings and geographic nuances.

- In patients with acute LBP, medications can play a meaningful role in reducing pain and restoring function.

- For patients with acute LBP, the choice of medication must be individualized and can include a skeletal muscle relaxant, an NSAID, and an opioid for patients with severe pain.

- For patients with chronic LBP, medications should be part of a program that also includes rehabilitation and possible spinal injections and/or psychological treatment.

- Opioids should be reserved for well-selected patients with severe and refractory LBP; careful follow-up is essential.

Annotated References

1. *Survey of Income and Program Participation 2008 Panel Wave 6 Topical Module Microdata File.* US Census Bureau. Washington, DC, 2014. Available at: http://www.census.gov/content/dam/Census/programs-surveys/sipp/tech-documentation/complete-documents/2008/SIPP%20 2008%20Panel%20Wave%2006%20-%20Topical%20 Module.pdf. Accessed February 21, 2017.

2. Brault MW: *Americans with Disabilities: 2010. Household Economic Studies: Current Population Reports.* US Department of Commerce Economics and Statistics Administration, US Census Bureau, 2012, pp 70-131.

Available at: http://www.census.gov/prod/2012pubs/p70-131.pdf. Accessed February 21, 2017.

This highly regarded resource provides specific data from the 2008 Survey of Income and Program Participation as it relates to the number of individuals with disability and severity prevalence by age, race, type, region, employment, and income level.

3. Ma VY, Chan L, Carruthers KJ: Incidence, prevalence, costs, and impact on disability of common conditions requiring rehabilitation in the United States: Stroke, spinal cord injury, traumatic brain injury, multiple sclerosis, osteoarthritis, rheumatoid arthritis, limb loss, and back pain. *Arch Phys Med Rehabil* 2014;95(5):986-995.e1.

This literature review of 82 articles reported data regarding the incidence, prevalence, costs, and effect of various medical conditions, including back pain. Results showed that back pain and arthritis are the most common conditions and the costliest.

4. Vos T, Flaxman AD, Naghavi M, et al: Years lived with disability (YLDs) for 1160 sequelae of 289 diseases and injuries 1990-2010: A systematic analysis for the Global Burden of Disease Study 2010. *Lancet* 2012;380(9859):2163-2196.

This article examines the renowned Global Burden of Disease study of 2010 and, specifically, the effect of 291 diseases on years lived with disability. The analysis revealed that back pain and neck pain are among the leading worldwide causes of disability.

5. Rizzo JA, Abbott TA III, Berger ML: The labor productivity effects of chronic backache in the United States. *Med Care* 1998;36(10):1471-1488.

6. Andersson G: *The Burden of Musculoskeletal Diseases in the United States: Prevalence, Societal and Economic Cost.* Rosemont, IL, American Academy of Orthopaedic Surgeons, 2008.

7. Katz JN: Lumbar disc disorders and low-back pain: Socioeconomic factors and consequences. *J Bone Joint Surg Am* 2006;88(suppl 2):21-24.

8. DeHaven T: *The Rising Cost of Social Security Disability Insurance.* Cato Institute Policy Analysis No. 733. August 6, 2013. Available at: https://object.cato.org/sites/cato.org/files/pubs/pdf/pa733_web.pdf. Accessed February 21, 2017.

9. US Social Security Administration: Office of Retirement and Disability Policy, Office of Research, Evaluation, and Statistics Annual Statistical Report on the Social Security Disability Insurance Program, 2013. Available at: http://www.socialsecurity.gov/policy/docs/statcomps/di_asr/2013/ Accessed February 21, 2017.

10. Goertz M, Thorson D, Bonsell J, et al; Institute for Clinical Systems Improvement: *Adult Acute and Subacute Low Back Pain.* Updated November 2012. Available at: https://www.icsi.org/_asset/bjvqrj/lbp.pdf. Accessed February 17, 2017.

This article provides a healthcare guideline with algorithmic presentation of the recommended care process for nonspecific LBP, radicular pain, and the identification of red flags. Full referencing, evidence-based grading, and recommendations are provided.

11. Pleis JR, Lucas JW, Ward BW: Summary health statistics for U.S. adults: National Health Interview Survey, 2008. *Vital Health Stat 10* 2009;242:1-157.

12. Patzkowski JC, Rivera JC, Ficke JR, Wenke JC: The changing face of disability in the US Army: The Operation Enduring Freedom and Operation Iraqi Freedom effect. *J Am Acad Orthop Surg* 2012;20(suppl 1):S23-S30.

    In this retrospective review of the entire US Army Physical Evaluation database, medically discharged individuals were identified to determine and compare disabling conditions. Back pain and osteoarthritis were the two most common causes of medical discharge during peacetime and war.

13. Brundage FJ, ed: Low back pain, active component, U.S. Armed Forces, 2000-2009. *Medical Surveillance Monthly Report* 2010;17(7):2-7. Available at http://www.health.mil/Reference-Center/Reports/2010/01/01/Medical-Surveillance-Monthly-Report-Volume-17-Number-7. Accessed February 21, 2017.

14. Blair JA, Patzkowski JC, Schoenfeld AJ, et al; Skeletal Trauma Research Consortium (STReC): Are spine injuries sustained in battle truly different? *Spine J* 2012;12(9):824-829.

    The authors examine the severity and prognosis of battlefield and nonbattlefield spine-related injuries from October 2001 to December 2009. Results showed comparatively disparate spine disorders in both populations, with vastly different long-term prognoses.

15. Jones GT, Macfarlane GJ: Epidemiology of low back pain in children and adolescents. *Arch Dis Child* 2005;90(3):312-316.

16. Watson KD, Papageorgiou AC, Jones GT, et al: Low back pain in schoolchildren: Occurrence and characteristics. *Pain* 2002;97(1-2):87-92.

17. Council for Disability Awareness: Chances of Disability. Updated July 3, 2013. Available at: http://www.disabilitycanhappen.org/chances_disability/disability_stats.asp. Accessed April 11, 2017.

18. Council for Disability Awareness: 2013 Long-Term Disability Claims Review. Available at: http://www.disabilitycanhappen.org/research/CDA_LTD_Claims_Survey_2013.pdf. Accessed April 11, 2017.

19. Schoen C, Osborn R, Squires D, Doty M: *Access, affordability, and insurance complexity are often worse in the United States compared to 10 other countries.* Health Affairs Web First. November 14, 2013. Available at: http://www.commonwealthfund.org/publications/in-the-literature/2013/nov/access-affordability-and-insurance. Accessed February 20, 2017.

    This article summarizes the results of a 2013 survey of 11 industrialized countries, including the United States, to determine adult perspectives on healthcare access, costs, and the utility of the insurance system. Adults in the United States are substantially more likely to complain about all of these factors as they relate to the current medical system and are much more likely to endorse sweeping healthcare reform.

20. Callahan CD, Adair D, Bozic KJ, Manning BT, Saleh JK, Saleh KJ: Orthopaedic surgery under national health reform: An analysis of power, process, adaptation, and leadership. AOA critical issues. *J Bone Joint Surg Am* 2014;96(13):e111.

    The authors present a general review of evolving healthcare reforms, barriers to success, and the driving factors that will force modifications to ensure affordability and appropriate use of available resources.

21. Mayer EA, Mayer TG: The interdisciplinary treatment of patients with chronic pain, in Rao RD, Smuck M, eds: *Orthopaedic Knowledge Update: Spine 4.* Rosemont, IL, American Academy of Orthopaedic Surgeons, 2012, pp 169-180.

    A comprehensive framework is described for managing patients with chronic pain by leveraging multiple disciplines in a process of care coordination that is objective and goal directed. Emphasis is placed on interprofessional communication and cooperation rather than care prescribed in a stepwise and fragmented manner.

22. Donovan M, Khan A, Johnston V: The effect of a workplace-based early intervention program on work-related musculoskeletal compensation outcomes at a poultry meat processing plant. *J Occup Rehabil* 2017;27(1):24-34.

    An 18% reduction in claims and an $831 average cost reduction per claim was achieved by implementing a program of early intervention, triage, reassurance, and onsite physiotherapy at an Australian poultry plant.

23. Porter ME: What is value in health care? *N Engl J Med* 2010;363(26):2477-2481.

24. Porter ME: Measuring health outcomes: The outcome hierarchy. Available at: http://www.academia.edu/2917824/Measuring_health_outcomes_the_outcomes_hierarchy. Accessed April 10, 2017.

25. Resnick DK, Tosteson AN, Groman RF, Ghogawala Z: Setting the equation: Establishing value in spine care. *Spine (Phila Pa 1976)* 2014;39(22 suppl 1):S43-S50.

    Determining value in spine care is complex and burdensome. Simplistic equations that consider a limited dataset related to individual patient outcomes are inadequate when the effect of medical management considers all stakeholders. Legislative actions that lead to meaningful and cost-effective reform must factor in the economic, occupational, and social effects on society.

26. Gore M, Sadosky A, Stacey BR, Tai KS, Leslie D: The burden of chronic low back pain: Clinical comorbidities, treatment patterns, and health care costs in usual care settings. *Spine (Phila Pa 1976)* 2012;37(11):E668-E677.

   This claim-based review of 101,294 patients with chronic LBP compared levels of comorbidity, treatment patterns, healthcare utilization, and direct medical cost with those of a control group. A substantial burden of comorbidity and a relatively higher rate of healthcare utilization and associated cost was found in the patients with chronic LBP compared with the control group.

27. Hoefsmit N, Houkes I, Nijhuis FJ: Intervention characteristics that facilitate return to work after sickness absence: A systematic literature review. *J Occup Rehabil* 2012;22(4):462-477.

   This systematic review examined evidence-based interventions that facilitate return to work after an injury or the onset of symptoms. Early intervention and multidisciplinary care had a positive effect on return to work.

28. Raines DS: *The Impact of the Clinical Nurse Leader/ Navigator on Clinical Outcomes and Patient Satisfaction.* Jacksonville, Florida, University of North Florida, 2013. Thesis.

   The effects of leveraging masters-level–educated nurses to offset the effects of higher patient-to-nurse ratios in a hospital setting are examined. Results showed a positive effect on readmissions and other indicators; however, patient satisfaction was not preserved with relatively lower patient-to-nurse ratios.

29. Foster NE, Mullis R, Hill JC, et al; IMPaCT Back Study team: Effect of stratified care for low back pain in family practice (IMPaCT Back): A prospective population-based sequential comparison. *Ann Fam Med* 2014;12(2):102-111.

   This prospective study compared usual medical management with risk-stratified care using a stratification tool that classified patients based on relative risk for disability. In the 922 patients reviewed, the risk-stratified cohort had less disability, less time off work, and lower costs at the 6-month follow-up compared with the patients who received usual medical management.

30. Whitehurst DG, Bryan S, Lewis M, Hay EM, Mullis R, Foster NE: Implementing stratified primary care management for low back pain: Cost-utility analysis alongside a prospective, population-based, sequential comparison study. *Spine (Phila Pa 1976)* 2015;40(6):405-414.

   A cost-utility analysis was used to compare usual medical management with stratified care of patients with LBP. Results showed cost savings and earlier return to work in the stratified care subgroup. Level of evidence: II.

31. Reiss-Brennan B, Brunisholz KD, Dredge C, et al: Association of integrated team-based care with health care quality, utilization, and cost. *JAMA* 2016;316(8):826-834.

   This retrospective cohort study examined patient outcomes, healthcare utilization, and costs associated with integrated primary care versus the usual care of 113,452 unique patients over a 3-year period. Results demonstrated higher levels of quality of some measures and lower rates of care utilization and costs in patients managed with an integrated primary care process.

32. Mayer TG, Gatchel RJ, Brede E, Theodore BR: Lumbar surgery in work-related chronic low back pain: Can a continuum of care enhance outcomes? *Spine J* 2014;14(2):263-273.

   This prospective cohort study compared socioeconomic and patient-reported outcomes in a workers' compensation patient population. Patients with chronic LBP were divided into two groups—those who had a lumbar fusion procedure and those who had nonfusion lumbar surgery prior to admission to a functional restoration program. Both groups received medically supervised functional restoration. Both groups had similar return-to-work rates and few differences relative to socioeconomic measures.

33. Artner J, Kurz S, Cakir B, Reichel H, Lattig F: Intensive interdisciplinary outpatient pain management program for chronic back pain: A pilot study. *J Pain Res* 2012;5:209-216.

   This retrospective pilot study reported on 160 patients with chronic LBP who underwent a program of comprehensive interdisciplinary care. Results showed significant improvements in pain and self-perceived disability after only 3 weeks of care.

34. Brede E, Mayer TG, Gatchel RJ: Prediction of failure to retain work 1 year after interdisciplinary functional restoration in occupational injuries. *Arch Phys Med Rehabil* 2012;93(2):268-274.

   The authors report on a prospective study of 1,850 patients with a chronic disabling occupational musculoskeletal disorder who underwent interdisciplinary functional restoration treatment. Predictive factors related to posttreatment work retention are identified.

35. Wilgenbusch CS, Wu AS, Fourney DR: Triage of spine surgery referrals through a multidisciplinary care pathway: A value-based comparison with conventional referral processes. *Spine (Phila Pa 1976)* 2014;39 (22 suppl 1):S129-S135.

   This retrospective review of the medical records of patients with LBP examined the likelihood of surgical recommendation in a cohort managed through a multidisciplinary care pathway versus a conventional referral process. The clinical differences between the groups and wait times for diagnostic and surgical considerations also were reviewed. Results showed that the multidisciplinary pathway delivered a greater proportion of surgical candidates and reduced wait times for MRI and surgical assessment. Level of evidence: III.

36. Kindrachuk DR, Fourney DR: Spine surgery referrals redirected through a multidisciplinary care pathway: Effects of nonsurgeon triage including MRI utilization. *J Neurosurg Spine* 2014;20(1):87-92.

The authors report on 87 consecutive patients managed through a process of triage to determine appropriate imaging, surgeon referrals, and cost savings. Results showed reduced rate of MRI use, less inappropriate surgeon referrals, and lower costs.

37. Kamper SJ, Apeldoorn AT, Chiarotto A, et al: Multidisciplinary biopsychosocial rehabilitation for chronic low back pain: Cochrane systematic review and meta-analysis. *BMJ* 2015;350:h444.

This systematic review and meta-analysis of randomized control trials evaluated the effects of multidisciplinary biopsychosocial rehabilitation in patients with chronic LBP. Results showed that this treatment paradigm was more effective than usual care and other therapies.

38. Norbye AD, Omdal AV, Nygaard ME, Romild U, Eldøen G, Midgard R: Do patients with chronic low back pain benefit from early intervention regarding absence from work? A randomized, controlled, single-center pilot study. *Spine (Phila Pa 1976)* 2016;41(21):E1257-E1264.

A single-center, randomized controlled trial that examined the effects of an early intervention for 58 patients with LBP reported that early intervention did not affect return to work and sick leave at a follow-up of 12 months. The authors advocate for a larger sample size of at least 382 patients in future studies.

39. Jensen C, Nielsen CV, Jensen OK, Petersen KD: Cost-effectiveness and cost-benefit analyses of a multidisciplinary intervention compared with a brief intervention to facilitate return to work in sick-listed patients with low back pain. *Spine (Phila Pa 1976)* 2013;38(13):1059-1067.

Multidisciplinary care versus a brief intervention for patients with LBP were compared in this randomized control trial. Outcome measures included costs, utilization of healthcare services, and sick leave benefits used. Results showed higher costs in the multidisciplinary patient group because of greater use of healthcare services by most patients; however, cost savings were observed in a high-risk subgroup of patients. Level of evidence: II.

40. Manning BT, Callahan CD, Robinson BS, Adair D, Saleh KJ: Overcoming resistance to implementation of integrated care pathways in orthopaedics. *J Bone Joint Surg Am* 2013;95(14):e100-e106.

The authors present a general review of evolving healthcare reforms, barriers to success, and forces that will encourage modifications to ensure affordability and appropriate use of available resources. An emphasis is placed on integrated care pathways as a means of mitigating quality degradation and achieving fiscal stability.

41. Fearns N, Kelly J, Callaghan M, et al: What do patients and the public know about clinical practice guidelines and what do they want from them? A qualitative study. *BMC Health Serv Res* 2016;16(1):74.

A survey study of 62 individuals from the general public showed low awareness and understanding of clinical guidelines. However, participants expressed strong interest in any process that would afford them a better understanding of treatment options and potential side effects.

42. Chou R, Qaseem A, Snow V, et al; Clinical Efficacy Assessment Subcommittee of the American College of Physicians; American College of Physicians; American Pain Society Low Back Pain Guidelines Panel: Diagnosis and treatment of low back pain: A joint clinical practice guideline from the American College of Physicians and the American Pain Society. *Ann Intern Med* 2007;147(7):478-491.

ACP and APS guidelines for managing acute and chronic LBP included early testing and imaging and early treatment with exercise, advice, and the administration of medications.

43. Savigny P, Watson P, Underwood M; Guideline Development Group: Early management of persistent non-specific low back pain: Summary of NICE guidance. *BMJ* 2009;338:b1805.

44. Koes BW, van Tulder M, Lin CW, Macedo LG, McAuley J, Maher C: An updated overview of clinical guidelines for the management of non-specific low back pain in primary care. *Eur Spine J* 2010;19(12):2075-2094.

45. Pillastrini P, Gardenghi I, Bonetti F, et al: An updated overview of clinical guidelines for chronic low back pain management in primary care. *Joint Bone Spine* 2012;79(2):176-185.

This systematic review of clinical guidelines published between 2002 and 2010 compared and contrasted recommendations related to the treatment of patients with chronic nonspecific LBP in a primary care setting. Results showed acceptable quality guidelines with patterns of diagnostic and treatment recommendations distinct from those related to acute LBP.

46. Chou R, Deyo R, Friedly J et al. *Noninvasive Treatments for Low Back Pain*. Comparative Effectiveness Review No. 169. AHRQ Publication No. 16-EHC004-EF. Rockville, MD, Agency for Healthcare Research and Quality, 2016. Available at: https://effectivehealthcare.ahrq.gov/ehc/products/553/2192/back-pain-treatment-executive-160922.pdf Accessed February 17, 2017.

This systematic review looked at the evidence for pharmacologic and other nonsurgical treatments of LBP. It is currently the most up-to-date systematic review.

47. Chen JJ, Yang RK: A look inside an interdisciplinary spine center at an academic medical center. *Iowa Orthop J* 2008;28:98-101.

48. Nancarrow SA, Booth A, Ariss S, Smith T, Enderby P, Roots A: Ten principles of good interdisciplinary team work. *Hum Resour Health* 2013;11:19.

This integrated report combined the results of a systematic review of the literature regarding interdisciplinary teamwork and feedback from 253 healthcare providers. Results of this study produced 10 distinct characteristics that can be attributed to highly effective interdisciplinary teams.

49. Blackmore CC, Mecklenburg RS, Kaplan GS: At Virginia Mason, collaboration among providers, employers, and health plans to transform care cut costs and improved quality. *Health Aff (Millwood)* 2011;30(9):1680-1687.

This article describes the integrated process of care developed and used at VMMC. This system resulted in enhanced quality as well as a reduction in unnecessary treatments and costs.

50. Sethi RK, Pong RP, Leveque JC, Dean TC, Olivar SJ, Rupp SM: The Seattle Spine Team approach to adult deformity surgery: A systems-based approach to perioperative care and subsequent reduction in perioperative complication rates. *Spine Deform* 2014;2(2):95-103.

This retrospective review reports on complication rates associated with adult spine deformity surgery in two groups of patients. One group received care via an interdisciplinary process, dual-attending surgeons, and an intraoperative protocol. The other group was managed in a traditional manner with the systematic approach just described. Complication rates were substantially lower in the systematically managed group.

51. Weinstein JN, Brown PW, Hanscom B, Walsh T, Nelson EC: Designing an ambulatory clinical practice for outcomes improvement: From vision to reality—the Spine Center at Dartmouth-Hitchcock, year one. *Qual Manag Health Care* 2000;8(2):1-20.

52. Wirth B, Ehrler M, Humphreys BK: First episode of acute low back pain: An exploratory cluster analysis approach for early detection of unfavorable recovery. *Disabil Rehabil* 2016;19:1-7.

In a cohort of 158 patients with acute LBP followed for 1 year, one-third of the patients did not fully recover. High pain intensity and high disability, particularly when there was minimal pain reduction in the first week tended to predict a poor outcome.

53. Cutforth G, Peter A, Taenzer P: The Alberta Health Technology Assessment (HTA) Ambassador Program: The development of a contextually relevant, multidisciplinary clinical practice guideline for non-specific low back pain: A review. *Physiother Can* 2011;63(3):278-286.

After discovering knowledge gaps in the primary care of patients with LBP, the authors reviewed published clinical care guidelines to construct a point-of-care algorithm that is intended to be "clinician friendly."

54. Williams CM, Maher CG, Latimer J, et al: Efficacy of paracetamol for acute low-back pain: A double-blind, randomised controlled trial. *Lancet* 2014;384(9954):1586-1596.

This important and well-executed study showed that acetaminophen was no more effective than placebo for acute LBP. The incorporation of the results of this study changed some guideline recommendations.

55. Kuritzky L, Samraj GP: Nonsteroidal anti-inflammatory drugs in the treatment of low back pain. *J Pain Res* 2012;5:579-590.

The authors offer a narrative review based on multiple systematic reviews on NSAIDs. They conclude that NSAIDs have a role in acute LBP management but response is not predictable. There are many potential adverse events associated with long-term use.

56. Wong JJ, Côté P, Ameis A, et al: Are non-steroidal anti-inflammatory drugs effective for the management of neck pain and associated disorders, whiplash-associated disorders, or non-specific low back pain? A systematic review of systematic reviews by the Ontario Protocol for Traffic Injury Management (OPTIMa) Collaboration. *Eur Spine J* 2016;25(1):34-61.

This review was commissioned by the Province of Ontario to examine the evidence for neck and LBP treatment after motor vehicle collisions. Some of the conclusions regarding the use of medications differ some from other guidelines as they suggest skeletal muscle relaxants as possible first-line treatment rather than secondary treatment. The study did not find good evidence for the use of NSAIDs for acute spine pain.

57. Friedman BW, Dym AA, Davitt M, et al: Naproxen with cyclobenzaprine, oxycodone/acetaminophen, or placebo for treating acute low back pain: A randomized clinical trial. *JAMA* 2015;314(15):1572-1580.

This prospective study has garnered a good deal of editorial responses that have emphasized the fact that the addition of skeletal muscle relaxants, low-dose opioid (oxycodone 5 or 10 mg every 8 hours), or placebo did not improve pain control compared with placebo at 1 week or 3 months after the onset of acute LBP. Unfortunately, there was no true placebo group and the dose of oxycodone was low and too infrequent. At 3 months, 25% of all groups still reported moderate to severe LBP.

58. Rasmussen-Barr E, Held U, Grooten WJ, et al: Non-steroidal anti-inflammatory drugs for sciatica. *Cochrane Database Syst Rev* 2016;10:CD012382.

The authors present a systematic review to determine efficacy of NSAIDs in patients with sciatica. Pain reduction was approximately equal in those receiving treatment or placebo. An increased risk for side effects was reported, even with short-term use.

59. Witenko C, Moorman-Li R, Motycka C, et al: Considerations for the appropriate use of skeletal muscle relaxants for the management of acute low back pain. *P T* 2014;39(6):427-435.

The authors present a detailed review of skeletal muscle relaxants, including evidence for their use, class overuse, and a detailed discussion of the individual drugs.

60. Abdel Shaheed C, Maher CG, Williams KA, McLachlan AJ: Efficacy and tolerability of muscle relaxants for low back pain: Systematic review and meta-analysis. *Eur J Pain* 2017;21(2):228-237.

This review evaluated skeletal muscle relaxants in patients with LBP. There was high-quality evidence that muscle relaxants provide clinically significant pain relief in the short term for acute LBP. There was no information on

3: Medical Management of Spine Disorders

long-term outcomes. For chronic LBP, the effects of skeletal muscle relaxants are not known. There was no evidence to support the efficacy of benzodiazepines in LBP.

61. Balakrishnamoorthy R, Horgan I, Perez S, Steele MC, Keijzers GB: Does a single dose of intravenous dexamethasone reduce symptoms in emergency department patients with low back pain and radiculopathy (SEBRA)? A double-blind randomised controlled trial. *Emerg Med J* 2015;32(7):525-530.

    Intravenous dexamethasone (8 mg) was compared with placebo in patients with LBP and radicular symptoms in the emergency department. A significant reduction in pain and emergency department length of stay was found. Although the effect on pain was statistically significant, the improvement did not appear clinically meaningful. Any benefit was gone at the 6-week follow-up. Dexamethasone may reduce the length of stay in the emergency department and pain somewhat, but results appear short-lived.

62. Eskin B, Shih RD, Fiesseler FW, et al: Prednisone for emergency department low back pain: A randomized controlled trial. *J Emerg Med* 2014;47(1):65-70.

    The authors report on 67 patients available for follow-up after having been seen in a single emergency department for acute LBP. The patients were randomized to receive prednisone 50 mg daily versus placebo. There were no significant differences between groups in level of pain, time to return to normal activity, or return to work.

63. Deyo RA, Von Korff M, Duhrkoop D: Opioids for low back pain. *BMJ* 2015;350:g6380.

    The authors review the use of opioids for acute and chronic LBP. There are no adequate studies for opioid use in acute LBP and benefits are inferred from their value in other acute painful musculoskeletal conditions. Because there are no controlled long-term studies, neither the effectiveness nor safety of long-term opioid analgesic therapy is known. The authors review some strategies for reducing risks to patients and the public health.

64. Abdel Shaheed C, Maher CG, Williams KA, Day R, McLachlan AJ: Efficacy, tolerability, and dose-dependent effects of opioid analgesics for low back pain: A systematic review and meta-analysis. *JAMA Intern Med* 2016;176(7):958-968.

    In this systematic review of only randomized controlled trials, the authors found moderate-quality evidence that opioid analgesics reduce pain in the short term, but the effect was only modest for doses recommended by guidelines. Approximately 50% of patients withdrew because of adverse side effects. Evidence on long-term efficacy is lacking.

65. Deyo RA, Hallvik SE, Hildebran C, et al: Association between initial opioid prescribing patterns and subsequent long-term use among opioid-naïve patients: A statewide retrospective cohort study. *J Gen Intern Med* 2017;32(1):21-27.

The authors examined death certificates of Oregon residents who filled opioid prescriptions and later died and hospital discharge records of those who filled opioid prescriptions and did not die. The correlation, if any, between early prescription use of opioids and long-term use also was examined. Of the 536,767 patients who filled an opioid prescription, 5% became long-term users. Those with the highest number of refills and those given higher doses or long-acting opioids were more likely to become chronic opioid users.

66. Nijs J, Apeldoorn A, Hallegraeff H, et al: Low back pain: Guidelines for the clinical classification of predominant neuropathic, nociceptive, or central sensitization pain. *Pain Physician* 2015;18(3):E333-E346.

    The authors believe there is sufficient evidence to accept the concept of neuropathic axial LBP. In this study, a method is tested that allows clinicians to differentiate nociceptive, neuropathic, and central sensitization forms of chronic LBP. Such knowledge might prove useful to clinicians.

67. Förster M, Mahn F, Gockel U, et al: Axial low back pain: One painful area. Many perceptions and mechanisms. *PLoS One* 2013;8(7):e68273.

    In a cohort of 1,083 patients, neuropathic components were detected in 12% of the patients. The authors thought the patient's description of pain and its severity were useful in discriminating between the two types of pain mechanisms.

68. Enthoven WT, Roelofs PD, Deyo RA, van Tulder MW, Koes BW: Non-steroidal anti-inflammatory drugs for chronic low back pain. *Cochrane Database Syst Rev* 2016;2:CD012087.

    This Cochrane review looked at randomized controlled trials that investigated NSAID use for chronic LBP. Fifty percent of the studies showed NSAIDs to be more effective than placebo, but the effect size was quite small and the level of evidence was low. No difference was found for any specific NSAID. Sufficient evidence was not available to judge whether NSAIDs are safe for long-term use.

69. Skljarevski V, Zhang S, Desaiah D, et al: Duloxetine versus placebo in patients with chronic low back pain: A 12-week, fixed-dose, randomized, double-blind trial. *J Pain* 2010;11(12):1282-1290.

    This randomized, double-blind, placebo-controlled study assessed efficacy and safety of duloxetine 60 mg once daily in 401 patients with nonneuropathic chronic LBP. Duloxetine-treated patients reported a significantly greater reduction in pain and had improved Roland Morris Disability Questionnaire reports. Fifteen percent of the duloxetine-treated patients discontinued use versus 7% in the placebo-treated patients. Some of the study authors were employed by the manufacturer of duloxetine drugs.

70. Fishbain DA, Cole B, Lewis JE, Gao J: What is the evidence that neuropathic pain is present in chronic low back pain and soft tissue syndromes? An evidence-based structured review. *Pain Med* 2014;15(1):4-15.

This review examined the evidence to determine whether neuropathic pain is present in patients with chronic LBP. In their review, neuropathic LBP was present in every study that looked for it, regardless of the method used for diagnosis. The aggregate presence was 36%. The authors emphasize that this is an important finding because it can influence and guide treatment.

71. Orita S, Yamashita M, Eguchi Y, et al: Pregabalin for refractory radicular leg pain due to lumbar spinal stenosis: A preliminary prospective study. *Pain Res Manag* 2016;2016:5079675.

    The effects of pregabalin in patients with neuropathic leg pain and intermittent claudication were evaluated using well-established outcome instruments. Pregabalin significantly improved pain, sleep, gait, and psychological dysfunction and showed a trend in improving distance before claudication.

72. Mathieson S, Maher CG, McLachlan AJ, et al: Trial of pregabalin for acute and chronic sciatica. *N Engl J Med* 2017;376(12):1111-1120.

    This randomized, prospective, blinded study examined the use of pregabalin for patients with sciatica. No differences were seen between the group treated with pregabalin and the placebo group. Level of evidence: I.

73. Muehlbacher M, Nickel MK, Kettler C, et al: Topiramate in treatment of patients with chronic low back pain: A randomized, double-blind, placebo-controlled study. *Clin J Pain* 2006;22(6):526-531.

74. Schofferman J: Long-term use of opioid analgesics for the treatment of chronic pain of nonmalignant origin. *J Pain Symptom Manage* 1993;8(5):279-288.

    In a longitudinal clinical study, 33 patients underwent a trial of long-acting or sustained release opioid medications. Five patients discontinued use because of side effects. Twenty-eight patients completed the trial, and significant improvement occurred in 21 patients. These patients were treated and followed for a mean of 32 months. Beneficial effects continued. No drug diversion, addictive behavior, or organ toxicity were noted. Dosing remained stable.

75. Allan L, Richarz U, Simpson K, Slappendel R: Transdermal fentanyl versus sustained release oral morphine in strong-opioid naïve patients with chronic low back pain. *Spine (Phila Pa 1976)* 2005;30(22):2484-2490.

76. Chaparro LE, Furlan AD, Deshpande A, Mailis-Gagnon A, Atlas S, Turk DC: Opioids compared to placebo or other treatments for chronic low-back pain. *Cochrane Database Syst Rev* 2013;8:CD004959.

    The authors performed a systematic review and meta-analysis to assess efficacy of opioids in chronic LBP. They concluded there is evidence of short-term efficacy (moderate for pain and small for function). The effectiveness and safety of long-term opioid therapy for treatment of chronic LBP remains unproved because of the lack of long-term studies, rather than because efficacy has been disproved.

77. Schofferman J, Fishman SM, Harden RN, Kirschner KL: Did we reach too far? The opioid epidemic and chronic pain. *PM R* 2014;6(1):78-84.

    This brief overview discusses some of the criteria that should be considered before undertaking long-term opioid analgesic therapy. In all medical decisions, clinicians must rely on the best available published evidence, which is not necessarily a very high level of evidence. Each patient must be considered individually.

78. Fishman S: *Responsible Opioid Prescribing*, ed 2. Washington, DC, Waterford Life Sciences, 2012.

    This short but extremely useful text reviews the value of opioid analgesics for some patients. It also reviews some of the ways to identify higher risk patients and the preferred way to follow patients on long-term opioid analgesic therapy.

79. Smith HS, ed: *Opioid Therapy in the 21st Century*. New York, New York, Oxford University Press, 2008.

3: Medical Management of Spine Disorders

Chapter 11
Therapeutic Exercise

Annie O'Connor MSPT, OCS, Cert. MDT   Thomas J. Lotus, DC, FACO, Cert. MDT

Abstract

Spine-related impairment is the primary cause of disability worldwide and has a negative effect on global wellness, productivity, and economics. It is important for care providers to ascertain the effects of spine pain on the patient's life and ability to function. Pathoanatomic diagnosis and imaging findings are not consistently relevant to the dominant pain mechanism and source of symptoms, and the degree of injury is not always equal to the intensity of pain. Healthcare providers should be fluent in the use of classification systems that are valid and reliable for subgrouping patients with spine pain based on their clinical presentation and provoking and relieving activities and motions. A better defined common language among spine care providers will advance the field and allow precise diagnoses and specific individualized treatments.

Keywords: conservative spine care; low back pain subgroups; pain mechanism classification system; patient education; therapeutic exercise

Introduction

Disability caused by spine-related pain is currently a major health problem, with approximately $600 billion spent annually in the United States for spine care.[1] A growing body of scientific literature has concluded that pathoanatomic diagnosis and MRI findings are not consistently relevant to the dominant pain mechanism and source of symptoms,[2,3] and the degree of injury may not equal the intensity of pain.[4] The literature also

supports the concept of using alternative classification systems[5,6] rather than relying solely on the pathoanatomic diagnosis. The use of classification systems to assist in making a diagnosis in patients with low back pain (LBP) is associated with better outcomes.[7] Treatment interventions performed without reference to a patient's specific presentation and without an attempt at classification into a subgroup can lead to suboptimal care, poorer outcomes, and decreased patient satisfaction.[8] A prolonged cycle of nonspecific treatment undertaken with the hope that one therapy will be effective can lead to frustration for both the patient and the healthcare provider.[8]

The choice of the specific classification or diagnostic system used should be made carefully by weighing the evidence and pros and cons regarding the clinician's practice and broader healthcare implications. An additional tool or system should be used to assess the psychosocial components of a patient's spine pain and potential barriers to recovery. The reliability of two systems, the classification of mechanical nociceptive spinal pain mechanisms using the McKenzie Method of Mechanical Diagnosis and Therapy (MDT; McKenzie Institute International)[9] and a treatment-based classification system (TBC), are supported by evidence in the literature.[10,11] The Pain Mechanism Classification System (PMCS) was developed in the late 1990s to address both nociceptive movement-dominated pain mechanisms and centrally mediated pain mechanisms related to the emotional, social, and sensorimotor dimensions of pain. More recently, the PMCS has been found to be a reliable classification system with good interrater and intrarater reliability and high specificity.[7,12-14] The PMCS also has a high likelihood ratio for identifying the dominant pain mechanism, with 95% of clinical characteristics covered and applicability across many pain locations, patient ages, and levels of neurologic and musculoskeletal disability.[7,15] Classification systems are important for directing specific interventions. The PMCS has been shown to effectively and efficiently guide and direct patient education and active care, especially on the patient's first clinical visit.[7,13,15] Regardless

3: Medical Management of Spine Disorders

of whether spine pain is acute or chronic, the PMCS, MDT, and TBC promote independence in self-care without the need for passive treatments performed in a rehabilitation setting.

Foundation Principles of Spine Classification Systems

Not all nociceptive spine-related symptoms are caused by structural, pathologic, mechanical, or chemical mechanisms. In 35% of patients with chronic pain, there is an underlying central nervous system (CNS)–mediated mechanism.[7] The PMCS, MDT, and TBC systems for spine-related conditions direct specific therapeutic exercise for LBP dominated by nociceptive pain mechanisms. The PMCS is unique in that it takes into account mechanical nociceptive and centrally mediated sources of pain that represent the cognitive, emotional, social, psychological, and sensorimotor dimensions of a patient's pain experience.[7,16] These three classification systems have evidence to support their effects on positive outcomes, decreased cost to the healthcare system, and help in selecting active therapeutic exercises.

Therapeutic exercise is a conservative intervention offered by many providers with various training backgrounds. Therapeutic exercise should include a strong patient education component for self-management of spine-related problems. Conservative care is an overarching term that includes the concepts of active treatment directed for immediate cure of a disease or management of an injury, causal treatment to prevent a disease, nonsurgical care to avoid radical medical therapeutic measures or surgical procedures, and empiric treatment that has proved to be beneficial.[17]

When a surgeon refers a patient to a provider of conservative care, the surgeon should ensure that the provider prioritizes patient education and active care before ordering procedures such as passive electrical modalities, tests, manual medicine interventions, and injections. Patient education and active exercise should be directed toward reducing or eliminating the mechanism of spine-related pain preventing the recurrence of pain. The care provider should use both patient- and clinician-rated validated outcome measures. The surgeon should assess the effects of conservative care interventions by reviewing results of the outcome measures and take responsibility for ensuring that all aspects of evidence-based medicine have been performed relative to the selected education and exercise intervention. This approach also provides the surgeon with an understanding of the services offered by therapeutic exercise providers and their contribution to disease management.

Patient Education

Appropriate Language

Education is an important aspect of patient recovery and self-maintenance. The healthcare provider must be cautious in the selection of words or statements used to educate a patient because some types of communication can be hurtful or harmful. In contrast, other words and statements can be helpful and may provide a patient with hope and a change in mind-set about a condition, diagnosis, or symptom.

Examples of words and statements that can be misleading or may conflict with appropriate conservative care include instructing a patient with pain to stop moving because it may be harmful, listing activities that the patient should never do, and indicating that the care provider is unsure of the best treatment and the patient must get accustomed to his or her pain. In contrast, other words and statements will promote a patient's engagement in his or her care. For example, a patient should be reassured that the pain is real, but that not all pain is bad. Understanding the behavior of pain during movements will determine the safety of the pain. A patient can be informed about the mechanism causing the pain (eg, a tight, trapped, or sensitive nerve) and the potential for recovery with the appropriate exercise therapy.[14,16] Reassurance that the patient is "not crazy" and referral to a medical professional who can help the patient cope with life stressors also is an example of positive communication.

Methods and Outcomes

Studies have shown the benefits of providing education to patients with LBP.[18-21] Advice to patients with LBP to exercise when back pain is at its worst has resulted in increased satisfaction and improved functional outcomes.[18] For example, patients can be given booklets with detailed exercise instructions after a medical consultation. Cognitive changes have been documented in patients who are given reassurance that exercise is not harmful.[19] Words can heal and have an immediate effect by physically altering the patient's perception of the meaning of pain; this may decrease the need for further interventions.[22] Activity guidelines have shown that the concept of movement-safe pain is critical to a successful outcome. Patients who read an educational book on self-treatment of back pain demonstrated long-term improvements and had fewer recurring pain episodes than those who did not read the book.[20] A reduction in fear-avoidance behaviors was found in patients with chronic back pain who were provided with information about the neurophysiology of pain mechanisms. This strategy decreased pain and improved outcomes.[21]

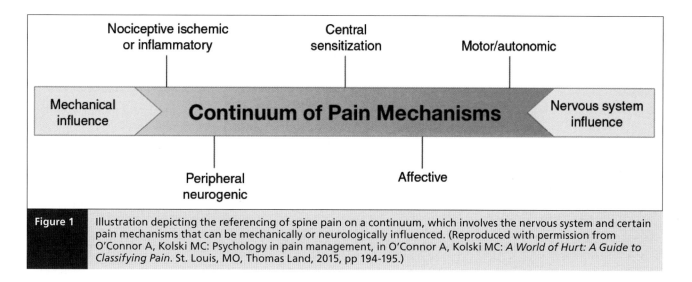

Figure 1 Illustration depicting the referencing of spine pain on a continuum, which involves the nervous system and certain pain mechanisms that can be mechanically or neurologically influenced. (Reproduced with permission from O'Connor A, Kolski MC: Psychology in pain management, in O'Connor A, Kolski MC: *A World of Hurt: A Guide to Classifying Pain*. St. Louis, MO, Thomas Land, 2015, pp 194-195.)

Advice given to a patient may translate into behavioral changes.[23] The clinician should be careful to use terms and phrases familiar to the patient and should remember that patient-friendly language is important.[24,25] Using a classification system such as the PMCS can efficiently and effectively guide patient education and provide activity guidelines and exercise prescriptions. The PMCS provides a common language and image that the patient and provider can use to enhance communication regarding the dominating pain mechanism.[16] Also, group education can be as effective as individual patient education. Consideration should be given to the development of short (<8 weeks) group interventions.[26]

Two-Point System of Patient Education

Patient education should be consistent across all touchpoints in the healthcare system. The PMCS allows providers to offer this consistency via the use of the following two-point system for patient education: (1) explain pain using a mechanism-based language common to the patient and the provider and (2) use an "activity traffic light," which is a guide to movement-safe pain. PMCS education may reduce the number of needed interventions such as surgical procedures, drugs, and injections by improving the patient's understanding of pain and the dominant mechanism causing symptoms.[16,22]

Explanation of Pain Mechanisms

The patient should be instructed that pain is an output of the brain, not an input from the body. This is an important topic because all patients with acute or chronic pain should understand the meaning of their symptoms and whether the brain is causing pain by interpreting a symptom as an alert of danger and the need to protect that area. Most symptomatic signals sent by the body are

related to some type of imbalance (ie, injury, directions, positions, deconditioning, poor coping, and negative emotions and thoughts); these signals are then interpreted by the brain. Based on a perceived threat to the body, the brain may interpret the signal as an indication of harm and the need for protection; this results in pain and nociceptive sensitivity. The actual symptoms of pain may be referred to the areas of signal generation or other areas based on past and current life experiences related to the interpretation of these signals of impending harm. Spine pain occurs on a continuum and involves mechanical influences signaling a state of imbalance. If allowed to persist, the signals involve the nervous system and related pain mechanisms that become neurologically influenced[16] (**Figure 1**). Nociceptive mechanical mechanisms of pain can include chemical or mechanical inflammation, ischemia, and peripheral neurogenic pain. Nervous system influences that are directly related to the central nervous system include central sensitization, affective, and motor/autonomic pain mechanisms. Patients with LBP should understand that their dominant pain mechanism lies somewhere on this continuum. This understanding is vital to patient education, which can affect therapeutic exercise selection and, ultimately, the patient's movement.

Activity Traffic Light: A Guide to Movement-Safe Pain

The second aspect of the two-point system of patient education is explaining what the signal means and whether it is indicating the need for protection or indicating that the pain is safe.[19] The best analytic tool is the activity traffic light. Education about movement-safe pain is not about what the patient feels, but more about how the pain behaves with respect to the patient's movement. Pain behavior may be a red light indicating harm is occurring and an activity should stop; a yellow light indicating that

Table 1

Activity Traffic Light: A Guide to Movement-Safe Pain

Traffic Light Color	Pain Behavior After Activity	Motion Analysis After Activity	Understanding Pain
Red	Severe pain that does not allow continued activity and persists for weeks	50% or greater loss of mobility from normal baseline movement	Potential harm/injury: seek medical advice, contact therapy team.
Yellow	Moderate to severe pain during and after an activity that returns to baseline pain levels within 24 to 48 hr	No loss of movement or ability from baseline levels	Indication that no harm has occurred and it is safe to continue activity. This behavior is indicative of doing too much too fast.
Green	Moderate to severe pain during activity that returns to baseline levels within 2 hr after activity	No change in range of motion during and after the activity	Indicative of safe pain; no harm has occurred and adding more activity is safe.

an activity is too much and too fast, but with the need to stay the course at an appropriate pace; or a green light indicating the need to continue an activity and confidently increase and intensify the activity. Interpretation of the activity traffic light involves considering the behavior of the symptoms during and after movements and the effect on range of motion (**Table 1**). This analytic skill will help a patient understand when pain is safe (no harm is occurring) and avoid pain flare-ups or reinjury as return to activity progresses. This understanding is key to successful self-management of pain for patients with any dominating mechanism and any recommended exercise intervention. It can prevent a patient from misinterpreting his or her pain as harmful and can discourage negative thoughts, which become an active trigger and cause misinterpretation and sensitization of the body's signals.

Validating the PMCS as a Subgrouping Classification System

The PMCS is a patient-centered biopsychosocial subgrouping method and language used to classify the dominant pain mechanism. The PMCS guides the provider in understanding relevant subjective and objective characteristics related to mechanical and neurologic pain mechanisms and focuses on the mechanical, cognitive, emotional, social, and sensorimotor manifestations of pain seen in clinical practice. In an analysis of data regarding clinical pain characteristics using kappa and percentage of agreement values, 68% and 95% of items on the clinical criteria checklist demonstrated clinically acceptable inter- and intra-examiner reliability, respectively, across multiple disciplines.[15] Inter- and intra-examiner agreement

associated with clinicians' identification of clinical criteria per pain mechanism involving low back and leg pain was substantial and almost perfect, respectively. These findings provided preliminary evidence supporting the reliability of clinical judgments associated with pain mechanism classification in patients with LBP and leg pain. A 2016 study reported good agreement between the PMCS category determined by trained therapists and the PMCS category assigned based on a computer-generated statistical model that used patients' signs and symptoms.[7] Cluster analysis involving five assumed groups found that 97% of patients could be classified by both models at the first visit. Sensitivity and specificity results (95% confidence interval) were calculated for the five categories using the PMCS categories assigned by the physical therapist as the criterion standard for approximately 38,000 patients receiving therapy for pain. The largest number of patients in the study were those with spine pain. Sensitivity for four categories of pain (inflammatory, ischemia, peripheral neurogenic, and central mechanisms) ranged from 72.4% (ischemia) to 98.8% (central mechanisms). This study provides empiric support that the PMCS can be used to accurately diagnose dominant pain mechanisms in all areas of the body at the first visit in an outpatient clinical pain practice.[7] The PMCS is a reliable and valid method for patient classification and can provide better predictable outcomes.

Pain Mechanism Education and Prescriptive Therapeutic Exercise

It is important to understand the involved pain mechanism, the type of therapeutic exercise to prescribe, and the overall effect of the therapeutic exercise. If an exercise is not effective, other pain mechanisms and exercise approaches should be considered. An ineffective therapeutic exercise regimen may result in greater patient dependency on the care provider and increase the risk that spine pain will result in disability.[27] Pain mechanism education and prescriptive therapeutic exercise for LBP can be classified into five exercise intervention subgroups that will ensure implementation of the correct type, frequency, and intensity dosage needed for treatment of the dominant pain mechanism.

Nociceptive Mechanical Inflammation Pain Mechanism and Directional Preference Exercise Subgroup

In the nociceptive mechanical inflammation pain mechanism and directional preference exercise subgroup, a nontraumatic mechanical mechanism is related to a position or cumulative movement that occurs over time and involves too much loading in the same direction without load reversal and movement in the opposite direction. The needed treatment involves a certain direction of movement. The clinician instructs the patient in an exercise that highlights a preferred direction of movement. The pain response is rapid because directional exercise restores the balance in movement and stops the receptor from signaling.[20] When the most prevalent nociceptive mechanical inflammatory signals can be eased by movement in a certain direction, the need for therapeutic exercise in a preferred direction is indicated to decrease the risk of irritating or worsening the condition.[28-33] The directional exercise will alleviate symptoms, and signs of centralization may occur with repeated movements in that direction.[28,29,32,33] The primary goal of exercise in this group is to abolish pain by using the directional preference.

Nociceptive Ischemia Pain Mechanism and Remodel Tight and Weak Tissue Exercise Subgroup

In the nociceptive ischemia pain mechanism and remodel tight and weak tissue exercise subgroup, there is not enough blood and oxygen to allow complete healing or restoration of full function to the tissues. This condition may occur during healing stages of repair and remodeling of connective tissues. Remodeling exercise is indicated when nociceptive mechanical ischemic signals indicate the need to increase mobility and strength in specific tissues (ie, muscle, ligament, tendon, cartilage, or bone).[8,24,34] The signals being sent are more related to a need to stretch tight or strengthen weak connective tissue. This type of pain is safe and necessary to stimulate further tissue healing and recovery.[20] The remodeling exercise is intended to produce and increase pain, but overall symptoms should be no worse after exercise (green light, safe to keep performing). The adage of "no pain, no gain" applies. The patient's condition will slowly respond over time as the tissue is remodeled, and improved health will be acheived.[8,24]

Nociceptive Ischemia Pain Mechanism and Restore Function Subgroup

Another type of nociceptive mechanical ischemic signal may indicate the need for better quality movement.[35] The pain signal means that a function or a posture should be performed differently. The therapeutic exercise needs to be specific and look like the patient's function. Incorporating motor control theories, developmental sequencing, and principles of applied physics into the human kinetic chain is the focus of exercise to restore function. Often symptoms may originate from a body part above or below the area of the presenting symptoms. For example, back hinging (flexing) to perform forward-directed movements will load a passive inert system. Teaching the patient how to use hip hinging for forward-directed movement will load an active muscular system. The patient's condition will slowly improve as performance of the movement pattern becomes more subconscious with continued practice of the new motor strategy. The success of therapeutic exercise in this subgroup depends on how well the patient integrates the new motor strategy or posture into his or her daily habits and functions. In this therapeutic exercise subgroup of ischemia, the function and quality of performance are more important than targeting the remodeling of a specific tissue. Subjective and objective characteristics and intervention guidelines[7,16] for the three most prevalent mechanical PMCS exercise subgroups can be found in **Table 2**.

Central Sensitization or Affective Pain Mechanisms and Gradual Exposure to Fearful and Pleasurable Activities Exercise Subgroup

In patients requiring gradual exposure to fearful or pleasurable activities, therapeutic exercise focuses on the dominant CNS pain mechanisms of central sensitization and affective pain. Often, the pain is an indication of the need for gradual exposure to either feared activities (when dominated by central sensitivity) or the reintroduction of pleasurable activities (when dominated by affective pain). Central sensitization occurs when the cognitive processes in the spinal dorsal root ganglion and brain misinterpret the signal from the body as harmful, causing ongoing sensitivity to the nociception and persistent pain[20] (**Figure 2**). Treatment for this pain mechanism includes specific pain education regarding the brain's role in pain as an interpretation of the incoming signal for the purpose of protection and the effect of signal misinterpretation on

Table 2

Pain Mechanism Classification System Exercise Subgroups

Findings	Nociceptive Inflammatory Mechanical and Directional Preference	Nociceptive Ischemia and Remodel Tight Weak Tissues	Nociceptive Ischemia and Restore Function
Subjective characteristics	Location: local/referred/radicular Frequency: constant/intermittent Onset: sudden, acute or chronic 24-hr behavior: AM/PM increase; as day goes on, pain improves; inconsistent and variable pain pattern Worse/better: patterns dependent on certain motions, directions, and positions	Location: localized axial or radicular (adherent nerve root) Frequency: intermittent Onset: postinjury, progressive, chronic (6 to 8 weeks) 24-hr behavior: pain produced as tissue is loaded Worse/better: consistent with painful activities; consistent pain and motion pattern	Location: localized, may involve more than one site/no referral pain Frequency: intermittent Onset: no apparent reason, progressive positional, cumulative activity 24-hr behavior: worse after prolonged activity of 1- to 3-hr duration Worse/better: consistent with painful function; change in posture during function may alleviate symptoms
Objective characteristics	Inconsistent/variable pain and motion pattern Pain during motion Obstruction in certain motions Neurologic examination may include sensory or motor loss, tension signs Repeated or sustained positions or movements reveal directional preference that centralizes symptoms and improves obstruction and function Rapid changes in symptoms Irreducible: unable to centralize symptoms, change motion or function	Loss of end-range movement Contractile: pain during active and resisted movement Articular: end-range pain; pain produced at end range Consistent pain presentation, unable to change pain during repeated movement examinations	Positional/cumulative stress causes symptoms No pathology No loss of motion, no pain with motion No neurologic loss or tension signs Repeated or sustained examination: no effect; no worsening or improvement in symptoms

the sensitivity of the receptors in the tissues. The activity traffic light guides movement-safe pain to retrain the cognitive interpretation of the brain to incoming signals. In addition, patients are gradually exposed to activities and movements or functions perceived as fearful or harmful, with monitoring of their cognitive reframing of movement-safe pain that desensitizes their pain alarm system. The affective pain mechanism occurs when the emotional and social pressures of life reach a level that affects the patient's coping ability. This inability to cope is a result of negative emotions and poor coping strategies. Negative impulses sensitize emotional centers of the brain in attempts at protection and referral of pain and other symptoms to certain areas of the body to distract focus from unpleasant circumstances.[20] The signals indicate an imbalance in emotional coping related to negative thoughts and emotions that occur in an effort to deal with past, present, or future circumstances that have caused or can result in pain.[16] Treatment for this pain mechanism involves gradual exposure to activities, movements, or functions perceived as pleasurable, meaningful, and enjoyable. This gradual process is geared toward a patient learning to think, cope, believe, and behave differently about his or her pain. Patient education regarding this mechanism involves understanding the brain's role in pain as a protective mechanism directly influenced by positive active coping. The brain causes pain in the body in an effort to distract from life issues and their resolution.

Table 2

Pain Mechanism Classification System Exercise Subgroups (*continued*)

Findings	Nociceptive Inflammatory Mechanical and Directional Preference	Nociceptive Ischemia and Remodel Tight Weak Tissues	Nociceptive Ischemia and Restore Function
Exercise treatment progression	Directional preference: prescribe direction/position that centralizes, localizes, and alleviates distal symptoms; establish repetition and frequency to maintain alleviated symptoms	Articular: identify limited directions, establish repetitions, loads, and frequency to remodel tissue	Education on postural correction
	Avoid/modify directions/positions that cause peripheralization of symptoms	Activity traffic light: a guide to movement-safe pain	Application of posture principles into daily occupational and recreational functions
	Progressive return to motion and function	Expectations for remodeling: therapeutic exercise 3 to 6 times daily for 6 to 8 wk	Motivate to change posture and perform function differently
	Mechanically unresponsive radiculopathy: unresponsive nerve root compromise; unable to centralize symptoms with direction strategy	Contractile: muscle—initiate isometric load, establish repetitions, loads, and frequency to remodel the tissue	
	Consider referral for physical medicine and rehabilitation/epidural steroid injection consultation	tendon—initiate eccentric load progress to end range; establish repetitions, loads, and frequency to remodel the tissue	
	Consider surgical referral if leg and/or motor symptoms present	Activity traffic light: a guide to movement-safe pain	
	Patient education regarding red flags	Expectations for remodeling: 3 to 6 times daily for 6 to 8 wk	

A patient's readiness to take a different approach and actively cope better will directly affect outcomes.

Motor/Autonomic Pain Mechanism and Sensorimotor Exercise Subgroup

The motor/autonomic pain mechanism is dominant when representation is lost in the area of the primary somatosensory cortex of the brain that represents all body parts. Symptoms are related to cortical disinhibition, and they present as a lack of awareness and decreased ability to recognize body parts.[20] Signs and symptoms involving the sympathetic and parasympathetic nervous system are manifested. This pain mechanism has been well recognized in complex regional pain syndrome affecting the extremities and phantom pain; however, it also has been reported in spine-related pain. The therapeutic exercise treatment is sensorimotor exercises directed at changing brain recognition of body areas. Sensorimotor exercises involve exercise to improve left-right discrimination,

and the use of imagery and mirror reflection therapy to encourage awareness of the affected body part. These exercises involve a specific protocol of exercises and education regarding the active mechanism occurring in the brain. After sensory and motor recognition is perfected, traditional movement-based therapies can be directed at the affected body part.

Classification System Terminology

The overarching PMCS covers all exercise subgroups previously discussed. Other nociceptive mechanical classification systems that aid in therapeutic exercise selection are the MDT and the TBC systems, which have limited application to certain central nervous system pain mechanisms. Directional preference has been recognized in all three classification systems; however, different descriptive terms are used. The MDT system uses the term derangement syndrome, the TBC system uses the term specific exercise classification, and the PMCS uses

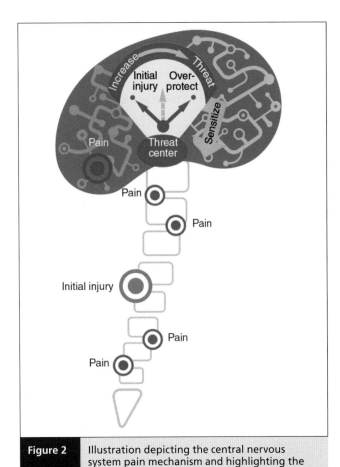

Figure 2 Illustration depicting the central nervous system pain mechanism and highlighting the input at the spinal cord level that affects the fear and threat centers with perceived threats that affect the descending inhibitory system and result in sensitization to the nociceptors. (Reproduced with permission from O'Connor A, Kolski MC: Central sensitization pain mechanism, in O'Connor A, Kolski MC: *A World of Hurt: A Guide to Classifying Pain*. St. Louis, MO, Thomas Land, 2015, pp 187-188.)

the term inflammation-mechanical. As a provider, it is helpful to determine the type of classification system used when communicating with a patient. Using multiple classification systems collaboratively for patients with LBP increases the strength of the therapeutic exercise prescription.

Mechanical Diagnosis and Treatment System

Derangement syndrome is reported to be the most common clinical presentation of spinal problems, and it is defined as internal displacement within a motion segment. Prevalence rates vary depending on chronicity, but trained therapists have reported rates of between 60% and 78% in the lumbar spine[28-33] and between 72% and 87% in the cervical spine.[30,36,37] Because of its high prevalence, the clinician should rule out this syndrome first when

making a diagnosis. Proper classification of patients in this subgroup is important because they will respond rapidly to end-range exercise using the correct directional preference. Therapeutic exercise performed in the wrong direction may worsen a patient's condition.[28,29,32,36,37]

Dysfunction syndrome is a mechanical deformation of impaired soft tissue(s) that may be caused by trauma, an inflammatory or degenerative process that results in contraction, scarring, adherence, adaptive shortening, and weakness. This pain mechanism is dominated by ischemia, which indicates the need for therapeutic exercise for remodeling of specific connective tissues.[24,34]

Posture syndrome is a mechanical deformation of soft tissue(s) resulting from prolonged end-range postures that deprive vascular transmission and cause ischemia. Joints, muscles, tendons, periosteal insertions, spinal disks, and peripheral nerves may be affected.[24,34]

Treatment-based Classification System

The most recent revision of the TBC system occurred in 2007,[8,10,11] but that revision did not acknowledge the biopsychosocial aspects of LBP.[35] This deficit in the TBC system illustrates the benefit of collaborative classification systems. The TBC has the following four main classification categories: manipulation, stabilization, specific exercise, and traction.[35]

Manipulation

Patients in the manipulation category meet the following criteria: recent onset of symptoms, symptoms localized to the back, hypomobility in the lumbar spine, and low scores on the Fear Avoidance Behavior Questionnaire.[35] A patient who meets the clinical prediction rule for lumbar manipulation also should be included in this category. Treatment includes mobilization and/or thrust manipulation followed by range-of-motion exercises.[35]

Stabilization

Patients in the stabilization category typically meet the following criteria: positive result on the prone instability test, the presence of aberrant motions, a straight leg raise test of greater than 90°, and recurrent episodes of spine pain.[35] Treatment includes exercises that focus on core strengthening and/or motor control.[35]

Specific Exercise

Patients in the specific exercise category meet the following criteria: symptoms that radiate into the lower extremity, a strong preference for either sitting or walking, and centralization and peripheralization of symptoms with repeated lumbar spine movements.[35] Treatment includes exercises or manual interventions that focus on centralizing and abolishing symptoms.[35] The most common treatment includes repeated and/or sustained lumbar extension; however, specific movements of flexion or lateral gliding are less commonly used directional preference exercises.[35]

Traction

Patients in the traction category meet the following criteria: pain radiating into the lower extremity, no directional preference, and a positive (crossed) straight leg raise test.[35] Treatment includes manual and/or mechanical lumbar traction.[35] The main goals of treatment are improvement in symptoms, function, and education to allow self-management of pain.[35]

Using Multiple Systems and Determining Risk Groups

The use of several classification systems (ie, PMCS, MDT, and TBC) is recommended to manage the risks associated with LBP across the entire pain continuum. The provider should determine which form of therapeutic exercise is appropriate for the patient and which classification system should be used to guide treatment. In general, patients with LBP should be triaged into one of four risk groups to guide referral to specialists and therapeutic exercise providers.

Risk Group 1

Risk group 1 includes patients with serious pathology, comorbidities, or red flags. Fewer than 5% of patients with spine pain are classified into this group.[38] The subjective information in the patient's history requires immediate medical management and referral to a specialist for diagnosis. Close monitoring should continue until an appropriate referral source is identified and care is transitioned. The objective evaluation shows symptoms that do not respond to repeated movements, positions, or provocation tests. The patient may demonstrate the following signs and symptoms: constant pain unrelated to position or movement and not relieved by rest, severe night pain unrelated to position or movement, recent unexplained weight loss, a history of direct blunt trauma, an appearance of acute illness, generalized weakness or malaise, abdominal pain that radiates to the groin and is associated with hematuria, sexual dysfunction, recent menstrual irregularities, bowel or bladder dysfunction, and anesthesia perineum.

Risk Group 2

Risk group 2 includes patients with disability resulting from pain and the presence of yellow flags. According to

the scientific literature, approximately 35% of patients are classified into this group (most have spine-related pain). All patients should be screened for potential yellow flags, which are characteristic of CNS pain mechanisms.[7,39,40] Instruments such as the Yellow Flag Risk Form (YFRF)[39,40] or the STarT Back Tool[41,42] can aid in screening for these central characteristics. Low scores on these types of assessment tools indicate a low occurrence of CNS characteristics and psychological distress; no uncontrolled comorbidities; and, typically, normal neurologic status.

The PMCS recommends that patients in this category be treated with education about CNS pain mechanisms (central sensitivity, affective, motor/autonomic), reassurance about movement-safe pain, and advice on certain active care procedures. The YFRF can be used to screen for pain disability risk and identify CNS pain characteristics to promote proper referral. The tool has 13 simple questions that highlight the four domains known to be key markers for transitioning to chronic pain and disability.[43] The four domains include (1) confidence and self-efficacy in mortality, pain control, and activity return; (2) emotional stability and balance, specifically affecting depression, anxiety, and sleep; (3) fear avoidance and catastrophizing related to activity and movement; and (4) the presence of nerve-related symptoms during the day or night.

The YFRF was created in the mid-1990s after previous peer-reviewed questionnaires were consolidated to simplify screening for yellow-flag domains.[39,40] This tool is appropriate for patients with pain in any part of the body. The higher the score, the greater the likelihood that central characteristics are present and CNS pain mechanisms are dominant. The recommended cutoff scores will guide referral to certain providers who can direct appropriate patient education and therapeutic exercise (**Table 3**). If a patient's score is less than 55, classification into risk groups 3 or 4 should be considered.

Risk Group 3

Risk group 3 includes patients whose condition may worsen with active care or exercise. Three situations exist in which active care can worsen the condition of a patient with a spine disorder. (1) If structural spine instability is present, the patient will exhibit progressive neurologic/structural instability signs. Surgical stabilization is required before active care can begin. A surgeon should be consulted. (2) If chemical inflammation is present, the patient is neurologically stable and has no structural abnormality; however, there will be objective findings of constant pain, with morning stiffness; noncentralization with movements or positions; worsening of pain in all positions and with repeated movements; and symptoms

Table 3

Yellow Flag Risk Form Pain Disability Cutoff Scores

Risks	Points	Recommended Classification System	Referral
Low	<55	Nociceptive mechanical classification system: PMCS, MDT, TBC	Refer to PMCS, MDT, TBC provider
Moderate	55-64	Subgroup: PMCS: central sensitization or affective or motor/autonomic MDT: other: chronic pain syndrome	PMCS: central sensitization—refer to cognitive behavioral therapy provider PMCS: affective—refer to psychological provider PMCS: motor/autonomic—refer to sensorimotor retraining provider
High	≥65	Subgroup: PMCS: central sensitization or affective or motor/autonomic MDT: other: chronic pain syndrome	PMCS: central sensitization—refer to cognitive behavioral therapy provider PMCS: affective—refer to psychological provider PMCS: autonomic/motor—refer to sensorimotor retraining provider

MDT = Mechanical Diagnosis and Therapy, PMCS = Pain Mechanism Classification System, TBC = treatment-based classification

not affected by traction. The patient should be referred to a physiatrist for an epidural steroid injection. After chemical inflammation is managed, directional preference exercise should be considered. (3) In patients with directional preference, one or two directions or positions will centralize and alleviate symptoms, and one or two directions or positions will cause peripheralization and worsen symptoms. The patient should be referred to a PMCS, MDT, or TBC provider for treatment.

Risk Group 4 For patients in risk group 4, active care has no effect. Because therapeutic exercise results in no improvement, a patient may attempt "provider jumping," which is defined as a history of attempted treatment with many different types of exercise providers and no substantial improvement. In patients with ischemia or peripheral neurogenic pain mechanisms, there is a risk that therapeutic exercise will have no effect.[16] Treatment failure occurs because the education and exercise prescription are not specific or intense enough to alleviate the pain mechanism or alter the patient's condition, function, or tissue status. In these patients, the exercise prescription must be specifically directed at the dominant pain mechanism and specific tissue and/or function. These patients experience moderate to low levels of pain that increase with certain movements and daily activities, but return to baseline levels when activity is stopped. Patients may report sudden and unexpected bouts of pain along with other pain-free periods. Active spinal movements are not obstructed and do not cause pain. Findings of decreased flexibility and poor motor control may exist, but there is no effect when treated with exercises and measured using functional outcome measures. The rehabilitation goal for these patients is proper classification of the pain

mechanism to allow guided patient education and active care. The patient should be referred to a PMCS, MDT, TBC, or progressive exercise provider.

Identified pain mechanisms in this risk group are described and treatment prescribed based on the classification system used because of overlap within the systems. Ischemia as defined in the PMCS requires aggressive intervention with remodeling exercises for the affected tissue or function. Subgroup classification of this pain mechanism allows a more specific therapeutic exercise prescription.[16]

Tissue dysfunction as defined in the MDT system is managed with progressive therapeutic exercise (achieving effort levels of 6 of 10 on effort scales, and pain levels of 4 to 7 on 10-point pain scales during exercise to achieve remodeling effects).[8,16,24] Exercise frequency is two to four times daily for 6 to 8 weeks to achieve 10% to 20% statistical improvement. Therapeutic exercises should be continued until pain is totally alleviated, which can take up to 24 months in some patients with chronic conditions.[7,16]

Functional loss from pain caused by pathologic ischemia is treated with therapeutic exercise(s) along with a holistic approach that includes weight management, improvement in cardiovascular health, general strength training, and balance exercises. The timeline to maximal improvement can be up to 24 months, depending on the patient's compliance and readiness for change in performance of the therapeutic exercise.[16] Setting goals to improve confidence and competence in a self-care program can affect overall success.

In patients with postoperative ischemia, therapeutic exercise is aimed at promoting healing of injured or repaired tissues. The timeline to maximal improvement

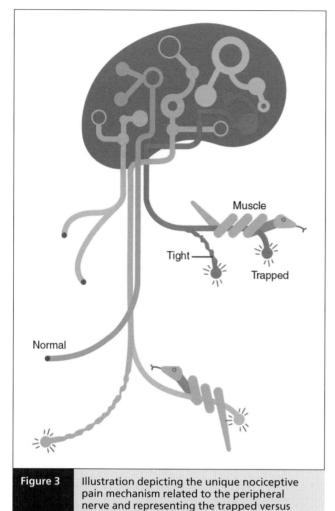

Figure 3 Illustration depicting the unique nociceptive pain mechanism related to the peripheral nerve and representing the trapped versus tight mechanical elements. (Reproduced with permission from O'Connor A, Kolski MC: Peripheral neurogenic pain mechanism, in O'Connor A, Kolski MC: *A World of Hurt: A Guide to Classifying Pain*. St. Louis, MO, Thomas Land, 2015, pp 105-106.)

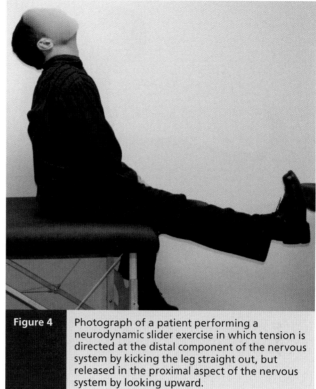

Figure 4 Photograph of a patient performing a neurodynamic slider exercise in which tension is directed at the distal component of the nervous system by kicking the leg straight out, but released in the proximal aspect of the nervous system by looking upward.

may be as little as 12 weeks or as long as 24 months, depending on the severity of tissue injury, healing complications, and the surgical procedures performed.[16] Patient compliance, readiness to change the performance of therapeutic exercise, and setting goals to improve confidence and competence in their self-care program are important areas that influence overall success.

Therapeutic exercise can be tailored to optimize management of ischemia related to poor physical performance of the kinetic chain (posture in the MDT system or stabilization in the TBC system) to achieve the ability to meet higher-level demands in sport- or job-related activities. The quality of movement is a primary concern. Biomechanical pitfalls can be identified by repeated functional testing and are associated with a preponderance of loading

of passive inert structures rather than establishing quality activation patterns of muscles. The predictors of success are consistent daily practice, recognition and correction of movement patterns, and recognition and prioritization of quality rather than quantity as the patient progresses to higher contextual applications of movement patterns.[16]

The risk of therapeutic exercise producing no effect is common in patients with peripheral neurogenic pain as defined by the PMCS.[16] The peripheral nerve often requires direct remodeling via neurodynamic exercise to alter the common peripheral neurogenic pain mechanism associated with spine-related conditions[20] (**Figure 3**). It is important to note that the primary goal of exercise in this group is to produce and increase nerve symptoms and pain to restore normal movement and health to the peripheral nerve associated with the entrapment or tightness related to the LBP. Aggressive therapeutic exercises are directed at the tissues of the peripheral nervous system (more specifically, the actual nerve). Subgrouping the peripheral neurogenic mechanism as "trapped" or "tight" will further refine the education and neurodynamic therapeutic exercise prescription.

For improvement in a patient with a trapped nerve, attention is needed to provide healthy movement for the tissues surrounding the nerve as well as the nerve itself. This requires a slider-type neurodynamic exercise with

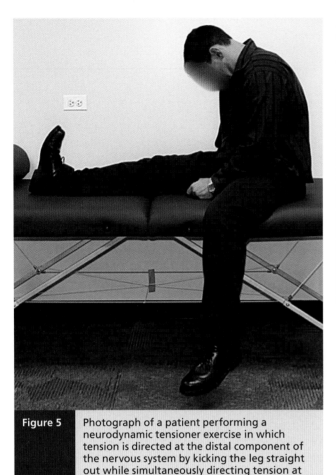

Figure 5 Photograph of a patient performing a neurodynamic tensioner exercise in which tension is directed at the distal component of the nervous system by kicking the leg straight out while simultaneously directing tension at the proximal aspect of the nervous system by looking downward.

one of the five pain mechanism and exercise subgroups. This classification helps direct patient education and the selection of the correct dosage of therapeutic exercise.

Key Study Points

- The PMCS, MDT, and TBC classification systems aid in determining the correct dosage of the conservative care interventions of patient education and therapeutic exercise.
- Patient education about the dominant pain mechanism as it relates to the exercise subgroup promotes better understanding of and compliance with the conservative care intervention.
- Therapeutic exercise for patients with LBP should be considered like a "movement pill," which requires understanding the correct dosage (intensity, frequency, and type of exercise).
- Pain mechanism education and prescriptive therapeutic exercise for LBP can be summarized into the following five pain mechanisms and exercise intervention subgroups: (1) nociceptive mechanical inflammation pain mechanism and directional preference, (2) nociceptive ischemia pain mechanism and remodel tight and weak tissues, (3) nociceptive ischemia pain mechanism and restore function, (4) central sensitization or affective pain mechanism and gradual exposure to fearful and pleasurable activities, and (5) motor/autonomic pain mechanism and sensorimotor retraining.

a focus on sliding the nerve through the interfacing tissue that is trapping the nerve. To restore health to the nerve, the nerve should slide through the interfacing tissue to promote movement in the neural container[14,16] (**Figure 4**). For a tight nerve, therapeutic exercise is aimed at improving the actual neural tissue and its movement characteristics of elasticity, tensile, and compressive loading. Remodeling requires a tensioner-type neurodynamic exercise in which movement is focused on the tensile properties of the nerve's tissues[14,16] (**Figure 5**).

Summary

To achieve the best outcome for patients with spine pain, it is vital to properly classify the dominant pain mechanism to guide patient education and therapeutic exercise. These interventions vary based on the risk group and subgroups within each risk group. The identification of the proper risk group for spine pain allows ease of categorization into

Annotated References

1. Vos T, Flaxman AD, Naghavi M, et al: Years lived with disability (YLDs) for 1160 sequelae of 289 diseases and injuries 1990-2010: A systematic analysis for the Global Burden of Disease Study 2010. *Lancet* 2012;380(9859):2163-2196.

   This systematic analysis for the Global Burden of Disease Study reported that the main disease contributors were mental and behavioral disorders, musculoskeletal disorders, and diabetes or endocrine diseases. The leading causes of years lived with disability (LBP, major depressive disorder, iron-deficiency anemia, neck pain, chronic obstructive pulmonary disease, anxiety disorders, migraine, diabetes, and falls) were approximately the same in 2010 as they were in 1990.

2. Matsumoto M, Okada E, Ichihara D, et al: Prospective ten-year follow-up study comparing patients with whiplash-associated disorders and asymptomatic subjects

using magnetic resonance imaging. *Spine (Phila Pa 1976)* 2010;35(18):1684-1690.

3. Matsumoto M, Okada E, Ichihara D, et al: Age-related changes of thoracic and cervical intervertebral discs in asymptomatic subjects. *Spine (Phila Pa 1976)* 2010;35(14):1359-1364.

4. Moseley GL: Teaching people about pain: Why do we keep beating around the bush? *Pain Manag* 2012;2(1):1-3.

    A clear and direct relationship does not exist among pain, nociception, and tissue damage. Pain is multifactorial and broadly fits within the following three categories: prioritization, meaning, and transmission/processing. Evidence shows tissue pathology does not equate to chronic pain. The goal is reconceptualization of pain before it becomes chronic pain.

5. Sembrano JN, Polly DW Jr: How often is low back pain not coming from the back? *Spine (Phila Pa 1976)* 2009;34(1):E27-E32.

6. Nijs J, Apeldoorn A, Hallegraeff H, et al: Low back pain: Guidelines for the clinical classification of predominant neuropathic, nociceptive, or central sensitization pain. *Pain Physician* 2015;18(3):E333-E346.

    Low back pain is a diverse condition that includes nociceptive, neuropathic, and central sensitization pain. The pain classification system for LBP is focused on these pain mechanisms and should be considered an addition to classification systems and diagnostic procedures.

7. Kolski MC, O'Connor A, Van Der Laan K, Lee J, Kozlowski AJ, Deutsch A: Validation of a pain mechanism classification system (PMCS) in physical therapy practice. *J Man Manip Ther* 2016;24(4):192-199.

    The authors provide validation that peripheral components of pain can be classified and the PMCS can be implemented into clinical practice. The study used cluster analysis; 97% of the patients were classified.

8. Fritz JM, Cleland JA, Childs JD: Subgrouping patients with low back pain: Evolution of a classification approach to physical therapy. *J Orthop Sports Phys Ther* 2007;37(6):290-302.

9. Clare HA, Adams R, Maher CG: Reliability of McKenzie classification of patients with cervical or lumbar pain. *J Manipulative Physiol Ther* 2005;28(2):122-127.

10. Delitto A, Erhard RE, Bowling RW: A treatment-based classification approach to low back syndrome: Identifying and staging patients for conservative treatment. *Phys Ther* 1995;75(6):470-485, discussion 485-489.

11. Burns SA, Foresman E, Kraycsir SJ, et al: A treatment-based classification approach to examination and intervention of lumbar disorders. *Sports Health* 2011;3(4):362-372.

    LBP is a common athletic injury resulting in missed play time. The TBC system allows the clinician to reliably classify the athlete's condition and apply the optimal intervention, with the potential to reduce lost participation time, disability, and pain.

12. Butler DS, Gifford LS: The integration of pain science into clinical practice. *J Hand Ther* 1997;10(2):86-95.

13. Smart KM, Curley A, Blake C, Staines A, Doody C: The reliability of clinical judgments and criteria associated with mechanisms-based classifications of pain in patients with low back pain disorders: A preliminary reliability study. *J Man Manip Ther* 2010;18(2):102-110.

14. Butler DS: *The Sensitive Nervous System*. Adelaide, Australia, NOI Group Publications, 2000.

15. Smart KM, Blake C, Staines A, Doody C: Clinical indicators of 'nociceptive', 'peripheral neuropathic' and 'central' mechanisms of musculoskeletal pain: A Delphi survey of expert clinicians. *Man Ther* 2010;15(1):80-87.

16. Kolski M, O'Connor A: *World of Hurt: A Guide to Classifying Pain* .St. Louis, MO, Thomas Land Publishers Inc, 2015, p 194.

    The authors select elements from two medical classification systems to create one useful and comprehensive guide for pain classification. An integrative approach to pain classification and practical guidance to the approach of diagnosis and treatment are presented.

17. Thomas CL: *Taber's Cyclopedic Medical Dictionary* ,ed 12. Philadelphia, PA, F.A. Davis Company, 1973, p T-62.

18. Little P, Roberts L, Blowers H, et al: Should we give detailed advice and information booklets to patients with back pain? A randomized controlled factorial trial of a self-management booklet and doctor advice to take exercise for back pain. *Spine (Phila Pa 1976)* 2001;26(19):2065-2072.

19. Cherkin DC, Deyo RA, Street JH, Hunt M, Barlow W: Pitfalls of patient education: Limited success of a program for back pain in primary care. *Spine (Phila Pa 1976)* 1996;21(3):345-355.

20. Udermann BE, Spratt KF, Donelson RG, Mayer J, Graves JE, Tillotson J: Can a patient educational book change behavior and reduce pain in chronic low back pain patients? *Spine J* 2004;4(4):425-435.

21. Fletcher C, Bradnam L, Barr C: The relationship between knowledge of pain neurophysiology and fear avoidance in people with chronic pain: A point in time, observational study. *Physiother Theory Pract* 2016;32(4):271-276.

    Patients who are more knowledgeable about the neurophysiology of pain exhibit less fear avoidance. Clinically, education can decrease fear avoidance and may be an effective strategy to decrease disability in patients with chronic pain.

22. Moseley GL: Evidence for a direct relationship between cognitive and physical change during an education

3: Medical Management of Spine Disorders

intervention in people with chronic low back pain. *Eur J Pain* 2004;8(1):39-45.

23. Roberts L, Little P, Chapman J, Cantrell T, Pickering R, Langridge J: The back home trial: General practitioner-supported leaflets may change back pain behavior. *Spine (Phila Pa 1976)* 2002;27(17):1821-1828.

24. McKenzie R, May S: *The Lumbar Spine: Mechanical Diagnosis & Therapy,* ed 2. Waikanae, New Zealand, Spinal Publications, 2003.

25. Moseley L: Unraveling the barriers to reconceptualization of the problem in chronic pain: The actual and perceived ability of patients and health professionals to understand the neurophysiology. *J Pain* 2003;4(4):184-189.

26. Randhawa K, Côté P, Gross DP, et al: The effectiveness of structured patient education for the management of musculoskeletal disorders and injuries of the extremities: A systematic review by the Ontario Protocol for Traffic Injury Management (OPTIMa) Collaboration. *J Can Chiropr Assoc* 2015;59(4):349-362.

    Little is known regarding the effectiveness of structured patient education concerning musculoskeletal disorders of the extremities. Two studies found that education used alone may be less effective than other interventions in patients with persistent lateral epicondylitis and patellofemoral syndrome.

27. Dagenais S, Caro J, Haldeman S: A systematic review of low back pain cost of illness studies in the United States and internationally. *Spine J* 2008;8(1):8-20.

28. Long A, Donelson R, Fung T: Does it matter which exercise? A randomized control trial of exercise for low back pain. *Spine (Phila Pa 1976)* 2004;29(23):2593-2602.

29. Long A, May S, Fung T: The comparative prognostic value of directional preference and centralization: A useful tool for front-line clinicians? *J Man Manip Ther* 2008;16(4):248-254.

30. May S: Classification by McKenzie mechanical syndromes: A survey of McKenzie-trained faculty. *J Manipulative Physiol Ther* 2006;29(8):637-642.

31. Hefford C: McKenzie classification of mechanical spinal pain: Profile of syndromes and directions of preference. *Man Ther* 2008;13(1):75-81.

32. Werneke MW, Hart DL, Cutrone G, et al: Association between directional preference and centralization in patients with low back pain. *J Orthop Sports Phys Ther* 2011;41(1):22-31.

    Findings of this study suggest that classification by pain pattern, directional preference, and centralization can improve the ability of a therapist to provide a short-term prognosis regarding function and pain outcomes. Directional preference and centralization should be considered independent classification variables. Level of evidence: Ib.

33. Otéro J, Bonne F: Low back pain: Prevalence of McKenzie's syndromes and directional preferences. *Kinésithérapie, la Revue* 2014;14(145):36-44.

    A high rate of derangement was found in the lumbar spine based on the McKenzie classification. Extension was the most prevalent directional preference, followed by lateral movement and flexion. Derangement was confirmed in 90% of cases, and directional preference changed in 26.5% of cases. Level of evidence: II.

34. McKenzie R: *The Cervical and Thoracic Spine: Mechanical Diagnosis and Therapy.* Waikanae, New Zealand, Spinal Publications, 1990.

35. Alrwaily M, Timko M, Schneider M, et al: Treatment-based classification system for low back pain: Revision and update. *Phys Ther* 2016;96(7):1057-1066.

    Use of the TBC system reduces disability and pain. The first level of classification is to determine if physical therapy is appropriate for the patient. The second level of classification determines the severity of the patient's condition and resulting disability. The third level of classification divides patients into four subgroups to direct treatment selection—manipulation, stabilization, specific exercise, and traction.

36. Edmond SL, Cutrone G, Werneke M, et al: Association between centralization and directional preference and functional and pain outcomes in patients with neck pain. *J Orthop Sports Phys Ther* 2014;44(2):68-75.

    Directional preference and centralization were associated with improved functional outcomes in patients with neck pain. Neither centralization nor directional preference was associated with pain outcomes.

37. Otéro J, Bonne F: Neck pain: Prevalence of McKenzie's syndrome and directional preferences. 2015. Available at: https://www.researchgate.net/publication/286875499_Neck_Pain_Prevalence_of_McKenzie%27s_Syndrome_and_Directional_Preference. Accessed June 5, 2017.

    The authors investigated the prevalence of centralization of pain and directional preference in patients with nonspecific neck pain and directional stability over time. A high rate of derangement syndrome was reported, with the classification confirmed 9 of 10 times. The directional preference changed in 41% of the cases. Level of evidence: III.

38. Leerar PJ, Boissonnault W, Domholdt E, Roddey T: Documentation of red flags by physical therapists for patients with low back pain. *J Man Manip Ther* 2007;15(1):42-49.

39. Liebenson CS, Yeomans SG: Yellow flags: Early identification of risk factors of chronicity in acute patients. *J Rehabil Outcomes Meas* 2000;4(2):31-40.

40. Liebenson CS, Yeomans SG: Identification of the patient at risk for persistent or recurrent low back trouble, in Yeomans SG, ed: *Application of Outcomes Assessment to Clinical Practice.* New York, NY, Appleton & Lange, 2000, pp 437-447.

41. Hill JC, Whitehurst DG, Lewis M, et al: Comparison of stratified primary care management for low back pain with current best practice (STarT Back): A randomised controlled trial. *Lancet* 2011;378(9802):1560-1571.

    LBP is a worldwide problem. A stratified and a nonstratified management model were compared. The results of the study show that the stratified approach has a general health benefit and cost savings.

42. Foster NE, Mullis R, Hill JC, et al; IMPaCT Back Study team: Effect of stratified care for low back pain in family practice (IMPaCT Back): A prospective population-based sequential comparison. *Ann Fam Med* 2014;12(2):102-111.

    Family practice use of stratified care for patients with LBP resulted in improvement in patient disability and a reduction in time off from work without an increase in healthcare costs. The mean time off work was 50% less and there was a 30% decrease in sickness certification in patients managed with stratified care compared with those given typical care.

43. Lentz TA, Beneciuk JM, Bialosky JE, et al: Development of a yellow flag assessment tool for orthopaedic physical therapists: Results from the Optimal Screening for Prediction of Referral and Outcome (OSPRO) Cohort. *J Orthop Sports Phys Ther* 2016;46(5):327-343.

    Assessment of yellow flags in outpatient therapy clinics is feasible. A yellow flag tool is a multidimensional tool that can be used to screen pain-associated psychological distress. Further research is needed to compare the results to risk assessment tools for treatment monitoring.

3: Medical Management of Spine Disorders

Chapter 12

Manual Medicine and Spine Care

Samuel A. Yoakum, DO   John M. Lavelle, DO

Abstract

Spinal manipulative treatment is a frequently used option for patients with acute or chronic low back pain. Understanding the variety of treatment techniques and the appropriate selection of patients is important for the successful use of osteopathic manipulative medicine. When used by the spine specialist or orthopaedic practitioner, manual medicine can provide a safe and beneficial treatment option.

Keywords: nonsurgical options; nonsurgical spine care; spinal manipulation

Introduction

The topic of spine care is exceedingly broad, largely because of the variety of problems that can result in a patient seeking care. A substantial amount of care provided for the spine is related to the nonspecific diagnosis of low back pain, as well as its equally vague associated diagnosis of neck pain. In the setting of serious spinal disorders, which can be traumatic, degenerative, or pathologic in nature, a theoretically finite number of presentations and causative agents exist, most of which can be paired with an appropriate workup and a range of reasonable treatment options. However, given the breadth of entities potentially responsible for axial low back pain or neck pain, particularly any chronic or subacute variety, the overworked practitioner may simply add the semispecific, virtually all-encompassing term "musculoskeletal" to the diagnosis. Irrespective of specialization in the spine, any practitioner who evaluates patients with such musculoskeletal problems recognizes the vast number of

patients with subjective discomfort caused not by fracture or neurocompression disorder, but rather by one of many potential muscular, soft-tissue, or articular dysfunctions. These issues are quite frequently included in the realm of manual medicine, and have been for many years.

Origins of Osteopathic Medicine

Osteopathic medicine was introduced in 1874 and based on several central tenets: structure and function are interrelated, the body has self-regulatory mechanisms (such as homeostasis), and the body is one interrelated unit; rational treatment of patients should consider these tenets. None of these concepts is particularly radical and would be considered reasonable by most physicians. The first students of osteopathic medicine learned to examine for dysfunction within the plasticity of the structure of the body, and when appropriate, sought to resolve the dysfunction and help reestablish homeostasis. This goal was accomplished by using one of many techniques classified under the general term manipulation. Manual medicine has been in use longer than American systems such as osteopathy, which regarded manipulation as an augmentation of medical treatment, or the more widely known chiropractic approach, which presented a complete alternative to medical care. These systems predominate in western medicine, and over time influenced greatly the day-to-day practices of physical therapy and massage.

Osteopathy in the Literature

Although a cursory PubMed search using terms such as "spinal manipulation" and "manual techniques" combined with "low back pain" or "spine pain" will result in thousands of citations, studies of sufficient size, breadth, and levels of blinding are limited. Some studies offer insight into the potential effectiveness of the use of manual medicine in spine care. A 1999 study on low back pain demonstrated that osteopathic spinal manipulation used fewer days for medication and physical therapy compared with standard medicine.[1] In 2003, a randomized controlled study demonstrated a similar reduction

3: Medical Management of Spine Disorders

in physical therapy days as well as a decrease in overall cost in patients with low back pain.[2] In 2004, a systematic review noted that in patients with acute low back pain, manipulation provided more short-term relief than several other physical therapy techniques.[3] When evaluating chronic low back pain, manipulation was found to have an effect essentially equal to that of NSAIDs and provided short-term relief equivalent to medical management and long-term relief similar to that of physical therapy. Although positive evidence was reported, none of these studies demonstrated overwhelming improvement when compared with other treatment modalities. A 2010 study in the United Kingdom examined a broad variety of both medical and pain-related ailments and found spinal manipulation to be effective for acute and chronic back pain as well as neck pain and cervicogenic headache.[4] Thoracic manipulation was found to improve cervical pain, but cervical manipulation alone was inconclusive. A 2011 study comparing structured exercise with manipulation found improvements to be equivalent in pain complaint and function at 8 weeks.[5]

Many studies have conclusions with familiar descriptions such as inconclusive, no worse than, and not superior to.[6-8] These results appear to be the most common; therefore, they are frequently used as evidence to discount any benefit from manual techniques in patients with spine problems. The most recently performed meta-analysis reported at least modest benefit with the use of spinal manipulative therapy in patients with acute back pain.[9] In this study, however, no specific modality, treatment type, or clinical operator could be identified as superior to another. One difficulty in developing specific, robust, evidence-based practice recommendations is the inadequate number of studies performed; however, it is necessary to consider why the studies that have been conducted have demonstrated little or no statistical difference among nonsurgical treatments. The challenge of interpreting outcomes and making recommendations in these studies is similar to the challenges faced by those investigating interventional pain procedures. Establishing evidence in interventional pain treatment and manual treatment is difficult because of confounding variables. Essentially, the categorization of these patients becomes vaguer, which results in inconclusive evidence. Similarly, each intervention must be performed by a clinician, who will have his or her own processes, techniques, and approaches, all of which are counterproductive for achieving a successful, repeatable investigation resulting in level I evidence. The reasonable conclusion that can be drawn from the available evidence is that manipulation may be one of many tools used against the vagaries of musculoskeletal axial spine complaints, and although a balanced approach is necessary, manipulation can be included as a worthwhile treatment for patients with acute and chronic neck- and back-related problems.

The Knowledge Gap Between Osteopathy and the Traditional Medical Approach

One of the barriers to understanding between physicians who practice manual medicine (as well as physical and occupational therapists, chiropractors, and licensed massage therapists) and most physicians is not a lack of knowledge but a lack of a common language. What exactly is the goal of manipulation? What is being treated aside from vague musculoskeletal problems? Manual practitioners should choose their techniques and focus areas based on the appropriate diagnosis of an injury. In osteopathic medicine, the problems being treated are referred to as somatic dysfunction, which means disrupted function of the body, typically at the local level. These disruptions most frequently occur in articular areas (such as facet joints), in muscles, and throughout the high-tension zones of the soft tissues.

Although some practitioners use generic, universal treatment routines for all patients with similar problems, this approach is similar to offering an epidural steroid injection for every patient who reports back pain: some patients will improve, but establishing a clear diagnosis before treatment is begun should result in a better, more efficient, and more economical outcome. The location of the individual's symptoms is of some value, and the patient history also helps, but most diagnoses in manual medicine result from primarily palpatory examinations.

Evaluation for somatic dysfunction relies largely on asymmetry (both static and with movement) and restriction of motion. In osteopathy, perfect alignment is not the actual goal because many patients have anatomic asymmetry as their baseline. Rather, freedom of motion and full range of motion within the anatomic limits is the goal; therefore, any restriction is primarily considered the starting point. In the axial spine, vertebral segments are first assessed as a group and then individually, considering the changing mechanics as the spine enters lordosis, transitions to kyphosis, eases through neutral, and then returns to lordosis. Tissue texture changes also are important clues (particularly in soft-tissue concerns and acute symptoms in the axial spine) and tenderness of the area also can be of value in making a diagnosis. In soft tissues, particularly the layers from the surface to the outer muscle layers, tissue texture changes (the so-called lumps and bumps) often are evidence of somatic dysfunction. The more acute the dysfunction or injury, the more acute the findings, including redness, local microedema, tautness, and warmth. Soft-tissue somatic dysfunction that is more chronic tends to produce findings that are more chronic, often described as ropey or stringy, and even a leathery feeling of the overlying dermis, which is typical with more dense soft tissue.

Indications for Treatment

Although practitioners who primarily focus on manipulation likely can find some type of subacute dysfunction to treat in almost any patient, certain patients and diagnoses are more appropriate for a manual treatment plan. Many common back and neck pain conditions can be treated effectively with osteopathic manipulation, particularly because it is used to maintain proper body mechanics and motion. The goal of treatment for all conditions is to improve function, and ultimately, quality of life, by means of treatment to relieve motion restrictions. This goal is accomplished via proper diagnosis of areas of restriction within the neuromusculoskeletal system and by restoring optimal tissue texture, body symmetry, and range of motion. By improving motion and flexibility within the spine by means of mobilization of the joints, muscles, fascia, muscle function, and spine mechanics can be optimized, allowing improvement in the patient's day-to-day activities and function.

Most spinal pain results from the complex interactions between the spine with normal age-related degeneration and the sensitivity and responsiveness of the nervous system, which regulates the consciousness of pain.[10] When pain is present, compensatory patterns often develop to alleviate the patients' pain, resulting in restrictions in joint motion, hypertonicity within muscles, and fascial strain patterns. These patterns also are identified as somatic dysfunction and can affectively be improved with osteopathic manipulative treatment resulting in the normalization of physiologic motion and decreased pain.

Osteopathic manipulative treatment also should be considered in patients with pain resulting from muscle strains/sprains or myofascial pain such as in athletic injuries, whiplash injuries, or even from performing housework. By applying osteopathic manipulative treatment techniques to the restricted joint, muscular and/or fascial motion can be restored more effectively, facilitating a return to normal mechanics, improvement in pain, and reduced use of oral medication.

In conditions such as spinal stenosis, disk herniations, radiculopathy, or scoliosis, osteopathic manipulative treatment can alleviate chronic somatic symptoms and potentially optimize tissue mechanics to improve back pain over time.[5,6,11-13] The likelihood of worsening a single-level disk herniation by means of spinal

manipulation is exceedingly low.[14] Although manipulation is unlikely to resolve underlying problems, there is value in potentially improving mobilization and function and reducing pain levels by treating somatic dysfunction with osteopathic manipulative treatment.[2,5,8]

When to Avoid or Modify Treatment

Certain patients and diagnoses respond well to manual treatment, whereas other patients and diagnoses are unlikely to improve after manipulation. In certain patients (specifically, patients with a history of cancer, acute fracture, osteomyelitis, discitis, severe osteoporosis, or rheumatoid arthritis), manipulation should be used with caution to prevent trauma or worsening dysfunction. Osteopathic manipulative treatment is not contraindicated in these patients, but the treatment technique and duration needs to be selected carefully. High velocity–low amplitude thrust techniques should be avoided because of the risk of fracture. In the setting of rheumatoid arthritis, a risk of spinal cord compromise exists with cervical manipulation if the cruciform ligament has sustained damage. Indirect techniques are recommended in these patients.

During osteopathic manipulative treatment, if progressive neurologic decline develops in a patient or associated constitutional symptoms such as night pain, fever, or bowel/bladder dysfunction occur, the appropriate workup with further diagnostic tests should be performed to determine the proper treatment course.

Technique

Many categories of techniques have been developed, with some targeting specific types of dysfunction and others offering multiple approaches for managing the same type of dysfunction. The osteopathic model has two major technique types: direct techniques that engage the restriction and indirect techniques that work away from the restrictive barrier to relieve tension and pressure. The choice of technique often relies as much on a practitioner's knowledge, experience, comfort level, and preference as it does the specific dysfunction because many dysfunctions can be approached either directly or indirectly. Information regarding osteopathic principles and techniques is abundantly available.[15,16]

Direct Techniques
Muscle Energy
The osteopathic term muscle energy is not used as extensively as activated stretching or contract-relax, both of which better describe the technique. The targeted somatic

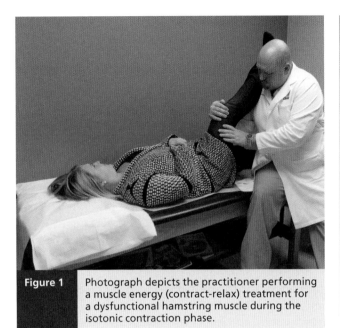

Figure 1   Photograph depicts the practitioner performing a muscle energy (contract-relax) treatment for a dysfunctional hamstring muscle during the isotonic contraction phase.

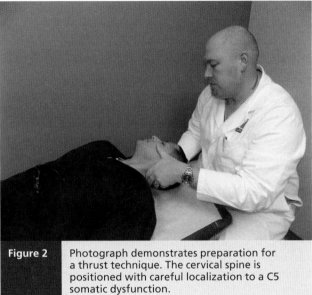

Figure 2   Photograph demonstrates preparation for a thrust technique. The cervical spine is positioned with careful localization to a C5 somatic dysfunction.

dysfunction may be in the muscle belly itself, or may be an articulating joint spanned by the muscle; in either case, the restrictive barrier is engaged, most frequently by stretching the muscle to the edge of tolerable range of motion and maintaining it in a static position. The patient is directed to activate that muscle in an isotonic contraction while the practitioner holds against that force (**Figure 1**). The contraction is held for 3 to 5 seconds, and the muscle is then allowed to relax. After a few seconds of elapse to allow complete relaxation of the muscle, the muscle is stretched further to the new edge of its range of motion. This is repeated until the restriction is gone or until no further improvement is obtained.

High Velocity–Low Amplitude
High velocity–low amplitude techniques are the thrust techniques most individuals think of in a discussion of manipulation. The purpose of a high velocity–low amplitude technique is to articulate a joint that is held in a dysfunctional pattern. This is similar to cracking a stiff proximal interphalangeal joint, and should be no more forceful or painful when applied appropriately. Some individuals use broad-range, high velocity–high amplitude techniques for the general treatment of an entire region, such as the whole cervical or lumbar spine, with a single technique. These shotgun techniques are quick and can be relatively successful in young patients, but the potential exists for unintended injury, so a more targeted approach is best. The low amplitude aspect of a high velocity–low amplitude technique implies a targeted, localized, and fine-tuned setup of a single vertebral segment pair

(**Figure 2**) or other joint to apply a short, brisk thrust. This technique should not be painful for the patient; pain implies a problem with the setup or technique chosen. Some patients may be uneasy and have strong apprehensive muscle tension. Patients should not be pushed through these techniques; rather, a different technique should be chosen.

Soft-Tissue Techniques
Soft-tissue techniques are most appropriately compared with massage both in appearance and effect. The techniques are typically direct (working into the restrictive barriers) but can be indirect (working with and away from the restriction) and are often alternating combinations of both. Often, a general area surrounding the specific somatic dysfunction is treated to reduce outside tension forces on the targeted somatic dysfunction. The techniques involve using the pads of the fingers and the heels of the hands to gently mobilize the soft tissues, typically in a lateral direction (**Figure 3**). Force is typically applied at 15° to 30° from horizontal and should not be particularly uncomfortable for the patient. As the restrictions are released, other techniques can be applied to treat the deeper dysfunction.

Indirect Techniques
Indirect techniques present minimal risk of injury or agitation because they are directed away from the restriction; however, the techniques are more challenging to perform because they require the palpatory capacity to feel the tissues release tension as they relax and the restriction dissipates.

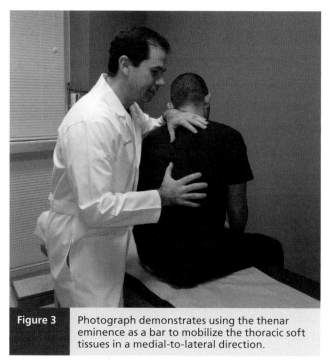

Figure 3 | Photograph demonstrates using the thenar eminence as a bar to mobilize the thoracic soft tissues in a medial-to-lateral direction.

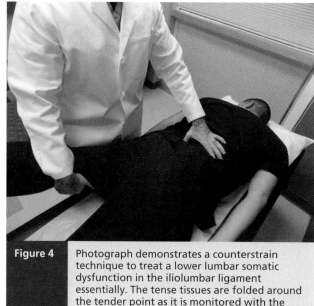

Figure 4 | Photograph demonstrates a counterstrain technique to treat a lower lumbar somatic dysfunction in the iliolumbar ligament essentially. The tense tissues are folded around the tender point as it is monitored with the second digit of the monitoring hand.

Counterstrain Technique

Counterstrain techniques, also called strain-counterstrain, is a somewhat broad category that focuses on treating individual areas of somatic dysfunction in the belly of individual muscles referred to simply as tender points. After a tender point is identified in an individual muscle, the muscle around the tender point is shortened by the practitioner while continuously palpating the tender point with a single digit, based on the directionality of the particular muscle fibers (**Figure 4**). Most commonly, patient feedback is elicited while a position of greatest comfort is attempted and held for a varied amount of time (novices are taught to hold this position for approximately 90 seconds). Ideally, complete resolution is achieved at this point. The concept of this technique is to reduce as much tension as possible from the fibers surrounding the tender area to completely reset muscle fiber length to baseline levels.

Facilitated Positional Release

Facilitated positional release techniques are similar to counterstrain techniques in most ways. Tender points, or dysfunctional segments, are palpated and focused on. The area is arranged in multiple planes to find a position of comfort, whether subjectively for the patient or relative to a balance point of neutral tension for the practitioner. After such a position is identified, a facilitating force is applied to the area (**Figure 5**), typically compression or distraction, to refine the amount of tension. The use of

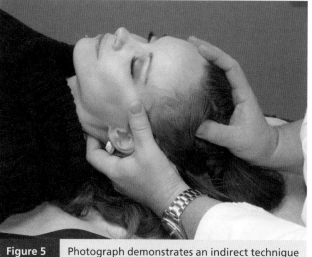

Figure 5 | Photograph demonstrates an indirect technique for the cervical spine, initially set up for either counterstrain or facilitated positional release. This position creates an axial load down the cervical spine to facilitate treatment.

this facilitating force typically requires control of both ends of the joint, which makes this maneuver easily executable for the cervical spine, wrists, and ankles, but more challenging for the lumbar spine and hips.

Myofascial Release

Myofascial techniques vary greatly by practitioner and by patient. Patients with high sensitivity to typical mobilization and exercise sometimes do better with myofascial techniques. Myofascial release, which is frequently performed in a direct fashion, typically focuses on the soft

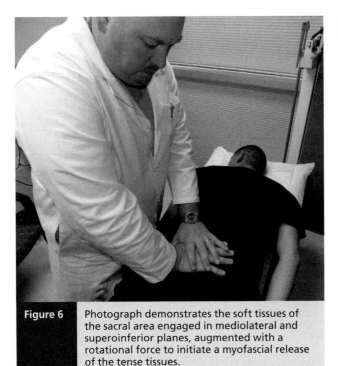

Figure 6 Photograph demonstrates the soft tissues of the sacral area engaged in mediolateral and superoinferior planes, augmented with a rotational force to initiate a myofascial release of the tense tissues.

tissues and follows tension lines to find positions of least tension (indirect) or most tension (direct). In general, tissues are manipulated in craniocaudal and mediolateral planes and augmented with rotational forces (**Figure 6**). These techniques are the most highly subjective, both for identification of somatic dysfunction and reassessment after treatment.

The Practitioner

Because the experience, capacity, proficiency, and setting of each practitioner of manipulation can vary greatly, the considered diagnosis and treatment selection are dependent on who performs the manipulation. Identified potential challenges that are not likely to improve with manipulation may require other attention or workup, and they can be worsened with the application of substantial manual force. Currently, subgroups of individuals licensed for body work, from traditional osteopathic physicians and chiropractors to most physical therapists (and more recently, licensed massage therapists and athletic trainers) are marketing themselves as experts in treating the same problems as orthopaedic surgeons and spine specialists. Sharing information and fully informing all members of the treatment team (irrespective of whether they work in the same organization) of the risks and benefits of any treatments provided is in the best interest of the patient.

Summary

Many patients who consult with orthopaedic surgeons have specific preferences, needs, and inherent biases, along with predetermined notions about their symptoms, expected diagnosis, and the type of treatment they are willing to undergo. Some patients may consider manipulation to be an intimidating treatment option. It is helpful if the orthopaedic surgeon or spine specialist has a general understanding of the terminology used by practitioners of manipulation and is familiar with the focus of the individual offering care involving manipulation. Although the literature has not demonstrated manipulation to be superior to other nonsurgical measures, many patients may be receptive to management of their spinal condition with a method that is considered as effective as NSAIDs. Spinal manipulation has been demonstrated to help in the management of symptoms of both acute and chronic back and neck pain, and it should be considered a reasonable option for managing appropriate spinal conditions.

Key Study Points

- Osteopathic manipulative treatment is the treatment of somatic dysfunction for removing restrictions in bodily function.
- Manipulative treatments are all based on the idea that the body possesses self-regulatory mechanisms that can be augmented or supported by manipulation just as they are by medical treatment.
- Spinal manipulative treatment has been demonstrated to be at least moderately effective in the treatment of acute low back pain.
- Injuries during manipulative treatment are rare and typically involve transient muscle irritation.
- For patients with mechanical spine pain who are hesitant to undergo standard medical treatments, appropriately directed manipulative treatment should be considered as a viable option.

Annotated References

1. Andersson GB, Lucente T, Davis AM, Kappler RE, Lipton JA, Leurgans S: A comparison of osteopathic spinal manipulation with standard care for patients with low back pain. *N Engl J Med* 1999;341(19):1426-1431.

2. Licciardone JC, Stoll ST, Fulda KG, et al: Osteopathic manipulative treatment for chronic low back pain: A

randomized controlled trial. *Spine (Phila Pa 1976)* 2003;28(13):1355-1362.

3. Bronfort G, Haas M, Evans RL, Bouter LM: Efficacy of spinal manipulation and mobilization for low back pain and neck pain: A systematic review and best evidence synthesis. *Spine J* 2004;4(3):335-356.

4. Bronfort G, Haas M, Evans R, Leininger B, Triano J: Effectiveness of manual therapies: The UK evidence report. *Chiropr Osteopat* 2010;18:3.

5. Standaert CJ, Friedly J, Erwin MW, et al: Comparative effectiveness of exercise, acupuncture, and spinal manipulation for low back pain. *Spine (Phila Pa 1976)* 2011;36(21suppl):S120-S130.

This multistudy analysis compared several interventions for back pain. The studies indicate that structured exercise and spinal manipulation therapy appear to have equivalent benefits in pain and functional improvement for those with chronic low back pain with clinical benefits evident within 8 weeks of care.

6. Rubinstein SM, van Middelkoop M, Assendelft WJ, de Boer MR, van Tulder MW: Spinal manipulative therapy for chronic low-back pain. *Cochrane Database Syst Rev* 2011;2:CD008112.

This Cochrane review analyzed a large group of studies, eliminating those with apparent risk of bias, and determined no difference between spinal manipulation and other nonsurgical care.

7. Chou R, Qaseem A, Snow V, et al; Clinical Efficacy Assessment Subcommittee of the American College of Physicians; American College of Physicians; American Pain Society Low Back Pain Guidelines Panel: Diagnosis and treatment of low back pain: A joint clinical practice guideline from the American College of Physicians and the American Pain Society. *Ann Intern Med* 2007;147(7):478-491.

8. Assendelft WJ, Morton SC, Yu EI, Suttorp MJ, Shekelle PG: Spinal manipulative therapy for low back pain: A meta-analysis of effectiveness relative to other therapies. *Ann Intern Med* 2003;138(11):871-881.

9. Paige NM, Miake-Lye IM, Booth MS, et al: Association of spinal manipulative therapy with clinical benefit and harm for acute low back pain: Systematic review and meta-analysis. *JAMA* 2017;317(14):1451-1460.

The effectiveness of spinal manipulative therapy for acute low back pain was reviewed. Modest improvements in pain and function were reported at up to 6 weeks.

10. Rainville J, Sobel J, Hartigan C, Monlux G, Bean J: Decreasing disability in chronic back pain through aggressive spine rehabilitation. *J Rehabil Res Dev* 1997;34(4):383-393.

11. Schneider M, Haas M, Glick R, Stevans J, Landsittel D: Comparison of spinal manipulation methods and usual medical care for acute and subacute low back pain: A randomized clinical trial. *Spine (Phila Pa 1976)* 2015;40(4):209-217.

In this randomized clinical trial, acute and subacute low back pain were treated with medical care, muscle energy techniques, or thrust techniques. All treatments resulted in some improvement, and the thrust techniques provided the best self-reported improvement in the short term. Level of evidence: II.

12. Senna MK, Machaly SA: Does maintained spinal manipulation therapy for chronic nonspecific low back pain result in better long-term outcome? *Spine (Phila Pa 1976)* 2011;36(18):1427-1437.

This small, single-blinded, placebo-controlled study examined baseline manipulation versus long-term maintenance treatment. The longer-term treatment was demonstrated to maintain improvements achieved during initial treatment phase.

13. Lau HM, Wing Chiu TT, Lam TH: The effectiveness of thoracic manipulation on patients with chronic mechanical neck pain: A randomized controlled trial. *Man Ther* 2011;16(2):141-147.

This randomized controlled trial reported on thoracic manipulation in patients with chronic neck pain with an initial treatment phase and follow-up at 8 weeks and 3 and 6 months. The patients with manipulation had substantially better self-reported improvement directly after treatment and at follow-up.

14. Oliphant D: Safety of spinal manipulation in the treatment of lumbar disk herniations: A systematic review and risk assessment. *J Manipulative Physiol Ther* 2004;27(3):197-210.

15. Chila A, ed: *Foundations of Osteopathic Medicine*, ed 3. Philadelphia, PA, Lippincott Williams & Wilkins, 2011.

This text provides a comprehensive description of most aspects of osteopathy.

16. DeStefano LA: *Greenman's Principles of Manual Medicine,* ed 5. Philadelphia, PA, Wolters Kluwer, 2017.

This text provides a practical hands-on application of the principles of manual medicine for use in the clinical setting.

3: Medical Management of Spine Disorders

Chapter 13

Alternative Medicine and Spine Care

Chi-Tsai Tang, MD   Craig Ziegler, MD

Abstract

Alternative medicine is gaining popularity within mainstream Western medical practice, and literature supporting various treatments is growing. Management of low back and neck pain include acupuncture, dry needling, cupping, chiropractic care, massage therapy, herbal medicines and supplements, yoga, and tai chi. Acupuncture involves inserting small needles in specific locations in the body, and dry needling can be viewed as a westernized form of acupuncture with a limited indication of managing myofascial pain. Acupuncture has the most evidence supporting it, and can provide improvements in pain and function immediately postintervention and potentially for several months in patients with chronic low back pain and neck disorders. Cupping provides suction to the skin to help increase blood circulation. Chiropractic care typically involves performing spinal manipulations using high-velocity, low-amplitude thrusts. Massage therapy involves manipulation of different layers of muscles and fascia. Several herbal medicines and supplements may be effective for managing acute or chronic low back pain. Yoga and tai chi are movement-based treatments that involve a meditative and breathing component, respectively.

Keywords: acupuncture; chiropractic care; complementary and alternative medicine; cupping; dry needling; herbal medicine; supplements; massage therapy; tai chi; yoga

Introduction

Complementary and alternative medicine (CAM) is a therapy that is not fully accepted in mainstream Western medical practice. Reasons include a lack of medical literature to support its use and an accepted mechanism of action. Many treatments that have been historically considered alternative in the United States are gaining popularity and acceptance. Professional athletes' use of alternative treatments, the desire for more natural treatments, and a lack of efficacy from standard mainstream treatments often are reasons for the use of CAM therapy. The medical literature supporting many alternative treatments is growing. A recent study showed that patients with lumbar disk herniations and radiating pain who received CAM therapy had significant improvements in pain and function. Eighty-seven percent of patients were highly satisfied or satisfied, and fewer than 10% went on to have surgery at 5-year follow-up.[1]

Alternative treatments of the spine can be categorized as (1) bioenergetic therapies, such as acupuncture or cupping; (2) biomechanical treatments, such as chiropractic care or massage therapy; (3) supplements and herbal products; and (4) mind-body therapies, such as yoga, tai chi, or hypnosis. Although a comprehensive review of alternative treatments is beyond the scope of this chapter, common treatments with supporting evidence are reviewed.

Acupuncture

Acupuncture is probably one of the most well-known alternative treatments in spine care. Treatment involves placing small (typically 30- to 36-gauge) solid filiform needles in several specific locations on the body. Acupuncture has its origins in traditional Chinese medicine, in which the ancient Chinese believed pain was a result of blockages in the flow of qi (life energy) and stagnation in the flow of blood. The Chinese believed that qi circulated along meridians, and that qi can be influenced by needling specific acupuncture points along the body.

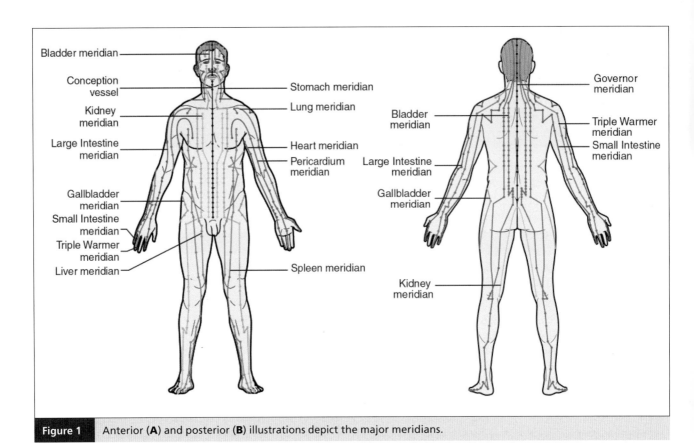

Figure 1 Anterior (**A**) and posterior (**B**) illustrations depict the major meridians.

There are 361 different acupuncture points along the body that are distributed along 12 principal meridians and 8 extraordinary meridians (**Figure 1**). The 12 principal meridians are named after traditional Chinese medicine organs and include the Gallbladder, Heart, Kidney, Large Intestine, Liver, Lung, Pericardium, Small Intestine, Spleen, Stomach, Urinary Bladder, and Triple Heater or San Jiao. The San Jiao does not have an analogous organ in Western medicine, but functions in metabolism and is located in the thoracic and abdominopelvic cavities. Specific acupuncture points are designated by the meridian on which they are located and a particular number. Many of the acupuncture points correlate with motor points of muscles, are over focal meeting points of superficial nerves, or are located along intermuscular connective tissue planes.[2,3] Studies of acupuncture points have found that many of the points have decreased resistance compared with surrounding tissue and there is less resistance when current is passed between points on the same meridian compared with control points.[4,5] Studies also have shown that certain acupuncture points may have a distinct effect distant from their site. For example, a study showed that electroacupuncture at Urinary Bladder 67 (an acupuncture point located at the distal tip of the fifth toe for which one of its classic functions is

related to the eyes) caused increased signal in Brodmann Areas 18 and 19 (areas in the brain empirically related to ophthalmic disorders) on functional MRI.[6] Meridians have not been found to correlate with any known nervous, vascular, or lymphatic channels; however, research has linked acupuncture meridians to myofascial pathways. For example, the Urinary Bladder meridian correlates well with the myofascial meridian of the posterior line and the myofascial sequence of retromotion.[7,8]

Some of the techniques used in acupuncture, such as needle rotation[9] and leaving the needles in place for a short period of time,[10] have been shown to have significant effects on the fibroblasts in the loose connective tissue, which can cause the tissues to change shape and expand. In addition to local tissue effects, acupuncture has been shown to have systemic effects, including the release of endogenous opioids, which are the body's own pain-inhibiting substances. For example, a study showed that needling the Large Intestine 4 acupuncture point can inhibit tooth pain, but this effect was nullified when naloxone, an opioid antagonist, was given.[11] This result indicates that acupuncture works in part because of endogenous opioid mechanisms.

A course of acupuncture will typically consist of a series of treatments performed once to twice per week for several weeks; more chronic conditions usually require more treatments. In modern medical acupuncture practice, there are numerous acupuncture practices and treatment paradigms. Some practices, such as Baldry and the Japanese style, involve superficial needling only, and this method is thought to be sufficient in alleviating pain and deactivating trigger points.[12] Other practices, such as Gunn Intramuscular Stimulation, involve needling into the deep paraspinal muscles and motor points of muscles. Gunn Intramuscular Stimulation proposes a radiculoneuropathic myofascial pain model in which silent myofascial lesions in the deep paraspinal muscles cause compression and dysfunction of the nerve root, which causes denervation supersensitivity down the myotomal chain.[13] Some treatments involve needling at the site of pain, whereas other treatments such as auricular acupuncture rely on supposed reflex mechanisms of action.[14] Other acupuncture treatments involve attaching electrical leads to the acupuncture needles and passing current between the needles; a commonly used method is called percutaneous electrical nerve stimulation.[15]

Patient safety is of the utmost concern when recommending a particular treatment. Acupuncture is a minimally invasive procedure that is safe when performed by properly trained individuals. Adverse events occur approximately 7% of the time, and the most common adverse events include pain, hematoma, and bleeding.[16] More serious events can include pneumothorax, infection, vasovagal reaction, hypertensive crisis, and peripheral nerve injury; however, these events are exceedingly rare and typically preventable.[17] Although many of the acupuncture points target peripheral nerves, the likelihood of injury to these nerves is limited because the needles have a pencil-like tip that splits tissues instead of a beveled cutting edge found in hypodermic needles (**Figure 2**).

There have been numerous studies on acupuncture for chronic low back pain. A recent systematic review and meta-analysis of 25 randomized controlled trials showed acupuncture had a clinically meaningful reduction in self-reported pain levels when compared with sham acupuncture treatment and improved function, both immediately postintervention and potentially up to 3 months postintervention, when compared with no treatment.[18] Function also clinically improved when acupuncture was provided in addition to usual care or when electroacupuncture was provided compared with usual care alone. Acupuncture was found to be slightly superior to medications (NSAIDs, muscle relaxers, analgesic medications) and usual care, but differences were small.

Two large-scale studies presenting level I evidence showed acupuncture was not significantly better than sham acupuncture but was significantly better than the usual care of physical therapy and medications in patients with chronic low back pain.[19,20] In a more recent study, 638 patients were randomized to receive individualized acupuncture (in which different points were specifically chosen for each patient based on individual symptoms and presentation), standardized acupuncture (in which the same back pain protocol was used on every patient), simulated acupuncture (using a toothpick and guide tube), or usual care.[20] The outcomes were measured with the Roland-Morris Disability Questionnaire score (0 to 24) and symptom bothersomeness scale (0 to 10). At 8 weeks posttreatment, the mean dysfunction scores for individualized, standardized, and simulated acupuncture groups had improved by 4.4, 4.5, and 4.4 points, respectively, compared with 2.1 points for patients receiving usual care ($P < 0.001$). Symptoms improved by 1.6 to 1.9 points in the treatment groups compared with 0.7 points in the usual care group ($P < 0.001$). The results also appeared durable at 1 year for function but not for symptoms. Individualized acupuncture was not found to be better than standardized acupuncture.[20] There also is some evidence that acupuncture can be helpful in nonspecific acute low back pain disorders.[21]

A recent Cochrane review on acupuncture for neck disorders (whiplash-associated disorders, chronic myofascial neck pain, arthritic neck pain, chronic nonspecific neck pain, and neck pain with radicular symptoms) reported overall moderate-quality evidence in favor of acupuncture.[22] Specifically, acupuncture is beneficial at immediate-term follow-up compared with sham acupuncture for reducing pain intensity, at short-term follow-up (1 day to 3 months) compared with sham or inactive management of pain intensity, at short-term follow-up compared with sham management of disability, and at short-term follow-up compared with a waitlist control group for pain intensity and neck disability. In a randomized controlled multicenter trial plus nonrandomized cohort study from general practices in Germany, 14,161 patients with chronic neck pain were randomized to acupuncture treatment or a control group receiving no acupuncture but including usual care.[23] At 3 months, neck pain and disability improved by 16.2 to 38.3 points in the acupuncture group on the Neck Pain and Disability Scale by Wheeler, compared with 3.9 to 50.5 points in the control group, with an average difference of 12.3 ($P < 0.001$). Treatment success was maintained through 6 months.

Several difficulties exist when analyzing acupuncture studies. What is the best control group to use when studying acupuncture? Some studies use sham acupuncture as the control, whereas others use usual treatment or no

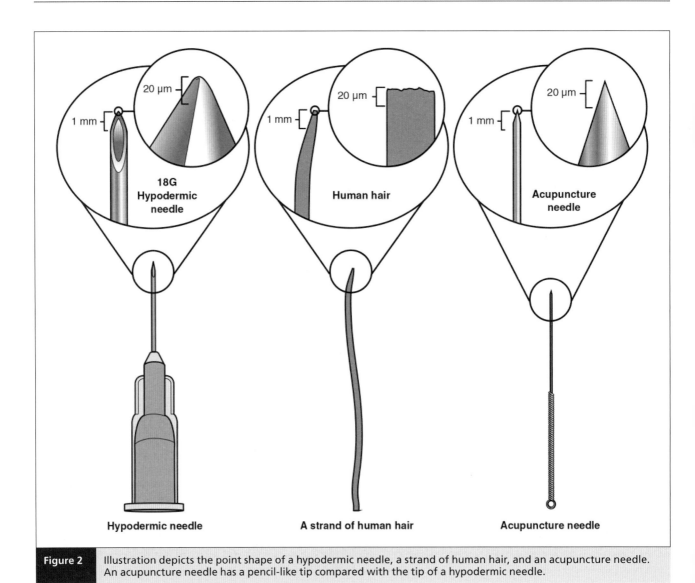

Figure 2 Illustration depicts the point shape of a hypodermic needle, a strand of human hair, and an acupuncture needle. An acupuncture needle has a pencil-like tip compared with the tip of a hypodermic needle.

treatment. If sham treatment is used, what is the most appropriate treatment method? Some studies have used superficial needling in nonacupuncture points as a sham treatment, but superficial needling in nonacupuncture points may not be a true sham treatment because there are physiologic effects from any type of needling. Another difficulty in analyzing acupuncture studies on low back pain is that most of the studies involve nonspecific chronic low back pain, and a structural diagnosis is not given. The lack of a diagnosis may limit the use of the literature in helping clinicians decide whether acupuncture is appropriate for a particular patient. New literature is emerging about acupuncture treatment of specific spinal conditions such as spinal stenosis; however, results currently are inconclusive.[24] Another issue regarding acupuncture is whether it is a placebo effect, because some of the major studies showed it was not better than sham acupuncture.

Acupuncture undoubtedly has a large placebo effect, as do other treatments. However, there is likely a true acupuncture effect. Using the Cohen effect size d index in which 0.8 is a large effect, 0.5 is a medium effect, and 0.2 is a small effect, one study estimated the acupuncture effect on chronic neck and low back pain was 0.55, with 0.22 the result of placebo or nonspecific effects and 0.23 the result of verum or specific effects.[25]

Dry Needling

Dry needling uses acupuncture or hypodermic needles to treat myofascial pain (nothing is injected), and often is performed by physical therapists or physiotherapists, whereas acupuncture is typically practiced by physicians or licensed acupuncturists. The safety profile for dry needling is nearly identical to that of acupuncture.[26] In many ways, dry needling can be thought of as a westernized form of acupuncture with a more limited indication. The points used in dry needling are tender points in the muscle or trigger points and are called ah shi points by acupuncturists. Trigger points are discrete hyperirritable nodules felt within skeletal muscle that have altered motor end plate activity.[27] Until recently, the only way to identify a trigger point was by palpation. However, in a recent study using ultrasound imaging and elastography, palpable myofascial trigger points were found to have nodular regions of hypo-echogenicity and show diminished vibration amplitude on external vibration, which is consistent with local regions of increased mechanical stiffness.[28]

A number of studies have reviewed the physiologic effects of needling a muscle. In a 2008 study observing trigger points, it was found that the chemical milieu at trigger points is abnormal with a decreased pH level and an increased number of inflammatory markers such as substance P, calcitonin gene-related peptide, bradykinin, 5-hydroxytryptamine receptors, norepinephrine, tumor necrosis factor-α, and interleukin-1b.[29] After needling the trigger point and eliciting a local twitch response, there is an immediate decrease in substance P and calcitonin gene-related peptide, but the duration of the decrease is unknown. It is thought that it is important to achieve a local twitch response after dry needling because it may cause a decrease in local inflammation and also normalize abnormal end plate activity.

Many published studies on efficacy of dry needling for low back or neck pain have been grouped with acupuncture studies, but there are several separate dry needling studies as well. A study of 66 patients with low back pain who responded positively to multifidus dry needling, defined as an improvement in Oswestry Disability Index at 1 week, found that these responders exhibited greater improvements in lumbar multifidi muscle contraction (as measured by the percent change in muscle thickness on ultrasound) and nociceptive sensitivity (as measured by assessing the pressure pain threshold) 1 week after treatment, but not immediately, when compared with nonresponders.[30] A separate study by the same author also found that increased low back pain with the multifidi lift test ($P = 0.01$) and no aggravation with standing ($P = 0.01$) were the two best predictors of improved disability with dry needling of lumbar multifidus.[31]

Cupping

Cupping is an ancient medical treatment that applies suction to the skin by use of a glass or plastic cup. A negative suction is created by heating the air in the glass cup, or using a manual pump to draw air out of the cup. There

are two main techniques used: wet cupping, in which skin incisions are made to allow blood and other body fluids to escape, and dry cupping, in which no incisions are made. Cupping can be helpful for numerous pain conditions, including neck pain and low back pain, and is thought to increase local blood circulation and thereby relieve painful muscle tension. Cupping also can be combined with massage techniques in which the cups are dragged along the skin while suction occurs.[32,33] Although cupping is considered safe, adverse events including vasovagal reaction, generalized body ache, increased local pain after cupping, pain during the procedure, skin laceration, and worsened headache and tinnitus have been reported.[32-34]

Cupping was shown to be more effective than waitlist control for managing pain and disability in the immediate term for chronic neck pain (moderate evidence). Several small and lower-quality studies showed a small clinical significance that cupping was more effective than medications (NSAIDs) in reducing pain and disability at immediate term for chronic low back pain (low evidence). Findings of large clinical significance indicated that cupping was more effective than usual care in treating pain and disability in the short term for chronic low back pain (moderate evidence).[33]

Chiropractic Care

Chiropractic care is one of the most widely used complementary health therapies for patients with spine-related pain. Some similarities exist between chiropractic and osteopathic treatments. Both treatments have philosophies that spinal alignment influences whole body health. Chiropractors tend to use more spinal manipulation techniques, whereas physical therapists or osteopathic physicians may use mobilizations and other techniques as well. Manipulation is active facilitation of a joint with the goal of movement beyond the physiologic barrier, whereas mobilization is active facilitation of a joint with the goal of movement to the physiologic barrier but not through it. Different types of treatments can accomplish either manipulation or mobilization. Approximately 8% to 9% of patients with low back pain seek chiropractic care.[35]

In general, chiropractic spinal manipulation is well tolerated and typically has mild side effects. Local discomfort occurs in more than 50% of patients.[36] Of those who experience discomfort, most report the severity as mild or moderate. Other common side effects include headache, tiredness, radiating discomfort, dizziness, nausea, and hot skin.

Although severe adverse events are rare after manipulation, such occurrences have been estimated to occur in 1:400,000 adjustments and may result in devastating injury. The greatest concern is the potential risk for cervical dissection of the vertebral artery or internal carotid artery after cervical manipulation therapy (CMT), which may result in stroke or death.[37] Several case-control studies have demonstrated an association between cervical spinal manipulations and cervical dissection, but critics argue that manipulation does not prove causation. Many investigators have sought to clarify the ambiguity between incidence and causation regarding cervical spinal manipulation, but studies are often flawed by reporting bias, selection bias, and the challenges associated with studying rare outcomes. A 2014 consensus statement from the American Heart Association and the American Stroke Association recommends that "although the incidence of CMT-associated cervical dissection in patients who have previously received CMT is not well established, and probably low...patients should be informed of the statistical association between cervical dissection and CMT prior to undergoing manipulation of the cervical spine."[38]

In a 2016 Cochrane review, 51 trials with 2,920 collective participants with chronic neck pain were reviewed.[39] For acute and subacute neck pain, the review found that cervical spine manipulation may result in greater improvements in pain relief than medications such as NSAIDs, opioids, or muscle relaxers. Cervical spine manipulation resulted in immediate pain relief, but not at short-term follow-up (up to 1 month) when compared with results of inactive control participants. There were similar results in improvements in pain relief, function, quality of life, and satisfaction when comparing cervical manipulation with mobilization. A 2016 randomized controlled trial reported improved cost-effectiveness of spinal manipulation with home exercise for adults older than 65 years with chronic neck pain compared with supervised exercise and home exercise or home exercise alone.[40]

In a 2011 Cochrane review, 12 randomized controlled trials with 2,887 collective participants with low back pain were reviewed.[41] For acute and subacute low back pain, chiropractic care improved short- and medium-term pain (less than 1 month and 1 to 6 months' duration, respectively), but no statistical difference was found in long-term pain (more than 6 months). In addition, short-term improvement in disability was seen in chiropractic care compared with other therapies. For chronic low back pain, there was no significant difference between chiropractic care and other treatments regarding improvement in pain or disability.

Massage Therapy

Massage therapy is the manipulation of superficial and deeper layers of muscle and connective tissue using various techniques to enhance function, aid in the healing process, decrease muscle reflex activity, inhibit motor-neuron excitability, and promote relaxation and well-being.[42] There are many types of massage therapies. In Swedish massage, the therapist uses long strokes, kneading, deep circular movements, vibration, and tapping. Petrissage and effleurage, techniques used to treat lymphedema, involve various ways of kneading and rolling and picking up the skin and muscles. Friction includes using the thumb, fingertips, or knuckles to apply deep, direct pressure to one site of muscular tension. Tapotement involves fast, stimulating, and percussion-type movements and can include cupping, hacking, and pounding. Sports massage combines techniques of Swedish massage and deep tissue massage to release chronic muscle tension, and it is adapted to the needs of athletes. Myofascial trigger point therapy focuses on trigger points.

Recent investigations undertaken to better understand the fascial system have led to the development of massage therapy techniques that incorporate more anatomic knowledge. Fascia has traditionally been thought of as a passive structure that envelops muscles; however, it is now evident that fascia is a dynamic tissue with complex vasculature and dense innervation. There is little consistency when referring to fascia; terms such as aponeurosis, retinaculum, fascia, and ligaments refer to some form of fascia. Fascia can be categorized as superficial or deep. Superficial fascia is formed by loosely packed interwoven collagen fibers mixed with abundant elastic fibers, is tightly connected with superficial veins and lymphatic vessels, and has functions of thermoregulation. Deep fascia refers to all the well-organized, dense fibrous layers that interpenetrate and surround muscles, bones, nerves, and blood vessels and bind them together into a continuous mass. When it covers bones, deep fascia is termed periosteum; around tendons it forms paratenon; and around vessels and nerves, it forms the neurovascular sheath.

There are two types of deep fascia: aponeurotic and epimysial. Aponeurotic fascia contains collagen fiber bundles that align along the main axis of the limbs in both longitudinal and oblique directions and function similar to a tendon by allowing force transmission along the limbs. Thoracolumbar fascia, which is considered aponeurotic fascia, has dense sensory innervation and is thought to be an important link in nonspecific low back pain.[43] Epimysial fascia is tightly adhered to underlying muscles via multiple fibrous septa that originate from the inner aspect and penetrate the muscle; therefore, it

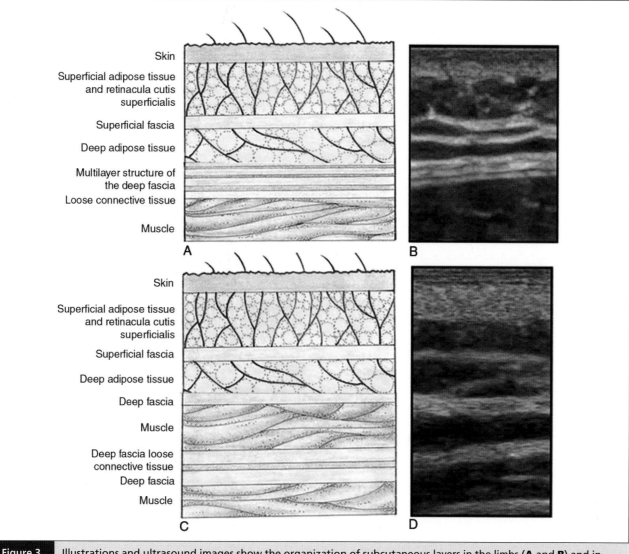

Figure 3 Illustrations and ultrasound images show the organization of subcutaneous layers in the limbs (**A** and **B**) and in the trunk (**C** and **D**). The superficial fascia divides the subcutaneous tissue into two adipose layers in the body: the superficial adipose tissue and the deep adipose tissue. Fibrous septa connect the superficial fascia to skin and to deep fascia, which form a three-dimensional network around fat lobules. The deep fascia shows different features according to the region. In the limbs, it is formed by two or three fibrous sublayers separated by hyaluronic acid, and in the trunk, the deep fascia only consists of one fibrous layer and thus, is thinner. (Adapted with permission from Stecco C, Tiengo C, Stecco A, et al: Fascia redefined: Anatomical features and technical relevance in fascial flap surgery. *Surg Radiol Anat* 2013:35[5]:369-376.)

is impossible to separate the function of epimysial fascia from that of muscle[44] (**Figure 3**).

Disorders of the fascia can account for many conditions that otherwise may be difficult to explain. Myofascial pain has been termed the great mimicker and can cause symptoms of numbness, tingling, and radiating pain in nondermatomal or myotomal distributions. Because superficial fascia is closely linked with lymphatics and blood vessels, alterations of superficial fascia can result in lymphedema, venous dilatation, changes in skin color, or chronic ischemia of the skin in the absence of measurable vascular or circulation problems. Disorders of aponeurotic deep fascia can result in myofascial pain.[44] Etiology of myofascial pain is typically thought of as multifactorial, with a notable contribution from peripheral tissues, specifically fascia. One functional characteristic of fascia is the sliding capability of fascial sublayers. Hyaluronic acid is commonly found between the fascial layers and provides a lubricating surface for fascia to glide smoothly over muscles and tendons. The biologic properties of hyaluronic acid vary depending on the size of their molecular chains. With a decreased pH level that can be seen after muscle exhaustion and lactic acid buildup, the molecular chains increase in size, and the viscosity of hyaluronic acid in the endomysium and perimysium can increase considerably.[45] This increased viscosity of hyaluronic acid can result in stiffness throughout the muscles and surrounding areas, which in normal situations disappears after rest. However, this same increased viscosity can result in dysfunction, poor gliding of the fascial layers, and myofascial pain.

Manipulation and massage of muscles and their associated fascia can increase local temperature and catalyze an inflammatory reaction, both of which facilitate breakdown of larger chains of hyaluronic acid, resulting in decreased hyaluronic acid viscosity and restoration of normal gliding of fascial layers. These results can be accomplished with a massage technique called fascial manipulation, which is deep compression and friction over specific points in the body that are thought to be commonly dysfunctional and densified. This technique can be performed with a knuckle or an elbow and is performed along a functional myofascial sequence.

A gentler massage technique called myofascial release involves applying low pressure and long-duration stretches to the myofascial complex that are intended to break up fascial adhesions, restore optimal length, decrease pain, and improve function.[46,47] Myofascial release can be performed directly at the site of restricted fascia with the use of knuckles, elbows, or tools to apply tension with a few kilograms of force to stretch the fascia. Alternatively, it can be performed indirectly by applying gentle pressure of a few grams, using the hands to follow the direction of fascial restriction, and holding the stretch to allow the fascia to unwind itself.

Images of the fascia reveal that increased thickness (specifically, an increase in loose connective tissue) correlates with increased pain. A recent study using ultrasonography found a correlation between a decrease in range of motion and increase in deep fascial thickness in the neck.[48] A value of 0.15 mm of sternocleidomastoid fascia was proposed as a cutoff value that allows the diagnosis of myofascial disease in patients with chronic neck pain. In addition, there are changes in both the histologic structure (increased inflammation and microcalcifications) and the degree of innervation (loss of nerve fibers) of the thoracolumbar fascia in patients with chronic low back pain, which indicate a possible role of fascia in lumbar pain.[49] A recent study found thoracolumbar fascia shear strain was approximately 20% lower in patients with low back pain, potentially implicating the intrinsic connective tissue pathology of decreased gliding in these patients.[50]

A Cochrane review of massage therapy for adults with nonspecific low back pain included 25 randomized controlled trials with more than 3,000 participants.[51] The quality of evidence was deemed low or very low because of bias and imprecision. Results showed that for acute low back pain, massage was better than inactive controls for pain, but not for function in the short term (less than 3 months). For subacute and chronic low back pain, massage was better than inactive controls for pain and function in the short term, but not in the long term (more than 3 months). However, when compared with active controls, which included manipulation, mobilization, transcutaneous electrical nerve stimulation, acupuncture, traction, relaxation, physical therapy, exercises, or self-care education, massage was better for pain both in the short- and long-term follow-ups, but no differences were found for function. There were no reports of serious adverse events in any of the massage therapy trials. Increased pain intensity was the most common adverse event reported in 1.5% to 25% of the participants.

A few trials have been performed to specifically analyze fascial manipulation. In a recent randomized controlled trial of 24 patients, the effectiveness of fascial manipulation with physical therapy was compared with physical therapy alone.[52] Results showed those receiving fascial manipulation had statistically and clinically significant improvement in the short term (end of treatment) for all outcomes (assessed with the visual analog scale and brief pain inventory, function with the Roland-Morris Disability Questionnaire, and state of well-being with the Medical Outcomes Study 36-Item Short Form Health Survey) and in the medium term (1 to 3 months; assessed with the visual analog scale and brief pain inventory) compared with physical therapy alone. Another study showed fascial manipulation may improve cervical range of motion more than standard therapy in patients with whiplash.[53] There also have been a few trials studying myofascial release. A recent study showed that dynamic ultrasound evaluation can be used to monitor effective sliding motion of fascial layers in vivo, and myofascial release is an effective manual technique to release the areas of impaired sliding fascial mobility and improve pain perception over a short term (3 days) in individuals with nonspecific neck pain or low back pain.[54] In a randomized, single-blinded, parallel group study of 59 patients with neck pain, 29 patients were treated with manual therapies and 30 patients were treated with myofascial release.[55] The study showed that after five sessions, the group treated with myofascial release had better advanced position of the head, better range of motion in side bending and rotation, and improved quality of life compared with the manual treatment group. Another study analyzed myofascial release compared with sham control for chronic low back pain, with both treatments used as an adjunct to specific back exercises.[56] The study found that the myofascial release group performed better than the control group after 8 weeks of treatment and at 12 weeks based on the McGill Pain Questionnaire and the Quebec Back Pain Disability Scale.

Herbal Medicines and Supplements

A recent Cochrane review of herbal medicines for low back pain included 14 randomized controlled trials with more than 2,000 participants with acute, subacute, and chronic low back pain.[57] The results of the included trials suggest that specific herbal medicines may be effective for short-term improvement in pain (4 to 6 weeks) and functional status for individuals with acute flare-ups of chronic, nonspecific low back pain. The review found that topical *Capsicum frutescens* (cayenne) had the best evidence for reducing pain more than placebo. Other herbal medicines, such as *Harpagophytum procumbens* (devil's claw), *Salix alba* (white willow bark), *Symphytum officinale* (comfrey), *Solidagochilensis* Meyen (Brazilian arnica), and lavender essential oil also seem to reduce pain more than placebo, although evidence for these supplements was of moderate quality at best. No substantial adverse events were noted in these trials, but a few patients reported mild gastrointestinal discomfort and skin irritation. *Capsicum*, better known as chili peppers, contains a chemical called capsaicin, which is a neurotoxin that irritates the skin to reduce pain by causing defunctionalization of nociceptive pain fibers. Devil's claw is an herb native to Africa that has fruit covered in hooks, and it contains chemicals that might decrease inflammation, swelling, and pain. White willow bark contains a chemical called salicin that acts similar to aspirin. Comfrey is a plant that contains allantoin, which is thought to stimulate cell growth and repair, while depressing inflammation. However, it also contains hepatotoxic chemicals called pyrrolizidine alkaloids and, therefore, should only be used topically. Brazilian arnica is a plant from the daisy family; the flower of the plant is used to make medicines with anti-inflammatory properties.

A review of randomized controlled trials analyzing cannabinoids for chronic pain associated with rheumatic conditions (back pain, fibromyalgia, osteoarthritis, rheumatoid arthritis) found that superiority of cannabinoids over controls (placebo, amitriptyline) was inconsistent. Cannabinoid receptors are widely distributed throughout the central and peripheral nervous systems and also may be found in peripheral nonnervous tissue. It is hypothesized that cannabinoids function to reduce sensitization of nociceptive sensory pathways and induce alterations in cognitive and autonomic processing in states of chronic pain. Engaging the system may provide therapeutic effects for pain and inflammation. Cannabinoids were generally well tolerated and safe during study duration despite some troublesome side effects. Currently, there is insufficient evidence for recommendation of any cannabinoid preparations for symptom management in patients with chronic pain associated with rheumatic diseases.[58] There are some limited clinical studies that show cannabis or cannabis derivative can improve symptoms of neuropathic pain in patients with HIV, general peripheral neuropathic pain, spasticity caused by multiple sclerosis or spinal cord injury, and central pain caused by multiple sclerosis.[59]

Yoga

Yoga is derived from the Sanskrit word *yug*, which means to put to active and purposeful use, and is described as a method of discipline.[60] Once solely an oral tradition, the yogic philosophy was transcribed into the *Yoga Sutra*, a manuscript teaching ways of dealing with the challenges of life. There are numerous styles of yoga, but among the most commonly practiced in the United States is Hatha yoga, which is the willful or forceful physical practice of yoga postures with the original purpose of preparing for meditation. Similar to other meditative exercises, the practice of yoga in the United States has grown significantly to 9.5% of adults and 3.1% of children in 2012.[35,61] Of those who practice yoga for specific health conditions, back pain is the most commonly cited (19.7%).[62] **Figure 4** demonstrates a few common yoga poses that patients with low back pain may find beneficial.

A recent systematic review evaluated 14 randomized controlled trials to assess the effectiveness of yoga on chronic low back pain.[63] Most of the studies reported beneficial effects for patients with low back pain, including improvements in pain relief, flexibility, function, depression, balance, and gait parameters. Yoga was more effective in reducing pain severity compared with control methods. A study among low-income populations with chronic low back pain found similar improvements in pain and function when comparing once-weekly yoga classes with twice-weekly yoga classes.[64]

Another systematic review evaluated three randomized controlled trials totaling 184 participants with chronic neck pain to assess the effectiveness of yoga.[65] Participants were assigned to yoga practice for either a 90-minute session weekly for 9 weeks or a 60-minute session 5 days per week for 3 months. Neck pain and functional disability were significantly lower

3: Medical Management of Spine Disorders

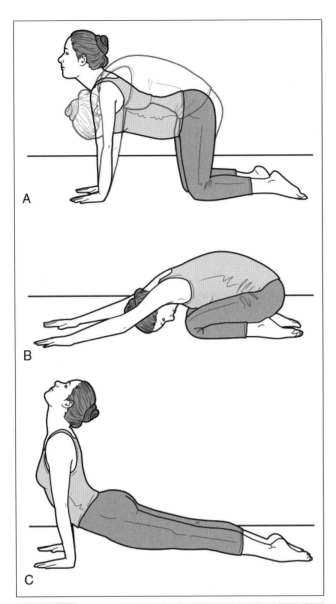

Figure 4 Illustrations show three common yoga posses found helpful by indviduals with low back pain. **A,** Cat-cow pose. **B,** Child's pose. **C,** Upward-facing dog.

principles of yin and yang. Tai chi involves deep breathing combined with a series of continuous, slow, graceful movements with the purpose of allowing qi to flow unencumbered throughout the body and promote better health. Tai chi is thought to be suitable for all age groups,[66] but there has been tremendous interest among older adults because of its beneficial effects for reducing falls, improving psychological well-being, and improving general health.[67] Although most studies have reviewed other aspects of health, there is some evidence for the use of tai chi for neck and back pain.

At 24-week follow-up, one study found that 12 weeks of tai chi or instruction in conventional neck exercises both provided patients with similar improvements in neck pain, disability, and physical functioning compared with a waitlist control group.[68] Both exercise groups had a progressive decline in group attendance over 12 weeks, but 68% of those practicing tai chi attended at least 80% of the sessions. A similar study found that 18 group sessions (40 minutes each) of tai chi at a community venue provided greater improvement in chronic low back pain, disability, and physical functioning at 10-week follow-up compared with results from a waitlist control group.[69]

Summary

With the increased use of alternative medicine treatments, orthopaedic practitioners should have some familiarity with the various treatments available. Acupuncture is safe when performed by properly trained individuals and has the most evidence supporting its use as a stand-alone or adjunctive treatment for patients with chronic low back pain and neck disorders. Dry needling has been shown to decrease local inflammation and normalize abnormal muscle electrical activity. Cupping can be effective for managing chronic low back and neck pain in the immediate and short term. Chiropractic care is one of the most widely used alternative treatments and can provide improvement in acute and subacute neck and low back pain. Patients should be aware of an association between cervical manipulation therapy and cervical dissection (vertebral artery or internal carotid artery), although the incidence is probably low. Massage therapy can provide effective management of acute, subacute, and chronic low back pain, although the quality of evidence is low. Recent research has shown that dysfunctional fascia with poor gliding may play a major role in chronic neck and low back pain. Several studies of herbal medicines and supplements show that specific compounds can provide short-term improvement in pain and function for patients with acute flare-ups of chronic low back pain. Clinical trials involving cannabinoids in chronic low back pain

among yoga participants versus the control group, which included no treatment, general exercise, or manual self-care. Adverse effects were generally mild, including transient worsening of neck pain, low back pain, muscle soreness, migraine, and vertigo.

Tai Chi

Tai chi is a Chinese martial art that has been practiced for several hundred years and is based on the balance and fibromyalgia showed inconsistent results, although there is some evidence that it may be effective in managing neuropathic pain and spasticity. Yoga and tai chi appear to improve pain and function in patients with chronic low back and neck pain, and the latter may be particularly suitable for elderly patients.

Key Study Points

- Acupuncture has moderate evidence supporting its use in chronic low back pain and neck disorders and may work in part by treating the myofascial meridians.

- Dry needling can be considered a Western medicine form of acupuncture and involves using acupuncture needles to deactivate trigger points.

- Chiropractic manipulations can provide immediate and medium-term relief of acute or subacute neck or low back pain, but there is a potential risk of carotid artery dissection with neck manipulations.

- Research on the fascial system is increasing, and fascia has been identified as a potential source of pain and dysfunction.

Annotated References

1. Shin JS, Lee J, Kim MR, et al: The short-term effect of integrated complementary and alternative medicine treatment in inpatients diagnosed with lumbar intervertebral disc herniation: A prospective observational study. *J Altern Complement Med* 2016;22(7):533-543.

   A prospective observational study of 524 patients with low back and leg pain hospitalized for lumbar intervertebral disk herniation reported good improvement in pain and function, with most patients receiving only complementary and alternative medicine treatments and a smaller percentage also receiving nonsurgical conventional medicine treatments. Level of evidence: IV.

2. Gunn CC, Ditchburn FG, King MH, Renwick GJ: Acupuncture loci: A proposal for their classification according to their relationship to known neural structures. *Am J Chin Med (Gard City N Y)* 1976;4(2):183-195.

3. Langevin HM, Yandow JA: Relationship of acupuncture points and meridians to connective tissue planes. *Anat Rec* 2002;269(6):257-265.

4. Hyvärinen J, Karlsson M: Low-resistance skin points that may coincide with acupuncture loci. *Med Biol* 1977;55(2):88-94.

5. Helms JM: An overview of medical acupuncture. *Altern Ther Health Med* 1998;4(3):35-45.

6. Siedentopf CM, Golaszewski SM, Mottaghy FM, Ruff CC, Felber S, Schlager A: Functional magnetic resonance imaging detects activation of the visual association cortex during laser acupuncture of the foot in humans. *Neurosci Lett* 2002;327(1):53-56.

7. Myers T: *Anatomy Trains: Myofascial Meridians for Manual and Movement Therapists*, ed 3. Tw M, ed. London, Churchill Livingstone Elsevier, 2014.

   This textbook, first published in 2001, describes functionally integrated body-wide continuities within the fascial webbing forming traceable meridians of myofascia.

8. Stecco L, Stecco C: *Fascial Manipulation Practical Part.* Padova, Italy, Piccin Nuova Libraria S.p.A, 2009.

9. Langevin HM, Bouffard NA, Badger GJ, Churchill DL, Howe AK: Subcutaneous tissue fibroblast cytoskeletal remodeling induced by acupuncture: Evidence for a mechanotransduction-based mechanism. *J Cell Physiol* 2006;207(3):767-774.

10. Langevin HM, Bouffard NA, Fox JR, et al: Fibroblast cytoskeletal remodeling contributes to connective tissue tension. *J Cell Physiol* 2011;226(5):1166-1175.

    The results of this original research study showed that the viscoelastic behavior of areolar connective tissue under tension is substantially affected by cellular activity.

11. Mayer DJ, Price DD, Rafii A: Antagonism of acupuncture analgesia in man by the narcotic antagonist naloxone. *Brain Res* 1977;121(2):368-372.

12. Baldry P: Superficial versus deep dry needling. *Acupunct Med* 2002;20(2-3):78-81.

13. Gunn CC: Chronic pain: Time for epidemiology. *J R Soc Med* 1996;89(8):479-480.

14. Oleson T: Auriculotherapy stimulation for neuro-rehabilitation. *NeuroRehabilitation* 2002;17(1):49-62.

15. Ghoname EA, Craig WF, White PF: Use of percutaneous electrical nerve stimulation (PENS) for treating ECT-induced headaches. *Headache* 1999;39(7):502-505.

16. Melchart D, Weidenhammer W, Streng A, et al: Prospective investigation of adverse effects of acupuncture in 97 733 patients. *Arch Intern Med* 2004;164(1):104-105.

17. Witt CM, Pach D, Reinhold T, et al: Treatment of the adverse effects from acupuncture and their economic impact: A prospective study in 73,406 patients with low back or neck pain. *Eur J Pain* 2011;15(2):193-197.

    A prospective observational study of 73,406 patients who received acupuncture for chronic low back or neck pain showed that adverse events occurred approximately 7%

3: Medical Management of Spine Disorders

of the time, with bleeding, hematoma, and pain the most common events. Level of evidence: IV.

18. Lam M, Galvin R, Curry P: Effectiveness of acupuncture for nonspecific chronic low back pain: A systematic review and meta-analysis. *Spine (Phila Pa 1976)* 2013;38(24):2124-2138.

    A systematic review of 32 studies, including a meta-analysis of 25 studies, of randomized controlled trials of acupuncture for nonspecific chronic low back pain showed that acupuncture may have a favorable effect on self-reported pain and functional limitations. Level of evidence: II.

19. Haake M, Müller HH, Schade-Brittinger C, et al: German Acupuncture Trials (GERAC) for chronic low back pain: Randomized, multicenter, blinded, parallel-group trial with 3 groups. *Arch Intern Med* 2007;167(17):1892-1898.

20. Cherkin DC, Sherman KJ, Avins AL, et al: A randomized trial comparing acupuncture, simulated acupuncture, and usual care for chronic low back pain. *Arch Intern Med* 2009;169(9):858-866.

21. Hasegawa TM, Baptista AS, de Souza MC, Yoshizumi AM, Natour J: Acupuncture for acute non-specific low back pain: A randomised, controlled, double-blind, placebo trial. *Acupunct Med* 2014;32(2):109-115.

    A prospective, randomized, parallel-group, double-blind, placebo-controlled trial of 80 men and women with acute nonspecific low back pain showed that Yamamato's new scalp acupuncture was more effective than sham treatment with regard to decrease in pain, NSAID use, and improvement in function and quality of life. Level of evidence: I.

22. Trinh K, Graham N, Irnich D, Cameron ID, Forget M: Acupuncture for neck disorders. *Cochrane Database Syst Rev* 2016;5:CD004870.

    This Cochrane review, which included 27 studies of acupuncture for neck pain (whiplash-associated disorders, chronic myofascial neck pain, chronic pain due to arthritis, chronic nonspecific neck pain, neck pain with radicular signs, and mechanical neck pain), reported moderate-quality evidence that acupuncture relieves pain and improves disability. Level of evidence: II. Study withdrawn.

23. Witt CM, Jena S, Brinkhaus B, Liecker B, Wegscheider K, Willich SN: Acupuncture for patients with chronic neck pain. *Pain* 2006;125(1-2):98-106.

24. Kim KH, Kim TH, Lee BR, et al: Acupuncture for lumbar spinal stenosis: A systematic review and meta-analysis. *Complement Ther Med* 2013;21(5):535-556.

    This systematic review and meta-analysis of acupuncture trials for lumbar spinal stenosis included six randomized controlled trials and six nonrandomized controlled clinical trials. There was no conclusive evidence of the effectiveness and safety of acupuncture for this diagnosis because of high or uncertain risk of bias and the limited generalizability of included studies. Level of evidence: III.

25. Vickers AJ, Cronin AM, Maschino AC, et al; Acupuncture Trialists' Collaboration: Acupuncture for chronic pain: Individual patient data meta-analysis. *Arch Intern Med* 2012;172(19):1444-1453.

    This systematic review was performed to identify randomized trials of acupuncture for chronic pain in which allocation concealment was adequate; 31 trials were included. Individual patient data meta-analysis was performed using data from 17,922 patients. Acupuncture was shown to be superior to both sham therapy and no acupuncture for nonspecific back or neck pain, chronic headache, and osteoarthritis. Level of evidence: II.

26. Brady S, McEvoy J, Dommerholt J, Doody C: Adverse events following trigger point dry needling: A prospective survey of chartered physiotherapists. *J Man Manip Ther* 2014;22(3):134-140.

    A prospective survey was undertaken of 39 physiotherapists who had completed David G. Simons Academy dry needling and trigger point therapy training to evaluate the incidence of adverse events. Common adverse events included bruising, bleeding, and pain; however, there were no significant adverse events. Level of evidence: IV.

27. Shah JP, Thaker N, Heimur J, Aredo JV, Sikdar S, Gerber L: Myofascial trigger points then and now: A historical and scientific perspective. *PM R* 2015;7(7):746-761.

    A narrative review of myofascial trigger points is presented.

28. Sikdar S, Shah JP, Gebreab T, et al: Novel applications of ultrasound technology to visualize and characterize myofascial trigger points and surrounding soft tissue. *Arch Phys Med Rehabil* 2009;90(11):1829-1838.

29. Shah JP, Gilliams EA: Uncovering the biochemical milieu of myofascial trigger points using in vivo microdialysis: An application of muscle pain concepts to myofascial pain syndrome. *J Bodyw Mov Ther* 2008;12(4):371-384.

30. Koppenhaver SL, Walker MJ, Su J, et al: Changes in lumbar multifidus muscle function and nociceptive sensitivity in low back pain patient responders versus non-responders after dry needling treatment. *Man Ther* 2015;20(6):769-776.

    A quasi-experimental study involving 66 volunteers with mechanical low back pain showed that patients who responded to a single dry needling treatment of the lumbar multifidus muscle with improved disability 1 week after treatment exhibited larger improvements in lumbar multifidi muscle contraction and nociceptive sensitivity 1 week after dry needling.

31. Koppenhaver SL, Walker MJ, Smith RW, et al: Baseline examination factors associated with clinical improvement after dry needling in individuals with low back pain. *J Orthop Sports Phys Ther* 2015;45(8):604-612.

    A quasi-experimental study involving 72 volunteers with mechanical low back pain showed that increased low back pain with the multifidus lift test on physical examination was the strongest predictor of improved disability

1 week after a single dry needling treatment of the lumbar multifidus.

32. Lauche R, Materdey S, Cramer H, et al: Effectiveness of home-based cupping massage compared to progressive muscle relaxation in patients with chronic neck pain: A randomized controlled trial. *PLoS One* 2013;8(6):e65378.

A randomized controlled trial of 61 patients with nonspecific neck pain showed that cupping massage was no more effective than progressive muscle relaxation for improving pain but may be better in improving well-being and decreasing pressure pain sensitivity. Level of evidence: I.

33. Yuan QL, Guo TM, Liu L, Sun F, Zhang YG: Traditional Chinese medicine for neck pain and low back pain: A systematic review and meta-analysis. *PLoS One* 2015;10(2):e0117146.

A systematic review and meta-analysis of traditional Chinese medicine treatments for neck pain and low back pain identified 75 randomized controlled trials involving 11,077 patients. Results showed moderate evidence that acupuncture was more effective than sham acupuncture in reducing pain immediately posttreatment for chronic neck pain, chronic low back pain, and acute low back pain. Level of evidence: II.

34. Kim TH, Kang JW, Kim KH, et al: Cupping for treating neck pain in video display terminal (VDT) users: A randomized controlled pilot trial. *J Occup Health* 2012;54(6):416-426.

A randomized controlled pilot trial of 40 individuals with neck pain who used video display terminals showed that cupping was more effective than a heating pad in improving pain and function. Level of evidence: II.

35. Clarke TC, Black LI, Stussman BJ, Barnes PM, Nahin RL: Trends in the use of complementary health approaches among adults: United States, 2002-2012. *Natl Health Stat Report* 2015;79:1-16.

This article, based on results from the National Health Interview Survey, provides statistical trends regarding the use of complementary and alternative medicine in the United States. It is a helpful review of the various other treatments that are sought outside the realm of traditional Western medicine.

36. Stevinson C, Ernst E: Risks associated with spinal manipulation. *Am J Med* 2002;112(7):566-571.

37. Thomas LC: Cervical arterial dissection: An overview and implications for manipulative therapy practice. *Man Ther* 2016;21:2-9.

38. Biller J, Sacco RL, Albuquerque FC, et al; American Heart Association Stroke Council: Cervical arterial dissections and association with cervical manipulative therapy: A statement for healthcare professionals from the American heart association/American stroke association. *Stroke* 2014;45(10):3155-3174.

Guidelines for cervical manipulative therapy were provided in a joint manner by the American Heart Association and American Stroke Association, specifically in regard to the risk for arterial dissection. This landmark article provides helpful recommendations for manual medicine practitioners and physicians who see patients treated with manual medicine techniques.

39. Gross A, Langevin P, Burnie SJ, et al: Manipulation and mobilisation for neck pain contrasted against an inactive control or another active treatment. *Cochrane Database Syst Rev* 2015;9:CD004249.

The authors provide a systematic review of cervical and thoracic manipulation versus active and inactive controls. Their review included 51 trials with 2,920 total participants. Their data include outcome measures for pain, function, and quality of life. Level of evidence: II.

40. Leininger B, McDonough C, Evans R, Tosteson T, Tosteson AN, Bronfort G: Cost-effectiveness of spinal manipulative therapy, supervised exercise, and home exercise for older adults with chronic neck pain. *Spine J* 2016;16(11):1292-1304.

The authors provide estimates on cost-effectiveness of common therapies for older patients with chronic neck pain, using data collected from a randomized controlled trial. This study provides helpful information about the cost-effectiveness and clinical outcomes for selected therapies after 1 year. Level of evidence: I.

41. Walker BF, French SD, Grant W, Green S: A Cochrane review of combined chiropractic interventions for low-back pain. *Spine (Phila Pa 1976)* 2011;36(3):230-242.

The authors provide a systematic review of lumbar chiropractic manipulations versus an active or inactive control. This review included 12 trials with 2,887 total participants. Their data include outcome measures for pain and disability. Level of evidence: II.

42. Chaitow L: Massage therapy: A profession in search of future directions? *J Bodyw Mov Ther* 2013;17(3):269-270.

An editorial from a leader in the field of bodywork and movement therapies is presented.

43. Tesarz J, Hoheisel U, Wiedenhöfer B, Mense S: Sensory innervation of the thoracolumbar fascia in rats and humans. *Neuroscience* 2011;194:302-308.

A basic science rat and human study showed that the thoracolumbar fascia in both is a densely innervated tissue with marked differences in the distribution of nerve endings over the fascial layers and presumably contains nociceptive fibers.

44. Stecco A, Stern R, Fantoni I, De Caro R, Stecco C: Fascial disorders: Implications for treatment. *PM R* 2016;8(2):161-168.

A narrative review of fascia research and treatment is presented.

45. Gatej I, Popa M, Rinaudo M: Role of the pH on hyaluronan behavior in aqueous solution. *Biomacromolecules* 2005;6(1):61-67.

46. Meltzer KR, Cao TV, Schad JF, King H, Stoll ST, Standley PR: In vitro modeling of repetitive motion injury and myofascial release. *J Bodyw Mov Ther* 2010;14(2):162-171.

47. Barnes JF: *Myofascial Release: The Search for Excellence. A Comprehensive Evaluatory and Treatment Approach.* Laurel, MD, Rehabilitation Services, 1990.

48. Stecco A, Meneghini A, Stern R, Stecco C, Imamura M: Ultrasonography in myofascial neck pain: Randomized clinical trial for diagnosis and follow-up. *Surg Radiol Anat* 2014;36(3):243-253.

    A study of 25 healthy patients and 28 patients with chronic neck pain found a difference in the thickness of the sternocleidomastoid fascia and the scalene fascia as measured using ultrasound between the two groups, with neck pain patients having thicker fascia. Level of evidence: III.

49. Bednar DA, Orr FW, Simon GT: Observations on the pathomorphology of the thoracolumbar fascia in chronic mechanical back pain: A microscopic study. *Spine (Phila Pa 1976)* 1995;20(10):1161-1164.

50. Langevin HM, Fox JR, Koptiuch C, et al: Reduced thoracolumbar fascia shear strain in human chronic low back pain. *BMC Musculoskelet Disord* 2011;12:203.

    A study involving 50 patients without low back pain and 71 patients with chronic low back pain showed that thoracolumbar fascia shear strain, as measured with ultrasound cine-recording and a motorized hinge table, was reduced in approximately 20% in the low back pain group. Level of evidence: III.

51. Furlan AD, Giraldo M, Baskwill A, Irvin E, Imamura M: Massage for low-back pain. *Cochrane Database Syst Rev* 2015;9:CD001929.

    A Cochrane review of massage therapy for low back pain included 25 trials and 3,096 participants. Little evidence was found that massage is an effective treatment for low back pain. Patients with acute, subacute, and chronic low back pain had improvements in pain outcomes from massage in the short term. Level of evidence: III.

52. Branchini M, Lopopolo F, Andreoli E, Loreti I, Marchand AM, Stecco A: Fascial Manipulation® for chronic aspecific low back pain: A single blinded randomized controlled trial. *F1000Res* 2015;4:1208.

    This single-blinded randomized controlled trial of 24 patients with chronic a specific low back pain showed that those receiving fascial manipulation and physiotherapy had statistically and clinically significant short- and medium-term improvements in pain and function compared with those receiving physiotherapy alone. Level of evidence: I.

53. Picelli A, Ledro G, Turrina A, Stecco C, Santilli V, Smania N: Effects of myofascial technique in patients with subacute whiplash associated disorders: A pilot study. *Eur J Phys Rehabil Med* 2011;47(4):561-568.

    A pilot randomized clinical trial of 18 patients with subacute whiplash-associated disorder found that fascial manipulation resulted in a statistically significant improvement in neck flexion immediately after treatment compared with conventional neck exercises and mobilization. Level of evidence: II.

54. Tozzi P, Bongiorno D, Vitturini C: Fascial release effects on patients with non-specific cervical or lumbar pain. *J Bodyw Mov Ther* 2011;15(4):405-416.

    In a study of 60 patients with nonspecific neck pain or low back pain evaluated before and after fascial techniques and compared with 30 control subjects given sham treatments, it was found that dynamic ultrasound topographic anatomy evaluation can be a valid instrument to assess effective sliding of fascial layers in vivo. Level of evidence: III.

55. Rodríguez-Fuentes I, De Toro FJ, Rodríguez-Fuentes G, de Oliveira IM, Meijide-Faílde R, Fuentes-Boquete IM: Myofascial release therapy in the treatment of occupational mechanical neck pain: A randomized parallel group study. *Am J Phys Med Rehabil* 2016;95(7):507-515.

    A randomized, single-blinded parallel group study of 59 patients with occupational neck pain showed that after five sessions, myofascial release therapy seemed to be more effective than manual therapy for correcting advanced position of the head, recovering range of motion in side bending and rotation, and improving quality of life. Level of evidence: I.

56. Ajimsha MS, Daniel B, Chithra S: Effectiveness of myofascial release in the management of chronic low back pain in nursing professionals. *J Bodyw Mov Ther* 2014;18(2):273-281.

    A randomized, controlled, single-blinded trial involving 80 nursing professionals with chronic low back pain showed that myofascial release as an adjunct to specific back exercises is more effective than sham myofascial release and specific back exercises in terms of reduction in pain and functional disability. Level of evidence: I.

57. Gagnier JJ, Oltean H, van Tulder MW, Berman BM, Bombardier C, Robbins CB: Herbal medicine for low back pain: A Cochrane review. *Spine (Phila Pa 1976)* 2016;41(2):116-133.

    This Cochrane review to determine the effectiveness of herbal medicines for nonspecific low back pain analyzed 14 randomized controlled trials involving 2,050 participants. Results showed that *Capsicum frutescens* reduced pain more than placebo. Several other compounds also may reduce pain, but quality of evidence was less for those compounds compared with that of *Capsicum frutescens*.

58. Fitzcharles MA, Baerwald C, Ablin J, Häuser W: Efficacy, tolerability and safety of cannabinoids in chronic pain associated with rheumatic diseases (fibromyalgia syndrome, back pain, osteoarthritis, rheumatoid arthritis): A systematic review of randomized controlled trials. *Schmerz* 2016;30(1):47-61.

A systematic review of cannabinoids in chronic pain returned three studies after screening, two of which were randomized controlled trials. The findings of superiority of cannabinoids over controls were not consistent. Level of evidence: III.

59. Leung L: Cannabis and its derivatives: Review of medical use. *J Am Board Fam Med* 2011;24(4):452-462.

The authors presented patient scenarios and suggested treatments for the use of cannabis and its derivatives, detailed the harms and challenges of using cannabis, and reviewed clinical studies of patients using cannabis and its derivatives for Tourette syndrome, glaucoma, and pain. Good results were reported in patients with HIV and multiple sclerosis.

60. Carrico M: A Beginner's Guide to the History of Yoga. Available at: http://www.yogajournal.com/yoga-101/the-roots-of-yoga. Accessed May 5, 2017.

61. Black LI, Clarke TC, Barnes PM, Stussman BJ, Nahin RL: Use of complementary health approaches among children aged 4-17 years in the United States: National Health Interview Survey, 2007-2012. *Natl Health Stat Report* 2015;78:1-19.

This article, based on results from the National Health Interview Survey, provides statistical trends regarding the use of complementary and alternative medicine in the United States. It is a helpful review of a variety of other treatments for pediatric patients that are outside of the realm of traditional Western medicine.

62. Cramer H, Ward L, Steel A, Lauche R, Dobos G, Zhang Y: Prevalence, patterns, and predictors of yoga use: Results of a U.S. nationally representative survey. *Am J Prev Med* 2016;50(2):230-235.

This article, based on results from the National Health Interview Survey, provides information regarding the use of yoga in the United States in 2012.

63. Chang DG, Holt JA, Sklar M, Groessl EJ: Yoga as a treatment for chronic low back pain: A systematic review of the literature. *J Orthop Rheumatol* 2016;3(1):1-8.

The authors present a systematic review of randomized controlled trials addressing yoga as a treatment for chronic low back pain. This article provided strong support for the use of yoga in reducing pain and disability. Level of evidence: II.

64. Saper RB, Boah AR, Keosaian J, Cerrada C, Weinberg J, Sherman KJ: Comparing once- versus twice-weekly yoga classes for chronic low back pain in predominantly low income minorities: A randomized dosing trial. *Evid Based Complement Alternat Med* 2013;2013:658030.

This randomized controlled trial demonstrates that once-weekly yoga classes are equally as effective in reducing pain and improving function as twice-weekly classes. For all patients, but especially those with limited resources, this is important to consider when creating a therapeutic exercise program for those with chronic low back pain.

65. Kim SD: Effects of yoga on chronic neck pain: A systematic review of randomized controlled trials. *J Phys Ther Sci* 2016;28(7):2171-2174.

This systematic review of three randomized controlled trials suggests a potential benefit for practicing yoga to manage chronic neck pain in regard to pain and functional disability. Level of evidence: II.

66. Uhlig T: Tai chi and yoga as complementary therapies in rheumatologic conditions. *Best Pract Res Clin Rheumatol* 2012;26(3):387-398.

This descriptive review provides a summarized overview of the historical treatment of rheumatoid arthritis and osteoarthritis with yoga and tai chi. This article may be helpful for providing a cultural reference and the benefits of these exercises for rheumatoid arthritis and osteoarthritis.

67. Lee MS, Ernst E: Systematic reviews of t'ai chi: An overview. *Br J Sports Med* 2012;46(10):713-718.

The authors of this article critically evaluate prior systematic reviews that evaluated the potential health benefits from participating in tai chi. Their findings support the use of tai chi for fall prevention and psychological health improvement.

68. Lauche R, Stumpe C, Fehr J, et al: The effects of tai chi and neck exercises in the treatment of chronic nonspecific neck pain: A randomized controlled trial. *J Pain* 2016;17(9):1013-1027.

The authors present a randomized controlled trial evaluating the effectiveness of three treatments: tai chi, conventional neck exercises, and waitlist controls. Both tai chi and conventional neck exercises produced similar improvements in pain and quality of life when compared with no treatment.

69. Hall AM, Maher CG, Lam P, Ferreira M, Latimer J: Tai chi exercise for treatment of pain and disability in people with persistent low back pain: A randomized controlled trial. *Arthritis Care Res (Hoboken)* 2011;63(11):1576-1583.

This randomized controlled trial demonstrates the increased effectiveness of tai chi on pain interference, pain severity, and disability when compared with outcomes in a waitlist control group. Level of evidence: II.

3: Medical Management of Spine Disorders

Chapter 14

Nonsurgical Care of the Spine: Procedures

Jason Friedrich, MD   Benjamin Marshall, DO

Abstract

In appropriately selected patients, percutaneous spine interventions can effectively reduce pain and disability resulting from a variety of painful spine conditions. Research supports the efficacy of transforaminal epidural steroid injections to manage lumbar radicular pain resulting from disk herniation and the efficacy of radiofrequency neurotomy to manage chronic pain in the spinal facet joint. Other spine interventions remain controversial because of inadequate or conflicting research. Meticulous diagnosis, patient selection, and technique are required to achieve optimal outcomes with the use of spine interventions.

Keywords: epidural steroid injection; percutaneous spine intervention; radiofrequency neurotomy; spine

Introduction

Most spine-related pain is effectively managed nonsurgically. When included in a comprehensive treatment regimen, percutaneous spine interventions can reduce pain, facilitate rehabilitation, reduce the need for surgery, and help predict surgical outcome. Whether spine interventional procedures are useful for certain conditions, such as discogenic low back pain (LBP) and spinal stenosis, remains controversial. Despite the limitations of the available literature, it is important to provide a rational, evidence-informed approach to the use of spine interventions.

Neither of the following authors nor any immediate family member has received anything of value from or has stock or stock options held in a commercial company or institution related directly or indirectly to the subject of this chapter: Dr. Friedrich and Dr. Marshall.

Optimizing Interventional Spine Care

Most surgeons agree that spine interventional procedures can relieve pain in well-selected patients who have back and neck pain and that these procedures will not be effective in all such patients. The importance of establishing the correct pathoanatomic diagnosis before proceeding with a therapeutic interventional procedure cannot be overemphasized.

The three most common sources of axial LBP among adults are the intervertebral disk, lumbar facet joint, and sacroiliac (SI) joint, with incidence rates of approximately 40%, 15% to 30%, and 20%, respectively.[1] Intervertebral disk involvement consists of internal disk disruption or nonhealing annular fissure. Insufficiency fracture, ankylosing spondylitis, Baastrup syndrome, painful lumbosacral junction pseudarthrosis, and pain related to surgical hardware each account for fewer than 5% of instances of LBP. Malignancy, spinal infection, and cauda equina syndrome contribute a combined 1%. After age 55 years, the risk for discogenic pain decreases, but the risk for spinal facet joint pain rises, especially in the absence of midline pain.[1] Compared with the lumbar spine, the spinal facet joint accounts for a greater percentage of cervical pain (55%).[2] Prevalence of SI joint pain increases in patients with lumbosacral fusion and pain below L5.[1,3]

Mechanical spine pain is often multifactorial; thus, a comprehensive approach to diagnosis should be used to account for biomechanical factors that should be targeted with appropriate physical rehabilitation. Such biomechanical factors include head-forward position, anterior sagittal imbalance, hip abductor weakness, altered gait pattern, muscular deconditioning, poor motor control, midrange segmental motion instability, hip flexion contracture, hamstring tightness, and poor ergonomics. A comprehensive musculoskeletal and neuromuscular examination is needed to evaluate for competing diagnoses such as hip or shoulder disorders and peripheral neuropathies. A multidisciplinary approach must be used to treat patients in whom psychosocial factors or central

3: Medical Management of Spine Disorders

---

sensitization are involved. Proceeding with interventional treatments while neglecting the biomechanical, neurophysiologic, and psychosocial aspects of spine pain will be a low-value endeavor and may cause harm.

Even after thorough analysis of the patient history, detailed physical examination, and diligent inspection of all pertinent diagnostic testing, the precise etiology of spine pain often remains unknown. Although imaging evaluation is critical in diagnosis, degenerative findings are nonspecific and can be misleading.[4] In patients in whom clinical and radiologic information yield at least a moderate or high pretest probability for chronic spine pain, carefully performed diagnostic procedures confirm the source of the pain in at least 80% of patients.[2,3] False-positive diagnostic injection occurs in up to 40% of patients after a single injection, so in patients in whom accurate diagnosis is imperative, the surgeon should take steps to reduce the risk for false-positive diagnostic injection.[5] To reduce the risk for false-positive results, the surgeon can perform a second block with an anesthetic of different duration of action and classify the patient's response by both percentage and duration of improvement. A concordantly positive response would be one in which the patient attains a predetermined level of pain relief for the expected duration of the anesthetic used.[5] After the pathoanatomic diagnosis is established, targeted interventional treatments can be used to reduce pain and disability. In some patients, targeted interventional treatment obviates the need for spinal surgery.

Rationale for Use of Spine Interventional Procedures

Understanding of the pathophysiology of the various causes of spine pain continues to evolve. Radicular pain can occur as a result of mechanical compression or a chemoinflammatory response, as occurs in the setting of an intervertebral disk herniation. An annular fissure exposes the highly antigenic nucleus pulposus, triggering an inflammatory cascade that contributes to local neural edema, altered nerve function, and sensitization.[6-8] Sensitizing chemicals and inflammatory mediators have been identified at the site of disk injury, along with upregulation of neuropeptide receptors in local pain generators, including the dorsal root ganglion (DRG), anulus fibrosus, and ligaments.[7] Placement of autologous nucleus pulposus around the DRG triggers sustained neural discharges that are consistent with nociception.[7] Neurogenic inflammation associated with spinal facet joint arthritis similarly produces peripheral sensitization (increased sensitivity of primary afferent neurons in the richly innervated joint capsule and synovial membrane) as well as central

sensitization (hyperexcitability of nociceptive interneurons in the central nervous system).[6]

Because of the chemoinflammatory and neural sensitization contributions to pain, corticosteroid and local anesthetic are rational treatment approaches to spine pain. Corticosteroid decreases inflammation via inhibition of prostaglandins in the arachidonic acid cascade, which may in turn improve microcirculation, capillary permeability, nerve root edema, and ischemia. Similar to the effect of local anesthetic, corticosteroid may also directly attenuate the excitation and sensitization of pain-generating C-fiber neurons. Lidocaine and bupivacaine are well-known direct inhibitors of sodium channel activation of peripheral nociceptive C-fibers and A-sigma fibers at the site of tissue injury, reducing peripheral sensitization. When local anesthetic is administered to the spinal epidural space, it can potentially inhibit N-methylaspartate–receptor currents critical to a component of central sensitization.[6] The precise mechanisms by which corticosteroid and local anesthetic act on spinal pain are not completely understood.

Technical Considerations

After it has been decided to proceed with therapeutic spine intervention, the surgeon must determine the procedural approach, medication, type of image guidance, timing, and frequency of repeat procedures. These considerations are especially important in the performance of epidural steroid injections (ESIs), by far the most widely used pain intervention.

Epidural Steroid Injection

Three approaches exist for entrance to the lumbar epidural space: caudal ESI, interlaminar ESI, and transforaminal ESI. The selection of approach is based on a patient's symptoms, anatomy, pathology, and treatment goals. For any elective spine procedure, image guidance is the standard of care to optimize safety, accuracy, and effectiveness. Without image guidance, at least 30% to 50% of interlaminar and caudal epidural injections fail to deliver medication to the intended epidural space.[9,10] Aspiration alone is insensitive for detecting potentially catastrophic intravascular needle placement.[5,7]

In a caudal ESI, the needle is directed toward the sacral hiatus and a relatively larger volume of medication is injected to distribute it cephalad, as high as L4-L5 (**Figure 1**). Caudal ESI is frequently used in patients with L4-L5 or L5-S1 pathology, in whom the anatomy prohibits interlaminar or transforaminal ESI. For example, patients who have severe scoliosis or who have previously undergone spine surgery may be treated via caudal ESI.

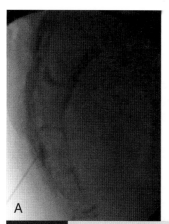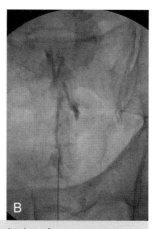

Figure 1   A, Lateral fluoroscopic view demonstrates epidural contrast injection into the sacral hiatus via a caudal approach. B, AP view demonstrates cephalad migration of the epidural contrast.

Interlaminar ESI can be performed at any spinal level at which a competent ligamentum flavum is present—typically, C6-C7 through L5-S1 (**Figure 2**). Most often, the needle enters the posterior epidural space via a paramedian approach, which makes use of a so-called loss of resistance technique. The injectant may travel several levels cephalad or caudad from the site of injection.[7] Interlaminar ESI is often considered in patients with bilateral symptoms related to spinal stenosis. This approach should be avoided at levels of prior posterior spinal surgery, severe stenosis, or inadequate posterior epidural space, all of which increase the risk for intrathecal placement.

In transforaminal ESI, the approach to the epidural space is made via an oblique angle to the lateral foramina. Transforaminal ESI can be performed at any level in the spine, is thought to be the most selective of all three approaches, and most consistently delivers medication to the ventral epidural space near an intervertebral disk herniation (**Figure 3**). Although this approach is the best studied, it carries the greatest risk of potentially catastrophic injection into a radicular artery. Image guidance is required and optimized with the use of contrast injection under live fluoroscopy and digital subtraction angiography. Transforaminal ESI is often performed to relieve radicular pain in the setting of intervertebral disk herniation or stenosis or to assist with diagnosis through more selective placement of local anesthetic on a specific nerve.

Radiofrequency Neurotomy

For managing spinal pain, radiofrequency neurotomy (RFN) is typically performed under biplanar fluoroscopy, with the goal of thermal coagulation of a nociceptor. Most commonly, the surgeon targets the medial branches of the primary dorsal rami innervating the spinal facet joint (**Figure 4**). In conventional RFN, radiofrequency energy is used to heat a needle tip to approximately 80°C to create a lesion measuring approximately 1 to 3 mm. The size of the lesion created is dependent on the size of the needle and duration of the stimulus. Outcomes of conventional RFN are highly dependent on technique; the best outcomes are achieved when the needle tip lies parallel to the target nerve.[5,11] Cooled RFN is a newer, more costly technique that has some advantages over conventional RFN. Cooled RFN uses a fluid pump that circulates sterile water to cool the needle tip and adjacent tissue. Because the probe tip temperature is 60°C, the coagulation time is longer (approximately 150 seconds), and the lesion size is larger than with conventional RFN. Moreover, the lesion created using cooled RFN extends farther beyond the needle tip, allowing easier needle placement, which is helpful in patients with complex anatomy or who are undergoing SI joint RFN.[12] The larger lesion size generated with cooled RFN warrants additional caution. After RFN, the coagulated nerves typically regenerate and can restore nociception to the joint. Although the duration of effect from RFN varies, at least 50% improvement in pain for at least 6 months constitutes a positive outcome.

Corticosteroid Selection

The types of corticosteroid commonly used in spine procedures are listed in **Table 1**. The US FDA has not approved the epidural use of corticosteroid and stated in 2014 that effectiveness and safety of epidural steroids has not been established.[13] Bristol-Myers Squibb, the maker of Kenalog (triamcinolone) changed its package label in 2011 to include a warning against epidural use of the steroid because of reports of serious medical events, including death.[14] Since 2011, epidural use of triamcinolone has declined, but off-label use of other corticosteroid brands persists.

Inadvertent intra-arterial injection of a particulate steroid during a transforaminal ESI can result in embolic infarct of the brain or spinal cord and cause stroke, blindness, paralysis, or death. Dexamethasone is the only corticosteroid that is essentially aqueous in solution and does not coagulate particles larger than red blood cells (**Table 1**). Theoretically, a particulate corticosteroid will linger at the site of injection to extend the duration of anti-inflammatory effect; most of the early efficacy studies on transforaminal ESIs used a particulate corticosteroid.[15] However, since 2011 multiple studies have demonstrated essentially equivalent effectiveness with dexamethasone compared with a

3: Medical Management of Spine Disorders

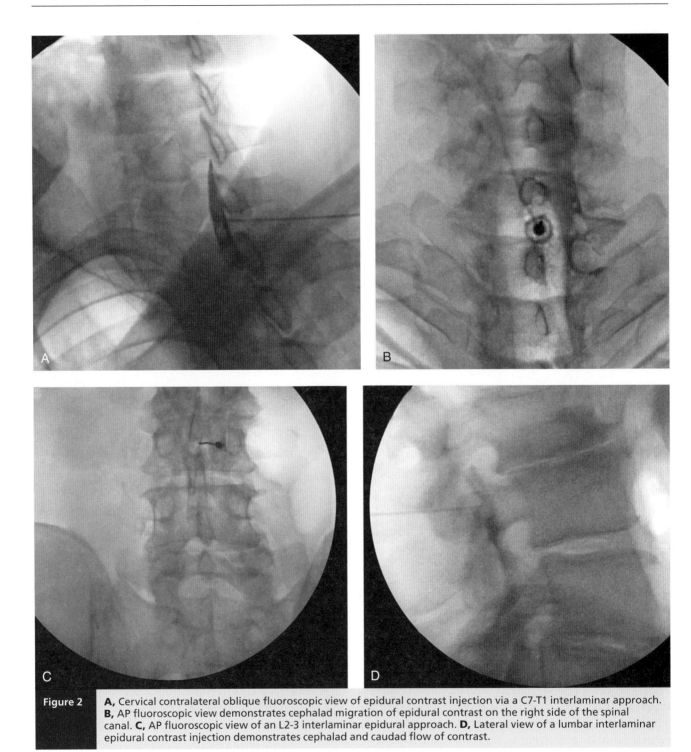

Figure 2   **A,** Cervical contralateral oblique fluoroscopic view of epidural contrast injection via a C7-T1 interlaminar approach. **B,** AP fluoroscopic view demonstrates cephalad migration of epidural contrast on the right side of the spinal canal. **C,** AP fluoroscopic view of an L2-3 interlaminar epidural approach. **D,** Lateral view of a lumbar interlaminar epidural contrast injection demonstrates cephalad and caudad flow of contrast.

particulate corticosteroid for transforaminal ESI.[16,17] A high-quality study showed that 10% to 15% of patients may require one additional injection to achieve optimal effect with dexamethasone compared with particulate steroid, but otherwise steroid selection did not predict outcome.[17] Based on the theoretic improved safety profile and equivalent effectiveness of dexamethasone compared with other corticosteroids, dexamethasone has been recommended as the first-line agent for transforaminal ESI.[16,17]

For procedures other than transforaminal ESI, corticosteroid selection tends to be based more on provider preference than safety concerns. Most effectiveness studies on interlaminar ESIs, caudal ESIs, and intra-articular injections used particulate steroids. A recent retrospective

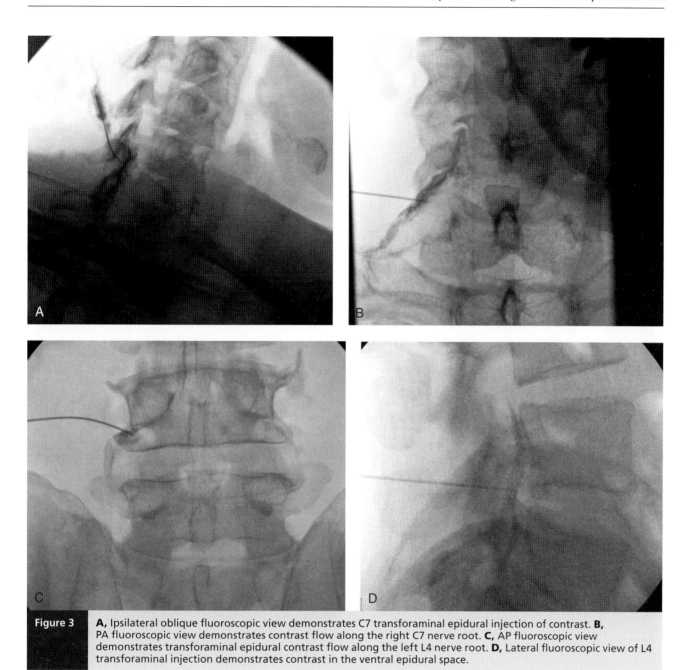

Figure 3 **A,** Ipsilateral oblique fluoroscopic view demonstrates C7 transforaminal epidural injection of contrast. **B,** PA fluoroscopic view demonstrates contrast flow along the right C7 nerve root. **C,** AP fluoroscopic view demonstrates transforaminal epidural contrast flow along the left L4 nerve root. **D,** Lateral fluoroscopic view of L4 transforaminal injection demonstrates contrast in the ventral epidural space.

series of 531 patients compared response to interlaminar ESI with either 40 mg triamcinolone or 4 mg dexamethasone and found twice the rate of positive outcomes at 1-month follow-up in the triamcinolone group.[18]

Timing and Frequency of Injections

Spinal injections should be performed only after treatment goals and expectations have been established and agreed on. There is no consensus on the timing and frequency of therapeutic spinal injections, and the historically used so-called series of three approaches has no scientific basis.

If a technically sound injection does not provide substantial improvement, then repeating the same injection is not recommended, because only 6% of patients are likely to respond to the repeat procedure.[19] If temporary improvement is obtained with the first injection, then a repeat injection between 2 and 4 weeks later can be considered. It may take 1 to 2 weeks to determine the effectiveness of the injection and 3 to 4 weeks for adrenal suppression to subside. Typically one or two injections are required to achieve optimal benefit, and patients rarely need a third injection to address radicular pain.[19] Spine injections should be limited to no more than three in a 6-month

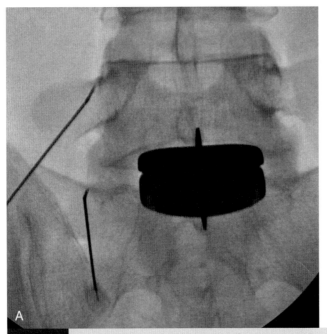 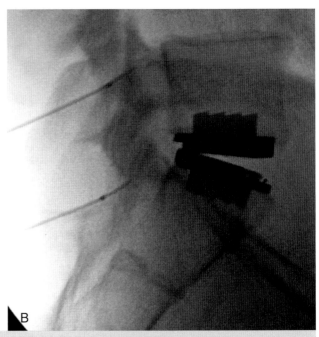

Figure 4 **A,** AP fluoroscopic view of needle placement for radiofrequency neurotomy of the left L4 medial branch of the primary dorsal ramus and the L5 primary dorsal ramus to denervate the right L5-S1 facet joint in a patient who had previously undergone L5-S1 disk arthroplasty. **B,** Lateral fluoroscopic view of the same patient confirms needle placement at the junction of the superior articular and transverse processes for denervation of the L4 medial branch of the primary dorsal ramus and the sacral ala for denervation of the L5 primary dorsal ramus.

Table 1

Commonly Injected Corticosteroids and Their Relative Particle Size

Corticosteroid	Equivalent Potency (mg)	Soluble	Maximum Particle Size (µM)
Methylprednisolone	40	No	>500
Triamcinolone	40	No	>500
Betamethasone	7.5	No	500
Dexamethasone	7.5	Yes	0.5
Red blood cell	NA	NA	8
Terminal vessels	NA	NA	60-100 (diameter)

NA = not applicable.

Adapted with permission from MacMahon PJ, Eustace SJ, Kavanagh EC: Injectable corticosteroid and local anesthetic preparations: A review for radiologists. *Radiology* 2009;252(3):647-661.

period and four in 1 year.[5,15] Successful RFN should not need repeating more often than every 6 months.

There is new research regarding the effect of corticosteroid injection around the time of spine surgery, including retrospective database analyses of more than 60,000 patients.[20,21] The following postoperative infection rates were reported for patients who did not undergo ESI preoperatively: 2% for posterior cervical surgery, 0.6% for anterior cervical diskectomy and fusion, and 0.8%

for lumbar decompression. If an ESI is performed within 3 months prior to surgery, postoperative infection rates rise to 4% for posterior cervical surgery, 0.8% for anterior cervical diskectomy and fusion, and 1.2% for lumbar decompression, which equates to numbers of 50, 500, and 250, respectively, needed to harm. Similar analyses of Spine Patient Outcomes Research Trial (SPORT) and Lumbar Spinal Stenosis Outcome Study (LSOS) cohorts reported conflicting results.[22,23] Patients in the SPORT cohort had an increased likelihood of crossover from surgical to nonsurgical treatment if they underwent an ESI compared with those who had no ESI (62% versus 33%, respectively); however, patients treated with ESI who eventually underwent surgery had fusion surgeries lasting an average of 26 minutes longer, longer hospital stays by 1 day, and overall poorer outcomes.[22] In contrast, the LSOS cohort demonstrated no negative or positive effects of preoperative ESI on postoperative outcomes.[23] Additional studies are needed to definitively determine if and when to avoid ESI around the time of spine surgery.

Image Guidance

Spine procedures may be performed under fluoroscopy, CT, or ultrasonography. Fluoroscopy is the most commonly used image guidance modality. Fluoroscopy was used in the highest quality studies on ESI. Fluoroscopy has the advantage of multiplanar and real-time visualization of contrast injection, which is important for reducing the risk of potentially catastrophic intravascular injection (especially during transforaminal ESIs). Although routine CT-guided procedures do not allow for real-time visualization of contrast injection and typically deliver increased amounts of radiation to the patient, axial CT views are useful in patients who require either transforaminal ESI in a region of severe spinal deformity (such as scoliosis) or intra-articular injection to severely arthritic joints (such as the lateral atlantoaxial joint). Musculoskeletal ultrasonography is a developing modality for spine interventions, with techniques described for most spine procedures.[24] When used by an experienced surgeon, ultrasonography is helpful in the effective delivery of medications to the target structure. However, the failure of ultrasonography to detect real-time intravascular flow limits its safety and utility for transforaminal epidural procedures. Safety and efficacy studies are needed to further define the role of ultrasonography for spine procedures.

Indications for Percutaneous Interventions

The potential benefits from spine interventional procedures are determined by the particular indication and the individualized treatment goals. As a diagnostic tool, spine intervention procedures can be used to confirm a suspected diagnosis, rule out a competing diagnosis, and predict patient response to more aggressive treatments, such as decompression surgery to manage radicular pain or RFN to manage facet joint pain. The short- or medium-term pain relief from percutaneous intervention may be highly beneficial to a patient for whom a

rehabilitation program is unsuccessful as a result of moderate or severe pain, or in a patient in whom the natural history of the painful condition is likely to improve with time, such as radicular pain resulting from an intervertebral disk herniation. With the exception of successful RFN for managing chronic facet joint pain, the benefits of percutaneous intervention in patients who have chronic stable pain but for whom no defined functional rehabilitation goals exist are less clear and less predictable. Although percutaneous spine procedures are beneficial for managing pain, they have not been widely demonstrated to improve other spine-related symptoms, such as weakness, numbness, and incoordination. The most common indications for spine interventions are lumbar radicular pain resulting from disk herniation, lumbar radicular pain or neurogenic claudication resulting from spinal stenosis, and cervical radicular pain.

Lumbar Radicular Pain Resulting From Disk Herniation

Lumbar radicular pain resulting from intervertebral disk herniation is the most common and well-accepted indication for ESI.[15,19] Evaluation of the efficacy of ESI is challenging because, historically, studies have included variable treatment protocols, patient selection, and outcome measures. In addition, early research focused on interlaminar ESI without image guidance. More recent research has been of higher quality and primarily studied fluoroscopically guided transforaminal ESIs. In 2013, the North American Spine Society published a consensus statement that included a grade A recommendation for transforaminal ESI to manage radicular pain resulting from lumbar intervertebral disk herniation.[15] The best level I study, which was published in 2010, included 150 patients who were deemed surgical candidates to manage lumbar intervertebral disk herniation in conjunction with acute or chronic radicular pain.[25] Patients treated with transforaminal ESI had substantially more responders (≥50% improvement in pain, improved function, decreased healthcare needs) at 1 month postinjection compared with patients treated with transforaminal normal saline, transforaminal local anesthetic, intramuscular steroid, or intramuscular normal saline. More than 50% of patients in the transforaminal ESI group responded at 1 month postinjection, and 25% responded at 1 year postinjection. The number needed to treat (NNT) for transforaminal ESI compared with transforaminal normal saline was 2 to 3 for response at 1 month postinjection and 4 to 5 for response at 3, 6, and 12 months postinjection. Pooled effectiveness data from multiple level I and II studies and reviews indicate that 60% to 70% of patients experience at least 50% pain relief for 1 to 2 months

3: Medical Management of Spine Disorders

postinjection, and 25% to 40% of patients experience this percentage of improvement at 1 year postinjection.[5,19]

No high-quality, prospective, placebo-controlled trials have been done on interlaminar ESIs and caudal ESIs. Level II and III studies of fluoroscopically guided interlaminar ESI and caudal ESI report short-term pain relief, with variable improvement beyond 1 month post-injection.[5] Furthermore, interlaminar injection with local anesthetic alone may provide pain relief equivalent to that of interlaminar ESI.[5,7] Low-quality prospective and retrospective comparison studies that include patients with lumbar radicular pain resulting from any cause do not show a difference in effectiveness between transforaminal ESI and interlaminar ESI; additionally, both transforaminal ESI and interlaminar ESI typically demonstrate better results than those of caudal ESIs.[5]

Patients most likely to respond to ESI for radicular pain include those who have a diagnosis of intervertebral disk herniation, higher initial Oswestry Disability Index scores, and electromyography-confirmed radiculopathy.[19,26,27] Results are better in patients with contained intervertebral disk herniations (75% success rate) than in patients who have extrusions with severe nerve compression.[5,19] Predictors of poorer response include duration of pain greater than 1 year, prior surgery, high preinjection anxiety, catastrophizing, fear avoidance, and low treatment expectations.[27] Expected outcomes of spine interventional treatments are included in **Table 2**.[5,7,11,12,15,17,19,25,28-44]

Lumbar Radicular Pain or Neurogenic Claudication Resulting From Spinal Stenosis

Many patients with lumbar spinal stenosis report stability of symptoms over years, with some periods of worsening and some periods of improvement. Theoretically, a nonsurgical treatment such as an ESI that can offer even temporary improvement during flare-ups may reduce the need for surgery in some patients.

Even though 25% of ESIs are performed for spinal stenosis, there are no level I trials assessing the efficacy of ESI for lumbar stenosis against a true placebo.[28] In 2013, the North American Spine Society reported that there is insufficient evidence to make a recommendation for or against the efficacy of transforaminal ESI to manage neuroforaminal stenosis or central canal stenosis.[15] A Cochrane review published that same year indicated that supportive evidence for ESI to manage lumbar spinal stenosis with neurogenic claudication is limited to low-quality evidence.[29] The authors of a higher quality multicenter study published in 2014 randomly assigned 400 patients to either any type of lumbar ESI or epidural injection of lidocaine.[28] At 6-week follow-up, patients in

both treatment groups achieved statistically significant improvements in pain and function. Specifically, 30% to 40% of patients achieved at least 30% improvement in Roland-Morris Disability Questionnaire scores, and 40% of patients achieved at least 50% improvement in leg pain. All patients had central canal stenosis, but it is unclear how many had multilevel stenosis or coexisting neuroforaminal stenosis or how many patients had leg pain resulting from neurogenic claudication versus monoradicular pain. Although small differences favored the corticosteroid group in physical function, patient satisfaction, and depression, there were no statistically significant differences in leg pain between the corticosteroid and local anesthetic-only group. In addition, there were no significant differences in outcomes between transforaminal ESI and interlaminar ESI. Similarly, neither SPORT nor LSOS cohorts experienced a significant positive effect on long-term outcome after ESI to manage spinal stenosis.[22,23] A trial of an epidural injection of corticosteroid and/or local anesthetic is a reasonable (albeit debatable) treatment option for carefully selected patients with moderate to severe leg pain from spinal stenosis.

Cervical Radicular Pain

Although cervical radiculopathy is less extensively studied than lumbar radiculopathy, nonsurgical management of this condition also has a similarly high success rate of approximately 80% to 90%, and cervical radicular pain can be responsive to cervical ESI.[30,31] No level I studies have been published. A clinically useful study compared cervical ESI to intramuscular tender-point injection with corticosteroid to manage cervical radicular pain that was unresponsive to physical therapy or NSAIDs.[32] This study included only 50 patients, and 8 of 25 patients in the intramuscular steroid group were excluded from the study. At 1-week follow-up, 44% of patients treated with ESI and 18% of patients treated with intramuscular steroid achieved at least 75% improvement (NNT = 3.8). Greater than 60% of patients treated with ESI achieved this outcome at 1-year follow-up (NNT = 2). Pooled data from multiple level II, III, and IV studies on cervical interlaminar ESI and cervical transforaminal ESI indicate at least 50% improvement in pain for a duration of 1 to 6 months, with one or two injections required. Response rates ranged from 40% to 70%.[30,31] Data indicate that a smaller percentage of patients experience improved pain for 12 months. Based on the available evidence, it remains unclear if cervical interlaminar ESI is more effective than cervical transforaminal ESI or if ESI is more effective than epidural injection of local anesthetic or saline.

Table 2

Effectiveness of Spine Interventional Treatments

Indication	Procedure	Estimated Percentage of Patients With ≥50% Improvement (Duration)	Grade of Evidence[b]	Comments
Radicular pain	Lumbar TFESI	60%-70% (1-2 mo) 25%-40% (1 yr)	A	The only Grade A recommendation for this procedure is for the management of radicular pain resulting from disk herniation
	Lumbar ILESI/ caudal ESI	50% (≥1 mo)	I	CS is not proven to be better than LA alone
	Cervical ILESI or TFESI	40%-70% (1-6 mo) 50% (1 yr)	C	Whether either procedure is better than placebo is unknown
	Pulsed RF to DRG	37.5% (3 mo)	I	Findings from a pilot study
Lumbar stenosis (leg pain)	Lumbar ESI (any type)	40% (6 wk)	I	CS is not proven to be better than LA alone Conflicting evidence
Spinal facet joint pain	Lumbar RFN	60%-80% (6-24 mo), if ≥80% improvement on dual MBBs; complete relief in 50% if complete relief achieved after MBBs	C	Better controlled trials are needed Outcome is dependent on technique and patient selection in high-quality observational studies
	Lumbar facet joint injection	18%-63% (unknown)	I	Low-quality studies with poor inclusion criteria
	Cervical RFN	75% (10-24 mo), if ≥80% improvement on dual MBBs; complete relief in 60%-75% if complete relief achieved after MBBs	C	Better controlled trials are needed Outcome is dependent on technique and patient selection in high-quality observational studies
	Cervical facet joint injection	20% (2-3 mo)	I	CS is not proven to be better than LA alone Few studies
Discogenic pain	ESI (any type)	25%-50% (6-52 wk)	I	Based on a small number of mostly level III studies
	Intradiscal methylene blue	40% experience ≥30% relief (6 mo)	I	Based on one small study
	Intradiscal platelet-rich plasma	47% (6 mo)	I	Based on one small level IV series only Adequate categorical data not provided by RCTs
	Intradiscal electrothermal annuloplasty (eg, IDET)	40% (6 mo) 50% do not respond at all	I	Conflicting studies; unclear whether the technique is better than a sham procedure
	Intradiscal biacuplasty	50% get ≥30% (3 mo) 36% get ≥30% (6 mo)	I	Better than placebo, but small effect and many nonresponders

3: Medical Management of Spine Disorders

Effectiveness of Spine Interventional Treatments (continued)

Indication	Procedure	Estimated Percentage of Patients With ≥50% Improvement (Duration)	Grade of Evidence[b]	Comments
Sacroiliac joint pain	Intra-articular sacroiliac joint injection	50% (6 wk), but improves to 70% if radiographic sacroiliitis	I	Best outcome from CS injection can be expected when patients have ≥75% improvement after injection of LA
	Sacral RFN	35%-70% (6-12 mo), if ≥50% on LBBs	I	Few/conflicting studies Cooled RFN was used in level I studies

a. Categorical data are not available for all spinal treatments.

b. Estimated level of evidence and grade are based on North American Spine Society definitions: A = good evidence (level I studies with consistent findings); B = fair evidence (level II or III studies with consistent findings); C = poor-quality evidence (level IV or V studies); I = insufficient or conflicting evidence.

CS = corticosteroid, DRG = dorsal root ganglion, ESI = epidural steroid injection, IDET = intradiscal electrothermal therapy, ILESI = interlaminar epidural steroid injection, LA = local anesthetic, LBB = lateral branch blocks, MBB = medial branch blocks, RCT = randomized controlled trial, RF = radiofrequency, RFN = radiofrequency neurotomy, TFESI = transforaminal epidural steroid injection.

Reducing the Need for Surgery

The role of injections in preventing the need for surgery, primarily as a secondary outcome measure, has been evaluated. According to a 2015 review, low-quality evidence suggests that ESI can prevent the need for surgery (at least in the short term) in one-third to one-half of patients considering surgery to manage radicular pain resulting from intervertebral disk herniation or stenosis.[33]

Whether ESI is a surgery-sparing treatment remains debatable. The only prospective study in which surgery was the primary outcome demonstrated that surgical candidates with radicular pain resulting from intervertebral disk herniation or lumbar spinal stenosis treated with up to four transforaminal ESIs had a significantly lower surgical rate than patients injected with local anesthetic only (29% and 67%, respectively; $P < 0.004$).[45] A 5-year follow-up study of those same patients reported that 81% of patients who avoided surgery at 1 year had avoided surgery at 5 years as well, irrespective of their initial treatment group.[45] These findings suggest that ESI may help patients by managing acute flares of pain, and radicular pain will subside in many patients over time. A single ESI does not affect surgical rates in patients with spinal stenosis,[23] which suggests that repeat injections are required to reduce the need for surgery in these patients.

Predicting Surgical Outcomes

Retrospective evidence suggests that fluoroscopically guided ESIs that produce at least 80% immediate improvement in radicular symptoms (local anesthetic effect) and at least 50% pain relief for at least 1 week (corticosteroid effect) are predictive of at least 50% pain relief with surgical decompression (positive predictive value of 85% to 91% and negative predictive value of 77%, irrespective of duration of symptoms).[3,7,34] A completely negative response to ESI reduces the likelihood of positive response to decompression surgery.[3,7,34]

Axial Discogenic Pain

Approximately 40% of all cases of LBP are believed to be discogenic.[1,8] Annular fissures and disk degeneration can be accompanied by nociceptive nerve ingrowth, and stimulation of these nerve endings via inflammatory mediators can result in pain.[8,35] Despite the high prevalence of discogenic LBP, no single interventional treatment has proved to be consistently effective or to have sustained benefits over time. As with surgery, emotional and psychological factors influence the perception of discogenic pain and affect percutaneous treatment outcomes. Diskography remains the preferred method for diagnosing discogenic pain; strict procedural guidelines must be followed.[3,5,8] MRI findings, including Modic type I or II end plate changes and high-intensity zone in the outer anulus fibrosus, can support a clinical diagnosis of discogenic pain.[5] Percutaneous techniques for managing discogenic pain have largely disappointed, including ESI, intradiscal injections, intradiscal neurolysis, and percutaneous diskectomy.

No high-quality level I or II trials of ESI for axial discogenic LBP or neck pain without radicular pain have been performed; therefore, it is not clear whether ESI is better than placebo for this condition. Findings from level II and III studies suggest that only 25% of patients with axial discogenic LBP and up to 50% of patients with neck pain will achieve at least 50% short-term improvement of pain.[5,7,8,36] Retrospective studies indicate that some patients report benefits lasting 1 to 2 years.[5,7]

Based on limited and conflicting evidence, it remains unclear whether intradiscal steroids are helpful for some patients; however, the risk of iatrogenic discitis, calcification, degeneration, and vertebral end plate necrosis remains a prohibitive concern for many surgeons.[35] Although animal models have suggested that intradiscal injection of tumor necrosis factor-α inhibitor (such as etanercept) administered around the time of intervertebral disk herniation can prevent onset of pain behavior and pathologic nerve root changes, clinical study in humans showed no efficacy compared with placebo at 1 month in patients with positive diskography findings.[5]

Both chymopapain and methylene blue showed promise for managing discogenic pain, but they have largely been abandoned in the United States. Chymopapain is a proteolytic enzyme that can have a neurolytic effect on annular nociceptors and can degrade the nucleus, thereby reducing intradiscal pressure in the setting of contained disk herniations. Although clinical results of this enzyme were mostly favorable, use in the United States halted in 1999 because of a series of severe anaphylactic reactions believed to occur in approximately 1% of patients, as well as even more rare cases of hemorrhage, transverse myelitis, and discitis.[46] Chymopapain remains in use elsewhere in the world.

Methylene blue can also act as a chemoneurolytic agent. Recent trials have been unable to replicate the remarkably positive results reported in a level I study that was published in 2010.[35,37,47] A feasibility trial published in 2016 indicated that 6 of 15 patients experienced 30% pain relief 6 months after treatment.[37] A placebo-controlled randomized controlled trial (RCT) based on these data is planned, but such a trial will likely require high numbers of patients to demonstrate substantial improvement compared with placebo. Of additional concern is the potential neurotoxic effect of methylene blue should extravasation occur into the epidural space.

Intradiscal injection of ozone was first proposed as a treatment for intervertebral disk herniation in the 1980s as a means of reducing the size of herniation through chemically induced nucleus degradation. Although intradiscal injection of ozone is frequently used in Europe and especially Italy, no level I trials exist for this indication. Observational and retrospective studies indicate a 75% success rate maintained for 10 years after injection of

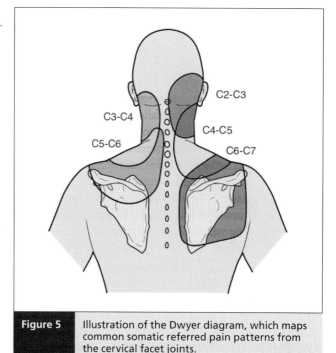

Figure 5 Illustration of the Dwyer diagram, which maps common somatic referred pain patterns from the cervical facet joints.

intradiscal ozone.[48] Controlled trials are needed to confirm treatment effect beyond the natural history of the condition.

Application of thermal energy to an injured disk has been proposed as a means to coagulate nociceptive nerve endings within the disk anulus fibrosus (or to target the ramus communicans). Although it has not been clinically proven, it may also be possible to use thermal energy to shrink collagen fibrils within the anulus fibrosus to reduce the size of annular fissures and intervertebral disk herniation. Thermal neurolysis techniques include intradiscal electrothermal annuloplasty, percutaneous intradiscal radiofrequency thermocoagulation, electrothermal ablation of ramus communicans, and intradiscal biacuplasty. These modalities have shown some therapeutic benefit compared with placebo in a small proportion of patients with discogenic pain.[1,5,8] Each study that shows positive effect has some pitfalls that limit generalizability to all patients with discogenic pain. A recent systematic review concluded that intradiscal electrothermal annuloplasty and percutaneous intradiscal radiofrequency thermocoagulation are likely ineffective for treating the general discogenic pain population and that ablation of the ramus communicans and intradiscal biacuplasty offer some promise in carefully selected patients.[35] Because of the limited or conflicting research, most payers consider these treatments investigational.

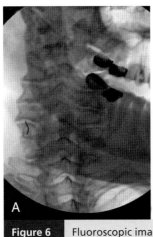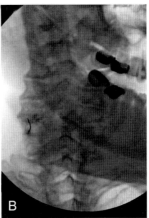

Figure 6 Fluoroscopic images show intra-articular injection to manage spinal facet joint pain. **A,** AP view demonstrates needle placement into the left C5-6 facet joint. **B,** AP view demonstrates the appearance of the contrast injection into the left C5-6 facet joint capsule.

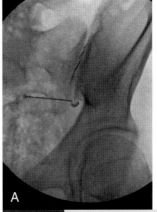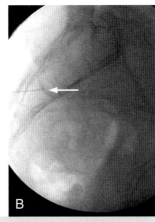

Figure 7 Fluoroscopic images show intra-articular injection to manage sacroiliac joint pain. **A,** AP view demonstrates needle placement in the inferior right sacroiliac joint, with intra-articular contrast flow cephalad. **B,** Lateral view demonstrates needle placement in the posteroinferior aspect of the joint as well as contrast filling the inferior recess of the joint (arrow).

Spinal Facet Joint Pain

Spinal facet joints, that is, zygapophyseal joints (Z-joints), are a well-known source of chronic axial spine pain, especially in patients with paracentral neck pain or LBP who are older than age 55 years and in all patients with chronic neck pain after a whiplash-type motor vehicle collision injury. The spinal facet joints are also often implicated in cervicogenic headaches and axial pain resulting from degenerative spondylolisthesis. In the cervical spine, the facet joints often cause pain in well-known distributions (**Figure 5**). Referral patterns from the lumbar spine are less specific. There are no historical features, physical examination maneuvers, or radiographic findings by which it is possible to specifically and definitively identify facet joint pain. Identification of mobile spondylolisthesis on radiography, increased uptake on single photon emission computed tomography, and/or increased signal in the perifacet bone marrow or intra-articular edema on T2-weighted or short tau inversion recovery MRI sequences can support a diagnosis of facet joint pain.[3,7] Nonetheless, the preferred method for diagnosis remains controlled anesthetic blocks to the specific joint or its nerve supply.

Percutaneous therapeutic treatment options for spinal facet joint pain include intra-articular injection and RFN. To date, no RCTs have used a dual anesthetic block protocol for patient selection to study the effectiveness of intra-articular facet joint injections. Although intra-articular facet joint injection is still used as a diagnostic tool, its therapeutic value is not supported in the literature. For some patients, intra-articular facet joint injection (**Figure 6**) may reduce pain, reduce frequency of cervicogenic headaches, and improve tolerability of active physical therapy; however, injection should not be used as a stand-alone treatment.[38,39]

Alternatively, RFN has been shown to be effective in studies that used rigorous selection criteria and anatomically correct techniques (**Table 2**). Positive results have been obtained in studies that selected patients on the basis of at least 80% improvement on two separate anesthetic injections in the lumbar spine and 100% improvement in the cervical spine. Only a small number (<20%) of patients selected for diagnostic medial branch blocks will meet these strict inclusion criteria.[5,9,38] Recent prospective cohort studies of patients carefully selected on the basis of 100% relief after dual anesthetic blocks reported greater than 50% success in the lumbar spine and greater than 60% success in the cervical spine after a single RFN treatment, with success defined as complete relief of pain for 6 months or more, complete restoration of activities of daily living, no need for further healthcare interventions, and return to work.[11,49] These studies used optimal technique with 16-gauge needles. Less rigorous selection and technical variation negatively affects outcomes in RFN.

Sacroiliac Joint Pain

The SI joint is the cause of chronic LBP in 15% to 30% of patients, with a higher prevalence in older patients as well as in patients with a history of lumbosacral fusion, spondyloarthropathy, and/or pain isolated below L5.[1] Although no single physical examination maneuver has a high predictive value for diagnosing SI joint pain, the following criteria predict a positive response to a diagnostic block in 70% to 80% of patients: maximal pain below L5 and positive findings on at least three of these six provocation tests—distraction; compression; thigh thrust; Gaenslen; flexion, abduction, external rotation; and sacral thrust.[40] Unless true sacroiliitis is present, imaging is of limited use in diagnosing presumed SI joint pain. The preferred method for diagnosing SI joint pain remains positive response to an image-guided intra-articular block with local anesthetic. As with facet joint injections, false-positive rates are high with single blocks (20% to 40%).[5]

After SI joint pain has been confirmed and physical rehabilitation has been unsuccessful, interventional treatment may be performed. Treatment options include intra-articular SI joint injection with corticosteroid (**Figure 7**), conventional RFN, and cooled RFN. All procedures should be performed under image guidance. Intra-articular injections should be confirmed with radiopaque contrast. Similar to the facet joint injection studies, most therapeutic SI joint injection trials suffer from loose patient selection criteria. The estimated therapeutic effectiveness of SI joint injection is shown in **Table 2**.

RFN may be considered for patients who have confirmed SI joint pain and who do not experience sustained improvement after intra-articular injection. Because of the complex innervation of the SI joint, positive response to diagnostic lateral branch blocks should be obtained before proceeding to RFN, even in patients who have a positive response to the intra-articular local anesthetic block. The most common protocol includes anesthetic blockade of the L5 dorsal ramus and lateral branches from S1-S3 (blocked at the lateral aspects of the S1, S2, and S3 sacral foramina). The ventral innervation of the joint is not accessible. Patients who experience a positive intra-articular block but have a negative response to lateral branch blocks may still have pain related to the SI joint ligament complex; however, these patients are not good candidates for RFN. Placebo-controlled trials using cooled RFN suggest NNT of 1.5 to 2 to achieve at least 50% pain relief for 3 to 9 months, if patients are selected on the basis of having experienced at least 50% to 75% relief from anesthetic blocks.[41,42] Further studies are needed to evaluate the effectiveness of conventional RFN in the management of SI joint pain.

Soft-Tissue Pain From Posterior Hardware

In a study that used a stringent diagnostic protocol, including the use of two local anesthetic blocks and a saline injection, approximately 2.9% (95% confidence interval, 1.3% to 6.7%) of patients with postfusion axial pain were found to have hardware-mediated pain.[1] There are currently no literature-supported percutaneous treatments for hardware-mediated pain.

Pseudoarticular Pain

Pseudoarticular pain is a rare cause of LBP, occurring in fewer than 3% of patients and may result from Baastrup disease or Bertolotti syndrome.[1] Diagnosis is easily confirmed on image-guided local anesthetic injection. Although the use of corticosteroid injection or RFN in such patients has not been rigorously studied, these modalities do provide pain relief in some patients.

Contraindications to and Risks of Spine Interventions

Absolute contraindications to most percutaneous spine interventions include bleeding disorder; infection; history of severe allergic reaction with any of the injected materials; tumor in the location of the injection; pregnancy; and inability to obtain informed consent, including reasonable patient expectations. Guidelines should be used for periprocedural management of anticoagulants and antiplatelet agents.[50] Other relative contraindications include uncontrolled diabetes mellitus; heart failure; mild pain that responds to less invasive treatments; pain in multiple regions of the body; and/or substantial preinjection anxiety, fear-avoidance, or catastrophizing.

Percutaneous procedural complications are rare, occurring in fewer than 1% of patients; however, complications can include infection (0.01% to 0.1% of injections), epidural hematoma (<0.0001% of epidural injections), anaphylaxis, air embolism, vasovagal syncope (1% to 2% for lumbar and 8% for cervical injections), and temporary or permanent nerve injury.[5,7,51] Risks particular to ESIs include dural puncture, spinal headache, nerve puncture, intrathecal injection, and intravascular injection. Intrathecal injection of local anesthetic can result in variable degrees of spinal block, which is potentially catastrophic in the cervical spine. Intrathecal injection of any substance, particularly corticosteroid, carries the risk for arachnoiditis. Intravenous injection is rarely dangerous; however, intra-arterial injection can cause catastrophic injury, with the potential for seizure, stroke, paralysis, or death.[31] Awareness of the risk for intra-arterial injection is particularly pertinent when performing cervical transforaminal ESI (because the vertebral and radicular arteries can reside in close proximity to the needle) and transforaminal ESI in the lower thoracic spine (and, more rarely, the lumbar spine) where the artery of Adamkiewicz

3: Medical Management of Spine Disorders

is located. The artery of Adamkiewicz provides the main blood supply to the anterior spinal artery and typically enters the spinal canal between T9 and L2; however, this artery can enter the spinal canal more caudally and on the right side. Inadvertent injection of particulate corticosteroid into this artery during transforaminal ESI has been linked to several cases of paraplegia.[51] Negative aspiration is inadequate for detecting intravascular penetration in 50% of epidural injections.[5,51] Fluoroscopically guided contrast injection can reduce the risk of intravascular injection, and use of digital subtraction angiography, if available, is an even better option.[5,7,51] Risks of corticosteroid injection can be substantial, including but not limited to osteoporosis, adrenal insufficiency, Cushing syndrome, and hyperglycemia.

RFN carries additional unique risks, including post-RFN neuritis, anesthesia dolorosa, and muscle injury/denervation. Risk to the dorsal and ventral nerve roots is low when correct technique is used. Post-RFN neuritis can occur even with perfect technique, and it typically involves painful dysesthesias in the distribution of the targeted nerve lasting days to several weeks. Segmental multifidus denervation occurs with successful RFN, but this finding is not clinically significant in the lumbar spine.[52] Cervical muscle weakness and kyphosis have been reported after multilevel cervical RFN. Added caution is needed when performing RFN at a site near posterior spinal hardware, because hardware temperatures can potentially heat to dangerous levels. [53]

Investigational Technologies

Some surgeons believe that pulsed radiofrequency to the DRG may be an alternative to ESI for managing refractory radicular pain. In pulsed radiofrequency, a conventional RFN needle is heated to 42°C and the target nerve is exposed to an electrical field in an attempt to suppress ectopic firing of nociceptive fibers, without coagulating the nerve. Limited early studies show small effect size compared with sham treatment, with an NNT of 6 to achieve at least 50% improvement in pain.[43] A large RCT is required to investigate the efficacy of this technique.

The Minimally Invasive Lumbar Decompression (mild; Vertos Medical) procedure involves percutaneous removal of redundant ligamentum flavum under fluoroscopic guidance. Most studies are industry sponsored, with the best study indicating stronger treatment effect than ESI through 12 weeks postprocedure.[54] The best systematic review indicates that the mild procedure appears to be generally safe, with some positive treatment effects after up to 1-year follow-up based on low-quality evidence.[54]

Plasma disk decompression involves percutaneous removal of nucleus pulposus through a 17-gauge needle with the goal of decompressing an intervertebral disk herniation. Industry-sponsored studies suggest a higher rate of responders at 2-year follow-up after treatment with plasma disk decompression compared with transforaminal ESI in patients in whom physical therapy, medications, and one ESI have been unsuccessful. Specifically, this study reported a 50% probability of needing a second procedural intervention (such as repeat injection or surgery) within 2 years in the group receiving plasma disk decompression versus an 80% probability in the group receiving a transforaminal ESI.[55] Level I trials are needed to determine the efficacy of this technique.

Biologic regenerative treatments for degenerative spine conditions, especially for discogenic pain, are of considerable interest currently. Although animal and in vitro models have shown promise for both platelet-rich plasma (PRP) and stem cells, published clinical trials are lacking and treatments remain experimental. One recent double-blind, placebo-controlled RCT reported positive mean outcomes of intradiscal PRP compared with injection of contrast at 8-week follow-up.[44] However, categorical data were provided for patient satisfaction only, with satisfaction rates of 55% after intradiscal PRP and 18% after contrast injection. Prospective case studies have demonstrated positive effects of intradiscal PRP, intradiscal autologous bone marrow aspirate for diskography-confirmed discogenic LBP, PRP injection for SI joint pain, and hyaluronic acid injection for lumbar facet joint pain.[56] An FDA-monitored phase II RCT assessed the safety and efficacy of allogeneic mesenchymal stem cells injected into a single mildly degenerative disk.[56] Preliminary results indicate a 69% response rate for at least 50% improvement in LBP, compared with a 33% response rate in the control group (NNT = 2.8). A phase III study is in development.

Missing Evidence

Currently, there is no evidence to support the widespread use of injections to manage thoracic pain, axial pain resulting from stenosis, or spondylolisthesis. No evidence exists that any interventional treatment, whether percutaneous or surgical, is better than therapeutic exercise for managing chronic nonspecific axial LBP.

Summary

In the current healthcare environment, procedural interventions are increasingly being judged on their ability to provide measurable population-based benefits. In other words, to add value to the system, therapeutic spine interventions must be effective in more than a small proportion of patients treated, facilitate restoration of function and increased return-to-work rates, decrease healthcare utilization, be cost-effective, and be better than placebo. The importance of accurate diagnosis and patient selection cannot be overstated. When used in the appropriate patient and with precise technique, percutaneous spine interventions remain a valuable part of a comprehensive treatment approach.

Key Study Points

- Of all percutaneous therapeutic spine interventions, the only grade A recommendation is for lumbar transforaminal ESI to manage radicular pain resulting from disk herniation.
- In carefully selected patients, RFN has proved to be effective for maintaining long-term improvement in chronic facet joint pain.
- Although some patients with spinal stenosis benefit from ESI, it remains unclear if corticosteroid is better than epidural injection of local anesthetic.
- No percutaneous intradiscal procedures have proved to be consistently effective in a majority of patients with axial discogenic pain.

Annotated References

1. DePalma MJ, Ketchum JM, Saullo T: What is the source of chronic low back pain and does age play a role? *Pain Med* 2011;12(2):224-233.

   The intervertebral disk is the most common cause of chronic low back pain in adults. Spinal facet pain and sacroiliac joint pain become more common with increased age.

2. Yin W, Bogduk N: The nature of neck pain in a private pain clinic in the United States. *Pain Med* 2008;9(2):196-203.

3. DePalma M, Laplant B: Interventional spine care, in Rao RD, Smuck M, eds: *Orthopaedic Knowledge Update: Spine*, ed 4. Rosemont, IL, American Academy of Orthopaedic Surgeons, 2012, pp 121-146.

   Interventional spine procedures can reveal the source of chronic spinal pain in 80% to 90% of patients. Procedures aimed at the appropriate pain generator can reduce pain and disability.

4. Brinjikji W, Luetmer PH, Comstock B, et al: Systematic literature review of imaging features of spinal degeneration in asymptomatic populations. *AJNR Am J Neuroradiol* 2015;36(4):811-816.

   Imaging findings of spine degeneration are present in high proportions of asymptomatic individuals, and these findings increase with age. Many imaging-based degenerative features likely are part of the normal aging process and are unassociated with pain.

5. Bogduk N, ed: *Practice Guidelines for Spinal Diagnostic and Treatment Procedures*, ed 2. San Francisco, CA, International Spine Intervention Society, 2013.

   Diagnostic and therapeutic spine interventions continue to evolve. Technical guidelines exist to optimize patient selection and performance.

6. Woolf CJ: Central sensitization: Implications for the diagnosis and treatment of pain. *Pain* 2011;152 (3 suppl):S2-S15.

   Nociceptive input from a disk, joint, or nerve can increase excitability and synaptic efficacy in central nociceptive pathways, which is representative of the neuroplasticity of the pain processing system.

7. Friedrich JM, Harrast MA: Lumbar epidural steroid injections: Indications, contraindications, risks, and benefits. *Curr Sports Med Rep* 2010;9(1):43-49.

8. Bogduk N, Aprill C, Derby R: Lumbar discogenic pain: State-of-the-art review. *Pain Med* 2013;14(6):813-836.

   This evidence-based review supports the pathophysiology of discogenic pain. Correctly performed diskography remains the standard for diagnosis.

9. Barham G, Hilton A: Caudal epidurals: The accuracy of blind needle placement and the value of a confirmatory epidurogram. *Eur Spine J* 2010;19(9):1479-1483.

10. Fredman B, Nun MB, Zohar E, et al: Epidural steroids for treating "failed back surgery syndrome": Is fluoroscopy really necessary? *Anesth Analg* 1999;88(2):367-372.

11. MacVicar J, Borowczyk JM, MacVicar AM, Loughnan BM, Bogduk N: Lumbar medial branch radiofrequency neurotomy in New Zealand. *Pain Med* 2013;14(5):639-645.

    This prospective outcome study of 106 patients reported that lumbar RFN can be effective when performed in a rigorous manner in appropriately selected patients. Level of evidence: IV.

12. Aydin SM, Gharibo CG, Mehnert M, Stitik TP: The role of radiofrequency ablation for sacroiliac joint pain: A meta-analysis. *PM R* 2010;2(9):842-851.

13. US FDA website. FDA Drug Safety Communication: FDA requires label changes to warn of rare but serious neurologic problems after epidural corticosteroid injections for pain. April 23, 2014. Available at: http://www.fda.gov/Drugs/DrugSafety/ucm394280.htm. Accessed February 15, 2017.

14. Bristol-Myers Squibb: Package insert for Kenelog®-40 Injection. Revised January 2016. Available at:

http://packageinserts.bms.com/pi/pi_kenalog-40.pdf. Accessed February 15, 2017.

15. Akuthota V, Bogduk N, Easa JE, et al: *Lumbar Transforaminal Epidural Steroid Injections: Review and Recommendation Statement.* Burr Ridge, IL, North American Spine Society, 2013. Available at: www.spine.org/Portals/0/Documents/ResearchClinicalCare/LTFESIReviewRecStatement.pdf. Accessed January 25, 2017.

Grade A evidence from level I trials supports the use of transforaminal epidural steroid injections in the management of radicular pain. Evidence is limited for other indications.

16. Feeley IH, Healy EF, Noel J, Kiely PJ, Murphy TM: Particulate and non-particulate steroids in spinal epidurals: A systematic review and meta-analysis. *Eur Spine J* 2016; Feb 12 [Epub ahead of print].

Particulate steroids are not demonstrably better for relieving pain compared with their nonparticulate steroid preparations in spinal epidural injections. Nonparticulate steroids may be safer than particulate steroids. Level of evidence: II.

17. Kennedy DJ, Plastaras C, Casey E, et al: Comparative effectiveness of lumbar transforaminal epidural steroid injections with particulate versus nonparticulate corticosteroids for lumbar radicular pain due to intervertebral disc herniation: A prospective, randomized, double-blind trial. *Pain Med* 2014;15(4):548-555.

There is no significant difference between nonparticulate and particulate steroids in outcomes after transforaminal epidural steroid injections to manage radicular pain. A small number of patients receiving nonparticulate steroids require an additional injection to obtain optimal benefit. Level of evidence: II.

18. Bensler S, Sutter R, Pfirrmann CW, Peterson CK: Is there a difference in treatment outcomes between epidural injections with particulate versus non-particulate steroids? *Eur Radiol* 2016;Jul 19 [Epub ahead of print].

The authors of this retrospective analysis of 597 patients who were treated with an interlaminar epidural steroid injection to manage radicular pain reported more favorable outcomes in patients who received particulate steroid injection compared with patients who received nonparticulate steroid injections. Level of evidence: III.

19. MacVicar J, King W, Landers MH, Bogduk N: The effectiveness of lumbar transforaminal injection of steroids: A comprehensive review with systematic analysis of the published data. *Pain Med* 2013;14(1):14-28.

In most patients with lumbar radicular pain resulting from disk herniation, transforaminal injection of corticosteroids is effective in reducing pain, restoring function, reducing the need for other health care, and avoiding surgery. Level of evidence: II.

20. Cancienne JM, Werner BC, Puvanesarajah V, et al: Does the timing of pre-operative epidural steroid injection affect infection risk after ACDF or posterior cervical fusion? *Spine (Phila Pa 1976)* 2016;Apr 23 [Epub ahead of print].

Preoperative cervical epidural steroid injection within 3 to 6 months of cervical surgery is independently associated with an increased rate of postoperative infection. Level of evidence: III.

21. Singla A, Yang S, Werner BC, et al: Preoperative lumbar epidural injections are associated with increased risk of infection after single level lumbar decompression: A nationwide database analysis of 62,241 cases. *Spine J* 2015;15(10):S126 Available at: http://www.thespinejournalonline.com/article/S1529-9430(15)00791-3/abstract. Accessed January 18, 2017.

Lumbar decompression within 3 months after epidural steroid injection may be associated with an increased rate of postoperative infection, although the incidence of infection remains low.

22. Radcliff K, Kepler C, Hilibrand A, et al: Epidural steroid injections are associated with less improvement in patients with lumbar spinal stenosis: A subgroup analysis of the Spine Patient Outcomes Research Trial. *Spine (Phila Pa 1976)* 2013;38(4):279-291.

Epidural steroid injections are associated with significantly less improvement at 4-year follow-up among all patients with spinal stenosis in SPORT. Such injections are also associated with longer surgical time and hospital stays.

23. Fekete T, Woernle C, Mannion AF, et al; LSOS Working Group: The effect of epidural steroid injection on postoperative outcome in patients from the Lumbar Spinal Stenosis Outcome Study. *Spine (Phila Pa 1976)* 2015;40(16):1303-1310.

Epidural steroid injections had no significant effect on surgical or nonsurgical outcomes in a cohort of 281 patients with lumbar stenosis. Level of evidence: III.

24. Hurdle MF: Ultrasound-guided spinal procedures for pain: A review. *Phys Med Rehabil Clin N Am* 2016;27(3):673-686.

Most spine procedures for managing pain can be performed under ultrasonographic guidance; however, clinical trials are lacking, and bone may obscure the surgeon's ability to detect intravascular injection when performing transforaminal epidural steroid injection.

25. Ghahreman A, Ferch R, Bogduk N: The efficacy of transforaminal injection of steroids for the treatment of lumbar radicular pain. *Pain Med* 2010;11(8):1149-1168.

26. Annaswamy TM, Bierner SM, Avraham R: Role of electrodiagnosis in patients being considered for epidural steroid injections. *PM R* 2013;5(5suppl):S96-S99.

Positive electrodiagnostic evaluation for radiculopathy is associated with increased odds of positive response to epidural steroid injection.

27. Sivaganesan A, Chotai S, Parker SL, Asher AL, McGirt MJ, Devin CJ: Predictors of the efficacy of epidural steroid injections for structural lumbar degenerative pathology. *Spine J* 2016;16(8):928-934.

Attributes associated with substantial positive functional outcomes after epidural steroid injection include a diagnosis of disk herniation, central stenosis, and increased initial disability. Negative responses were predicted by prior surgery, longstanding symptoms, and preinjection anxiety.

28. Friedly JL, Comstock BA, Turner JA, et al: A randomized trial of epidural glucocorticoid injections for spinal stenosis. *N Engl J Med* 2014;371(1):11-21.

For management of lumbar spinal stenosis, epidural injection of corticosteroid plus lidocaine offered minimal or no short-term benefit compared with epidural injection of lidocaine alone. Level of evidence: II.

29. Ammendolia C, Stuber KJ, Rok E, et al: Nonoperative treatment for lumbar spinal stenosis with neurogenic claudication. *Cochrane Database Syst Rev* 2013;8(8):CD010712.

The authors of this study present low-quality evidence that epidural steroid injections provide short-term benefit compared with exercise. Moderate- and high-quality evidence for nonsurgical management of spinal stenosis is lacking.

30. Easa JE, Kreiner DS, Ghogawala Z, et al: *Cervical Epidural Steroid Injections: Review and Recommendation Statement.* Burr Ridge, IL, North American Spine Society, 2011. Available at: https://www.spine.org/Portals/0/Documents/ResearchClinicalCare/CESIReviewRec Statement.pdf. Accessed January 18, 2017.

Grade C recommendation state that transforaminal and interlaminar epidural steroid injections can provide short- and long-term relief in patients who have cervical radiculitis. Grade B recommendation state that better outcomes are predicted by cervical disk herniation as well as central or foraminal stenosis.

31. Engel A, King W, MacVicar J; Standards Division of the International Spine Intervention Society: The effectiveness and risks of fluoroscopically guided cervical transforaminal injections of steroids: A systematic review with comprehensive analysis of the published data. *Pain Med* 2014;15(3):386-402.

This study reports low-quality evidence suggesting that 50% of patients experience 50% relief of radicular pain with cervical transforaminal epidural steroid injection and that injection may obviate the need for surgery in some patients.

32. Stav A, Ovadia L, Sternberg A, Kaadan M, Weksler N: Cervical epidural steroid injection for cervicobrachialgia. *Acta Anaesthesiol Scand* 1993;37(6):562-566.

33. Bicket MC, Horowitz JM, Benzon HT, Cohen SP: Epidural injections in prevention of surgery for spinal pain: Systematic review and meta-analysis of randomized controlled trials. *Spine J* 2015;15(2):348-362.

Epidural steroid injections have a small to moderate surgery-sparing effect (noted in up to 50% of patients), at least in the short term (less than 1 year). Only studies using surgery as the primary outcome demonstrated long-term effects of injection. Level of evidence: II.

34. Costandi SJ, Azer G, Eshraghi Y, et al: Cervical transforaminal epidural steroid injections: Diagnostic and therapeutic value. *Reg Anesth Pain Med* 2015;40(6):674-680.

Registry analysis of 64 patients indicates that 70% of patients treated with cervical transforaminal epidural steroid injections avoided surgery for cervical radiculopathy. Of those who needed surgery, patients who had a positive initial response to an injection tended to have more favorable surgical outcomes compared with those who did not respond to the injection. Level of evidence: III.

35. Lu Y, Guzman JZ, Purmessur D, et al: Nonoperative management of discogenic back pain: A systematic review. *Spine (Phila Pa 1976)* 2014;39(16):1314-1324.

Proven generalizable nonsurgical management for discogenic low back pain is lacking. Level of evidence: II.

36. Lee JH, Lee SH: Comparison of clinical efficacy between interlaminar and transforaminal epidural injection in patients with axial pain due to cervical disc herniation. *Medicine (Baltimore)* 2016;95(4):e2568.

A study of 108 patients treated with interlaminar or transforaminal approaches to manage axial pain reported an overall 53% rate of successful pain relief at 8-week follow-up. Level of evidence: III.

37. Kallewaard JW, Geurts JW, Kessels A, Willems P, van Santbrink H, van Kleef M: Efficacy, safety, and predictors of intradiscal methylene blue injection for discogenic low back pain: Results of a multicenter prospective clinical series. *Pain Pract* 2016;16(4):405-412.

Of 15 consecutive patients treated with intradiscal methylene blue injection for the management of discogenic low back pain, 40% reported at least 30% pain relief 6 months after injection. Level of evidence: IV.

38. Barnsley L, Lord SM, Wallis BJ, Bogduk N: Lack of effect of intraarticular corticosteroids for chronic pain in the cervical zygapophyseal joints. *N Engl J Med* 1994;330(15):1047-1050.

39. Dreyfuss PH, Dreyer SJ; NASS: Lumbar zygapophysial (facet) joint injections. *Spine J* 2003;3(3 suppl):50S-59S.

40. Laslett M: Evidence-based diagnosis and treatment of the painful sacroiliac joint. *J Man Manip Ther* 2008;16(3):142-152.

41. Cohen SP, Hurley RW, Buckenmaier CC III, Kurihara C, Morlando B, Dragovich A: Randomized placebo-controlled study evaluating lateral branch radiofrequency denervation for sacroiliac joint pain. *Anesthesiology* 2008;109(2):279-288.

3: Medical Management of Spine Disorders

42. Patel N, Gross A, Brown L, Gekht G: A randomized, placebo-controlled study to assess the efficacy of lateral branch neurotomy for chronic sacroiliac joint pain. *Pain Med* 2012;13(3):383-398.

 This study randomized 51 patients on a 2:1 basis to lateral branch neurotomy or sham treatment. At 3-month follow-up, at least 50% reduction in pain was achieved in 47% of the patients treated with neurotomy versus 12% in the patients who underwent sham treatment. Level of evidence: I.

43. Shanthanna H, Chan P, McChesney J, Thabane L, Paul J: Pulsed radiofrequency treatment of the lumbar dorsal root ganglion in patients with chronic lumbar radicular pain: A randomized, placebo-controlled pilot study. *J Pain Res* 2014;7:47-55.

 Outcomes at 3-month follow-up demonstrated small effect sizes of treatment compared with placebo. Level of evidence: I.

44. Tuakli-Wosornu YA, Terry A, Boachie-Adjei K, et al: Lumbar intradiskal platelet-rich plasma (PRP) injections: A prospective, double-blind, randomized controlled study. *PM R* 2016;8(1):1-10, quiz 10.

 In this trial of 47 patients treated with either intradiscal PRP or intradiscal injection of contrast, mean improvement in pain and function and categorical improvement in patient satisfaction was achieved in the treatment group at 8-week follow-up. Level of evidence: I.

45. Riew KD, Park JB, Cho YS, et al: Nerve root blocks in the treatment of lumbar radicular pain: A minimum five-year follow-up. *J Bone Joint Surg Am* 2006;88(8):1722-1725.

46. Varshney A, Chapman JR: A review of chymopapain for chemonucleolysis of lumbar disc herniation. *Curr Orthop Pract* 2012;23(3):203-208.

 This review examined the available evidence on chymopapain injection for treatment of symptomatic lumbar disk herniation. It was concluded that chymopapain is more effective than placebo injection, but probably not more effective than surgery.

47. Peng B, Pang X, Wu Y, Zhao C, Song X: A randomized placebo-controlled trial of intradiscal methylene blue injection for the treatment of chronic discogenic low back pain. *Pain* 2010;149(1):124-129.

48. Buric J, Rigobello L, Hooper D: Five and ten year follow-up on intradiscal ozone injection for disc herniation. *Int J Spine Surg* 2014;8:17.

 This retrospective review of 108 patients indicated that 75% of patients benefited from the intervention. Of those patients who avoided surgery, improved outcomes persisted in more than 80% 5 and 10 years after the intervention. Level of evidence: III.

49. MacVicar J, Borowczyk JM, MacVicar AM, Loughnan BM, Bogduk N: Cervical medial branch radiofrequency neurotomy in New Zealand. *Pain Med* 2012;13(5):647-654.

 This high-quality study demonstrated successful outcomes in 61% to 74% of carefully selected patients treated with RFN. Relief persisted 17 to 20 months after one treatment. Repeat treatments were also effective in most patients. Level of evidence: IV.

50. Narouze S, Benzon HT, Provenzano DA, et al: Interventional spine and pain procedures in patients on antiplatelet and anticoagulant medications: Guidelines from the American Society of Regional Anesthesia and Pain Medicine, the European Society of Regional Anaesthesia and Pain Therapy, the American Academy of Pain Medicine, the International Neuromodulation Society, the North American Neuromodulation Society, and the World Institute of Pain. *Reg Anesth Pain Med* 2015;40(3):182-212.

 Guidelines for anticoagulant use around the time of spine interventions are presented, indicating measurable increased cardiovascular risk associated with anticoagulant cessation and the need for shared decision making with patients.

51. Bogduk N, Dreyfuss P, Baker R, et al: Complications of spinal diagnostic and treatment procedures. *Pain Med* 2008;9(suppl 1):S11-S34.

52. Dreyfuss P, Stout A, Aprill C, Pollei S, Johnson B, Bogduk N: The significance of multifidus atrophy after successful radiofrequency neurotomy for low back pain. *PM R* 2009;1(8):719-722.

53. Lamer TJ, Smith J, Hoelzer BC, Mauck WD, Qu W, Gazelka HM: Safety of lumbar spine radiofrequency procedures in patients who have posterior spinal hardware. *Pain Med* 2016;17(9):1634-1637.

 Posterior spinal hardware can heat to dangerous levels during RFN. Temperature monitoring with a probe on the hardware surface is recommended. Level of evidence: IV.

54. Kreiner DS, MacVicar J, Duszynski B, Nampiaparampil DE: The mild® procedure: A systematic review of the current literature. *Pain Med* 2014;15(2):196-205.

 The current body of evidence addressing the Minimally Invasive Lumbar Decompression (mild) procedure is of low quality. High-quality studies independent of industry sponsorship are needed.

55. Gerszten PC, Smuck M, Rathmell JP, et al; SPINE Study Group: Plasma disc decompression compared with fluoroscopy-guided transforaminal epidural steroid injections for symptomatic contained lumbar disc herniation: A prospective, randomized, controlled trial. *J Neurosurg Spine* 2010;12(4):357-371.

56. DePalma MJ, Gasper JJ: Cellular supplementation technologies for painful spine disorders. *PM R* 2015;7(4suppl):S19-S25.

 Animal models support biologic therapies for degenerative spine conditions. Clinical trials are beginning to address discogenic low back pain.

Section 4

Surgical Management of Degenerative Spine Disorders

SECTION EDITOR:

Charles A. Reitman, MD

Chapter 15

Cervical Degenerative Disease

Patrick B. Morrissey, MD   Alan S. Hilibrand, MD

Abstract

Cervical degenerative disease, the most common cause of spinal cord impairment worldwide, affects up to 180 of every 100,000 people, and its treatment comprises a large portion of surgical spinal pathology. Cervical degenerative disease encompasses several pathologic processes such as cervical disk derangement (herniated or protruding disks), spondylosis, and ossification of the posterior longitudinal ligament; these processes can result in symptomatic cervical radiculopathy and/or myelopathy. A wide range of treatment options, both surgical and nonsurgical, exists for symptomatic cervical degenerative disorders, depending on the specific compressive pathology. Surgical treatment is typically recommended for patients with myelopathy, and for those with persistent pain or worsening neurologic findings. Cervical fusion, disk arthroplasty, and laminoplasty are all commonly used, effective techniques, each with specific advantages and disadvantages. Complications and sequelae of surgical intervention for cervical degenerative disease are adjacent-segment disease, pseudarthrosis, neurologic injury, postoperative kyphosis, and infection. It is important to understand the epidemiology, pathophysiology, diagnosis, and management of cervical degenerative disease and its complications.

Dr. Hilibrand or an immediate family member has received royalties from Aesculap/B. Braun, Amedica, and Biomet; has stock or stock options held in Amedica, Benvenue Medical, Lifespine, Nexgen, Paradigm Spine, PSD, Spinal Ventures, and Vertiflex; and serves as a board member, owner, officer, or committee member of the American Academy of Orthopaedic Surgeons, the Cervical Spine Research Society, and the North American Spine Society. Neither Dr. Morrissey nor any immediate family member has received anything of value from or has stock or stock options held in a commercial company or institution related directly or indirectly to the subject of this chapter.

Keywords: adjacent-segment disease; anterior cervical diskectomy and fusion; C5 nerve palsy; cervical disk replacement; cervical spondylosis; disk herniation; laminectomy; laminoplasty; myelopathy; ossification of the posterior longitudinal ligament; pseudarthrosis; radiculopathy

Introduction

Patients with degenerative disease of the cervical spine, the most common cause of spinal cord impairment, comprise a large population of surgically treated spine patients, both nationally and internationally. The term cervical degenerative disease encompasses a wide variety of different pathologies. Initial treatment is usually nonsurgical; however, in instances of spinal cord or symptomatic nerve root compression, surgical management may be recommended. Degenerative cervical myelopathy, commonly called cervical spondylotic myelopathy (CSM), has an incidence of 605 per 1 million people and accounts for 4.04 hospitalizations per 100,000 person-years.[1] Cervical radiculopathy is much more common, with incidences that range from 63.5 to 179 per 100,000 person-years; up to 26% of these patients ultimately require surgical intervention.[2,3] It is important to understand the variety of nonsurgical and surgical treatment techniques available to optimize patient outcomes while minimizing patient risks.

Cervical Spondylotic Myelopathy and Cervical Radiculopathy

The pathoanatomy of CSM involves both static and dynamic components. Age-related disk degeneration, associated spondylosis, and hypertrophy of the ligamentum flavum all contribute to static narrowing of the spinal canal and compression of the spinal cord[4] (**Figure 1**). The compressive effect of these anatomic changes can be compounded further by segmental instability secondary to degeneration of the facet joints and degradation

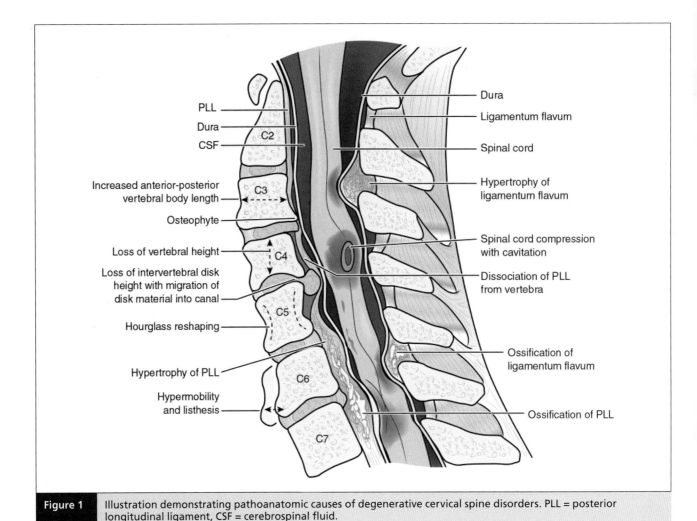

| Figure 1 | Illustration demonstrating pathoanatomic causes of degenerative cervical spine disorders. PLL = posterior longitudinal ligament, CSF = cerebrospinal fluid. |

of the ligamentous stabilizers, particularly the posterior longitudinal ligament (PLL) and ligamentum flavum. Chronic compression can result in cord ischemia and a proinflammatory environment that activates apoptotic pathways and triggers progressive neuronal cell death.[1]

As with its myelopathic counterpart, cervical radiculopathy also involves a substantial degenerative process, although the specific pathoanatomy is slightly different. Degeneration of the intervertebral disks decreases the height of the neuroforamen, and osteophytic formation at both the uncovertebral and zygoapophyseal joints can further decrease space for the exiting nerve roots. This compression results in an ischemic environment that, when coupled with the release of multiple proinflammatory cytokines, can result in sensitization and irritation of the nociceptive fibers within the dorsal root ganglion and, with persistent insult, apoptotic death of these nerve fibers.[2]

Clinical Evaluation

Thorough and accurate clinical evaluation of the patient with degenerative cervical disk disease is paramount in diagnosing these conditions. Initial evaluation should consist of a detailed history, specifically focusing on reports of progressive weakness, problems with fine motor tasks, gait and balance disturbances, and bowel or bladder dysfunction. A complete neurologic examination should be performed, with particular attention given to the presence of upper motor neuron signs including hyperreflexia, the Hoffman sign, the inverted radial reflex, the Babinski reflex, sustained clonus, and gait ataxia because these suggest compressive myelopathy and the need for surgical decompression. In addition, the presence of dermatomal or myotomal neurologic changes should be documented and correlated with relevant radiographic findings.

Radiographic Workup

The radiographic evaluation of degenerative cervical disease must only be used to confirm the findings of the

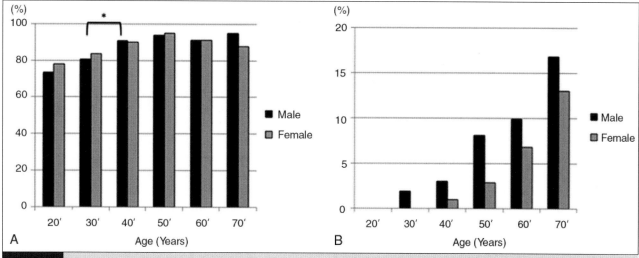

4: Surgical Management of Degenerative Spine Disorders

Figure 2 Graphs demonstrating the age-based incidence of cervical disk bulges (**A**) and spinal cord compression (**B**) seen on magnetic resonance images obtained from asymptomatic control subjects. Asterisk indicates *P* <0.05. (Adapted and reprinted with permission from Nakashima H, Yukawa Y, Suda K, Yamagata M, Ueta T, Kato F: Abnormal findings on magnetic resonance images of the cervical spines in 1211 asymptomatic subjects. *Spine* 2015;40[6]: 392-398.)

history and physical examination because of the relatively high prevalence of radiologic abnormalities among asymptomatic individuals. Workup should include plain radiographs of the cervical spine, with flexion and extension views obtained to evaluate for dynamic instability. Noncontrast MRI assists in the evaluation and quantification of neural compression and is a necessary diagnostic tool. CT myelography can be used in patients who are unable to undergo MRI. CT also can provide additional information when treating patients with ossification of the PLL or the ligamentum flavum, allowing better quantification of these pathologies to assist in both patient counseling and surgical decision making.

Although these studies contribute greatly to the evaluation of a patient, care must be taken during their interpretation. Several studies have highlighted the presence of abnormal imaging in asymptomatic individuals of all ages[5-7] (**Figure 2**). Given the high rate of asymptomatic degenerative findings, all abnormal imaging findings should be interpreted carefully in conjunction with the patient's history and examination when devising an appropriate treatment strategy.

Surgical Intervention

Indications
Of patients with cervical radiculopathy secondary to degenerative disease, more than 70% will respond to nonsurgical treatment modalities including anti-inflammatory medications, physical therapy, and epidural steroid injections. Surgical intervention is reserved for patients who do not improve after 6 to 12 weeks of nonsurgical treatment, those with a progressive neurologic deficit, and those with a persistent functionally limiting static deficit.

Surgical intervention for patients with CSM is much more common, with nonsurgical treatment reserved only for those with extremely mild symptoms and no functional impairment or for those who are medically unsuitable for surgical intervention. Since the 1950s, the natural history of CSM has been recognized as a progressive, stepwise deterioration of neurologic function.[8] Therefore, individuals undergoing nonsurgical treatment should be counseled appropriately regarding signs of disease progression to limit their potential for neurologic morbidity. Surgical intervention should be recommended for most patients with CSM. The urgency of treatment ("soon," but rarely emergent) is based on the severity of symptoms and the rapidity of disease progression; acute declines in neurologic function should be treated sooner.

Many options exist for the treatment of degenerative cervical disease, depending on the symptoms, compressive pathoanatomy, deformity, and other anatomic considerations. It is important to customize the treatment plan for each patient's situation. Different surgical techniques have relative advantages and disadvantages in the treatment of degenerative cervical disorders.

Intraoperative and Perioperative Considerations
In addition to the surgical technique, several perioperative factors can influence patient outcomes. In patients with severe myelopathy, awake fiberoptic intubation

should be considered. The patient should be positioned without excessive neck extension and postpositioning motor-evoked potentials should be considered to minimize positioning-related complications. In addition, the anesthesia team should ensure adequate spinal cord perfusion by maintaining mean arterial pressure higher than 85 mm Hg. Intraoperative neuromonitoring of somatosensory-evoked and motor-evoked potentials is helpful in avoiding intraoperative spinal cord injuries that can occur during distraction and instrumentation of the cervical spine.

Anterior Surgery: Cervical Fusion and Cervical Disk Arthroplasty

Anterior decompression is the cervical spine procedure most commonly performed for the treatment of degenerative cervical radiculopathy and myelopathy. Anterior decompression provides a relatively safe, simple anatomic approach to the cervical spine and has a high likelihood of relieving radicular complaints and preventing myelopathic symptom progression. Currently, two primary variations exist for anterior surgery: the more traditional anterior cervical diskectomy and fusion (ACDF) and the newer, motion-sparing option of anterior cervical total disk arthroplasty (TDA).

A Cochrane review compared outcomes of ACDF versus TDA for single-level radiculopathy, myelopathy, or both and found statistically but not clinically significant differences in favor of TDA.[9] The review analyzed data from nine randomized controlled trials with follow-up intervals of up to 2 years. Arthroplasty resulted in a significant reduction in both arm and neck pain according to visual analog scale (VAS) scores and improvements in both neck function (Neck Disability Index [NDI]) and global function (Medical Outcomes Study 36-Item Short Form [SF-36]). However, despite these statistically significant differences, no outcome was clinically significant, suggesting overall equivalency between the two procedures in short- and midterm follow-up. A long-term randomized controlled trial with 7-year follow-up further demonstrated equivalency between ACDF and TDA with no significant differences in improvement of NDI, SF-36, and VAS scores for both the arm and neck. However, there was a significant difference in the need for secondary surgery; revision surgery rates were 18% in the ACDF group and 7% in the TDA group.[10] Ultimately, regarding single-level cervical degenerative disease, both ACDF and TDA provide excellent clinical results with good longevity. Although TDA may demonstrate some superior outcomes, it is not suitable for all patients with degenerative cervical disk disease. Some relative contraindications to TDA in this population include degenerative instability, osteoporosis, loss of more than 50% of disk height, and facet arthropathy.

For patients with multilevel cervical degenerative disease, a few additional options exist for treatment. For two-level disease, surgeons have suggested two-level ACDF, corpectomy and fusion, two-level TDA, and hybrid constructs (ACDF at one level and TDA at another).

Regarding anterior fusion surgery, multilevel ACDF and corpectomy are two effective treatment options (**Figure 3**), each with its own advantages. Multilevel ACDF has potentially reduced blood loss, better ability to restore sagittal alignment, and the opportunity for segmental fixation in the middle vertebral body. Corpectomy allows decompression behind the vertebral body and fewer graft-host interfaces at risk for pseudarthrosis. A systematic review compiled the results of 10 studies that compared multilevel ACDF, multilevel corpectomy, and ACDF-corpectomy hybrid procedures performed for CSM and found that all procedures offered significant improvements in clinical outcomes (VAS neck, VAS arm, NDI, and Japanese Orthopaedic Association [JOA] scores).[11] However, evidence supported superior improvements with multilevel ACDF compared with both multilevel corpectomy and ACDF-corpectomy hybrid. Multilevel ACDF also allowed better restoration of sagittal alignment. The results of this review suggest that when patient pathology allows a choice in anterior fusion technique, multilevel ACDF is likely the best option.

With respect to two-level fusion versus two-level TDA, 4-year follow-up data from an FDA-approved prospective clinical trial was recently published with results that favor TDA.[12] Both cohorts demonstrated significant improvements in symptoms postoperatively and had similar safety profiles. However, the TDA group had significantly greater improvements in NDI, SF-12 physical component summary scores, and patient satisfaction. Revision surgery rates at the index levels were significantly lower in the TDA group (4.0%) compared with the fusion group (15.2%); the most common reason for reoperation in the fusion group was symptomatic pseudarthrosis. The presence of radiographic adjacent-segment disease was significantly higher in the fusion group, but the reoperation rates secondary to these radiographic findings were not reported. Overall, these data suggest the potential clinical superiority of two-level TDA compared with anterior fusion at medium-term follow-up.

The final option for anterior surgery in multilevel CSM is a hybrid procedure in which one level is treated with ACDF and the other with TDA. This concept was examined from both biomechanical and clinical perspectives in a systematic review.[13] From a biomechanical aspect, hybrid procedures had the capability to maintain the

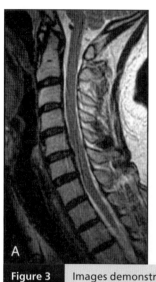
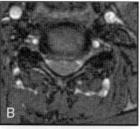
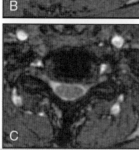
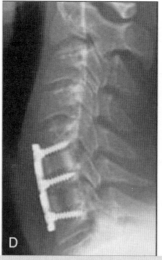
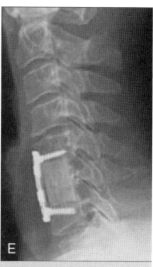

Figure 3 Images demonstrating anterior surgical options for multilevel cervical spondylotic myelopathy. Preoperative sagittal (**A**) and axial (**B** and **C**) magnetic resonance images show compressive pathology at C5-6 and C6-7. The postoperative lateral radiographs demonstrate two different treatment approaches: a two-level diskectomy and fusion (**D**) or a C6 corpectomy and fusion (**E**).

combined motion of the surgical levels; therefore, it had no adverse effects on spinal kinematics, intradiscal pressure of adjacent segments, or facet joint force. From a clinical aspect, hybrid surgery demonstrated equivalent significantly improved outcomes in NDI, VAS neck, and VAS arm scores, except for one study that demonstrated better recovery in NDI and VAS neck scores for two-level hybrid surgery compared with two-level ACDF. These results suggest a potential role for hybrid surgery in the management of multilevel CSM; however, no definitive conclusions can be made without further prospective studies.

Posterior Surgery: Decompression With Fusion and Laminoplasty

Posterior approaches are typically chosen for multilevel CSM in patients with neutral or maintained cervical lordosis. Specific indications for the use of posteriorly based procedures can include the presence of posterior compressive pathology or concern regarding the safety or feasibility of an anterior approach. Posterior surgery allows for direct decompression through the expansion or removal of the posterior elements, and an indirect decompressive effect by allowing the spinal cord to float away from any anterior pathology. Historically, multiple cervical laminectomies have a high incidence of postoperative kyphosis, cervical instability, and subsequent neurologic deterioration. As a result, cervical laminectomy has been replaced by either motion-preserving laminoplasty or posterior cervical laminectomy and fusion (**Figure 4**).

Decompressive laminoplasty relieves spinal cord compression by elevating the posterior spinal elements en bloc while preserving the posterior tension band and providing an anatomic restraint against postoperative deformity. The results of laminoplasty for CSM have been good in the mid to long term. A study with more than 20 years of patient follow-up indicated that JOA and neurologic recovery scores were maintained at 10 years, but demonstrated a decline in these measures at the most recent evaluation. However, these declines often were a result of other unrelated spinal and nonspinal pathology; therefore, laminoplasty is supported as a viable and long-lasting treatment for CSM.[14]

Compared with laminoplasty, posterior cervical decompression and fusion performed for CSM removes the static components of compression by means of a traditional laminectomy and eliminates the dynamic component of the disease, lessening the risk of postoperative kyphosis, halting spondylotic progression, and decreasing further neurologic insult secondary to pathologic motion.

Skip laminectomy is another posteriorly based technique that is not widely used.[15] This procedure was initially developed as a less invasive alternative to laminoplasty and is based on the premise of preserving the posterior tension band through maintenance of the semispinalis and multifidus attachments to each spinous process. In this technique, every other lamina is removed after the associated spinous process is longitudinally divided and removed from the lamina at the spinolaminar junction. After decompression is complete, the split processes are then reapproximated, restoring the posterior soft-tissue

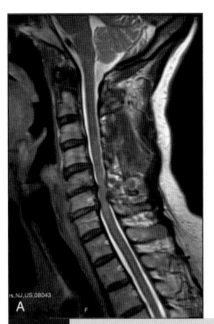 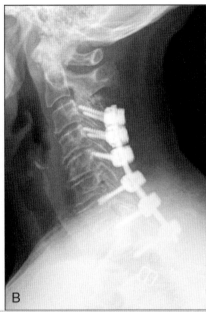 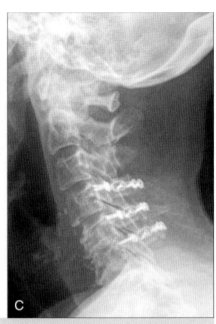

Figure 4 Images demonstrating posterior surgical options for multilevel cervical spondylotic myelopathy. The preoperative magnetic resonance image (**A**) shows compressive cervical degenerative disease at multiple levels. Note the preservation of cervical lordosis. The postoperative lateral radiographs demonstrate two different treatment approaches: a posterior cervical decompression and fusion (**B**) or cervical laminoplasty (**C**).

restraint. A literature review of alternative treatment options for CSM compared skip laminectomy with traditional laminoplasty and showed no difference in clinical outcomes of JOA, VAS neck, or SF-12 scores. However, radiographic range of motion was better preserved in the skip laminectomy group compared with traditional laminoplasty, which suggests a possible benefit.[16] Overall, definitive evidence is lacking to recommend for or against skip laminectomy as a laminoplasty alternative.

When comparing posterior surgical options, a systematic literature review found that both laminoplasty and combined laminectomy and fusion are equally efficacious in the treatment of CSM.[17] The review involved four retrospective cohort studies and demonstrated no definitive differences in neurologic outcomes, neck pain scores, and postoperative kyphosis. Recent data from the AOSpine North America and International study groups corroborated these findings in a prospective multicenter study group and demonstrated no difference between laminoplasty and combined laminectomy and fusion in NDI scores, SF-36 scores, Nurick grades, modified JOA scores, and complication rates.[18] Given these data, no recommendation can be made for either procedure over the other in the treatment of CSM.

Anterior Versus Posterior Surgery

With multiple options available to surgically treat CSM and cervical radiculopathy, choosing the appropriate procedure can be difficult. Most discussion regarding surgical tactics has not centered on specific surgical techniques, but rather the surgical approach. A systematic review of eight level III retrospective cohort studies investigated anterior and posterior approaches for the treatment of CSM.[19] No difference in JOA and neck pain scores was noted among cohorts and complication rates were not significantly different. An individualized approach to treatment was recommended based on patient pathoanatomy, preoperative deformity, and focal or diffuse nature of the disease. Data from the AOSpine North America CSM study group agreed with this recommendation after a retrospective review of 264 surgically treated cases of CSM in which the surgeon selected the approach based on patient pathology.[20] The general guiding principles of approach selection were to approach from the side of the pathology (anterior for ventral compression and vice versa), to use anterior procedures only when compression exists at three levels or fewer, and to use an anterior approach if restoration of cervical lordosis is needed. Using these principles, no difference in improvement was demonstrated in NDI, SF-36, and Nurick scores. Notably, significantly more improvement was seen in modified JOA scores in the posterior group, but after accounting for baseline disease characteristics, this difference was no longer significant. Complication rates were similar between patient cohorts.

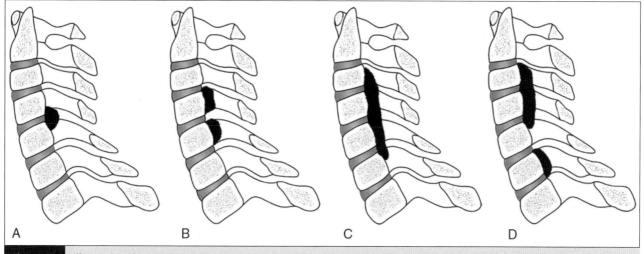

Figure 5 Illustration depicting the common morphologic presentations of ossification of the posterior longitudinal ligament: localized (**A**), segmental (**B**), continuous (**C**), and mixed (**D**). (Reproduced from An HS, Al-Shihabi L, Kurd M: Surgical treatment for ossification of the posterior longitudinal ligament in the cervical spine. *J Am Acad Orthop Surg* 2014;22[7]:420-429.)

Ossification of the Posterior Longitudinal Ligament

Ossification of the PLL is a specific pathologic entity in CSM that requires special consideration when discussing surgical treatment options. Ossification of the PLL is estimated to occur in up to 4.3% of patients with cervical spine disorders in eastern Asian countries and up to 1.7% of patients in North America.[21] The disease process is characterized by degenerative changes within the PLL that ultimately result in replacement of the normal collagen structure with lamellar bone. The disease can be localized, involving one level; segmental, involving several levels in a discontiguous manner; or continuous (**Figure 5**). Most patients present with symptoms in the fifth or sixth decade of life and up to 39% have myelopathy at the time of initial presentation.[21]

Decision making for surgical or nonsurgical treatment is the same as for other patients with degenerative cervical spine disease; prophylactic surgery plays no role in asymptomatic patients. A recent study compared outcomes of surgical intervention for CSM caused by ossification of the PLL with other causes and demonstrated equivalent clinical outcomes, although ossification of the PLL was associated with a higher risk of perioperative complications, specifically, superficial infection, new neck pain, and dural tears.[22] No changes were recommended to surgical decision making other than the technical considerations necessitated by the pathoanatomy of the disease, and decompression was advocated in the same manner as for other more common forms of CSM.

When properly selected, both anterior and posterior approaches are effective in the treatment of CSM secondary to ossification of the PLL. Anterior surgery is most commonly performed for localized disease (fewer than three levels), for patients with symptoms of radiculopathy that predominate over symptoms of myelopathy, and in instances of cervical kyphosis. In addition to restoring lordosis, another advantage to anterior surgical intervention is the ability to directly treat the compressive pathology. The primary disadvantage of anterior surgical intervention in ossification of the PLL is a high rate of dural tears, which can range from 6.7% to 31.8%[22] secondary to adhesions and/or ossification of the dura, which can occur in up to 15% of cases.[21]

Posterior surgical intervention consists of indirect decompression by means of either laminoplasty or combined laminectomy and fusion and typically is recommended for patients with more extensive disease (greater than three levels), for patients with a congenitally stenotic canal, and for patients with preserved cervical lordosis. To determine if an acceptable amount of cervical lordosis exists for posterior intervention, a kyphosis line (K-line) should be drawn from the center of the C2 canal to the center of the C7 canal. If the K-line passes through the PLL ossification mass, posterior surgical intervention should be avoided because outcomes were significantly inferior to outcomes in patients in whom the K-line passed posterior to the compressive pathology[23] (**Figure 6**).

Combined anterior-posterior approaches are another option for the treatment of ossification of the PLL, specifically in instances of multilevel disease in the setting of cervical kyphosis. A limited anterior procedure can help restore cervical lordosis, which allows the multilevel posterior procedure to indirectly decompress the neural elements (**Figure 7**). This approach avoids the problems

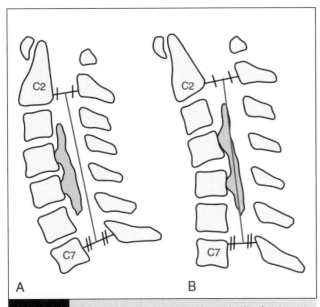

Figure 6 Illustrations demonstrate how the kyphosis line (K-line; blue line) can help predict the effectiveness of posterior surgical decompression in patients with cervical spondylotic myelopathy secondary to ossification of the posterior longitudinal ligament by determining if enough lordosis exists to allow the spinal cord to float away from the posterior longitudinal ligament mass. **A,** If the K-line passes posterior to the ossification mass, the patient is a good candidate for posterior surgical intervention. **B,** If the K-line passes through the posterior longitudinal ligament ossification mass, surgical intervention should be avoided.

excellent outcomes were more common in patients with a greater degree of cervical lordosis.[25]

Complications of Surgical Intervention

The literature on surgical decompression for CSM has repeatedly shown significantly more favorable patient functional outcomes in surgical cohorts compared with their nonsurgical counterparts. Given the high incidence of disease progression and neurologic decline, the consensus for surgical treatment is almost universal. However, some risks need to be considered, especially in the patient with myelopathy. A recent retrospective review of the American College of Surgeons National Surgical Quality Improvement Program database showed that patients with myelopathy undergoing ACDF had a ninefold greater likelihood of mortality, were 1.8 times more likely to experience a severe adverse event, and were 1.5 times more likely to experience any adverse event than patients without myelopathy.[26] A recent multicenter prospective study by the AOSpine North America group reported an overall rate of 18.7% for postoperative adverse events; the three most commonly reported were dysphagia (3.6%), superficial infection (2.9%), and cardiopulmonary events (2.5%).[27]

Intraoperative Complications

Several complications are associated with surgical decompression for CSM, ranging from dental injury during intubation to intraoperative spinal cord injury. The exact rates of these complications are difficult to determine, given the differences in reporting practices, although a 2015 study meticulously collected adverse event data for a cohort of 104 patients with CSM who underwent decompression using various surgical approaches.[28] An intraoperative adverse event rate of 13.5% was reported, the most common of which was intraoperative hardware-related issues: 4.9% of patients required revision surgery for either malposition or bone-implant interface failure. Other reported complications include spinal cord injury (1.0%) and dural tear (1.9%).

Other commonly cited intraoperative complications include vascular injury involving the vertebral or carotid arteries, tracheoesophageal injury, recurrent laryngeal nerve injury, and injury to the cervical sympathetic nerves with resultant Horner syndrome. The specific mechanisms of and management strategies for these complications are beyond the scope of this chapter; however, management of recurrent laryngeal nerve injury warrants attention. It is not uncommon to encounter a patient who has undergone prior cervical surgery, either for a previous spinal intervention or for a thyroid, a throat, or

associated with extensive anterior dissection and maximizes the efficacy of the posterior decompression by correcting the sagittal deformity. Posterior fixation also can be useful as a salvage surgery in cases of pseudarthrosis resultant from a prior anterior procedure.

Outcome differences in approach have been highlighted in several clinical studies. One study evaluated 5-year outcomes of patients with CSM secondary to ossification of the PLL treated with either ACDF or laminoplasty.[24] The preoperative cervical alignment and the degree of canal compromise were important considerations. In patients with more than 50% canal compromise from ossification of the PLL, ACDF resulted in significantly superior neurologic outcomes compared with laminoplasty. Regarding alignment, patients with preoperative kyphosis demonstrated a significantly higher neurologic recovery rate in the ACDF group than did those in the laminoplasty group. A retrospective study of patients with ossification of the PLL occupying greater than 60% of the canal had significantly better outcomes when treated with ACDF. In addition, in patients treated with laminoplasty, good or

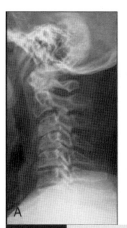
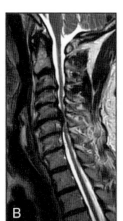
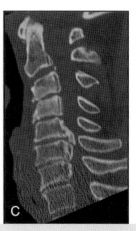
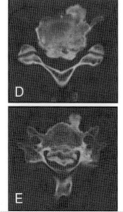
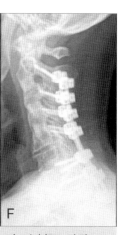

Figure 7 Preoperative lateral radiograph (**A**), sagittal magnetic resonance image (**B**), and sagittal (**C**) and axial (**D** and **E**) CT scans obtained from a patient with severe cervical spondylotic myelopathy in the setting of ossification of the posterior longitudinal ligament. Given the kyphotic alignment of the cervical spine, an isolated posterior approach is not suitable. This patient underwent a combined anterior-posterior procedure using a multilevel anterior cervical diskectomy and fusion to restore cervical lordosis followed by a posterior cervical decompression and fusion for indirect decompression of the spinal cord. The postoperative lateral radiograph (**F**) demonstrates a solid fusion with correction of preoperative kyphosis.

a vascular disorder. In these patients, the possibility of previous recurrent laryngeal nerve injury exists, and preoperative laryngoscopic evaluation should be performed to determine the status of vocal cord function. If evidence of dysfunction exists, the surgical approach must be performed on the side of the deficit to avoid the risk of bilateral vocal cord paralysis, despite the difficulties associated with revision surgery.

Postoperative Complications

In contrast to intraoperative complications, the incidence of postoperative and late adverse events in the surgical treatment of CSM is much better defined in the literature. In a recent study,[28] postoperative or late complications occurred in 37.5% of patients. During the 3-year study period, the most common complications were persistent dysphagia (13.5%) and postoperative neuropathic pain (7.7%). Other complications included neurologic deterioration (4.8%) and wound problems (3.9%).

Revision surgery rates in surgically treated CSM have recently been reported at 3.3% across all approaches at follow-up greater than 4 years; the revision surgery rate was 2.5% for anterior procedures, 7.9% for posterior laminoplasty, and 12.5% for posterior laminectomy and fusion. In addition to differences seen on the basis of approach, male sex, diabetes, and associated comorbidities were significantly associated with a higher rate of revision surgery.[29] Increased age and diabetes were associated with an increased risk for adverse events. Surgical risk factors identified as predictive of perioperative complications included longer surgical time and performing a two-stage anterior-posterior procedure, although

these were considered indicators of increased case complexity and therefore associated with many confounding variables. The authors were unable to comment on the differences between anterior and posterior approaches, with the exception of noting more axial neck pain in laminoplasty versus ACDF.[30]

Adjacent-Segment Disease

Perhaps the most discussed and debated late complication after surgery for cervical degenerative disease is the development of adjacent-segment disease. Adjacent-segment disease is defined as the development of radicular or myelopathic symptoms as a result of degenerative changes adjacent to a previously decompressed level. This differs from adjacent-segment degeneration, which is simply radiographic change in the absence of new symptoms.[31] This differentiation is clinically important because the incidence of radiographic degeneration has been reported as high as 92% at follow-up greater than 5 years; however, in that study, only 6.1% of patients required reoperation secondary to their disease.[32]

In the classic natural history study, the rate of adjacent-segment disease after ACDF was found to be relatively constant at 2.9% per year over the first 10 years following surgery (**Figure 8**); two-thirds of these patients ultimately required revision surgery.[31] A more recent retrospective review of 672 patients treated with ACDF demonstrated a revision rate of 7% for adjacent-segment disease at an average follow-up of 34 months;[33] the index procedures for these revisions included single-level fusion (43%), two-level fusion (53%), and three-level fusion (2%). For patients who have undergone initial revision surgery for adjacent-segment disease, the likelihood of a second revision surgery is significantly higher than after the initial procedure (27% versus 12.2%) and the time between second and third revision surgery is significantly shorter than the time between the index procedure and the first revision surgery (30 versus 47 months).[34]

Prevention of adjacent-segment disease is another controversy, particularly relative to ACDF versus cervical TDA and whether motion preservation of TDA results in lower rates of adjacent-segment disease. A meta-analysis of six prospective, randomized controlled trials found no significant difference in rates of reoperation at 2.5 years for adjacent-segment disease following ACDF (6.9%) compared with TDA (5.1%). The annual rate of revision for adjacent-segment disease was 2.4% in ACDF and 1.1% in TDA.[35]

Pseudarthrosis

An absence of solid fusion at sites of decompression can predispose patients to continued or worsening symptoms and the need for revision surgical procedures. Revision can consist of a repeat of the index procedure with revision instrumentation, use of a different graft material (such as autograft), or augmentation by means of a different approach (the addition of supplemental anterior or posterior fixation).

Although fusion rates in the cervical spine are historically good, the incidence of pseudarthrosis is significant. A recent evaluation of revision rates for ACDF demonstrated a 7% revision surgery rate for pseudarthrosis. Of these, 18% of patients initially underwent one-level procedures, 80% underwent two-level procedures, and 2% underwent three-level procedures.[33]

Numerous technical and host factors may determine whether fusion will ultimately occur in a patient following an ACDF, but modifiable risk factors such as smoking are given the most attention in the literature. The effect of smoking on single-level ACDF was recently published from a cohort of 573 patients.[36] An overall fusion rate of 91.4% was observed, with a rate of 91.6% in nonsmokers and 91.0% in smokers, with no significant difference. However, in multilevel procedures, smokers have a significantly lower rate of fusion; 81% of nonsmokers achieved stable arthrodesis compared with only 62% of smokers. Further subanalysis demonstrated that this effect was not present in a group of patients undergoing subtotal corpectomy and strut grafting, with equivalent fusion rates between cohorts. This finding suggests that in patients who are unable or unwilling to cease tobacco use, corpectomy may be a superior surgical option when treating multilevel disease.[37]

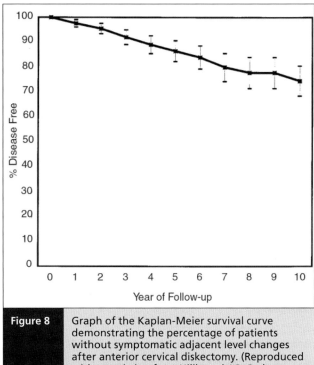

| Figure 8 | Graph of the Kaplan-Meier survival curve demonstrating the percentage of patients without symptomatic adjacent level changes after anterior cervical diskectomy. (Reproduced with permission from Hilibrand AS, Carlson GD, Palumbo MA, Jones PK, Bohlman HH: Radiculopathy and myelopathy at segments adjacent to the site of a previous anterior cervical arthrodesis. *J Bone Joint Surg Am* 1999;81[4]:519-528.) |

Alignment and Balance

When considering an anterior versus posterior surgical approach, it is important to include cervical sagittal balance in treatment decision making. In particular, cervical kyphosis places the cervical spinal cord at risk by increasing intramedullary pressure and decreasing cervical blood flow, which amplifies the effects of other compressive pathologies and accelerates neuronal loss.[38]

The influence of postoperative cervical alignment on surgical outcomes is not yet completely clear, perhaps secondary to the difficulty in determining what portion of the treatment effect results from restoration of alignment versus decompression. However, a study initially designed to investigate outcome differences between lordotic and parallel interbody grafts in ACDF found that, although graft morphology did not influence clinical outcome, maintenance of or improvement in segmental sagittal alignment resulted in significantly greater improvements in SF-36 physical component summary and NDI scores.[39] This finding highlights the importance of sagittal alignment and balance in the surgical treatment of degenerative cervical disease.

Anterior cervical procedures are best for the restoration of cervical lordosis and reestablishment of cervical sagittal balance in patients with preoperative kyphotic deformity. When posterior procedures are indicated, it is imperative to avoid substantial postoperative kyphotic deformity. A recent study that compared laminoplasty with laminectomy and fusion in the treatment of ossification of the PLL found that, although patients in both groups demonstrated a loss of lordosis over time, patients in the fusion group demonstrated better preservation of lordosis. Patients who underwent fusion also maintained cervical sagittal balance, which suggests that posterior cervical fusion best helps to avoid significant problems in patients at risk for postoperative sagittal malalignment.[40] In contrast, a retrospective radiographic review of a new laminoplasty technique among patients with 33-month follow-up demonstrated a 1.8° increase in lordosis, which suggests that changes in technique may allow better preservation of cervical alignment.[41]

Predicting which patients with preserved cervical lordosis are at risk for postoperative kyphosis can be difficult. One study investigated the preoperative risk factors for kyphosis after laminoplasty in 174 patients and determined that patients with significant sagittal imbalance (defined as a cervical sagittal vertical axis of greater than 42 mm) and those older than 75 years were at greater risk for the development of kyphotic deformity despite preserved preoperative lordosis.[42] The overall rate of postoperative kyphosis was 5.2%.

Cervical Nerve Root Palsy

Cervical nerve root palsy is another complication encountered in the surgical treatment of the degenerative cervical spine. This complication is encountered in both posteriorly and anteriorly based procedures. The most widely accepted mechanism of injury is stretch placed on the anatomically shorter C5 nerve root as the spinal cord moves following decompression; however, foraminal stenosis, root ischemia, and reperfusion injury also can play a role.[43] Cervical nerve root palsy manifests as clinical weakness in the deltoid muscles and occasionally the biceps brachii. The incidence of C5 palsy in CSM is 5.8% in ACDF,[44] 5.3% in laminoplasty,[45] and as high as 10.6% in laminectomy and fusion. Neurologic involvement is unilateral in 92% of patients. Proposed surgical risk factors for C5 nerve palsy include a wider laminectomy trough, increased posterior cord drift, wide asymmetric anterior decompression, and stretch injury secondary to substantial restoration of lordosis.

A 2014 study demonstrated that patients with a postoperative C5 palsy had significantly wider C5 laminectomy troughs (17.9 versus 15.2 mm) than their counterparts without C5 palsy, and they also had significantly more posterior spinal cord drift at the C3 through

C6 levels.[46] These results were recently challenged by a 2016 retrospective review that demonstrated no difference between laminectomy widths at C5 when comparing cohorts with and without palsy.[47]

With anterior surgery, wide and asymmetric decompression, as well as substantial restoration of cervical lordosis, has been shown to result in a higher incidence of C5 nerve palsy. A 2013 retrospective review showed that decompressions greater than 15 mm and those that have a substantial side-to-side difference significantly increased the risk of patients for the development of nerve palsy, resulting in the recommendation of smaller, more symmetric decompressions in CSM.[48] Another retrospective review examined restoration of cervical lordosis as a risk factor for C5 palsy and showed that the nerve palsy cohort had a significantly larger increase in lordosis. The study authors hypothesized that this injury is likely a result of increased tension on the cord coupled with iatrogenic foraminal stenosis.[44] Potential strategies for mitigating these problems include avoiding overdistraction and overcorrection at the intervertebral space and performing a prophylactic foraminotomy during decompression.

With respect to foraminal stenosis and C5 nerve palsy, a retrospective study of laminoplasty patients identified a significantly smaller foraminal diameter for those in the palsy group compared with those without palsy (1.99 versus 2.76 mm).[45] No conclusions were made regarding the role of prophylactic foraminotomy based on these data alone; however, another study investigated its effect by prospectively reviewing the results of patients treated with laminoplasty and bilateral prophylactic C4/C5 foraminotomy.[49] Of 141 consecutive patients, the rate of C5 palsy was 1.4%, which was significantly improved from the 6.4% rate of nerve palsy in a historical control group without foraminotomies. These results suggest that foraminal stenosis plays an important role in the pathology of postoperative C5 nerve palsy and should be considered in surgical planning.

Despite the significant functional morbidity associated with this neurologic deficit, most patients recover with observation and nonsurgical treatment measures: 71% of severe cases (manual muscle strength, 2 or less) and 96% of mild cases (manual muscle strength, 3 to 4) have demonstrated functional recovery without the need for further intervention.[44]

Postoperative Infection

Infection rates after spinal fusion surgery range from 2% to 13%,[50] which is a substantial problem for the patient and the treating surgeon. In the cervical spine, significant differences in the risk of infection exist between approaches; posterior procedures have a much higher incidence of infection. In addition to standard measures to help control perioperative infection, surgeons have investigated additional means to reduce the rate of post-operative infection. Two specific interventions are the use of topical vancomycin powder and surgical drains.

Vancomycin powder is a low-cost intervention that provides a high concentration of local antibiotic with coverage of methicillin-resistant *Staphylococcus aureus* when applied directly to the surgical wound bed. There is evidence supporting its clinical efficacy in cervical spine surgery, with a retrospective cohort study of patients undergoing posterior cervical fusion demonstrating a significant decrease in surgical site infection (from 10.9% to 2.5%) with the addition of 1 g of vancomycin powder to the wound bed.[50] In another study, a retrospective review of infection rates reported a reduction in wound infection rates from 1.83% to zero following the implementation of a protocol utilizing suprafascial drains in obese patients and routine application of 500 mg of vancomycin powder in all patients.[51]

Summary

Cervical degenerative disease comprises a wide range of compressive pathologies that can result in substantial patient morbidity and even mortality. Surgical decompression is an effective treatment and indicated in cases of neurologic impairment. Surgical strategy varies widely based on pathoanatomy, and the choice of a specific approach and technique should be determined based on the number of levels involved, predominant symptoms (radiculopathy versus myelopathy), and sagittal alignment. Complications include adjacent-segment disease, pseudarthrosis, neurologic injury, postoperative deformity, and infection. Despite the complexity of this problem and the numerous different treatment options, careful attention to patient symptoms, specific pathology, and surgical strategy will result in an optimal outcome for affected individuals.

Key Study Points

- Cervical radiculopathy is often a self-limited process for which almost three-fourths of patients can be treated nonsurgically.
- CSM is a progressive neurologic disorder with substantial morbidity and possible mortality if untreated. Surgical decompression effectively preserves neurologic function and is indicated in most patients who are able to undergo surgery.
- For patients with cervical kyphosis, posteriorly based procedures performed with and without fusion have inferior results compared with anterior approaches. If the pathology necessitates a posterior approach in a patient with kyphosis, a combined anterior-posterior procedure should be considered.
- Postoperative adjacent-segment disease commonly develops at a rate of approximately 2.9% per year. Currently, no identifiable differences exist between adjacent segment revision rates in ACDF versus TDA.
- C5 nerve palsy can occur in 4% to 10% of patients undergoing surgical intervention for CSM. Proposed prevention strategies include limited laminectomy width, avoidance of aggressive restoration of cervical height and lordosis, and prophylactic foraminotomy.

Annotated References

1. Nouri A, Tetreault L, Singh A, Karadimas SK, Fehlings MG: Degenerative cervical myelopathy: Epidemiology, genetics, and pathogenesis. *Spine (Phila Pa 1976)* 2015;40(12):E675-E693.

   This comprehensive review reports on the different manifestations of degenerative cervical myelopathy including the epidemiology, pathoanatomy, and genetics of the disease. Level of evidence: V.

2. Woods BI, Hilibrand AS: Cervical radiculopathy: Epidemiology, etiology, diagnosis, and treatment. *J Spinal Disord Tech* 2015;28(5):E251-E259.

   This comprehensive review of cervical radiculopathy includes epidemiology, pathoanatomy, diagnostic workup, and treatment options. In this study, 75% to 90% of patients experienced resolution of symptoms with nonsurgical treatments including immobilization, anti-inflammatory medications, physical therapy, and epidural steroid injections.

3. Wong JJ, Côté P, Quesnele JJ, Stern PJ, Mior SA: The course and prognostic factors of symptomatic cervical

disc herniation with radiculopathy: A systematic review of the literature. *Spine J* 2014;14(8):1781-1789.

This systematic review discusses the course and prognosis of cervical radiculopathy secondary to cervical disk herniation. Symptomatic improvements were noted in 4 to 6 months; 83% of patients recovered in 24 to 36 months. Workers' compensation patients had a poorer prognosis for recovery.

4. Fehlings MG, Tetreault LA, Wilson JR, Skelly AC: Cervical spondylotic myelopathy: Current state of the art and future directions. *Spine (Phila Pa 1976)* 2013;38(22suppl 1):S1-S8.

This narrative overview of 15 current publications on CSM summarizes the clinical questions and evidence-based treatment recommendations. The importance of early identification of CSM and the rapid establishment of an appropriate treatment course was stressed.

5. Boden SD, McCowin PR, Davis DO, Dina TS, Mark AS, Wiesel S: Abnormal magnetic-resonance scans of the cervical spine in asymptomatic subjects: A prospective investigation. *J Bone Joint Surg Am* 1990;72(8):1178-1184.

6. Matsumoto M, Fujimura Y, Suzuki N, et al: MRI of cervical intervertebral discs in asymptomatic subjects. *J Bone Joint Surg Br* 1998;80(1):19-24.

7. Nakashima H, Yukawa Y, Suda K, Yamagata M, Ueta T, Kato F: Abnormal findings on magnetic resonance images of the cervical spines in 1211 asymptomatic subjects. *Spine (Phila Pa 1976)* 2015;40(6):392-398.

This cross-sectional population study reported on cervical spine MRI findings in 1,211 subjects without clinical evidence of cervical disease; 87.6% demonstrated radiographic findings of degenerative disease. All findings increased significantly with patient age. Level of evidence: II.

8. Clarke E, Robinson PK: Cervical myelopathy: A complication of cervical spondylosis. *Brain* 1956;79(3):483-510.

9. Boselie TF, Willems PC, van Mameren H, de Bie RA, Benzel EC, van Santbrink H: Arthroplasty versus fusion in single-level cervical degenerative disc disease: A Cochrane review. *Spine (Phila Pa 1976)* 2013;38(17):E1096-E1107.

This systematic review of nine randomized controlled trials compared TDA with fusion in the treatment of degenerative cervical disorders. Significant differences existed in favor of arthroplasty for arm pain, neck pain, and functional status; none were clinically significant. Level of evidence: I.

10. Janssen ME, Zigler JE, Spivak JM, Delamarter RB, Darden BV II, Kopjar B: ProDisc-C total disc replacement versus anterior cervical discectomy and fusion for single-level symptomatic cervical disc disease: Seven-year follow-up of the prospective randomized U.S. Food and Drug Administration investigational device exemption study. *J Bone Joint Surg Am* 2015;97(21):1738-1747.

This 7-year multicenter randomized controlled trial compared TDA with ACDF. Equivalency was found in neck pain, arm pain, functional status, and adverse events. Patients who underwent TDA were less likely to undergo secondary surgery compared with patients who underwent ACDF. Level of evidence: I.

11. Shamji MF, Massicotte EM, Traynelis VC, Norvell DC, Hermsmeyer JT, Fehlings MG: Comparison of anterior surgical options for the treatment of multilevel cervical spondylotic myelopathy: A systematic review. *Spine (Phila Pa 1976)* 2013;38(22suppl 1):S195-S209.

This systematic review of 10 studies compared diskectomy, corpectomy, and hybrid options for the treatment of multilevel CSM. Multiple diskectomies result in superior clinical outcomes and correction of sagittal alignment, and are preferred when possible.

12. Davis RJ, Nunley PD, Kim KD, et al: Two-level total disc replacement with Mobi-C cervical artificial disc versus anterior discectomy and fusion: A prospective, randomized, controlled multicenter clinical trial with 4-year follow-up results. *J Neurosurg Spine* 2015;22(1):15-25.

This 4-year follow-up of a prospective randomized study compared two-level TDA with ACDF. Significantly greater improvements were noted in NDI, SF-12 physical component summary, and patient satisfaction scores for the TDA group. Revision surgery was performed less commonly after TDA. Level of evidence: I.

13. Jia Z, Mo Z, Ding F, He Q, Fan Y, Ruan D: Hybrid surgery for multilevel cervical degenerative disc diseases: A systematic review of biomechanical and clinical evidence. *Eur Spine J* 2014;23(8):1619-1632.

This systematic review of biomechanical and clinical studies investigated hybrid surgery in the treatment of degenerative cervical pathology. Biomechanical data support preservation of segment motion with reduced effect on adjacent levels. Clinical studies support significant improvements in functional outcome scores.

14. Kawaguchi Y, Nakano M, Yasuda T, et al: More than 20 years follow-up after en bloc cervical laminoplasty. *Spine (Phila Pa 1976)* 2016;41(20):1570-1579.

This retrospective review reported on long-term clinical outcomes in patients treated with laminoplasty for cervical degenerative disease. JOA scores and neurologic recovery rates improved postoperatively and were maintained at 10-year follow-up, but subsequently deteriorated as spinal degeneration progressed. Level of evidence: IV.

15. Shiraishi T, Fukuda K, Yato Y, Nakamura M, Ikegami T: Results of skip laminectomy-minimum 2-year follow-up study compared with open-door laminoplasty. *Spine (Phila Pa 1976)* 2003;28(24):2667-2672.

16. Traynelis VC, Arnold PM, Fourney DR, Bransford RJ, Fischer DJ, Skelly AC: Alternative procedures for the treatment of cervical spondylotic myelopathy: Arthroplasty, oblique corpectomy, skip laminectomy: evaluation

of comparative effectiveness and safety. *Spine (Phila Pa 1976)* 2013;38(22suppl 1):S210-S231.

In this systematic review of alternative treatment options for CSM, insufficient evidence exists to preferentially recommend TDA over ACDF or skip laminectomy over open-door laminoplasty. Oblique corpectomy is not recommended as a first-line treatment, given its high morbidity.

17. Yoon ST, Hashimoto RE, Raich A, Shaffrey CI, Rhee JM, Riew KD: Outcomes after laminoplasty compared with laminectomy and fusion in patients with cervical myelopathy: A systematic review. *Spine (Phila Pa 1976)* 2013;38(22suppl 1):S183-S194.

This systematic review of four retrospective cohort studies compared laminectomy and fusion with laminoplasty in the treatment of CSM. Both procedures were equally efficacious regarding neurologic outcomes, pain, and complication rates. Level of evidence: III.

18. Fehlings MG, Santaguida C, Tetreault L, et al: Laminectomy and fusion versus laminoplasty for the treatment of degenerative cervical myelopathy: Results from the AOSpine North America and International prospective multicenter studies. *Spine J* 2017;17(1):102-108

This international multicenter prospective cohort study compared results of laminoplasty with laminectomy and fusion in the treatment of CSM. Both procedures significantly improved modified JOA, NDI, and SF-36 scores with no difference in degree of improvement. Complication rates were equivalent. Level of evidence: II.

19. Lawrence BD, Jacobs WB, Norvell DC, Hermsmeyer JT, Chapman JR, Brodke DS: Anterior versus posterior approach for treatment of cervical spondylotic myelopathy: A systematic review. *Spine (Phila Pa 1976)* 2013;38(22suppl 1):S173-S182.

This systematic review compared anterior and posterior surgical intervention in multilevel CSM. Improvements in JOA scores were equivalent and postoperative C5 palsy rates were similar. Anterior surgery resulted in fewer infections and posterior surgery resulted in a lower rate of dysphagia. Level of evidence: III.

20. Fehlings MG, Barry S, Kopjar B, et al: Anterior versus posterior surgical approaches to treat cervical spondylotic myelopathy: Outcomes of the prospective multicenter AOSpine North America CSM study in 264 patients. *Spine (Phila Pa 1976)* 2013;38(26):2247-2252.

This prospective observational cohort study compared anterior and posterior approaches for CSM. Improvement in modified JOA scores was lower in the anterior group, although baseline impairment was less. Improvements in Nurick Scale, NDI, and SF-36 scores showed no difference between groups. Level of evidence: III.

21. An HS, Al-Shihabi L, Kurd M: Surgical treatment for ossification of the posterior longitudinal ligament in the cervical spine. *J Am Acad Orthop Surg* 2014;22(7):420-429.

This comprehensive review reported on the epidemiology, pathoanatomy, natural history, and treatment options for ossification of the PLL.

22. Nakashima H, Tetreault L, Nagoshi N, et al: Comparison of outcomes of surgical treatment for ossification of the posterior longitudinal ligament versus other forms of degenerative cervical myelopathy: Results from the prospective, multicenter AOSpine CSM-international study of 479 patients. *J Bone Joint Surg Am* 2016;98(5):370-378.

This prospective cohort study compared treatment outcomes in CSM patients with and without ossification of the PLL. No differences were found in improvements of modified JOA, Nurick scale, NDI, and SF-36 scores. A higher complication rate was reported in the group with ossification of the PLL. Level of evidence: II.

23. Fujiyoshi T, Yamazaki M, Kawabe J, et al: A new concept for making decisions regarding the surgical approach for cervical ossification of the posterior longitudinal ligament: The K-line. *Spine (Phila Pa 1976)* 2008;33(26):E990-E993.

24. Sakai K, Okawa A, Takahashi M, et al: Five-year follow-up evaluation of surgical treatment for cervical myelopathy caused by ossification of the posterior longitudinal ligament: A prospective comparative study of anterior decompression and fusion with floating method versus laminoplasty. *Spine (Phila Pa 1976)* 2012;37(5):367-376.

This prospective cohort study compared ACDF with laminoplasty when treating CSM caused by ossification of the PLL. At 5-year follow-up, anterior surgery had superior results when the ossification of the PLL mass occupied more than 50% of the canal or the patient had preoperative kyphotic alignment. Level of evidence: II.

25. Fujimori T, Iwasaki M, Okuda S, et al: Long-term results of cervical myelopathy due to ossification of the posterior longitudinal ligament with an occupying ratio of 60% or more. *Spine (Phila Pa 1976)* 2014;39(1):58-67.

This retrospective review compared ACDF with laminoplasty for CSM resulting from ossification of the PLL. ACDF had significantly higher recovery rates when the ossification of the PLL lesion occupied more than 60% of the spinal canal. In the posterior group, there was a significant association between increasing cervical lordosis and good or excellent outcomes. Level of evidence: III.

26. Lukasiewicz AM, Basques BA, Bohl DD, Webb ML, Samuel AM, Grauer JN: Myelopathy is associated with increased all-cause morbidity and mortality following anterior cervical discectomy and fusion: A study of 5256 patients in American College of Surgeons National Surgical Quality Improvement Program (ACS-NSQIP). *Spine (Phila Pa 1976)* 2015;40(7):443-449.

This retrospective cohort study investigated morbidity and mortality differences in ACDF for patients with and without CSM. For patients with myelopathy, a significant increase was noted in all-cause morbidity and a ninefold increase was noted in the likelihood of mortality. Level of evidence: III.

27. Fehlings MG, Wilson JR, Kopjar B, et al: Efficacy and safety of surgical decompression in patients with cervical spondylotic myelopathy: Results of the AOSpine North America prospective multi-center study. *J Bone Joint Surg Am* 2013;95(18):1651-1658.

This prospective cohort study evaluated the safety and efficacy of surgical decompression for CSM. At 1-year follow-up, modified JOA, Nurick grade, NDI, and SF-36 scores all improved significantly. The overall complication rate was 18.7%, with a 2.2% rate of revision surgery. Level of evidence: II.

28. Hartig D, Batke J, Dea N, Kelly A, Fisher C, Street J: Adverse events in surgically treated cervical spondylopathic myelopathy: A prospective validated observational study. *Spine (Phila Pa 1976)* 2015;40(5):292-298.

This prospective observational study evaluated surgical complications in the treatment of CSM. The adverse event rate was 42.3%. The number of preoperative comorbidities, anterior approach, and number of levels fused were all significantly associated with an increased rate of adverse events. Level of evidence: III.

29. Park MS, Ju Y-S, Moon S-H, et al: Reoperation rates after surgery for degenerative cervical spine disease according to different surgical procedures: National population-based cohort study. *Spine (Phila Pa 1976)* 2016;41(19):1484-1492.

This retrospective cohort study evaluated revision surgery rates following surgery for cervical degenerative disease. The overall revision surgery rate was 3.31%; the rate was higher for posteriorly based procedures. Male sex, diabetes, and the number of comorbidities all significantly increased the rate. Level of evidence: III.

30. Tetreault L, Ibrahim A, Côté P, Singh A, Fehlings MG: A systematic review of clinical and surgical predictors of complications following surgery for degenerative cervical myelopathy. *J Neurosurg Spine* 2016;24(1):77-99.

This systematic review investigated the predictors of surgical complications in CSM treatment. Increased patient age, longer surgical time, and two-stage surgery were associated with an increased complication rate. Body mass index, smoking status, and baseline symptom severity did not increase complications. Level of evidence: III.

31. Hilibrand AS, Carlson GD, Palumbo MA, Jones PK, Bohlman HH: Radiculopathy and myelopathy at segments adjacent to the site of a previous anterior cervical arthrodesis. *J Bone Joint Surg Am* 1999;81(4):519-528.

32. Goffin J, Geusens E, Vantomme N, et al: Long-term follow-up after interbody fusion of the cervical spine. *J Spinal Disord Tech* 2004;17(2):79-85.

33. van Eck CF, Regan C, Donaldson WF, Kang JD, Lee JY: The revision rate and occurrence of adjacent segment disease after anterior cervical discectomy and fusion: A study of 672 consecutive patients. *Spine (Phila Pa 1976)* 2014;39(26):2143-2147.

This retrospective cohort study evaluated the occurrence of adjacent-segment disease in patients undergoing ACDF. The overall revision surgery rate was 15% at 31-month follow-up, with 7% for adjacent-segment disease. The annual incidence of adjacent-segment disease was 4%. Level of evidence: III.

34. Xu R, Bydon M, Macki M, et al: Adjacent segment disease after anterior cervical discectomy and fusion: Clinical outcomes after first repeat surgery versus second repeat surgery. *Spine (Phila Pa 1976)* 2014;39(2):120-126.

This retrospective observational study evaluated adjacent-segment disease following ACDF over a 20-year period; 12.2% of patients required revision surgery for symptomatic adjacent-segment disease after the index procedure. This rate increased to 25% after a second cervical fusion. Level of evidence: III.

35. Verma K, Gandhi SD, Maltenfort M, et al: Rate of adjacent segment disease in cervical disc arthroplasty versus single-level fusion: Meta-analysis of prospective studies. *Spine (Phila Pa 1976)* 2013;38(26):2253-2257.

This meta-analysis of six randomized controlled trials compared rates of adjacent-segment disease in patients who underwent ACDF (6.9%) and TDA (5.1%). The difference was not significant. Level of evidence: I.

36. Luszczyk M, Smith JS, Fischgrund JS, et al: Does smoking have an impact on fusion rate in single-level anterior cervical discectomy and fusion with allograft and rigid plate fixation? Clinical article. *J Neurosurg Spine* 2013;19(5):527-531.

This retrospective cohort study investigated the effect of smoking on fusion rates following single-level ACDF. Fusion rates were equivalent for nonsmokers (91.6%) and smokers (91.0%). Level of evidence: III.

37. Hilibrand AS, Fye MA, Emery SE, Palumbo MA, Bohlman HH: Impact of smoking on the outcome of anterior cervical arthrodesis with interbody or strut-grafting. *J Bone Joint Surg Am* 2001;83(5):668-673.

38. Ames CP, Blondel B, Scheer JK, et al: Cervical radiographical alignment: Comprehensive assessment techniques and potential importance in cervical myelopathy. *Spine (Phila Pa 1976)* 2013;38(22suppl 1):S149-S160.

This comprehensive review reported on cervical alignment parameters, normative values, and methods for quantifying cervical alignment. Cervical alignment was discussed relative to global cervical-pelvic parameters, and weight-bearing 3-foot lateral radiographs should be considered as part of preoperative planning.

39. Villavicencio AT, Babuska JM, Ashton A, et al: Prospective, randomized, double-blind clinical study evaluating the correlation of clinical outcomes and cervical sagittal alignment. *Neurosurgery* 2011;68(5):1309-1316, discussion 1316.

This prospective randomized trial evaluated differences in sagittal alignment when using lordotic versus parallel grafts in ACDF. Graft choice made no difference, but

4: Surgical Management of Degenerative Spine Disorders

maintenance or improvement in cervical sagittal alignment resulted in greater improvements in SF-36 physical component summary and NDI scores. Level of evidence: I.

40. Lee C-H, Jahng T-A, Hyun S-J, Kim K-J, Kim H-J: Expansive laminoplasty versus laminectomy alone versus laminectomy and fusion for cervical ossification of the posterior longitudinal ligament: Is there a difference in the clinical outcome and sagittal alignment? *Clin Spine Surg* 2016;29(1):E9-E15.

   This retrospective review reported on posterior surgery for CSM resulting from ossification of the PLL. All groups lost cervical lordosis and C2-C7 sagittal vertical axis was maintained only in the fusion group. Fusion was recommended for patients with a sagittal vertical axis greater than 40 mm. Level of evidence: III.

41. Machino M, Yukawa Y, Hida T, et al: Cervical alignment and range of motion after laminoplasty: Radiographical data from more than 500 cases with cervical spondylotic myelopathy and a review of the literature. *Spine (Phila Pa 1976)* 2012;37(20):E1243-E1250.

   This prospective radiographic study reported on cervical alignment and range of motion following double-door laminoplasty for treatment of CSM. At 33.3-month follow-up, patients had a mean 1.8° increase in cervical lordosis and preservation of 87.9% of preoperative range of motion. Level of evidence: IV.

42. Sakai K, Yoshii T, Hirai T, et al: Cervical sagittal imbalance is a predictor of kyphotic deformity after laminoplasty in cervical spondylotic myelopathy patients without preoperative kyphotic alignment. *Spine (Phila Pa 1976)* 2016;41(4):299-305.

   This retrospective cohort study investigated the influence of preoperative cervical alignment on postoperative kyphosis following laminoplasty. The overall rate of deformity was 5.2%. Age older than 75 years and a cervical sagittal vertical axis greater than 42 mm were significant risk factors. Level of evidence: IV.

43. Sakaura H, Hosono N, Mukai Y, Ishii T, Yoshikawa H: C5 palsy after decompression surgery for cervical myelopathy: Review of the literature. *Spine (Phila Pa 1976)* 2003;28(21):2447-2451.

44. Kim S, Lee S-H, Kim E-S, Eoh W: Clinical and radiographic analysis of c5 palsy after anterior cervical decompression and fusion for cervical degenerative disease. *J Spinal Disord Tech* 2014;27(8):436-441.

   This retrospective cohort study evaluated radiographic parameters associated with C5 palsy after ACDF. A substantial increase in lordosis seen in the palsy group suggests that aggressive restoration of cervical lordosis can cause traction injury and contribute to C5 dysfunction. Level of evidence: III.

45. Katsumi K, Yamazaki A, Watanabe K, Ohashi M, Shoji H: Analysis of C5 palsy after cervical open-door laminoplasty: Relationship between C5 palsy and foraminal stenosis. *J Spinal Disord Tech* 2013;26(4):177-182.

   This retrospective cohort study evaluated the influence of foraminal stenosis on the development of C5 nerve palsy following laminoplasty for CSM treatment. Patients with palsy had significantly smaller foramen than those without (1.99 versus 2.76 mm). Level of evidence: III.

46. Radcliff KE, Limthongkul W, Kepler CK, et al: Cervical laminectomy width and spinal cord drift are risk factors for postoperative C5 palsy. *J Spinal Disord Tech* 2014;27(2):86-92.

   This retrospective case-control study evaluated the effect of laminectomy width and spinal cord drift on C5 palsy rates after laminectomy and fusion for CSM. Patients in the palsy group had both increased spinal cord drift and increased laminectomy width compared with control subjects. Level of evidence: III.

47. Klement MR, Kleeman LT, Blizzard DJ, Gallizzi MA, Eure M, Brown CR: C5 palsy after cervical laminectomy and fusion: Does width of laminectomy matter? *Spine J* 2016;16(4):462-467.

   This retrospective case-control study evaluated the influence of laminectomy width on C5 nerve palsy. Postoperative CT scans showed no significant difference in laminectomy width between the groups with and without palsy. Level of evidence: III.

48. Odate S, Shikata J, Yamamura S, Soeda T: Extremely wide and asymmetric anterior decompression causes postoperative C5 palsy: An analysis of 32 patients with postoperative C5 palsy after anterior cervical decompression and fusion. *Spine (Phila Pa 1976)* 2013;38(25):2184-2189.

   This retrospective case-control study evaluated the effect of decompression width and asymmetry on C5 nerve palsy in ACDF for CSM. Decompression on the palsy side was significantly larger and overall decompression width was increased in the palsy group. Level of evidence: IV.

49. Katsumi K, Yamazaki A, Watanabe K, Ohashi M, Shoji H: Can prophylactic bilateral C4/C5 foraminotomy prevent postoperative C5 palsy after open-door laminoplasty?: A prospective study. *Spine (Phila Pa 1976)* 2012;37(9):748-754.

   A prospective cohort study evaluated the effect of prophylactic C4/C5 foraminotomy on C5 nerve palsy rates in patients undergoing laminoplasty for CSM. Patients in the foraminotomy group had a palsy rate of 1.4% compared with 6.4% in those not undergoing foraminotomy. Level of evidence: III.

50. Strom RG, Pacione D, Kalhorn SP, Frempong-Boadu AK: Decreased risk of wound infection after posterior cervical fusion with routine local application of vancomycin powder. *Spine (Phila Pa 1976)* 2013;38(12):991-994.

   This retrospective cohort study evaluated the effect of vancomycin powder on infection rates in posterior cervical laminectomy and fusion. Routine vancomycin powder application reduced the infection rate from 10.9% to 2.5%. Level of evidence: II.

51. Pahys JM, Pahys JR, Cho SK, et al: Methods to decrease postoperative infections following posterior cervical spine surgery. *J Bone Joint Surg Am* 2013;95(6):549-554.

This retrospective review evaluated the effect of alcohol foam prep, suprafascial drains, and vancomycin powder on infection rates in posterior cervical surgery and reported that infection rates reduced from 1.86% to zero. Level of evidence: III.

Chapter 16

Degenerative Disease of the Thoracic Spine

Christopher G. Furey, MD

Abstract

Clinically relevant degenerative disease of the thoracic spine is relatively uncommon because of the inherent stability provided by the rib cage. However, disk herniation or spinal stenosis can cause spinal cord compression with resulting severe neurologic consequences. When indicated, surgery can be effective in relieving pain and preserving or restoring function. Various surgical strategies can be used in the thoracic spine and are based on the type and location of the compressive pathology, the clinical history of the patient, and the experience of the treating surgeon.

Keywords: disk; disk herniation; myelopathy; spine surgery; stenosis; thoracic spine

Introduction

Although the thoracic spine is susceptible to the same degenerative cascade that occurs throughout the spinal column, clinically relevant disk herniations and spinal stenosis are much less common than in the cervical and lumbar spines. The relative protection of the thoracic spine arises mainly from the inherent stability afforded by the rib cage. However, compression of the thoracic spinal cord can result in severe symptoms and progressive neurologic dysfunction. Given the relatively infrequent occurrence of thoracic pathology, a high index of suspicion is required for prompt, appropriate diagnosis. When indicated, thoracic spine surgery is technically challenging

Dr. Furey or an immediate family member serves as a board member, owner, officer, or committee member of the American Academy of Orthopaedic Surgeons Board of Councilors, the North American Spine Society, and the Ohio Orthopedic Society.

because of the vulnerability of the thoracic spinal cord and the array of surgical approaches and techniques available (**Figure 1**). Nonetheless, with the appropriate indications and technique, surgery can result in a predictably high degree of symptomatic relief and neurologic improvement.

Anatomy

The unique features of the thoracic spine provide greater proportionate stability than elsewhere in the spinal column. The anterior articulation of the ribs with the sternum provides substantial rigidity in flexion and extension. However, the caudal third of the thoracic spine is less rigid. Ribs 8 through 10, the "false ribs," articulate by using elongated costal cartilage attached to the inferior sternum. The free-floating 11th and 12th ribs have no sternal articulation. In addition, the facets become more coronally oriented in the lower thoracic spine, similar to the lumbar facets. Together, these anatomic differences allow proportionately greater motion in the lower thoracic spine. Degenerative changes and clinically relevant thoracic disk herniations and spinal stenosis are proportionately more common.

Several anatomic features make the spinal cord more susceptible to injury in the thoracic region. The spinal cord occupies a greater proportion of the thoracic spinal canal than within the cervical spine, which makes it more susceptible to extrinsic compression from pathologic processes. The thoracic canal is especially narrow cranially to T6 and gradually increases in diameter toward the thoracolumbar junction.[1] Congenital thoracic stenosis has a prevalence of 1% and is less common than in the cervical or lumbar spine, but similarly predisposes individuals to extrinsic compression.

The kyphotic alignment of the thoracic spine predisposes the spinal cord to drape over ventrally located disk pathology. The blood supply of the thoracic spinal cord is relatively tenuous compared with that of the cervical spine, especially in the watershed region of T4 through

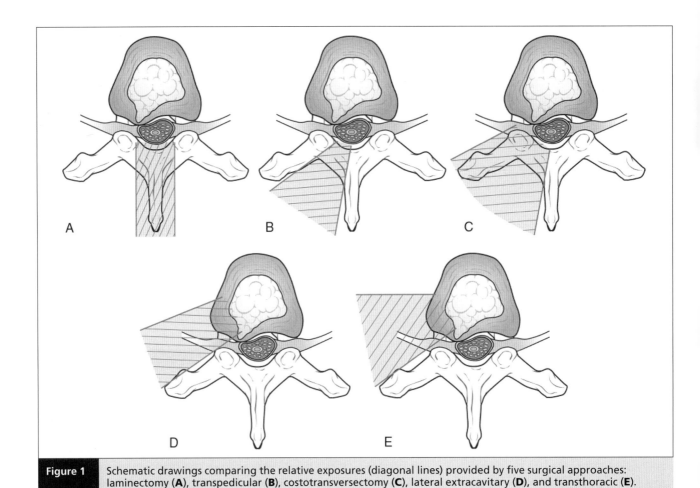

Figure 1 Schematic drawings comparing the relative exposures (diagonal lines) provided by five surgical approaches: laminectomy (**A**), transpedicular (**B**), costotransversectomy (**C**), lateral extracavitary (**D**), and transthoracic (**E**). As the exposure angle becomes more anterior and visualization of the ventral structures improves, the amount of dissection increases. (Reproduced from Gebhauer G, Vaccaro A: Thoracic disk herniation and stenosis, in Rao RD, Smuck M, eds: *Orthopaedic Knowledge Update Spine 4*. Rosemont, IL, American Academy of Orthopaedic Surgeons, 2012, pp 324-328.)

T9, resulting in a proportionately greater susceptibility to mechanical and vascular insult.

Although tandem stenosis of the cervical and lumbar spines is common, with a prevalence of up to 25%, tandem stenosis of the thoracic and lumbar spines has an estimated prevalence of less than 2%.[2] Nonetheless, advanced thoracic imaging should be considered in patients with symptomatic congenital lumbar stenosis and symptoms that suggest thoracic pathology.

Thoracic Disk Herniation

Thoracic disk herniation is common and found incidentally in 40% of asymptomatic individuals.[3] Although one study estimated that symptomatic thoracic disk herniation occurs in only one in 1 million people,[4] most spine practitioners will encounter patients with this rare but potentially serious condition. No sex or race predilection appears to exist for the development of thoracic disk herniation, although most symptomatic cases occur in patients in the fourth through sixth decades of life. The size of a disk herniation and the extent of spinal cord compression do not always correlate with the presence or magnitude of the patient's symptoms. Most symptomatic thoracic disk herniations occur caudal to the T8 level because of the proportionally greater motion within this region. Between 30% and 70% of thoracic disk herniations are calcified, although the pathophysiology of this phenomenon is not clear. Calcific disks are more likely to be symptomatic and more susceptible to adherence to the dura, increasing the potential morbidity associated with their resection. Up to 10% of calcific disk herniations are intradural, although this can be difficult to visualize or diagnose, even with advanced imaging.[5]

Clinical Presentation
Patients with thoracic disk herniation may present with axial back pain, thoracic radiculopathy, or myelopathy.

A combination of signs and symptoms is not uncommon, and patients can report back pain or radiculopathy, but exhibit more severe objective myelopathic features. The infrequent nature of thoracic disk pathology and the lack of a characteristic clinical presentation can contribute to a delay in recognition. Axial pain is the most common presenting complaint and can be acute and spontaneous in origin or more chronic in nature. Radiculopathy generally occurs with pain or paresthesia in a dermatomal fashion in the chest or abdomen that is either unilateral or bilateral, depending on the level and location of the disk herniation. The onset of myelopathy may be obvious and acute or subtle and insidious. Patients may experience weakness, gait difficulty, and frequent falls. When pain is not a major symptom, a patient's presentation can be delayed until substantial compromise of function and neurologic deficit occur. Objective lower extremity weakness, hyperreflexia, and clonus may be present. Bowel and bladder dysfunction can occur in up to 25% of patients with myelopathy, including acute incontinence or urinary retention and constipation. Concurrent thoracic and lumbar pathology is not uncommon, although the true incidence is not known. Symptoms of lumbar radiculopathy and neurogenic claudication arising from lumbar spine disease can overshadow the more subtle but serious features of concurrent thoracic myelopathy. A high index of suspicion is necessary in patients presenting with documented lumbar pathology who have subjective or objective evidence of myelopathy, especially those with radiographic evidence of congenital stenosis.

Because of the relative infrequency of thoracic disk herniation, the true natural history is difficult to define. Most, if not all, asymptomatic herniations remain asymptomatic; new onset of symptoms is uncommon. In symptomatic patients whose only symptoms are radicular, the prognosis is generally favorable and progression to myelopathy is uncommon.[6] Patients with myelopathy may be severely affected on initial presentation and the need for rapid surgical intervention makes it difficult to truly assess the potential of spontaneous improvement. In the setting of advanced thoracic myelopathy, resolution or improvement without surgical intervention is unlikely.

Imaging

MRI is the gold standard for the detection and evaluation of thoracic disk pathology. MRI (or CT myelography) is indicated with persistent thoracic back pain and radiculopathy or with the presence of even subtle myelopathic features. However, given the high incidence of clinically silent thoracic disk herniations, clinical correlation with MRI findings is essential.

The location of the displaced fragment within the canal affects the likelihood of neural element compression, and thus, subsequent symptoms. Central disk herniations are generally larger and more likely to result in cord compression and myelopathy. Lateral or foraminal disk herniations are likely to result in thoracic radiculopathy. Thoracic disk calcification is relatively common; therefore, the threshold to obtain CT should be low if calcification cannot be determined using plain radiography or MRI because this can affect management as well as surgical planning. Direct visualization with an anterior surgical approach is often necessary for safe, thorough removal of a calcified anterior disk herniation.

Treatment

Nonsurgical management is indicated for most patients. Management of axial back pain or radiculopathy initially consists of activity modification; NSAIDs; judicious, short-term use of muscle relaxants or opiate analgesics; and physical therapy. Patients with mild myelopathy undergo nonsurgical treatment, although close observation and careful patient education are essential. Patients with profound or progressive myelopathic features should be considered surgical candidates at the time of initial presentation. The goals of surgical management for thoracic disk herniation include thorough spinal cord decompression, maintenance or restoration of stability, and prevention of recurrence. The surgical approach is selected based on the patient's body habitus and medical comorbidities, the location and size of the herniation, the presence of calcification, and the surgeon's experience level.

Anterior Surgical Approaches

The anterior approach to the thoracic spine provides the most direct visualization of the disk space. Large central disk herniations and calcified disk herniations that are susceptible to dural adherence are most often removed safely and effectively using an anterior approach because posterior approaches may not allow enough exposure to thoroughly remove the compressed material or it can result in unsafe degrees of dural manipulation (**Figure 2**). When clinically indicated, multiple levels can be treated without substantial change in the extent of the anterior exposure. Following diskectomy, reconstruction with structural bone graft and anterior instrumentation should be considered to enhance stability, lessen the likelihood of kyphosis, or mitigate pain that can be associated with disk space collapse. No consensus exists regarding the need for adjunctive interbody fusion or the likelihood for the development of kyphosis or substantial axial back pain in the absence of fusion. The relative time and effort needed to perform interbody fusion is minimal, and multiple

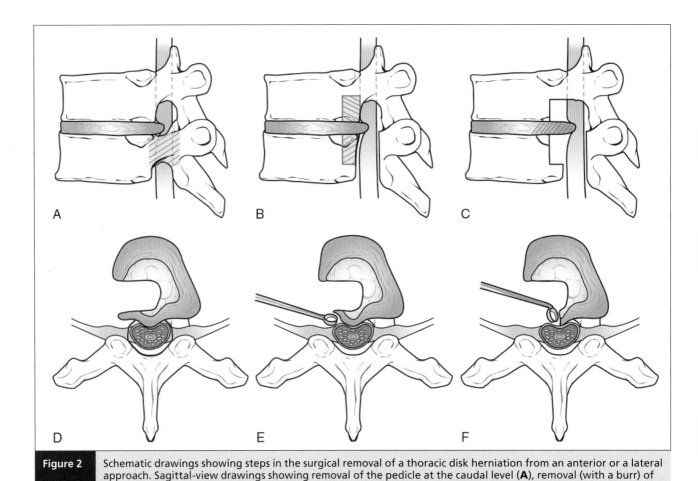

Figure 2 Schematic drawings showing steps in the surgical removal of a thoracic disk herniation from an anterior or a lateral approach. Sagittal-view drawings showing removal of the pedicle at the caudal level (**A**), removal (with a burr) of the posteroinferior aspect of the cranial vertebral body and the posterosuperior aspect of the caudal vertebral body to allow a plane to be developed between the disk and the spinal cord (**B**), and removal of the disk anterior to the herniation (**C**). Axial-view drawings showing the initial cavity created in the central portion of the disk (**D**), the disk elevated anteriorly off the curet (**E**), and the far side of the disk herniation elevated anteriorly using a reverse-angled curet (**F**). (Reproduced from Gebhauer G, Vaccaro A: Thoracic disk herniation and stenosis, in Rao RD, Smuck M, eds: *Orthopaedic Knowledge Update Spine 4*. Rosemont, IL, American Academy of Orthopaedic Surgeons, 2012, pp 324-328.)

series have reported successful radiographic healing and associated clinical improvement.[7,8]

The disadvantages of this approach relate primarily to morbidity associated with thoracotomy such as the need for a chest tube and the risk of pneumothorax, parenchymal lung injury, or intercostal neuralgia. Deconditioned patients or those with compromised pulmonary function may not be suitable candidates for an anterior approach.

Thoracotomy provides satisfactory exposure to the spinal column from T3 through L1. In most cases, a left-side approach is preferred because the thick wall of the aorta is less susceptible to injury than the more fragile vena cava. However, if the predominant disk pathology is to the right of the midline, a right-side approach may be preferable. At the thoracolumbar junction, the presence of the liver also favors a left-side approach. For the infrequently occurring upper thoracic disk herniation, a

right-side approach avoids the heart and subclavian and carotid arteries.

Thoracotomy for spine surgery is performed with the patient in the lateral position, with all body prominences well padded. A double-lumen tube is used to facilitate deflation of the ipsilateral lung to help expose the spinal column. The localization of the target level is of greatest importance. Intraoperative long radiographs that include the sacrum can assist with proper localization. These intraoperative images can be compared with long, preoperative sagittal images to ensure accurate, reliable identification of the surgical level. Alternatively, preoperative placement of a localizing marker while the patient is in the radiology suite can safely expedite surgery at the proper level.

The incision should be made one or two rib levels cephalad to the target level. A partial rib resection may be necessary, but is not essential if the intercostal space can be opened adequately and maintained to provide sufficient visualization. The parietal pleura over the rib head and vertebral body is incised and reflected. The rib head is resected at its insertion to identify the pedicle of the caudal level. The caudal pedicle is removed to reveal the spinal canal and disk space. An annulotomy is performed and the bulk of the disk material is removed to create a cavity within the disk space. The compressed disk material is delivered into the cavity using fine-angled curets in a ventrally directed manner. A plane is carefully created between the disk material and the dura to lessen the risk of durotomy. Partial resection of either adjacent vertebral body may be necessary for complete decompression, especially with extruded or migrated fragments. Partial vertebrectomy should be considered with giant disk herniation (one that occupies greater than 40% of the spinal canal), given that the size and propensity for calcification requires greater space and visualization for safe removal.[9]

If interbody fusion is planned following successful disk removal, the cartilaginous end plates are removed and the bony end plates are decorticated before placement of the structural graft to create an optimal environment for solid arthrodesis.

Most patients who undergo a transthoracic approach have had predictably favorable clinical outcomes. More than 90% of patients in two series who underwent open transthoracic diskectomy for large central disk herniations with myelopathy experienced neurologic improvement and symptomatic relief.[10,11]

Mini-open thoracotomy techniques have been introduced to use direct visualization while minimizing the morbidity associated with open thoracotomy. Proponents describe this as the shortest, most direct approach to the thoracic spine that also avoids violation of the pleural cavity.[12] A smaller skin incision and a limited rib osteotomy (instead of resection) is used followed by a blunt retropleural dissection directed toward the spinal column. The rib head articulation is identified and resected and the disk space entered in a manner similar to that of the open thoracotomy approach. Even extraordinarily large calcified disks have been effectively removed using these mini-open thoracotomy approaches.[12]

Even less invasive techniques such as those using dual-blade or tubular retractors inserted via the intercostal space and docked on the thoracic spine use direct visualization of the anterior approach and minimize soft-tissue dissection and rib resection. Access to the spine can be retropleural to avoid lung deflation and chest tube placement, thus limiting the potential for pulmonary complications.[13] Laterally based tubular systems, which have been widely used in the lumbar spine, also have been used in thoracic diskectomy, interbody fusion, and anterior instrumentation.[13,14] A potential disadvantage of a tubular-based approach is the increased distance from the surgeon's hands to the patient's spine, which can make surgical maneuvers more difficult and possibly less safe.[15]

Video-assisted thoracoscopic surgery, widely used by thoracic surgeons for diseases of the lung and pleural cavity, has been used in the treatment of thoracic disk herniation. Thoracoscopic techniques provide superior visualization of the transthoracic approach and are associated with minimal chest wall- or pulmonary-related complications. The illumination and visualization of thoracoscopy, especially using angled endoscopes, is superior to that of open or minimally invasive anterior techniques. A systematic meta-analysis of 545 patients who underwent thoracoscopic diskectomy reported almost 80% improvement and a 24% complication rate, although most complications were minor (most notably intercostal neuralgia and atelectasis).[16] Single-center studies have reported favorable outcomes in most patients undergoing thoracoscopic diskectomy for both radiculopathy and myelopathy.[17,18] Combining three-dimensional intraoperative image guidance with thoracoscopic techniques has been described as particularly safe and effective.[19] Disadvantages of thoracoscopic diskectomy include difficult access in obese patients or those with large thoracic cavities. Bone graft and anterior instrumentation placement and the management of incidental durotomies are also more difficult. With relatively few indications, it is unlikely that many surgeons would achieve the level of skill to routinely use thoracoscopic approaches.[20]

Posterolateral Surgical Approaches

The use of laminectomy for thoracic disk herniations has largely been stopped because of universally poor results and high rates of neurologic complications.[21] In a kyphotic spinal region, laminectomy alone does not alter the ventral force of the thoracic disk herniation. The propensity for kyphosis following laminectomy adds further mechanical insult to a spinal cord draped over the spinal column.

Relevant posterolateral approaches to the thoracic spine include costotransversectomy and transpedicular, transfacet pedicle-sparing, and lateral extracavitary approaches. Each technique ultimately provides lateral access to the disk space. Although posterolateral approaches do not provide the optimal direct visualization afforded by an anterior approach, they avoid morbidity associated with transthoracic techniques and are familiar to surgeons. Given the relative limited visualization and because dural sac manipulation is inadvisable, posterolateral techniques are most suitable for lateral disk herniations.

Patients are placed in the prone position with all body prominences well padded. Patients should be securely immobilized, especially if intraoperative rotation of the table is planned to facilitate the surgeon's line of vision. Intraoperative spinal cord monitoring is used routinely and is particularly valuable in patients with a compromised thoracic spinal cord. Motor-evoked potentials are reported to be more sensitive than somatosensory-evoked potentials in the early detection of neurologic injury.[22] Obtaining baseline traces before the patient is positioned may be useful in confirming that no neurologic injury has occurred as a result of patient positioning. In addition, careful attention should be given to maintain safe blood pressure parameters, which avoid unsafe fluctuations that can adversely affect the tenuous spinal cord. Before the procedure begins, it is essential to confirm that there will be access to reliable intraoperative radiography or fluoroscopy, which will allow visualization of the entire spinal column from the target level to the sacrum, thus ensuring accurate localization. When performing an accompanying instrumented fusion, placement of pedicle screws before the planned decompression can minimize potential iatrogenic spinal cord injury.

For the transpedicular approach, the posterior elements are exposed lateral to the facet joints in a subperiosteal fashion (**Figure 3**). A hemilaminectomy can be performed to improve visualization of the dorsolateral dura. The ipsilateral facet is resected to expose the caudal pedicle, which is removed to the level of the vertebral body. An annulotomy is performed and disk material is removed from a projection lateral to the thecal sac. As with other techniques, a central cavity is created within the disk space and fine-angle reverse elevators and curets are used in a ventral direction to push disk material within the cavity, which is subsequently removed using pituitary rongeurs.

The transfacet pedicle-sparing technique is an alternative to the transpedicular technique in which a portion of the medial facet is removed to expose the lateral aspect of the dura and disk space. Cadaver studies have shown that similar degrees of lateral access to the disk space can be obtained with either the transpedicular or transfacet techniques, despite less bone removal and soft-tissue dissection when the pedicle is maintained.[23] Preservation of the pedicle has been reported to be associated with less axial pain and better postoperative function.[24,25] Intraoperative ultrasonography has been used to assess the adequacy of ventral decompression in posterolateral thoracic diskectomies to circumvent the limited visualization associated with these approaches. Ultrasonography is a simple, safe tool that has been shown to accurately assess the dural-disk interface with both transpedicular and transfacet pedicle-sparing techniques.[26,27]

Costotransversectomy was originally described to treat the anterior pathology of Pott disease and provides a large, more ventral access than the transpedicular approach. This approach provides excellent exposure for lateral disk herniations. A midline or paramedian skin incision is made and wide soft-tissue exposure performed to achieve exposure lateral to the rib articulation. Portions of the rib, rib head, and transverse process are resected. The rib that articulates with the target disk is resected (the eighth rib articulates with the T7 and T8 vertebrae and crosses the T7-8 disk space). The caudal pedicle is removed to gain lateral access to the disk space. As with the transpedicular approach, a plane is carefully created between the disk and the dura, an annulotomy is performed laterally, and disk material is pushed in a ventral direction and removed. Reliable symptomatic improvement and neurologic recovery has been reported even for central disk herniations and for disks with intradural erosion.[28] The wider lateral exposure is associated with a larger area for visualization and more room for surgical instruments. The disadvantages of the more extensive lateral soft-tissue dissection and bone resection is the potential for pleural violation or intercostal neurovascular injury.

The lateral extracavitary approach (LECA) provides more expansive exposure to the posterior and ventrolateral thoracic spine than either the transpedicular or costotransversectomy approach. Originally designed for traumatic conditions for which extensive bone resection and reconstruction was planned, the LECA provides excellent visualization for lateral disk herniations and also access for placement of structural graft or devices in the interbody space when preferred. As with other posterolateral approaches, posterior supplemental fixation also can be performed via the same incision. Midline, hockey stick, or paramedian and curvilinear incisions have been described for these techniques.[28,29] The paraspinal musculature is exposed and either reflected and mobilized or transected to increase exposure. Transection of the musculature may afford better visualization laterally, but requires direct repair of the muscle belly before fascial closure. A medial portion of the rib is resected along with the rib head articulation. During exposure and removal of the rib, care should be taken to identify and protect the intercostal nerve, which can be followed to the neural foramen. Meticulous attention to the nerve can reduce the likelihood of postoperative neuralgia associated with the more lateral exposure provided by the LECA.[29] The transverse process and caudal pedicle are removed, the lateral disk space entered, and the diskectomy is performed. As with the costotransversectomy, various amounts of vertebral end plate can be removed to facilitate removal of migrated disk material. The greater lateral expanse to

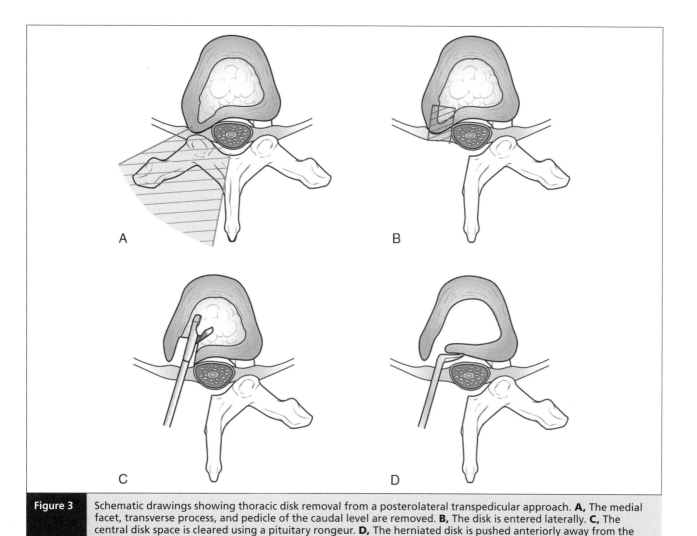

Figure 3 Schematic drawings showing thoracic disk removal from a posterolateral transpedicular approach. **A,** The medial facet, transverse process, and pedicle of the caudal level are removed. **B,** The disk is entered laterally. **C,** The central disk space is cleared using a pituitary rongeur. **D,** The herniated disk is pushed anteriorly away from the spinal cord and into the cavity at the center of the disk space, using a reverse-angled curet. (Reproduced from Gebhauer G, Vaccaro A: Thoracic disk herniation and stenosis, in Rao RD, Smuck M, eds: *Orthopaedic Knowledge Update Spine 4*. Rosemont, IL, American Academy of Orthopaedic Surgeons, 2012, pp 324-328.)

the disk space provided by the extracavitary approach is more amenable to safe insertion of a structural graft or cage device. A study of 65 patients undergoing LECA emphasized the benefit of excellent visualization provided by the greater lateral exposure and reported excellent neurologic improvement but a not insignificant risk of pulmonary complications.[30]

Posterior minimally invasive techniques also have been described in the thoracic spine. A tubular retractor system mounted to the operating table is introduced with minimal soft-tissue retraction and docked in a paraspinal location. Minimal bone resection of the lateral portion of the facet to expose the exiting nerve root is performed. The disk space is accessed just caudal to the nerve, which allows partial diskectomy with minimal dural retraction. Effective, safe use has been reported in a small series of patients undergoing minimally invasive thoracic diskectomy.[31]

The role of adjunctive spine fusion with thoracic diskectomy is controversial. When segmental instability exists, an instrumented fusion is indicated if excessive kyphosis is anticipated or if bilateral facetectomies are performed. In particular, fusion should be considered when substantial facetectomies are performed in the more mobile regions of the lower thoracic spine below the T8 level. Pedicle screw fixation has been performed in one small series, and high rates of fusion and minimal complication rates were reported.[27] Although the need for concomitant fusion in patients undergoing limited facet resections continues to be debated, adjunctive fusion appears to be indicated when removal of the entire facet is necessary. Surgical exposure should not be compromised by limited facet removal to avoid instability. An analysis of 13,837 patients who underwent thoracic disk surgery from 2000 to 2010 reported a dramatic shift in surgical trends: almost one-half of patients underwent accompanying instrumented fusion, compared with the prior decade in which two-thirds of all procedures involved disk excision only.[32] Such a substantial shift in surgical practice may reflect greater familiarity with the use of thoracic pedicle screw instrumentation as well as the presumed collective belief among spine surgeons that stability is essential for better clinical outcomes following thoracic diskectomies.[32] To date, no studies to compare thoracic disk surgery performed with and without fusion have been published. Several small observational studies have reported that instrumented fusion reduces postoperative instability and diminishes the potential of axial back pain.[33,34] Specifically, interbody fusion has been proposed to provide additional stability when bilateral facetectomies are necessary to treat large central disk herniations.[35] Transforaminal interbody fusions with posterior instrumentation and either structural allograft or autograft have been reported to be safe and effective, with high fusion rates and minimal adverse neurologic events.[24,35,36]

Comparative Studies

Because thoracic disk disease is relatively uncommon, no large prospective or randomized studies have evaluated various surgical approaches or techniques. Generally, the relevant literature consists of nonrandomized outcome studies that compare distinct surgical approaches (anterior versus posterior; open versus minimally invasive) or related techniques with various modifications (transpedicular versus pedicle-sparing approach; costotransversectomy versus LECA).

In a comprehensive evaluation of more than 25,000 patients from the Nationwide Inpatient Sample, anterior approaches were associated with longer hospitalization times, greater cost, and higher mortality rates (primarily a result of pulmonary problems).[37] One study evaluated four techniques (transthoracic, lateral extracavitary, transpedicular, and transfacet pedicle-sparing approaches) used to treat large calcified disk herniations and noted equivalent symptomatic improvement and restoration of neurologic function, but greater morbidity with the open transthoracic approach, although this did not adversely affect the ultimate outcome.[25] This study is representative of most pertinent literature because it is retrospective, it compares cohorts of wide-ranging numbers of patients, and the selection criteria for the surgical techniques used are unclear. Although open thoracotomy appears to have a predictably higher complication rate, less invasive anterior techniques seem to mitigate this without compromising efficacy. A 2014 study compared the use of mini-open transthoracic diskectomy for large calcified central herniations with transpedicular diskectomy for lateral herniations and found that duration of surgery, surgical blood loss, incidence of complications, and length of hospital stay were greater with the anterior approach, but both approaches had a similar likelihood for successful clinical outcomes.[20] A 2007 study compared mini-thoracotomy and thoracoscopic techniques for central disk herniations and found no significant difference in surgical duration, perioperative complication rate, or ultimate clinical outcome, although the thoracoscopic technique was noted to have a higher learning curve.[38] A 2005 study on giant densely calcified herniations reported superior results and fewer neurologic complications with open thoracotomy compared with thoracoscopy, because of the ability to leverage large calcified fragments with an open approach that would not have been safely possible thoracoscopically.[9] The literature is scarce in comparisons of the different posterolateral approaches. A retrospective study of small, unequal cohorts who underwent a costotransversectomy, LECA, transpedicular approach, or transfacet approach noted no difference in clinical outcome, neurologic improvement, or complication rate.[34] When surgeons are inexperienced with an anterior approach, posterolateral approaches are safe and effective. A 2012 study compared the LECA with costotransversectomy and found longer surgical times and greater blood loss with the more extensive ventral exposure of the LECA, but no difference was noted in clinical outcome or frequency of complications.[29] Another study found that the reported rates of morbidity and mortality associated with transpedicular approach, costotransversectomy, and LECA are virtually identical.[39] Given the array of techniques available, high-quality prospective studies are needed to better evaluate the true efficacy and best indications for each surgical approach.

Thoracic Spinal Stenosis

Thoracic spinal stenosis is much less common than either cervical or lumbar stenosis. However, thoracic spinal stenosis can cause disabling symptoms and severe neurologic dysfunction. Most frequently, stenosis results from degenerative changes of the intervertebral disk and facet joints along with ligamentum flavum hypertrophy. Ossification of the posterior longitudinal ligament or ossification of the ligamentum flavum also can result in thoracic spinal stenosis. Although rare, when ossifications of the posterior longitudinal ligament and of the ligamentum flavum coexist, severe stenosis and spinal cord compression result. Other conditions in which thoracic spinal stenosis can manifest include Scheuermann kyphosis,

Paget disease, achondroplasia, and diffuse idiopathic skeletal hyperostosis. Thoracic spinal stenosis affects men predominantly, especially after the sixth decade. As with disk herniations, thoracic spinal stenosis occurs more frequently below the T8 level. Patients with symptomatic thoracic stenosis are more likely to have concomitant cervical or lumbar stenosis.[40] Such scenarios can create diagnostic challenges, particularly when prominent symptoms of lumbar radiculopathy or neurogenic claudication obscure more subtle features of thoracic myelopathy.

As with thoracic disk herniation, the clinical presentation of thoracic spinal stenosis varies and can consist of individual or combined features of axial back pain, radiculopathy, or myelopathy. The diagnosis is made with advanced imaging, either MRI or CT myelography. These advanced imaging modalities should include the entire thoracic spine because spinal cord compression can occur at multiple, potentially noncontiguous levels. Patients with predominant symptoms of back pain or radiculopathy are best treated nonsurgically with exercise, analgesic medications, and nerve-modifying agents such as gabapentin or pregabalin. Epidural steroid injections should not be considered if evidence of spinal cord compression exists. Patients with mild, static myelopathy can be monitored with close clinical surveillance for any neurologic deterioration. Patient education should be provided. For advanced cases of myelopathy, surgery is the treatment of choice.

Decompression laminectomy is the preferred surgery for symptomatic thoracic spinal stenosis. All levels with substantial stenosis and spinal cord compression should be treated. Because of the tenuous nature of the compressed thoracic spinal cord, spinal cord monitoring is recommended, and baseline signals should be obtained before the patient is positioned for surgery. As with thoracic disk surgery, preoperative imaging of the thoracic spine should include reference points such as the sacrum or cervicothoracic junction to enable accurate intraoperative radiographic localization. Surgery is performed with the patient in the prone position. A midline approach is used with subperiosteal dissection of the levels intended for decompression. If no fusion is planned, care should be taken to minimize disruption of the facet joints during exposure. Laminectomy is performed with a high-speed burr, creating a trough at the junction of the lamina and facet joint down to the level of the ventral cortex. The laminectomy is completed with Kerrison microrongeurs (1 or 2 mm), which also can be used to remove the ligamentum flavum. The lamina can be elevated and removed en bloc. Great care should be taken to avoid unnecessary tension on the dural sac or any excessive manipulation of instruments within the spinal canal.

When ossification of the ligamentum flavum is present, particular attention should be given to avoid forceful removal, which can result in durotomies. Alternatively, if the calcified ligamentum is determined to be completely incorporated with the dura, direct resection of that portion of the ligamentum should be avoided. Adherent or incorporated areas of ligamentum can be decompressed at the periphery in a circumferential fashion and left as an island to float dorsally with the surrounding decompressed dura.

Small series of patients undergoing laminectomy alone for thoracic spinal stenosis with myelopathy have had generally good results: 80% to 90% of patients noted some degree of symptomatic relief and neurologic improvement.[41,42] Partial medial facetectomy may be necessary to allow thorough posterior decompression, although this will result in increased segmental motion by up to 30%.[43] Resection of greater than 50% of the surface area of the facet complex at a segment will markedly increase the potential for instability and requires instrumented fusion. Adjunctive spinal fusion is recommended when excessive resection of the facet joint complex is necessary or when multiple-level laminectomies are performed in patients with excessive kyphosis or preoperative instability. The stability provided by instrumented fusion is theorized to provide neural protection by decreasing the propensity for further kyphosis following laminectomy and the draping of the spinal cord that would result. No prospective randomized studies have compared laminectomy alone and laminectomy with fusion in the treatment of thoracic stenosis; however, relief of axial back pain and favorable neurologic outcomes have been reported following decompression laminectomy and instrumented fusion.[44] To provide additional interbody support, transforaminal lumbar interbody fusion has been described in a small series to achieve predictable positive outcomes and minimal morbidity, despite the more extensive approach and the need to work ventral to the spinal cord.[45] Transforaminal lumbar interbody fusion has the potential for better correction of kyphosis, greater stability, and increased likelihood of solid arthrodesis.

The use of spinal monitoring accurately identifies adverse neurologic events in thoracic stenosis surgery, especially when both somatosensory-evoked and motor-evoked potential monitoring are used.[46] Cerebrospinal fluid leaks are not infrequent, especially when ossified ligamentum flavum is present. Small linear defects can be repaired primarily. The extent of the durotomy must be accurately defined and the edges freed of any remaining bone to allow accurate approximation and repair. When a large, complex dural defect occurs, closure with a patch graft is indicated. A fascial autograft, allograft, or synthetic patch can be used and secured with interrupted sutures around the entire periphery. Adjunctive sealing with fibrin glue can be used to supplement the repair. Diversion of cerebrospinal fluid using an intrathecal drain can reduce the likelihood for recurrent leak, but is associated with a small risk of infection.

Summary

Thoracic disk herniation and thoracic spinal stenosis are relatively uncommon, largely because of the relative stability of the thoracic spinal column. However, both herniation and spinal stenosis can cause severe symptoms and neurologic dysfunction. A high degree of clinical suspicion often is necessary because pain may not be an obvious symptom and myelopathic features can progress slowly. In addition, symptoms related to coexistent lumbar or cervical stenosis can obscure those related to thoracic pathology. The presence of thoracic back pain and any objective or subjective features of myelopathy warrant advanced imaging. Surgical intervention is indicated for most cases of myelopathy and when radiculopathy and back pain have not improved with nonsurgical management. With the appropriate surgical approach, careful correlation of preoperative and intraoperative imaging for accurate localization, and skillful technique, surgery can be predictably safe and effective. For disk herniation, the size, location, and presence of any calcification determines which approach is most suitable, along with the patient's general health, particularly any pulmonary compromise that would make an anterior approach less favorable. Both anterior and posterior minimally invasive techniques provide the potential benefit of less soft-tissue compromise and more rapid recovery, although no prospective comparative studies exist. For stenosis, a decompression laminectomy is appropriate, and instrumented fusion may be indicated.

Key Study Points

- Thoracic disk herniations and spinal stenosis are relatively uncommon compared with degenerative disease in the cervical and thoracic spine.
- The inherent stability of the thoracic spine is largely provided by articulation with the rib cage; this results in substantially less clinically relevant neural compression than elsewhere in the spinal column.
- A high index of suspicion is necessary to diagnose thoracic pathology because coexistent neural compression in the cervical or lumbar spine often exists.
- Careful preoperative planning and meticulous technique are essential to ensure successful surgical outcomes and minimize adverse events.
- Various surgical techniques can be used effectively. The appropriate surgical strategy is based on the location of the neural compression, the patient's clinical presentation, and the surgeon's experience.

Annotated References

1. Bajwa NS, Toy JO, Ahn NU: Establishment of parameters for congenital thoracic stenosis: A study of 700 postmortem specimens. *Clin Orthop Relat Res* 2012;470(11):3195-3201.

   In this study, 700 cadaver spines were evaluated. Congenital thoracic stenosis was defined as a sagittal plane diameter less than 15 mm or an interpedicle distance less than 18.5 mm.

2. Bajwa NS, Toy JO, Ahn NU: Is lumbar stenosis associated with thoracic stenosis? A study of 1,072 human cadaveric specimens. *Spine J* 2012;12(12):1142-1146.

   Of 1,072 cadaver spines that were evaluated, concurrent lumbar and thoracic stenosis had a prevalence of 1.42%.

3. Wood KB, Blair JM, Aepple DM, et al: The natural history of asymptomatic thoracic disc herniations. *Spine (Phila Pa 1976)* 1997;22(5):525-529, discussion 529-530.

4. Arce CA, Dohrmann GJ: Herniated thoracic disks. *Neurol Clin* 1985;3(2):383-392.

5. Stillerman CB, Weiss MH: Management of thoracic disc disease. *Clin Neurosurg* 1992;38:325-352.

6. Brown CW, Deffer PA Jr, Akmakjian J, Donaldson DH, Brugman JL: The natural history of thoracic disc herniation. *Spine (Phila Pa 1976)* 1992;17(6suppl):S97-S102.

7. Ayhan S, Nelson C, Gok B, et al: Transthoracic surgical treatment for centrally located thoracic disc herniations

presenting with myelopathy: A 5-year institutional experience. *J Spinal Disord Tech* 2010;23(2):79-88.

8. Bohlman HH, Zdeblick TA: Anterior excision of herniated thoracic discs. *J Bone Joint Surg Am* 1988;70(7):1038-1047.

9. Hott JS, Feiz-Erfan I, Kenny K, Dickman CA: Surgical management of giant herniated thoracic discs: Analysis of 20 cases. *J Neurosurg Spine* 2005;3(3):191-197.

10. Quraishi NA, Khurana A, Tsegaye MM, Boszczyk BM, Mehdian SM: Calcified giant thoracic disc herniations: Considerations and treatment strategies. *Eur Spine J* 2014;23(suppl 1):S76-S83.

    In this study, 13 patients with giant calcified thoracic disk herniations underwent transthoracic diskectomy (6 of whom also underwent interbody fusion): 77% improved at least one Frankel grade and there were 4 complications (3 durotomies and 1 recurrent herniation). Level of evidence: IV.

11. Zhao Y, Wang Y, Xiao S, Zhang Y, Liu Z, Liu B: Transthoracic approach for the treatment of calcified giant herniated thoracic discs. *Eur Spine J* 2013;22(11):2466-2473.

    In this study, 15 patients with central or lateral thoracic disk herniations underwent transthoracic decompression and interbody fusion. All patients reported symptomatic improvement, 12 had neurologic improvement, and a low rate of complications was noted. Level of evidence: IV.

12. Moran C, Ali Z, McEvoy L, Bolger C: Mini-open retropleural transthoracic approach for the treatment of giant thoracic disc herniation. *Spine (Phila Pa 1976)* 2012;37(17):E1079-E1084.

    In this study, 17 patients with myelopathy underwent mini-open retropleural transthoracic diskectomy without rib resection. Of these, 13 had neurologic improvement of one or more Frankel grade, 3 had no neurologic improvement, and 1 patient died postoperatively of pneumonia.

13. Uribe JS, Smith WD, Pimenta L, et al: Minimally invasive lateral approach for symptomatic thoracic disc herniation: Initial multicenter clinical experience. *J Neurosurg Spine* 2012;16(3):264-279.

    In this study, 60 patients in five different centers underwent a mini-open lateral approach in which a blade retractor was introduced in a retropleural fashion and docked to the spine: 80% had an excellent result, with relief of myelopathy, radiculopathy, axial back pain, and bowel and/or bladder dysfunction. Major complications occurred in 6.7% of cases.

14. Deviren V, Kuelling FA, Poulter G, Pekmezci M: Minimal invasive anterolateral transthoracic transpleural approach: A novel technique for thoracic disc herniation. A review of the literature, description of a new surgical technique and experience with first 12 consecutive patients. *J Spinal Disord Tech* 2011;24(5):E40-E48.

    In this study, 12 patients underwent successful single-level anterior thoracic diskectomy and instrumented fusion with a minimally invasive tubular system. Approach-related morbidity was limited. Level of evidence: IV.

15. Angevine PD, McCormick PC: Thoracic disc. *J Neurosurg Spine* 2012;16(3):261-262, discussion 262-263.

    The authors present a critique of mini-open lateral thoracic diskectomy with a blade retraction system, with comments about increasing the surgical distance and limiting the working angles when using a tubular system in the thoracic spine.

16. Elhadi AM, Zehri AH, Zaidi HA, et al: Surgical efficacy of minimally invasive thoracic discectomy. *J Clin Neurosci* 2015;22(11):1708-1713.

    This meta-analysis reviewed 545 surgical patients from 12 articles on thoracoscopic diskectomy. Complete resolution of symptoms occurred in 79%, partial improvement in 10%, no change in 10%, and worsening in 1%. The overall complication rate was 24%.

17. Cornips EM, Janssen ML, Beuls EA: Thoracic disc herniation and acute myelopathy: Clinical presentation, neuroimaging findings, surgical considerations, and outcome. *J Neurosurg Spine* 2011;14(4):520-528.

    In this study, eight patients with acute myelopathy resulting from thoracic disk herniation underwent thoracoscopic microdiskectomy. Each patient improved at least one Frankel grade and all regained both continence and the ability to ambulate; four transient, mild complications occurred. Level of evidence: IV.

18. Wait SD, Fox DJ Jr, Kenny KJ, Dickman CA: Thoracoscopic resection of symptomatic herniated thoracic discs: Clinical results in 121 patients. *Spine (Phila Pa 1976)* 2012;37(1):35-40.

    In this study, 121 patients underwent thoracoscopically assisted thoracic diskectomy during a 15-year period. Improvement or resolution of myelopathy, radiculopathy, and axial back pain improved at rates of 91%, 97%, 86%, respectively; 97% of patients were willing to undergo surgery again. Complication rates were low and acceptable. Level of evidence: IV.

19. Johnson JP, Drazin D, King WA, Kim TT: Image-guided navigation and video-assisted thoracoscopic spine surgery: The second generation. *Neurosurg Focus* 2014;36(3):E8.

    Video-assisted thoracoscopic surgery was used in conjunction with image-guided surgical techniques to effectively treat eight patients with thoracic disk herniations. Level of evidence: IV.

20. Arts MP, Bartels RH: Anterior or posterior approach of thoracic disc herniation? A comparative cohort of mini-transthoracic versus transpedicular discectomies. *Spine J* 2014;14(8):1654-1662.

    In this comparative study, 56 patients with a central, calcified disk herniation underwent mini-transthoracic diskectomy and 44 patients with a lateral soft-disk herniation underwent transpedicular diskectomy. Surgical duration, blood loss, length of hospital stay, and complication risk

4: Surgical Management of Degenerative Spine Disorders

were greater in the mini-transthoracic cohort, although clinical outcomes were equivalent. Level of evidence: III.

21. Russell T: Thoracic intervertebral disc protrusion: Experience of 67 cases and review of the literature. *Br J Neurosurg* 1989;3(2):153-160.

22. Khoo LT, Smith ZA, Asgarzadie F, et al: Minimally invasive extracavitary approach for thoracic discectomy and interbody fusion: 1-year clinical and radiographic outcomes in 13 patients compared with a cohort of traditional anterior transthoracic approaches. *J Neurosurg Spine* 2011;14(2):250-260.

   In this study, 13 patients who underwent a minimally invasive LECA thoracic diskectomy and interbody fusion were compared with 11 patients who underwent transthoracic diskectomy. Symptomatic relief was superior in the LECA approach, and neurologic improvement at 1 year was equivalent. Level of evidence: III.

23. Stillerman CB, Chen TC, Day JD, Couldwell WT, Weiss MH: The transfacet pedicle-sparing approach for thoracic disc removal: Cadaveric morphometric analysis and preliminary clinical experience. *J Neurosurg* 1995;83(6):971-976.

24. Yang X, Liu X, Zheng Y: Surgical treatment of thoracic disc herniations using a modified transfacet approach. *Indian J Orthop* 2014;48(2):158-162.

   In this study, posterior decompression with laminectomy and transfacet diskectomy and instrumented fusion were effective in treating 33 patients with thoracic disk herniation. For ossification of the posterior longitudinal ligament or of the ligamentum flavum, the lamina was replanted and secured with suture fixation. Level of evidence: IV.

25. Stillerman CB, Chen TC, Couldwell WT, Zhang W, Weiss MH: Experience in the surgical management of 82 symptomatic herniated thoracic discs and review of the literature. *J Neurosurg* 1998;88(4):623-633.

26. Tan LA, Lopes DK, Fontes RB: Ultrasound-guided posterolateral approach for midline calcified thoracic disc herniation. *J Korean Neurosurg Soc* 2014;55(6):383-386.

   In this case report and literature review, ultrasonography was used to assess the efficacy of thoracic diskectomy in a posterior decompression with a modified pedicle-sparing technique.

27. Nishimura Y, Thani NB, Tochigi S, Ahn H, Ginsberg HJ: Thoracic discectomy by posterior pedicle-sparing, transfacet approach with real-time intraoperative ultrasonography: Clinical article. *J Neurosurg Spine* 2014;21(4):568-576.

   Of 16 patients, intraoperative ultrasonography effectively assisted with transfacet pedicle-sparing thoracic diskectomy; 15 patients showed neurologic improvement. Level of evidence: IV.

28. Young S, Karr G, O'Laoire SA: Spinal cord compression due to thoracic disc herniation: Results of microsurgical posterolateral costotransversectomy. *Br J Neurosurg* 1989;3(1):31-38.

29. Lubelski D, Abdullah KG, Mroz TE, et al: Lateral extracavitary vs. costotransversectomy approaches to the thoracic spine: Reflections on lessons learned. *Neurosurgery* 2012;71(6):1096-1102.

   In this retrospective review at a single institution, LECA was compared with costotransversectomy for a variety of thoracic pathologies including disk herniation. LECA was used for pathology that required more extensive anterior decompression and was associated with longer surgical times and greater blood loss, although overall complication rates were similar. Level of evidence: IV.

30. Foreman PM, Naftel RP, Moore TA II, Hadley MN: The lateral extracavitary approach to the thoracolumbar spine: A case series and systematic review. *J Neurosurg Spine* 2016;24(4):570-579.

   In this study, 23 patients with thoracic disk herniation underwent LECA for diskectomy. Most patients experienced neurologic improvement. A systematic review of similarly treated patients showed an equivalent level of improvement, but a substantially lower complication rate than reported in the literature (3% compared with 32%). Level of evidence: IV.

31. Cho JY, Lee SH, Jang SH, Lee HY: Oblique paraspinal approach for thoracic disc herniations using tubular retractor with robotic holder: A technical note. *Eur Spine J* 2012;21(12):2620-2625.

   In this study, endoscopic transforaminal diskectomy using a tubular retractor system was effective for five patients with thoracic disk herniation. No complications occurred. Level of evidence: IV.

32. Jain A, Menga EN, Hassanzadeh H, Jain P, Lemma MA, Mesfin A: Thoracic disc disorders with myelopathy: Treatment trends, patient characteristics, and complications. *Spine (Phila Pa 1976)* 2014;39(20):E1233-E1238.

   This study evaluated 13,837 patients from the Nationwide Inpatient Sample database who were treated surgically from 2000 to 2010 for myelopathy resulting from thoracic disk herniation. Posterior decompression with fusion was performed in more than one-half of patients. Complication and mortality rates were significantly higher in patients who underwent an anterior transthoracic procedure.

33. Arnold PM, Johnson PL, Anderson KK: Surgical management of multiple thoracic disc herniations via a transfacet approach: A report of 15 cases. *J Neurosurg Spine* 2011;15(1):76-81.

   The authors report on 15 patients with 32 lateral disk herniations treated with a hemilaminectomy and ipsilateral facetectomy followed by partial diskectomy; 2 patients also underwent an instrumented fusion. Nearly uniform success was reported in relief of pain, improved ambulation, and return to work; relief of sensory disturbance was effective, although less frequent. Level of evidence: IV.

34. Börm W, Bäzner U, König RW, Kretschmer T, Antoniadis G, Kandenwein J: Surgical treatment of thoracic disc herniations via tailored posterior approaches. *Eur Spine J* 2011;20(10):1684-1690.

    In this comparison of five posterolateral techniques for thoracic disk herniation, 27 patients experienced improvement, although specific indications for the choice of surgical approach used was not explicitly explained. Level of evidence: III.

35. Yamasaki R, Okuda S, Maeno T, Haku T, Iwasaki M, Oda T: Surgical outcomes of posterior thoracic interbody fusion for thoracic disc herniations. *Eur Spine J* 2013;22(11):2496-2503.

    In this study, 11 patients with thoracic disk herniation underwent posterior decompression using bilateral facet resection, diskectomy, and interbody and posterior instrumented fusion; 10 patients improved at least one Frankel grade and had radiographic healing of fusion. Level of evidence: IV.

36. Bransford R, Zhang F, Bellabarba C, Konodi M, Chapman JR: Early experience treating thoracic disc herniations using a modified transfacet pedicle-sparing decompression and fusion. *J Neurosurg Spine* 2010;12(2):221-231.

37. Yoshihara H, Yoneoka D: Comparison of in-hospital morbidity and mortality rates between anterior and nonanterior approach procedures for thoracic disc herniation. *Spine (Phila Pa 1976)* 2014;39(12):E728-E733.

    In this analysis, 25,413 patients from the Nationwide Inpatient Sample who had thoracic disk herniation underwent surgery from 2000 to 2009. Patients undergoing an anterior approach had higher complication and mortality rates as well as longer hospitalizations and increased hospital costs.

38. Bartels RH, Peul WC: Mini-thoracotomy or thoracoscopic treatment for medially located thoracic herniated disc? *Spine (Phila Pa 1976)* 2007;32(20):E581-E584.

39. Fessler RG, Sturgill M: Review: Complications of surgery for thoracic disc disease. *Surg Neurol* 1998;49(6):609-618.

40. Hitchon PW, Abode-Iyamah K, Dahdaleh NS, et al: Risk factors and outcomes in thoracic stenosis with myelopathy:
A single center experience. *Clin Neurol Neurosurg* 2016;147:84-89.

    In this study, 44 consecutive patients with thoracic stenosis and myelopathy had a high predominance of patients older than 70 years and a common concurrence of cervical and/or lumbar stenosis. Surgical decompression with laminectomy was associated with predictably favorable outcomes. Level of evidence: IV.

41. Shiokawa K, Hanakita J, Suwa H, Saiki M, Oda M, Kajiwara M: Clinical analysis and prognostic study of ossified ligamentum flavum of the thoracic spine. *J Neurosurg* 2001;94(2suppl):221-226.

42. Zhong ZM, Wu Q, Meng TT, et al: Clinical outcomes after decompressive laminectomy for symptomatic ossification of ligamentum flavum at the thoracic spine. *J Clin Neurosci* 2016;28(28):77-81.

    In this study, decompression laminectomies were performed in 22 patients with thoracic stenosis and ossification of the ligamentum flavum. Clinical improvement was significant and neurologic improvement was good or excellent in 17 patients; 8 patients had intraoperative complications of dural tears, epidural hematoma, and infection. Level of evidence: IV.

43. Oda I, Abumi K, Cunningham BW, Kaneda K, McAfee PC: An in vitro human cadaveric study investigating the biomechanical properties of the thoracic spine. *Spine (Phila Pa 1976)* 2002;27(3):E64-E70.

44. Li F, Chen Q, Xu K: Surgical treatment of 40 patients with thoracic ossification of the ligamentum flavum. *J Neurosurg Spine* 2006;4(3):191-197.

45. Liu FJ, Chai Y, Shen Y, Xu JX, Du W, Zhang P: Posterior decompression with transforaminal interbody fusion for thoracic myelopathy due to ossification of the posterior longitudinal ligament and the ligamentum flavum at the same level. *J Clin Neurosci* 2013;20(4):570-575.

    In this study, 13 patients with thoracic stenosis resulting from concurrent ossification of the posterior longitudinal ligament and of the ligamentum flavum underwent decompression and transforaminal interbody fusion. Neurologic improvement occurred in 12, and all patients had radiographic healing of fusion. Level of evidence: IV.

46. Eggspuehler A, Sutter MA, Grob D, Porchet F, Jeszenszky D, Dvorak J: Multimodal intraoperative monitoring (MIOM) during surgical decompression of thoracic spinal stenosis in 36 patients. *Eur Spine J* 2007;16(suppl 2):S216-S220.

Chapter 17

Lumbar Disk Herniations

Ilyas S. Aleem, MD, MSc, FRCSC   Rakesh D. Patel, MD   Ahmad Nassr, MD

Abstract

Lumbar disk herniations are common in the adult population and may be associated with substantial patient morbidity as well as personal and societal costs. Surgical treatment provides effective relief in carefully selected patients with severe or ongoing symptoms or in those who do not improve with nonsurgical care. The goal of surgical treatment is to provide adequate nerve root decompression and minimize soft-tissue damage without resultant spinal instability. Treatment of recurrent disk herniation is controversial but generally consists of revision diskectomy, with fusion reserved for multiple recurrences or instability.

Keywords: diskectomy; lumbar disk herniation; lumbar posterior ring apophyseal fracture; radiculopathy

Introduction

Symptomatic lumbar disk herniations have an estimated prevalence of 2% in the general adult population and may be associated with substantial patient morbidity

---

as well as billions of dollars in personal and societal costs.[1,2] Although lumbar disk herniation is generally considered a soft-tissue annular disruption associated with degenerative disease, it has been found that patients with a lumbar posterior ring apophyseal fracture (limbus fracture) account for up to 8% of all patients with lumbar disk herniation, with higher rates in adolescents and young adults.[3,4] Patients typically have a radicular pattern of pain, sensory loss, or weakness. Effective relief can be provided with surgical treatment in carefully selected patients who have severe or ongoing symptoms or in those who do not improve after nonsurgical treatment. Conventional open and minimally invasive surgery (MIS) techniques aim to decompress neural elements while minimizing the likelihood of developing instability and damage to soft tissues.[5]

In 2011, the North American Spine Society collaborated on a joint project that provided evidence-based recommendations to address key clinical questions surrounding the diagnosis and treatment of lumbar disk herniation with radiculopathy.[6] A thorough clinical evaluation, appropriate imaging, and carefully selected nonsurgical or surgical treatment is mandatory in the care of patients with this common spinal pathology.

History and Physical Examination

The clinical evaluation of patients with lumbar disk herniation starts with a thorough clinical evaluation, consisting of a history and physical examination. Classically, patients describe a period of intractable low back pain followed by unilateral or bilateral radiculopathy. Presenting symptoms and physical examination findings typically include any combination of paravertebral muscle spasm and tenderness, positive tension signs, sensory disturbance, motor weakness, and loss of deep tendon reflexes. A high index of suspicion must be maintained for patients presenting with bladder or bowel dysfunction, saddle anesthesia, and acute motor or sensory loss. In patients presenting with cauda equina symptoms, prompt evaluation with emergent imaging and surgical decompression is required.[7]

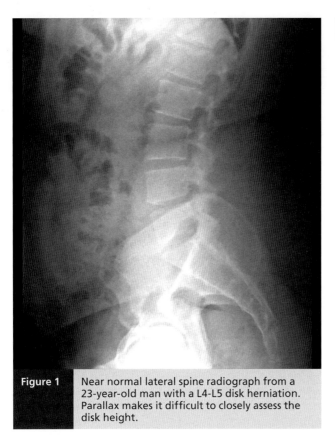

Figure 1 Near normal lateral spine radiograph from a 23-year-old man with a L4-L5 disk herniation. Parallax makes it difficult to closely assess the disk height.

Imaging

Radiographic assessment begins with weight-bearing AP and lateral plain radiographs to assess overall spinal alignment and the presence of degenerative disk disease, spondylolisthesis, or any other bony abnormalities (**Figure 1**). The presence of a transitional vertebra such as a lumbarized S1 or sacralized L5 must be appreciated preoperatively to ensure surgery at the correct level. In some instances, a symptomatic disk herniation will result in coronal plane deformity, the so-called sciatic scoliosis. This lateral shift of the upper spine generally occurs opposite to the side of the disk herniation and is differentiated from other forms of scoliosis primarily by lack of rotation of the vertebral bodies. This deformity is functional and resolves as radicular symptoms improve. In symptomatic patients, root compression from a herniated nucleus pulposus is confirmed with MRI[8] (**Figure 2**). For patients who cannot undergo MRI, CT myelography is preferred, but disk displacement often can be seen on plain CT if intrathecal dye is contraindicated. However, given the favorable natural history of herniated nucleus pulposus and the high rate of irrelevant findings in asymptomatic patients, up to 6 weeks of nonsurgical care is generally recommended before advanced imaging. Exceptions exist, and the presence of neurologic deficits justifies earlier advanced imaging, particularly if the deficits are progressive or consistent with cauda equina syndrome (**Figure 3**).

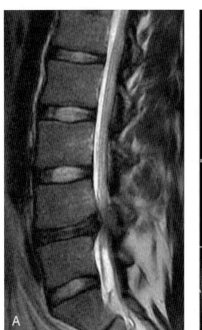
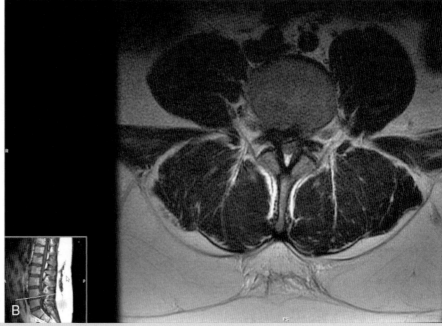

Figure 2 Sagittal (**A**) and axial (**B**) T2-weighted spine magnetic resonance images demonstrate a central and right posterolateral L4-L5 disk protrusion in a 23-year-old man. Inset depicts the level at which the axial image was obtained.

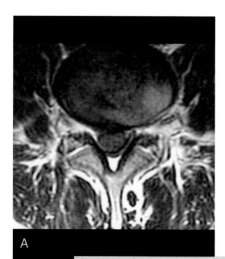
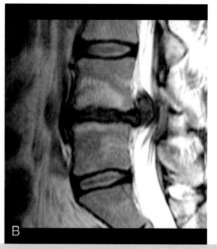
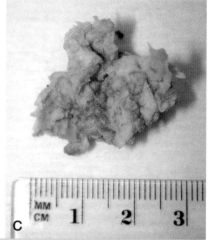

Figure 3 Images from a patient who presented with acute onset of back and bilateral leg pain and urinary incontinence. Axial (**A**) and sagittal (**B**) T2-weighted magnetic resonance images of large central disk herniation at the L4-L5 level. **C,** Clinical photograph of disk material removed from the patient. (Reproduced from Spector LR, Madigan L, Rhyne A, Darden B II, Kim D: Cauda equina syndrome. *J Am Acad Orthop Surg* 2008;16[8]:471-479.)

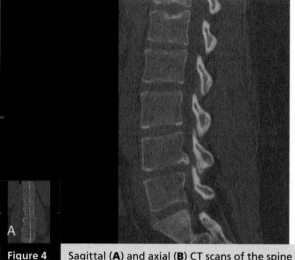
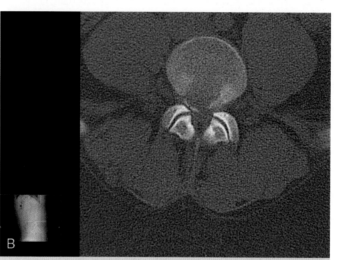

Figure 4 Sagittal (**A**) and axial (**B**) CT scans of the spine demonstrate L4-L5 disk herniation and a limbus fracture in a 23-year-old man. Insets depict levels at which respective images were obtained.

Evaluation of the bony anatomy using CT can help evaluate for the presence of a lumbar posterior ring apophyseal (or limbus) fracture, which may accompany lumbar disk herniation, particularly in young or more active patients[3] (**Figure 4**). The apophyseal fracture is characterized by separation of an osseous fragment at the posterior cephalad or caudal edge of the adjacent vertebral body.

Nonsurgical Treatment

Most patients with lumbar disk herniations respond to nonsurgical treatment consisting of symptomatic pain control, avoidance of activities that exacerbate symptoms, weight loss, a structured exercise program,[6] and time.

Evidence regarding the efficacy of other interventions such as spinal manipulation and traction remains limited. The use of spinal injections for symptomatic lumbar disk herniation is becoming common.[9] A systematic review compared three anatomic approaches to epidural injections and reported high-quality evidence to support the use of epidural injections to alleviate the pain and disability of lumbar disk herniation in the short term (less than 6 months) and moderate-quality evidence to support their use for long-term effects (6 months or longer).[10] The primary and secondary outcomes were pain relief and functional outcomes measured by disability scores, respectively.

Surgical Treatment

In carefully selected patients with lumbar disk herniation confirmed by using imaging and by leg symptoms persisting for at least 6 weeks, surgical diskectomy provides faster pain relief and resolution of symptoms compared with nonsurgical treatment. The Spine Patient Outcomes Research Trial (a randomized trial with a concurrent observational cohort involving 13 medical centers in 11 states) recently published 8-year results for surgical versus nonsurgical treatment of lumbar disk herniation.[11] Primary outcome measures were the Medical Outcomes Study 36-Item Short Form Health Survey and the Oswestry Disability Index. Although advantages were seen for surgery in intent-to-treat analyses for the randomized cohort for most primary and secondary outcomes, substantial nonadherence to treatment was noted: 49% of patients assigned to nonsurgical therapy underwent surgery versus 60% of patients assigned to surgery. The observed effects were relatively small for primary outcomes. However, comparison of secondary outcomes such as sciatica discomfort, satisfaction with symptoms, and self-rated improvement was significantly greater for surgery. Patients who underwent surgery for lumbar disk herniation achieved greater improvement compared with nonsurgically treated patients, with no degradation of outcomes at 8 years.[11]

The goal of surgical treatment is to provide adequate nerve root decompression and minimize soft-tissue damage and iatrogenic destabilization. Many techniques have been used successfully to access the disk space and decompress the roots. Prior to any surgical intervention, anatomic location of the disk herniation must be considered carefully. Most disk herniations are posterolateral, impinging the anterolateral traversing nerve root. The traversing nerve root also may be affected by central disk herniations. Foraminal and extraforaminal (far lateral) herniations are less common and impinge on the exiting nerve root at that level. Sequestered fragments, in which the disk material herniates through the anulus fibrosus and is no longer contiguous with the disk space, may result in superior or inferior migration of the fragment, resulting in a neurologic pattern based on the compression caused by the herniated fragment. Knowledge of the anatomic location of the disk herniation, nerve root involved, and pattern of pain and neurologic deficit is essential in surgical planning. If an apophyseal fragment is present, this should be identified and removed intraoperatively.

For posterolateral or central disk herniations, most surgeons currently perform standard image-guided microdiskectomy, which involves a 1- to 2-inch midline incision over the spinal segments of interest. It is important to correctly center the incision over the target pathology. Although most disk herniations occur at the level of the disk space in the cranial-to-caudal direction, an inferiorly migrated disk may require an approach slightly caudal to the level of the disk space to gain access to the pathology. The spine can be conceptually divided into three stories (disk level, foraminal level, and pedicle level).[12] This model allows the surgeon to preoperatively plan the degree and direction of laminotomy required to access the disk fragment. The muscles on the side of the disk herniation are then detached from their respective spinous processes and subperiosteal dissection is performed over the side of the planned decompression. A combination of a high-speed burr and/or curets and Kerrison rongeurs is used to perform a hemilaminectomy and partial facetectomy on the side of the pathology. Care is taken to preserve at least 50% of the facet joint and 8 to 12 mm of bone from the lateral edge of the decompression to the edge of the pars interarticularis to avoid iatrogenic instability. The ligamentum flavum is removed and the common dural tube and traversing nerve root are identified. The key to intraoperative localization of the disk and nerve root is the pedicle inferior to the targeted disk. After the ligamentum flavum is removed, the pedicle and corresponding nerve root, which runs from medial to lateral, is identified using an angled ball-tip probe or Woodson elevator. The disk lies just cephalad to the pedicle. The nerve root is gently mobilized medially to identify the disk herniation, and an annulotomy is made if necessary to access the disk fragment. The defect in the anulus fibrosus is probed for any additional, loose disk fragments that may herniate from the defect if left in place. These fragments are removed using a combination of pituitary rongeurs and curved microcurets. In more centrally located disk herniations, a Woodson elevator may be used to palpate the annular defect and ensure no further compression medially. The Woodson elevator also may be used through the annulotomy site to probe the disk space and remove any disk fragments located more centrally. The surgeon should be extremely cautious regarding the duration and extent to which the thecal sac is retracted to minimize traction injury. The defect is irrigated and the wound is closed after meticulous hemostasis is achieved. The nerve root should be freely mobile at the conclusion of the procedure. After completion of the procedure, some surgeons may wish to inject 1.0 mL of methylprednisolone acetate 40 mg/mL over the decompressed nerve root.[13]

The same procedure can be performed through a slightly smaller incision using a muscle-sparing approach with a tubular retractor system. This approach preserves the multifidus muscle attachments on the spinous processes. To date, no convincing evidence supports a meaningful long-term benefit with this approach. The advantages of this technique include decreased dissection time and blood loss. In addition, even in somewhat obese patients, the incision is not different, only the length of the tube is different. The disadvantages are primarily related to the learning curve, decreased direct visualization, and the need for fluoroscopy to dock the tube. Precise docking of the tube also is necessary because of the small diameter of the working window, which is typically 18 to 22 mm.

For extraforaminal (far lateral) disk herniations, a paramedian intertransverse approach via the interval between the multifidus and longissimus muscles is used. The key to identifying the extraforaminal disk fragment is the transverse process, which leads to the pedicle. However, unlike central or posterolateral disk herniations, the key pedicle is the one superior to the disk herniation. The skin incision is approximately 3 to 5 cm lateral to the midline. Careful dissection is performed in the interval between the multifidus and longissimus muscles. A combination of blunt and sharp dissection is performed until the two transverse processes can be palpated and a deep retractor blade is placed. The superior transverse process is identified and the intertransverse ligament is detached from the inferior surface of the superior transverse process, the superior surface of the inferior transverse process, and more medially, from the edge of the pars. The intertransverse ligament flap is gently retracted laterally, and the pedicle is palpated medially. This facilitates locating the nerve root, which is identified at the inferior and medial edges of the pedicle. Protecting the nerve, the disk space is identified (in general, caudal to the root), and the migrated disk fragment should be visible and removed as described previously. To access the disk space, the superior aspect of the facet joint also may need to be removed using a burr, especially at L5-S1. The nerve root is vulnerable with this approach, particularly the dorsal root ganglion, which is highly susceptible to injury, even from minor manipulation. Therefore, extreme diligence is required to limit any pressure or tension applied to the root.

Alternatively, the MIS version of this technique requires docking the tube to the pedicle inferior to the disk space. Because of the tubular retractor's small working window, the nerve is not directly visualized. The tube is docked through a paramedian incision onto the lateral aspect of the facet of the disk space of interest. Foraminal and extraforaminal disk herniations often occur at the level of the disk space. After the facet is identified, a high-speed burr or Kerrison rongeur is used to remove the overhanging lateral aspect of the superior articular process of the facet, allowing palpation of the superior and lateral borders of the pedicle inferior to the disk space. Depending on the medial-lateral location of the herniation, some of

the lateral pars intra-articularis may need to be removed. The disk space is directly superior to the superior margin of the pedicle. The disk herniation can then be removed without direct visualization of the nerve root. The amount of disk material removed should be carefully scrutinized and correlate with preoperative imaging to avoid disk fragment retention, resulting in continued neural compression and symptoms. Sometimes, both a traditional hemilaminectomy and extraforaminal approach may be used to work from both inside and outside the foramen to access the pathology. Care must be taken to avoid excessive bone removal and iatrogenic destabilization.

An additional alternative technique for foraminal and extraforaminal disk herniations involves a true foraminal approach to the disk space using endoscopic techniques. A more lateral incision is made, through which an approximately 7-mm cannula is docked into the neural foramen. This technique allows direct removal of the disk herniation with the smallest amount of bony resection, but requires a specialized set of instruments and endoscope. The technical demands and specialized equipment necessary for this technique have resulted in a high threshold for use by most spine surgeons (**Figure 5**).

The recent focus in spine surgery on these MIS techniques has sought to achieve the goals of surgery with a smaller skin incision and to be less destructive and traumatic to soft tissues.[14] Although MIS approaches may accelerate functional recovery, reduce pain, and decrease blood loss and length of hospital stay, the greater technical expertise required and increased risks of neurologic injury, incidental durotomy, and revision surgery challenge their usefulness compared with conventional open approaches.[5] Several recent studies have compared open techniques with minimally invasive diskectomy. A meta-analysis that included 10 randomized trials of 1,159 patients undergoing lumbar diskectomy concluded that low- to moderate-quality evidence suggests that a risk-benefit ratio does not support the routine use of MIS procedures.[15] A recent Cochrane review was performed to compare microdiskectomy or open diskectomy with minimally invasive diskectomy (percutaneous endoscopic interlaminar or transforaminal lumbar diskectomy, transmuscular tubular microdiskectomy, and automated percutaneous lumbar diskectomy) in adults with lumbar radiculopathy secondary to lumbar disk herniation.[16] Primary outcomes measured included pain and function; secondary outcomes included surgical complications, length of hospital stay, postoperative opioid use, quality of life, and overall patient satisfaction. Of 11 randomized controlled trials and quasirandomized controlled trials with 1,172 patients, 7 studies were found to have high overall risk of bias. Small and likely clinically insignificant

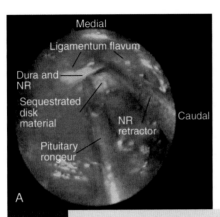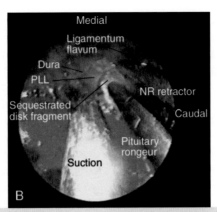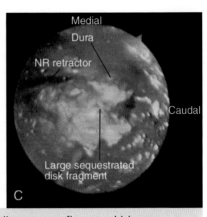

Figure 5 **A,** Endoscopic image shows the nerve root (NR) and dura with the covering ligamentum flavum, which were medially retracted. The tip of the extruded disk material is grasped with a pituitary rongeur. **B,** Endoscopic image shows part of the migrated fragment as it is grasped with the help of suction, a nerve root retractor, and a pituitary rongeur. **C,** Endoscopic image shows the extraction of large, migrated disk extrusion from under the dura. PLL = posterior longitudinal ligament. (Reproduced from Hussein M: Minimal incision, multifidus-sparing microendoscopic diskectomy versus conventional microdiskectomy for highly migrated intracanal lumbar disk herniations. *J Am Acad Orthop Surg* 2016;24[11]:805-813.)

differences were found between conventional and MIS techniques. Advantages of MIS included lower risk of infection and potentially shorter hospital stay.[16] Additional high-quality randomized trials evaluating clinically significant differences are required to appropriately define indications for MIS, clearly reporting the influence of surgeon expertise on patient-important outcomes.

Postoperative Assessment and Complications

After surgery, relief of symptoms often correlates with the preoperative duration of symptoms.[17] Younger patients with recent onset of symptoms (<6 months) generally have rapid and substantial improvement in radicular symptoms. Patients with long-standing or chronic symptoms may have less predictable improvement. Analgesic medications are provided acutely as required. When comfortable, patients are encouraged to resume mobility and are restricted from any heavy bending, lifting, or twisting activities for at least 6 weeks. Patients are discharged from the hospital when comfortable and rarely require physical therapy postoperatively.

Although lumbar diskectomy is largely successful in improving symptoms, more than 10% of patients undergoing primary diskectomy for radiculopathy may experience recurrent lumbar disk herniation.[18] Gadolinium-enhanced MRI is the imaging modality of choice for evaluating recurrent lumbar disk herniation and other processes such as epidural fibrosis, arachnoiditis, abscess, and hematoma.[19] Recurrent disk herniation often presents as a mass with smooth margins that has low signal on T1- and T2-weighted magnetic resonance images and

no enhancement after contrast enhancement. This distinguishes it from epidural scar, which has irregular margins and heterogenous enhancement secondary to vascularity.[20] One reason for recurrence is failure to adequately remove the primary herniation at the index procedure. After the completion of diskectomy, it is important to assess the findings, and at minimum to be assured that intraoperative findings were consistent with those expected based on imaging. Possible reasons for inconsistencies could include failure to remove the sequestered fragment, wrong-site surgery, or patient imaging that is not current. This should prompt additional intraoperative evaluation to ensure that the technical goals of the surgery have been properly achieved.

The extent of intraoperative diskectomy is controversial and has been correlated with back pain and recurrence risk. Limited diskectomy involves only removing the herniated fragment and any other loose fragments, whereas subtotal diskectomy involves removing a larger portion of the intervertebral disk. Limited diskectomy has the advantages of improved pain relief, patient satisfaction, and a theoretically decreased rate of degenerative disk disease at the cost of higher recurrence rates. Subtotal diskectomy has the advantages of decreased recurrence rates at the cost of greater loss of disk height, back pain, and theoretically increased rate of degenerative disk disease.[21] A systematic review of 13,359 patients showed that limited diskectomy was associated with 2.5-fold decrease in the incidence of long-term back and/or leg pain and a twofold increase in the incidence of recurrent disk herniation.[22] Patients with recurrent back or leg pain should undergo a detailed history, physical examination, and radiographic imaging as with their preoperative workup. This will help delineate disk recurrence with other causes of pain such as infection, degeneration at other levels, or instability. If the workup is consistent with a recurrent disk herniation, an initial course of nonsurgical treatment consisting of physical therapy and symptomatic pain control is recommended because symptoms may improve with time.

Back pain after diskectomy also can occur after surgery. Axial lower back pain can be related to discogenic pain, facet arthritis, or segmental instability.[20] Additional workups, including flexion and extension radiographs, should be performed. Translation of 3 to 5 mm or 10° of angulation relative to the adjacent vertebrae indicate segmental instability.[20] Postoperative discitis also should be included in the differential diagnosis. Although the incidence of discitis is low, it should always be considered in patients who have persistent back pain that does not respond to conventional nonsurgical treatment.[23] In the longer term, postoperative progressive degenerative disk disease may develop that, as with recurrent disk herniations, may prompt consideration of fusion in the absence of improvement with nonsurgical treatment.

Patients also may have persistent or even increased dysesthesias after diskectomy. Although the exact mechanism is not well understood, it may be a result of nerve damage from the original disk herniation, or a result of iatrogenic tension on the root during surgery, particularly at the dorsal root ganglion.[24,25] Most patients with these symptoms improve with time, but this condition can be quite debilitating and difficult to treat.

The surgical treatment of recurrent lumbar disk herniation is controversial. A survey of 2,560 orthopaedic surgeons and neurosurgeons in the United States (18% response rate) showed substantial variation in the surgical treatment of recurrent disk herniations.[26] Surgeons in practice for more than 15 years were more likely to perform revision microdiskectomy compared with surgeons in practice for fewer years, who were more likely to perform revision diskectomy with fusion. In the absence of instability, conventional open diskectomy as revision surgery for recurrent lumbar disk herniation has shown satisfactory results comparable with those of primary diskectomy.[27] Although not firmly established by the literature, many surgeons in the United States prefer to perform fusion for patients with two-time recurrent disk herniation,[26] or demonstrated instability, or disk space collapse greater than 50% after primary diskectomy.

Summary

Symptomatic lumbar disk herniations are common in the adult population and may be associated with substantial patient morbidity. Although most patients respond to nonsurgical treatment, surgical treatment is effective in providing relief in carefully selected patients with severe or ongoing symptoms or if nonsurgical treatment has been unsuccessful. Preoperative planning is key to performing lumbar diskectomy with minimal soft-tissue trauma and bone resection. The concept of the three-story anatomy of the spine helps localize the disk in a cephalad-caudal direction. The central canal, foraminal, and extraforaminal zones divide the spine in the medial-lateral direction. Clinical examination findings must correlate closely with radiographic imaging. The treatment of recurrent back or leg pain after diskectomy is controversial. Postoperative instability must be assessed carefully. In the absence of instability, revision diskectomy has shown good results, with fusion reserved for patients with multiple recurrences or instability.

Key Study Points

- Symptomatic lumbar disk herniations are common and may be associated with substantial patient morbidity.
- Although most patients respond to nonsurgical treatment, surgical treatment is effective in providing relief in patients with severe or ongoing symptoms.
- The goal of surgical treatment is to provide adequate nerve root decompression and minimize soft-tissue damage without resultant spinal instability.
- Treatment of recurrent disk herniation is controversial but generally consists of revision diskectomy, with fusion reserved for patients with multiple recurrences or instability.

Annotated References

1. Cenic A, Kachur E: Lumbar discectomy: A national survey of neurosurgeons and literature review. *Can J Neurol Sci* 2009;36(2):196-200.

2. Bruggeman AJ, Decker RC: Surgical treatment and outcomes of lumbar radiculopathy. *Phys Med Rehabil Clin N Am* 2011;22(1):161-177.

The authors review the epidemiology, pathophysiology, surgical treatment options, and outcomes in patients with lumbar radiculopathy.

3. Wu X, Ma W, Du H, Gurung K: A review of current treatment of lumbar posterior ring apophysis fracture with lumbar disc herniation. *Eur Spine J* 2013;22(3):475-488.

   This study reported that lumbar posterior ring apophysis fractures are an uncommon disorder, which typically occur in adolescents and young athletes and are frequently accompanied by disk herniations. Various modalities of classifications and surgical options exist.

4. Akhaddar A, Belfquih H, Oukabli M, Boucetta M: Posterior ring apophysis separation combined with lumbar disc herniation in adults: A 10-year experience in the surgical management of 87 cases. *J Neurosurg Spine* 2011;14(4):475-483.

   This retrospective study distinguishes characteristics between adults with and without posterior ring apophysis separation with lumbar disk herniation, including younger age, male sex, military affiliation, symptom duration, and anatomic location.

5. Kamper SJ, Ostelo RW, Rubinstein SM, et al: Minimally invasive surgery for lumbar disc herniation: A systematic review and meta-analysis. *Eur Spine J* 2014;23(5):1021-1043https://www.ncbi.nlm.nih.gov/pubmed/?term=24442183.

   This meta-analysis of randomized trials showed moderate-to low-quality evidence of no differences in clinical outcomes between MIS and conventional microdiskectomy.

6. Kreiner DS, Hwang SW, Easa JE, et al; North American Spine Society: An evidence-based clinical guideline for the diagnosis and treatment of lumbar disc herniation with radiculopathy. *Spine J* 2014;14(1):180-191.

   This is a report of the official North American Spine Society evidence-based recommendations regarding the diagnosis and treatment of lumbar disk herniation with radiculopathy.

7. McLain RF, Agrawal BM, Silverstein MP: Acute cauda equina syndrome caused by a disk herniation: Is emergent surgery the correct option? Surgical decompression remains the standard of care. *Spine (Phila Pa 1976)* 2015;40(9):639-641.

   Surgical decompression remains the standard of care for acute cauda equina syndrome caused by disk herniation.

8. Li Y, Fredrickson V, Resnick DK: How should we grade lumbar disc herniation and nerve root compression? A systematic review. *Clin Orthop Relat Res* 2015;473(6):1896-1902.

   The authors conclude that the Combined Task Force and the van Rijn classifications are the most reliable systems for describing lumbar disk herniation and nerve root compression.

9. Manchikanti L, Knezevic NN, Boswell MV, Kaye AD, Hirsch JA: Epidural injections for lumbar radiculopathy and spinal stenosis: A comparative systematic review and meta-analysis. *Pain Physician* 2016;19(3):E365-E410.

   Epidural corticosteroid injections with lidocaine alone or lidocaine with steroids were significantly effective for pain control for radiculopathy or spinal stenosis.

10. Manchikanti L, Benyamin RM, Falco FJ, Kaye AD, Hirsch JA: Do epidural injections provide short- and long-term relief for lumbar disc herniation? A systematic review. *Clin Orthop Relat Res* 2015;473(6):1940-1956.

    This systematic review reported the efficacy of three anatomic approaches (caudal, interlaminar, transforaminal) for epidural injections in the treatment of disk herniation.

11. Lurie JD, Tosteson TD, Tosteson AN, et al: Surgical versus nonoperative treatment for lumbar disc herniation: Eight-year results for the spine patient outcomes research trial. *Spine (Phila Pa 1976)* 2014;39(1):3-16.

    This 8-year follow-up of the Spine Patient Outcomes Research Trial showed little to no degradation of outcomes in patients surgically or nonsurgically treated for disk herniation. Level of evidence: II.

12. McCulloch JA, Young PH, eds: *Essentials of Spinal Microsurgery.* Philadelphia, PA, Lippincott-Raven, 1998.

13. Rasmussen S, Krum-Møller DS, Lauridsen LR, et al: Epidural steroid following discectomy for herniated lumbar disc reduces neurological impairment and enhances recovery: A randomized study with two-year follow-up. *Spine (Phila Pa 1976)* 2008;33(19):2028-2033.

14. Smith N, Masters J, Jensen C, Khan A, Sprowson A: Systematic review of microendoscopic discectomy for lumbar disc herniation. *Eur Spine J* 2013;22(11):2458-2465.

    This systematic review comparing open versus minimally invasive diskectomy found no significant difference in Oswestry Disability Index scores between study groups at any point.

15. Evaniew N, Khan M, Drew B, Kwok D, Bhandari M, Ghert M: Minimally invasive versus open surgery for cervical and lumbar discectomy: A systematic review and meta-analysis. *CMAJ Open* 2014;2(4):E295-E305.

    This meta-analysis of MIS versus open surgery for cervical and lumbar diskectomy showed no evidence to support the routine use of MIS.

16. Rasouli MR, Rahimi-Movaghar V, Shokraneh F, Moradi-Lakeh M, Chou R: Minimally invasive discectomy versus microdiscectomy/open discectomy for symptomatic lumbar disc herniation. *Cochrane Database Syst Rev* 2014;9:CD010328.

    This Cochrane systematic review demonstrated that minimally invasive diskectomy may be inferior to open diskectomy in leg pain relief, low back pain relief, and rehospitalization; however, differences in pain relief were small and may not be clinically important.

17. Schoenfeld AJ, Bono CM: Does surgical timing influence functional recovery after lumbar discectomy? A systematic review. *Clin Orthop Relat Res* 2015;473(6):1963-1970.

    This systematic review demonstrated that longer symptom duration, possibly beyond 6 months after symptom onset, had an adverse effect on results after lumbar diskectomy.

18. Ambrossi GL, McGirt MJ, Sciubba DM, et al: Recurrent lumbar disc herniation after single-level lumbar discectomy: Incidence and health care cost analysis. *Neurosurgery* 2009;65(3):574-578, discussion 578.

19. An HS, Nguyen C, Haughton VM, Ho KC, Hasegawa T: Gadolinium-enhancement characteristics of magnetic resonance imaging in distinguishing herniated intervertebral disc versus scar in dogs. *Spine (Phila Pa 1976)* 1994;19(18):2089-2094, discussion 2095.

20. Lee JK, Amorosa L, Cho SK, Weidenbaum M, Kim Y: Recurrent lumbar disk herniation. *J Am Acad Orthop Surg* 2010;18(6):327-337.

21. Carragee EJ, Spinnickie AO, Alamin TF, Paragioudakis S: A prospective controlled study of limited versus subtotal posterior discectomy: Short-term outcomes in patients with herniated lumbar intervertebral discs and large posterior anular defect. *Spine (Phila Pa 1976)* 2006;31(6):653-657.

22. McGirt MJ, Ambrossi GL, Datoo G, et al: Recurrent disc herniation and long-term back pain after primary lumbar discectomy: Review of outcomes reported for limited versus aggressive disc removal. *Neurosurgery* 2009;64(2):338-344, discussion 344-345.

23. Basu S, Ghosh JD, Malik FH, Tikoo A: Postoperative discitis following single-level lumbar discectomy: Our experience of 17 cases. *Indian J Orthop* 2012;46(4):427-433.

    A retrospective review of 17 cases of postoperative discitis demonstrated that most patients do well with nonsurgical treatment, with transpedicular fixation and débridement reserved for severe cases.

24. Swartz KR, Trost GR: Recurrent lumbar disc herniation. *Neurosurg Focus* 2003;15(3):E10.

    Recurrent disk herniation can occur in 5% to 15% of patients with lumbar disk herniation. Revision surgery requires meticulous surgical technique.

25. Cho JY, Lee SH, Lee HY: Prevention of development of postoperative dysesthesia in transforaminal percutaneous endoscopic lumbar discectomy for intracanalicular lumbar disc herniation: Floating retraction technique. *Minim Invasive Neurosurg* 2011;54(5-6):214-218.

    Postoperative dysesthesia caused by dorsal root ganglion injury is a unique complication of transforaminal percutaneous endoscopic lumbar diskectomy. The floating retraction technique can help avoid this complication.

26. Mroz TE, Lubelski D, Williams SK, et al: Differences in the surgical treatment of recurrent lumbar disc herniation among spine surgeons in the United States. *Spine J* 2014;14(10):2334-2343.

    Substantial differences exist among US spine surgeons in the surgical treatment of recurrent lumbar disk herniations.

27. Suk KS, Lee HM, Moon SH, Kim NH: Recurrent lumbar disc herniation: Results of operative management. *Spine (Phila Pa 1976)* 2001;26(6):672-676.

4: Surgical Management of Degenerative Spine Disorders

Chapter 18

Lumbar Stenosis and Degenerative Spondylolisthesis

Jad G. Khalil, MD   Jeffrey S. Fischgrund, MD   Richard V. Roberts, MD

Abstract

The management of spinal stenosis and spondylolisthesis has evolved over the years. Nonsurgical management is typically attempted first, including activity modification, use of NSAIDs, a structured physical therapy regimen, epidural steroid injections, and patient education on the benefits of a healthy lifestyle (eg, control of diabetes, weight loss programs, exercise, cessation of nicotine consumption). Several surgical options are available for managing lumbar spinal stenosis with or without spondylolisthesis in appropriately selected patients. Techniques include open laminectomy, open arthrodesis, and minimally invasive surgery. Options for anterior column support include posterior lumbar interbody fusion, transforaminal lumbar interbody fusion, lateral lumbar interbody fusion, and anterior lumbar interbody fusion. No clear consensus exists that one technique is superior to another. Anterior column support and interbody fusion are used at the surgeon's discretion because of the lack of strong data to support better clinical outcomes. Minimally invasive techniques have shown promising results of faster rehabilitation, lower infection rates, and faster return to function.

Keywords: degenerative spondylolisthesis; interbody fusion; lumbar laminectomy; lumbar spinal stenosis; minimally invasive surgery; posterolateral fusion

Introduction

Lumbar spinal stenosis is a primarily age-related degenerative condition, and narrowing of the spinal canal is its cardinal feature. This narrowing results in nerve root compression, or cauda equina syndrome, at one or more levels. Spinal stenosis and its accompanying symptoms are sometimes dismissed as part of the normal aging process by patients and physicians. However, symptoms can become debilitating in some patients; thus, adequate recognition and management of this condition is essential.

Patients who have lumbar degenerative spondylolisthesis often have spinal stenosis as well. Degenerative spondylolisthesis may be primary or secondary. Primary spondylolisthesis is a degenerative condition that results from arthritic changes in the intervertebral disk space and facet joints. It most commonly affects the L4-L5 level. Secondary spondylolisthesis typically occurs at a level cephalad to a prior lumbar fusion.

The cause of spinal stenosis is often multifactorial. Degenerative changes such as spondylosis, facet arthropathy, facet orientation, disk degeneration, synovial cyst

Dr. Khalil or an immediate family member is a member of a speakers' bureau or has made paid presentations on behalf of LDR Spine, Spine Wave, and Stryker; serves as a paid consultant to LDR Spine and Stryker; has stock or stock options held in Johnson & Johnson; and has received research or institutional support from Centinel Spine. Dr. Fischgrund or an immediate family member has received royalties from Stryker; serves as a paid consultant to ISTO Technologies, Relievant, and Stryker; has stock or stock options held in understand.com; has received research or institutional support from Smith & Nephew and Stryker); and serves as a board member, owner, officer, or committee member of the Cervical Spine Research Society and the Lumbar Spine Research Society. Neither Dr. Roberts nor any immediate family member has received anything of value from or has stock or stock options held in a commercial company or institution related directly or indirectly to the subject of this chapter.

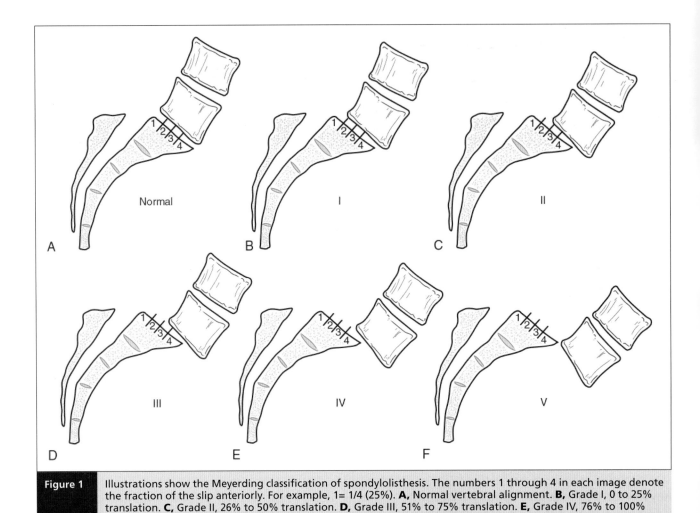

Figure 1   Illustrations show the Meyerding classification of spondylolisthesis. The numbers 1 through 4 in each image denote the fraction of the slip anteriorly. For example, 1= 1/4 (25%). **A,** Normal vertebral alignment. **B,** Grade I, 0 to 25% translation. **C,** Grade II, 26% to 50% translation. **D,** Grade III, 51% to 75% translation. **E,** Grade IV, 76% to 100% translation. **F,** Grade V, spondyloptosis.

formation, scoliosis, and spondylolisthesis all contribute to the development of spinal stenosis.[1]

Diagnosis

Degenerative spondylolisthesis is typically diagnosed based on upright lateral lumbar radiographs. On the standing (weight-bearing) lateral radiograph, a dynamic component of the slip can be revealed that would otherwise be partially or fully reduced with the patient in a supine position. Therefore, the surgeon who relies on supine MRI alone may miss the diagnosis of spondylolisthesis. The severity of spondylolisthesis is commonly determined using the Meyerding classification, in which grades are assigned based on the percentage of anterior translation of the vertebral body relative to the immediately caudal vertebra[2] (**Figure 1**).

Not only may supine sagittal MRI alone be insufficient to diagnose degenerative spondylolisthesis, but it also may not be necessary to obtain both flexion-extension and standing lateral radiographs to make the diagnosis. To test that hypothesis, the authors of a 2015 study began by determining the incidence of degenerative spondylolisthesis identified on dynamic flexion-extension radiographs but not on MRI.[3] Next, they compared the flexion-extension radiographs with standing lateral radiographs. Compared with flexion-extension radiographs, standing lateral radiographs were sufficient to make the diagnosis. Although the authors of that study agree that use of sagittal MRI alone can potentially result in an underdiagnosis of degenerative spondylolisthesis, they also modified their imaging protocol to forego obtaining routine flexion-extension radiographs and instead rely solely on a neutral lateral radiograph to identify degenerative spondylolisthesis.

Symptomatology
Patients who have lumbar spinal stenosis exhibit a typical constellation of symptoms consistent with radiculopathy and/or neurogenic claudication. This presentation is

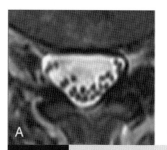 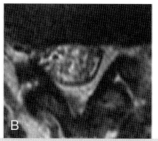 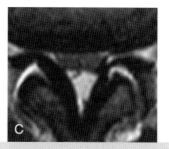 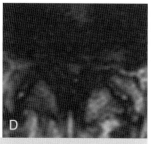

Figure 2 Grading of dural sac stenosis based on morphology seen via axial T2-weighted MRI. **A,** Grade A, minimal or no stenosis. Cerebrospinal fluid (CSF) is noticeably visible and is seen as the white area inside the dural sac. **B,** Grade B, moderate stenosis. Nerve rootlets occupy the entirety of the dural sac but can still be individualized. Some CSF is present and gives a grainy appearance to the dural sac. **C,** Grade C, severe stenosis. No nerve rootlets can be recognized, and the dural sac demonstrates a homogeneous gray signal with no CSF signal visible. Epidural fat is visualized posteriorly. **D,** Grade D, extreme stenosis. No recognizable nerve rootlets can be seen, and there is no epidural fat posteriorly. (Adapted with permission from Schizas C, Theumann N, Burn A, et al: Qualitative grading of severity of lumbar spinal stenosis based on the morphology of the dural sac on magnetic resonance images. *Spine [Phila Pa 1976]* 2010;35[21]:1919-1924.)

characterized by unilateral or bilateral buttock, thigh, and calf discomfort as well as pain or weakness that is precipitated by prolonged standing or walking.[4] Such symptoms often have a substantial effect on functional ability, quality of life, and independence because of the decreased distance of pain-free walking and decreased ability to maintain an erect posture. Patients who have neurogenic claudication often find relief via forward flexion at the waist (eg, sitting and leaning forward).

The presentation of patients who have spinal stenosis and spondylolisthesis is very similar to the presentation of patients who have spinal stenosis alone; most of the patients with stenosis and spondylolisthesis present with symptoms of radiculopathy or neurogenic claudication and/or back pain. Because spondylolisthesis may be asymptomatic, it may be an incidental finding.[5]

Imaging

The spinal canal cross-sectional area and foraminal size are substantially reduced in extension and increased with flexion.[6] As noted previously, multiple encroaching structures may contribute to spinal stenosis.[1] MRI is the most frequently used modality to assess the degree of spinal stenosis. Dural sac cross-sectional area (DSCA) is a useful radiologic method for measuring the degree of spinal stenosis. A DSCA of 76 to 100 mm[2] indicates relative spinal stenosis, and a DSCA less than 75 mm[2] indicates substantial stenosis.[7] In clinical practice, however, it is common for physicians to assess stenosis according to morphology rather than DSCA.[8] Because clinicians rely on their own visual, morphology-based assessment, a classification system was developed in which the appearance of the dural sac on axial T2-weighted MRI—specifically, the nerve rootlet/cerebrospinal fluid ratio—is assigned a morphologic grade of A, B, C, or D[7,8] (**Figure 2**). The

space available for the rootlets within the cerebrospinal fluid in the dural sac determines the grade, from no or minor stenosis (grade A) to extreme stenosis (grade D). Although a positive MRI finding is important in the diagnosis of spinal stenosis, there is not necessarily a correlation between the severity of DSCA and the severity of symptoms.[7] Thus, the value of a classification system is mainly in supporting the decision-making process rather than determining treatment decisions based on the classification alone.[7]

A 2010 study reported on a radiographic test for lumbar spinal stenosis that can differentiate between nonspecific low back pain (LBP) and symptomatic lumbar spinal stenosis.[9] In patients without lumbar spinal stenosis, there was sedimentation of the lumbar nerve roots of the dorsal part of the dural sac on supine MRI scans; in patients with symptomatic and morphologic central lumbar spinal stenosis, this sedimentation was rarely seen.[9] This phenomenon was designated as the sedimentation sign and defined the absence of the sedimentation of nerve roots as a positive sign for the diagnosis of lumbar spinal stenosis. A 2016 analysis, however, concluded that the nerve root sedimentation sign was not able to differentiate symptomatic lumbar spinal stenosis from nonspecific LBP after adjusting by the DSCA.[10] In addition, it appears that the sedimentation sign is most sensitive in defining severe cases of lumbar spinal stenosis, and it may not aid in differentiating lumbar spinal stenosis from LBP or vascular claudication.[11] Furthermore, the sedimentation sign may not add any specific diagnostic information beyond that provided by the traditional history, physical examination, and imaging studies that are currently standard in diagnosing lumbar spinal stenosis diagnosis, although the sign was shown to have a high intrarater reliability and acceptable interrater reliability.[11]

The value of dynamic imaging remains debatable. There are studies that show value in incorporating flexion-extension imaging in the decision-making process.[6] Some studies have shown that comparing supine MRI studies with upright radiographs might be a more sensitive technique to detect intervertebral translation.[6,12]

Nonsurgical Management

A trial of nonsurgical management is always recommended for patients with spinal stenosis with or without spondylolisthesis. Treatment modalities include activity modification, NSAIDs, a structured physical therapy regimen, and epidural steroid injections. Patients also are educated about the overall benefit of a healthy lifestyle, including control of diabetes, weight loss programs, exercise, and cessation of nicotine consumption. Patients who smoke tobacco experience less improvement than nonsmokers after surgical intervention to manage lumbar spinal stenosis.[13,14] An analysis of a subgroup of the Spine Patient Outcomes Research Trial (SPORT) reported that the baseline Oswestry Disability Index value and tobacco smoking were the two factors with the greatest magnitude of effect in outcomes after surgery to manage lumbar spinal stenosis.[15] A different study concluded that tobacco smoking is associated with delayed and impaired spinal fusion as well as pseudarthrosis after spinal instrumentation.[16]

Although surgeons often recommend a course of physical therapy to manage neurogenic claudication before considering surgical management, a systematic review published in 2012 found considerable variation in what constitutes physical therapy and therefore reported a lack of evidence to support a course of physical therapy.[4] Exercise was a common denominator in the therapy protocols evaluated in the systematic review, and compared with no treatment, exercise seemed to provide a short-term benefit with regard to leg pain and function. The study indicated that a supervised exercise program focused on improving lumbar spine strength and range of motion might be more effective than a home-based program.

Most patients who have spinal stenosis are evaluated first by their primary care physician, some of whom prescribe a course of opioid pain medications for patients with back pain and neurogenic claudication. However, prolonged use of narcotics can result in the development of opioid-related adverse drug events as well as overuse and subsequent dependence.[17] The use of opioids as part of nonsurgical management typically is not recommended.

Corticosteroid injections are often used as a treatment adjunct in the form of epidural steroid injections. These include injections in the interlaminar space or transforaminal nerve root and also are referred to as selective nerve root injections.[1] However, evidence is lacking regarding the effectiveness of epidural steroid injection for managing symptoms of spinal stenosis.[1] Despite the lack of convincing data, one study reported that approximately 25% of all epidural spinal injections performed in the Medicare population are for spinal stenosis,[18] and 74% of all epidural spinal injections performed in the Veterans Affairs system are for spinal stenosis.[19]

A 2012 study on data from the SPORT reported that certain patient variables are associated with a better outcome after surgical management compared with nonsurgical management. These variables include male sex, shorter duration of symptoms, higher level of education, higher income level, nonsmoking status, better overall mental health, no diabetes mellitus, and few medical comorbidities.[15]

Surgical Management

Patients in whom symptoms do not improve after a course of nonsurgical treatment may benefit from surgical treatment. For patients in whom surgery is indicated, several factors must be considered when selecting the appropriate procedure, including the pathology itself as well as patient-specific goals and overall functional status.[20]

Lumbar Spinal Stenosis

Simple decompressive laminectomy is often the preferred method for managing single-level or multilevel lumbar spinal stenosis. Laminectomy alone is recommended for patients who do not have spondylolisthesis and in patients who have low-grade, static spondylolisthesis.[21] The three components of a successful decompression are central laminectomy or bilateral hemilaminotomy, lateral recess decompression, and foraminotomy. Central laminectomy, or bilateral hemilaminotomy, is performed and extended in a side-to-side manner from pedicle to pedicle. Next, the lateral recess is decompressed, taking care to ensure complete bony removal of the medial part of the facet joint complex along with the ligamentum flavum. Foraminotomies are then performed as appropriate, taking care to achieve full decompression of the exiting and traversing nerve roots. The surgeon must preserve most of the facet joint and at least 8 mm of the pars interarticularis.[22] Overzealous decompression can result in iatrogenic disruption of the facet joint or the pars interarticularis, which could in turn result in either accelerated degeneration or spondylolisthesis, respectively.[23] Although decompression of all levels with substantial stenosis is advocated, advanced patient age or marked comorbidities may preclude an extended surgical procedure. In such patients, decompression of only the critically stenotic levels that are believed to contribute to the patient's symptoms is recommended. In patients who have unilateral symptomatology, especially if the symptoms are radicular rather than the result of claudication, hemilaminotomy with or without foraminotomy is usually a viable option.[24]

According to studies published in the past few decades, surgical management of lumbar stenosis results in favorable outcomes.[23,25] The SPORT demonstrated considerably more improvement in all primary outcomes after surgical management compared with nonsurgical management when an as-treated analysis was performed; this substantial improvement was sustained for 4 years.[23] In an 8- to 10-year follow-up of patients from the Maine Lumbar Spine Study, LBP relief, improvement of the predominant symptom, and patient satisfaction were found to be similar irrespective of management (surgical or nonsurgical).[25] However, patients who underwent surgical treatment experienced better pain relief in the leg and a greater improvement in back-related functional status.

The incidence of clinically significant lumbar spinal stenosis is increasing as the population ages, and the rising economic burden of managing this condition further highlights the need to optimize effective treatment strategies. In patients with clear documentation of focal spinal stenosis and debilitating neurogenic claudication, age alone should not be a contraindication for surgical treatment, because patient-reported outcomes have been shown to be similar between younger and older patients.[26]

Degenerative Spondylolisthesis

Historically, surgeons were advised to perform arthrodesis at the decompressed levels in patients who had both spinal stenosis and spondylolisthesis. Recently, however, increased emphasis has been placed on assessing the stability of listhetic segments to determine whether arthrodesis is necessary. Traditionally, preoperative flexion-extension standing lateral radiographs have been used to assess the potential for progression of the slip if decompression alone is performed without a fusion.[3] One study reviewed the results of patients who had spondylolisthesis considered to be stable based on dynamic radiographs (less than 4 mm of translation and 10° of angulation) and concluded that fusion may not be necessary.[23] However, if preoperative imaging shows a dynamic component to the spondylolisthesis, a fusion procedure should be considered. Other factors that reportedly increase the risk of slip progression include sagittal facet orientation, disk height, and the presence of fluid in the facet joints.[3,20,27]

Two recent studies looked at the outcomes of laminectomy versus laminectomy and fusion for lumbar spinal stenosis.[28,29] A randomized controlled trial showed that in patients with lumbar spinal stenosis, with or without degenerative spondylolisthesis, decompression plus fusion surgery did not result in better clinical outcomes at 2 years and 5 years than did decompressive surgery alone.[28] These results seem to differ from another recent study[29] as well as those of some previous landmark studies.[24,30] In a 2016 study comparing the effectiveness of laminectomy with instrumented lumbar fusion with laminectomy alone for lumbar stenosis with spondylolisthesis, it was reported that among patients with degenerative grade I spondylolisthesis, treatment with laminectomy with fusion was associated with slightly greater but clinically meaningful improvement in overall physical health-related quality of life than treatment with laminectomy alone.[29] A substantially higher revision rate during the follow-up period in the decompression-alone group than that of the fusion group (34% versus 14%, respectively) also was reported.[29] Also noted was that the addition of lumbar fusion to laminectomy was associated with substantially greater increases in the Medical Outcomes Study 36-Item Short Form physical component summary score at 2, 3, and 4 years after surgery; this signified a sustained difference between treatments over time.[29] It is recommended that patients with lumbar spinal stenosis and mobile degenerative spondylolisthesis are best treated with decompression and fusion.[20]

Outcomes after posterolateral fusion are improved in patients in whom successful arthrodesis was achieved.[23,30] Subanalyses of the SPORT trial reported that surgery for the management of degenerative spondylolisthesis showed that cost per quality-adjusted life year gained at 2-year follow-up was $115,600.[31] However, at 4-year follow-up, the surgical management became more cost-effective, with a cost per quality-adjusted life year gained of $64,300. A similar analysis of 45 patients after posterior interbody fusion for degenerative spondylolisthesis reported a value for cost per quality-adjusted life year gained of $42,854.[32] These cost-effectiveness findings compare favorably to other well-accepted cost-effective treatments such as total hip arthroplasty and total knee arthroplasty. An analysis of the Nationwide Inpatient Sample Database identified 48,911 patients who underwent surgical treatment for lumbar degenerative spondylolisthesis from 2001 through 2010.[33] Posterolateral fusion with posterior interbody fusion was the most frequently performed procedure, irrespective of geographic location, hospital size, and whether the hospital was a teaching institution (41,051 patients [83.9%]).[33]

Some controversy exists regarding treatment of patients who have multilevel stenosis and single-level spondylolisthesis. The posterior ligamentous complex helps provide spinal stability, and central decompression above a fused segment affects the integrity of that complex.[23] Because of the disruption of this posterior ligamentous complex, the fused caudal segment may place additional stress on the adjacent unstable segment, which could result in segmental instability.[34-39] However, fusion of multiple segments may result in increased stress on adjacent levels, thereby increasing the risk for adjacent-segment disease (ASD).[40-43] In the SPORT, many surgeons limited fusion to the level that demonstrated instability at the time of surgery, but some surgeons performed longer fusions to prevent adjacent-segment instability.[23] A subgroup analysis reported no clinically significant differences between multilevel fusion and single-level fusion; however, patients who underwent multilevel fusion experienced increased intraoperative blood loss and a longer surgical time compared with patients who underwent single-level fusion.[23] During the 4-year follow-up period, the revision rate was higher in patients who underwent single-level fusion than in those who underwent multi-level fusion.[23] Because of the additional surgical time and increased blood loss associated with multilevel fusions, multilevel fusion might not be advisable in older patients or those in poor health.[23]

The use of interbody fusion in the surgical management of spondylolisthesis is a topic of debate. Options for anterior column support include posterior lumbar interbody fusion, transforaminal lumbar interbody fusion (TLIF), lateral lumbar interbody fusion, and anterior lumbar interbody fusion. Interbody fusion is usually supplemented by interbody devices such as bone spacers, metallic cages, carbon fiber cages, and polyetheretherketone. Proposed benefits of interbody fusion include graft placement along the weight-bearing axis of the spine, improved spinal alignment, indirect decompression of the neural foramen, increased likelihood of fusion, improved reduction of the spondylolisthesis, and improved restoration of lordosis.[44,45]

Although studies showed increased fusion rates when interbody fusion was performed in addition to posterolateral fusion, patient outcomes were not substantially improved.[45] In fact, the routine addition of interbody fusion increases the cost of surgery, increases the surgical time of the procedure, and may increase the complication rate. One study reported an increased incidence of adjacent-segment degeneration at 5-year follow-up.[45,46]

Complications

Dural tear is among the most common complications associated with decompressive laminectomy, with an incidence rate of 4% to 9%.[47] Facet cysts, degenerative spondylolisthesis, and severe stenosis are known risk factors for dural tear. Historically, primary repair was considered the standard management. However, in a case series published in 2014, patients who were not treated with primary suture repair had outcomes similar to those of patients who underwent primary suture repair.[48] Older studies suggested that patients who sustained incidental durotomy during index surgery experienced long-term clinical sequelae.[49] However, a study published in 2016 reported that incidental durotomy did not have negative long-term effects on patient outcomes.[50]

Despite excellent primary outcomes in patients undergoing surgery for spinal stenosis and spondylolisthesis, revision surgery may be needed. Short-term causes of revision include infection and implant malposition. Long-term causes include revision surgery for same-segment disease or ASD. In a 2015 study of patients who underwent surgical management of degenerative spondylolisthesis, revision surgery for same-segment disease was much higher in patients who underwent laminectomy alone than in patients who underwent laminectomy and fusion.[51] These results confirm the findings of earlier studies that reported superior outcomes for laminectomy and instrumented fusion in the management of degenerative spondylolisthesis.[23,30]

The incidence of ASD may be increased in patients with prior arthrodesis because of alteration of the normal spine biomechanics. Factors that may increase this risk are a higher body mass index, preoperative facet and disk degeneration, and sagittal balance.[52,53] In addition, ASD occurs more frequently in patients with longer fusion constructs. These results indicate that surgeons should limit the number of fusion levels.[54]

Minimally Invasive Surgery

Minimally invasive surgery (MIS) techniques have recently gained popularity in the management of lumbar spinal stenosis and spondylolisthesis. Decompressive laminectomy can be performed using tubular retractor systems under either surgical loupe or microscope magnification. Even accounting for the learning curve associated with minimally invasive laminectomy, recent studies have shown positive outcomes of the minimally invasive method compared with open laminectomy. In a meta-analysis published in 2015, minimally invasive laminectomy was associated with reduced blood loss, shorter length of hospital stay, and a similar complication profile compared with open laminectomy.[55] The authors of that study postulated that MIS may be more cost-effective than open surgery because of the shorter length of stay and faster return to work after MIS. A 2015 cohort study of data from the Norwegian Registry for Spine Surgery reported comparable outcomes at 1-year follow-up after either MIS or open surgery.[56]

Minimally invasive adjunct arthrodesis techniques also have evolved and gained in popularity. MIS-TLIF is one of the most commonly used techniques for posterior instrumented arthrodesis. This technique allows for tubular decompression, typically via bilateral laminotomies, after which interbody arthrodesis and percutaneous pedicle screw placement are performed. One limitation of MIS-TLIF is the steep learning curve for most surgeons trained on open techniques.[57,58] Outcomes are mixed. In a 2013 study comparing MIS with open TLIF, clinical outcomes and fusion rates were comparable at 5-year follow-up.[59] Decreased postoperative pain scores, decreased blood loss, shorter hospitalization times, and earlier rehabilitation have been reported after MIS fusion.[59,60] However, other studies have failed to find strong clinical evidence favoring MIS over open techniques.[61]

In a healthcare climate in which medical care costs are increasingly scrutinized, MIS may be increasingly used should it prove to carry a lower cost of care. A 2014 study comparing MIS with open technique reported a lower total hospital cost after MIS over a 60-day perioperative period.[62] A meta-analysis of six studies addressing the subject showed no substantial difference in cost-effectiveness between MIS and traditional approaches.[63] These conclusions are limited by the current paucity of high-quality evidence in the literature.[64]

Summary

The mainstay of surgical treatment of lumbar spinal stenosis is decompressive laminectomy. In patients with same-level spondylolisthesis, posterolateral arthrodesis of the decompressed levels also is recommended. This leads to improved clinical outcomes and lower revision rates. Although interbody fusion leads to improved fusion rates, it has not been found to directly correlate with improved clinical outcomes. Newer techniques such as MIS show promising short-term advantage over traditional techniques. Longer-term follow-up studies are needed to detect clinical difference in outcomes.

Key Study Points

- If nonsurgical treatment is unsuccessful, surgical treatment can result in improved outcomes in patients with lumbar spinal stenosis with degenerative spondylolisthesis.
- Although the type of imaging required is debatable, obtaining a standing lateral radiograph in addition to MRI will detect mobile spondylolisthesis.
- Limiting the necessary number of levels involved in a fusion while providing a stable and solid construct is crucial to potentially minimizing the incidence of adjacent-segment disease.
- Although there is a learning curve in MIS for spinal stenosis, it offers a multitude of obtainable benefits for both the patient and surgeon.

Annotated References

1. Friedly JL, Bresnahan BW, Comstock B, et al: Study protocol: Lumbar Epidural Steroid Injections for Spinal Stenosis (LESS). A double-blind randomized controlled trial of epidural steroid injections for lumbar spinal stenosis among older adults. *BMC Musculoskelet Disord* 2012;13:48.

   A multicenter, double-blind randomized controlled trial is being conducted to evaluate the success of ESI for improving pain and function in patients with lumbar spinal stenosis. Safety and practicality also were evaluated.

2. Lasanianos NG, Triantafyllopoulos GK, Pneumaticos SG: Spondylolisthesis grades, in Lasanianos NG, Kanakaris NK, Giannoudis P, eds: *Trauma and Orthopaedic Classifications: A Comprehensive Overview*. London, England, Springer-Verlag, 2015, pp 239-242.

   This illustrative textbook reports trauma and orthopaedic classification systems currently used in clinical settings.

3. Segebarth B, Kurd MF, Haug PH, Davis R: Routine upright imaging for evaluating degenerative lumbar stenosis: Incidence of degenerative spondylolisthesis missed on supine MRI. *J Spinal Disord Tech* 2015;28(10):394-397.

   Standing lateral radiographs should be standard practice of care to identify degenerative spondylolisthesis. Up to 33% of spondylolisthesis is undiagnosed with supine MRI.

4. Ammendolia C, Stuber K, de Bruin LK, et al: Nonoperative treatment of lumbar spinal stenosis with neurogenic claudication: A systematic review. *Spine (Phila Pa 1976)* 2012;37(10):E609-E616.

   The authors discuss the need for large, high-quality trials to determine the efficacy of nonsurgical treatment of patients with lumbar spinal stenosis with neurogenic claudication.

5. Pearson A, Blood E, Lurie J, et al: Predominant leg pain is associated with better surgical outcomes in degenerative spondylolisthesis and spinal stenosis: Results from the Spine Patient Outcomes Research Trial (SPORT). *Spine (Phila Pa 1976)* 2011;36(3):219-229.

    Based on results of the Spine Patient Outcome Research Trial, the authors ranked outcomes according to the location of pain and treatment received. Better outcomes were found in patients with predominant leg pain who underwent surgery, followed by those with predominant LBP pain who underwent surgery, then by those with predominant LBP who were treated nonsurgically.

6. Inufusa A, An HS, Lim TH, Hasegawa T, Haughton VM, Nowicki BH: Anatomic changes of the spinal canal and intervertebral foramen associated with flexion-extension movement. *Spine (Phila Pa 1976)* 1996;21(21):2412-2420.

7. Lønne G, Ødegård B, Johnsen LG, Solberg TK, Kvistad KA, Nygaard ØP: MRI evaluation of lumbar spinal stenosis: Is a rapid visual assessment as good as area measurement? *Eur Spine J* 2014;23(6):1320-1324.

    DSCA and morphologic grading have a strong intercorrelation that can be used to evaluate lumbar spinal stenosis using MRI.

8. Schizas C, Theumann N, Burn A, et al: Qualitative grading of severity of lumbar spinal stenosis based on the morphology of the dural sac on magnetic resonance images. *Spine (Phila Pa 1976)* 2010;35(21):1919-1924.

9. Barz T, Melloh M, Staub LP, et al: Nerve root sedimentation sign: Evaluation of a new radiological sign in lumbar spinal stenosis. *Spine (Phila Pa 1976)* 2010;35(8):892-897.

10. Zhang L, Chen R, Liu B, Zhang W, Zhu Y, Rong L: The nerve root sedimentation sign for differential diagnosis of lumbar spinal stenosis: A retrospective, consecutive cohort study. *Eur Spine J* 2016; Feb 13 [Epub ahead of print].

    The authors present an evaluation of the sensitivity and specificity for diagnosing lumbar spinal stenosis using the sedimentation sign on MRI stratified by the DSCA. It was concluded that, after adjusting for the DSCA, the sedimentation sign could not be used to differentiate symptomatic lumbar spinal stenosis from nonspecific LBP.

11. Tomkins-Lane CC, Quint DJ, Gabriel S, Melloh M, Haig AJ: Nerve root sedimentation sign for the diagnosis of lumbar spinal stenosis: Reliability, sensitivity, and specificity. *Spine (Phila Pa 1976)* 2013;38(24):E1554-E1560.

    The authors discuss assessing the sensitivity and benefit of using the sedimentation sign to differentiate lumbar spinal stenosis from LBP or vascular claudication. Level of evidence: IV.

12. Anderson DG, Limthongkul W, Sayadipour A, et al: A radiographic analysis of degenerative spondylolisthesis at the L4-5 level. *J Neurosurg Spine* 2012;16(2):130-134.

    A cohort of patients with degenerative lumbar spondylolisthesis at the L4-L5 level demonstrated wide variations in the height of the disk, angulation, and translation at the L4-L5 level as well as angular and translational movement on flexion and extension.

13. Sandén B, Försth P, Michaëlsson K: Smokers show less improvement than nonsmokers two years after surgery for lumbar spinal stenosis: A study of 4555 patients from the Swedish Spine Register. *Spine (Phila Pa 1976)* 2011;36(13):1059-1064.

    Tobacco smokers have less improvement after surgery for lumbar spinal stenosis compared with nonsmokers and have a lower health-related quality of life at baseline.

14. Gulati S, Nordseth T, Nerland US, et al: Does daily tobacco smoking affect outcomes after microdecompression for degenerative central lumbar spinal stenosis? A multicenter observational registry-based study. *Acta Neurochir (Wien)* 2015;157(7):1157-1164.

    Although smokers had considerable improvement after microdecompression for lumbar spinal stenosis at 1-year follow-up, nonsmokers experienced a larger improvement.

15. Pearson A, Lurie J, Tosteson T, Zhao W, Abdu W, Weinstein JN: Who should have surgery for spinal stenosis? Treatment effect predictors in SPORT. *Spine (Phila Pa 1976)* 2012;37(21):1791-1802.

    A combined prospective randomized controlled trial and observational cohort study of lumbar spinal stenosis with an as-treated analysis showed patients improved more with surgery than with nonsurgical treatment.

16. Lau D, Berger MS, Khullar D, Maa J: The impact of smoking on neurosurgical outcomes. *J Neurosurg* 2013;119(5):1323-1330.

    The authors of this study found good evidence that smoking is associated with higher rates of perioperative complications after neurologic interventions.

17. Oderda G: Challenges in the management of acute postsurgical pain. *Pharmacotherapy* 2012;32(9suppl):6S-11S.

    A review of risks associated with opioid analgesics and the development of opioid-related adverse drug events is presented. Strategies for avoiding adverse drug events also are discussed.

18. Friedly J, Chan L, Deyo R: Increases in lumbosacral injections in the Medicare population: 1994 to 2001. *Spine (Phila Pa 1976)* 2007;32(16):1754-1760.

19. Friedly J, Nishio I, Bishop MJ, Maynard C: The relationship between repeated epidural steroid injections and subsequent opioid use and lumbar surgery. *Arch Phys Med Rehabil* 2008;89(6):1011-1015.

20. Schroeder GD, Kepler CK, Kurd MF, et al: Rationale for the surgical treatment of lumbar degenerative spondylolisthesis. *Spine (Phila Pa 1976)* 2015;40(21):E1161-E1166.

    A survey of members of the Lumbar Spine Research Society and AOSpine found that the most common surgical treatment for degenerative spondylolisthesis is decompression and fusion; a personalized surgical plan is required.

21. Epstein NE: Decompression in the surgical management of degenerative spondylolisthesis: Advantages of a conservative approach in 290 patients. *J Spinal Disord* 1998;11(2):116-122, discussion 123.

22. Sengupta DK, Herkowitz HN: Lumbar spinal stenosis: Treatment strategies and indications for surgery. *Orthop Clin North Am* 2003;34(2):281-295.

23. Smorgick Y, Park DK, Baker KC, et al: Single- versus multilevel fusion for single-level degenerative spondylolisthesis and multilevel lumbar stenosis: Four-year results of the Spine Patient Outcomes Research Trial. *Spine (Phila Pa 1976)* 2013;38(10):797-805.

    A subanalysis study of 207 patients with degenerative spondylolisthesis found similar primary and secondary outcome measures in patients who underwent a decompression and single-level fusion and those treated with a decompression and multilevel fusion.

24. Park JH, Hyun SJ, Roh SW, Rhim SC: A comparison of unilateral laminectomy with bilateral decompression and fusion surgery in the treatment of grade I lumbar degenerative spondylolisthesis. *Acta Neurochir (Wien)* 2012;154(7):1205-1212.

    The authors of this retrospective analysis concluded that unilateral laminectomy and bilateral decompression versus fusion had similar clinical outcomes overall; however, radiologic degeneration was not as serious after unilateral laminectomy and bilateral decompression than it was after fusion.

25. Atlas SJ, Keller RB, Wu YA, Deyo RA, Singer DE: Long-term outcomes of surgical and nonsurgical management of lumbar spinal stenosis: 8 to 10 year results from the Maine Lumbar Spine Study. *Spine (Phila Pa 1976)* 2005;30(8):936-943.

26. Aleem IS, Rampersaud YR: Elderly patients have similar outcomes compared to younger patients after minimally invasive surgery for spinal stenosis. *Clin Orthop Relat Res* 2014;472(6):1824-1830.

    Age alone should not deter the consideration of surgical treatment in patients with focal lumbar spinal stenosis if surgery is otherwise indicated. Level of evidence: III.

27. Enyo Y, Yoshimura N, Yamada H, Hashizume H, Yoshida M: Radiographic natural course of lumbar degenerative spondylolisthesis and its risk factors related to the progression and onset in a 15-year community-based cohort study: The Miyama study. *J Orthop Sci* 2015;20(6):978-984.

    The identified risk factors for slip progression in degenerative spondylolisthesis were identified as age younger than 60 years, female sex, the lumbar axis sacral distance, facet sagittalization, and the existence of slip at the baseline examination.

28. Försth P, Ólafsson G, Carlsson T, et al: A randomized, controlled trial of fusion surgery for lumbar spinal stenosis. *N Engl J Med* 2016;374(15):1413-1423.

    This randomized controlled trial from Sweden evaluated the efficacy of fusion in addition to decompressive laminectomy versus decompressive laminectomy alone in patients with lumbar spinal stenosis. The treatments were determined to be equally effective.

29. Ghogawala Z, Dziura J, Butler WE, et al: Laminectomy plus fusion versus laminectomy alone for lumbar spondylolisthesis. *N Engl J Med* 2016;374(15):1424-1434.

    This randomized controlled trial evaluated the outcome of adding fusion to decompressive lumbar laminectomy for lumbar spinal stenosis. In patients with degenerative grade 1 spondylolisthesis, adding lumbar spinal fusion to laminectomy resulted in clinically meaningful improvement compared with laminectomy alone.

30. Fischgrund JS, Mackay M, Herkowitz HN, Brower R, Montgomery DM, Kurz LT: Degenerative lumbar spondylolisthesis with spinal stenosis: A prospective, randomized study comparing decompressive laminectomy and arthrodesis with and without spinal instrumentation. *Spine (Phila Pa 1976)* 1997;22(24):2807-2812.

31. Tosteson AN, Tosteson TD, Lurie JD, et al: Comparative effectiveness evidence from the Spine Patient Outcomes Research Trial: Surgical versus nonoperative care for spinal stenosis, degenerative spondylolisthesis, and intervertebral disc herniation. *Spine (Phila Pa 1976)* 2011;36(24):2061-2068.

    For patients with spinal stenosis, degenerative spondylolisthesis, and intervertebral disk herniation, a cost-effectiveness analysis showed good value for surgery compared with nonsurgical care over a 4-year period.

32. Adogwa O, Parker SL, Davis BJ, et al: Cost-effectiveness of transforaminal lumbar interbody fusion for grade I degenerative spondylolisthesis. *J Neurosurg Spine* 2011;15(2):138-143.

    After 6 to 12 months of nonsurgical care, 45 patients underwent TLIF for grade I degenerative spondylolisthesis-associated back and leg pain. An improvement in pain, disability, and quality of life was reported, which suggests that TLIF is a cost-effective treatment of lumbar spondylolisthesis.

33. Norton RP, Bianco K, Klifto C, Errico TJ, Bendo JA: Degenerative spondylolisthesis: An analysis of the Nationwide Inpatient Sample Database. *Spine (Phila Pa 1976)* 2015;40(15):1219-1227.

    Analysis of the Nationwide Inpatient Sample database found that, even through the different variations in surgical management of degenerative spondylolisthesis, in the acute phase after surgery, posterolateral fusion procedures reduced the length of hospital stay, hospital charges, and postoperative complications. Level of evidence: III.

34. Hopp E, Tsou PM: Postdecompression lumbar instability. *Clin Orthop Relat Res* 1988;227:143-151.

4: Surgical Management of Degenerative Spine Disorders

35. Johnsson KE, Willner S, Johnsson K: Postoperative instability after decompression for lumbar spinal stenosis. *Spine (Phila Pa 1976)* 1986;11(2):107-110.

36. Katz JN, Lipson SJ, Larson MG, McInnes JM, Fossel AH, Liang MH: The outcome of decompressive laminectomy for degenerative lumbar stenosis. *J Bone Joint Surg Am* 1991;73(6):809-816.

37. Lu WW, Luk KD, Ruan DK, Fei ZQ, Leong JC: Stability of the whole lumbar spine after multilevel fenestration and discectomy. *Spine (Phila Pa 1976)* 1999;24(13):1277-1282.

38. Subramaniam V, Chamberlain RH, Theodore N, et al: Biomechanical effects of laminoplasty versus laminectomy: Stenosis and stability. *Spine (Phila Pa 1976)* 2009;34(16):E573-E578.

39. Tai CL, Hsieh PH, Chen WP, Chen LH, Chen WJ, Lai PL: Biomechanical comparison of lumbar spine instability between laminectomy and bilateral laminotomy for spinal stenosis syndrome: An experimental study in porcine model. *BMC Musculoskelet Disord* 2008;9:84.

40. Hsu K, Zucherman J, White A: The long-term effect of lumbar spine fusion: Deterioration of adjacent motion segments, in Yonenobu K, Ono K, Takemitsu Y, eds: *Lumbar Fusion and Stabilization* .Tokyo, Japan, Springer, 1993, pp 54-64.

41. Chow DH, Luk KD, Evans JH, Leong JC: Effects of short anterior lumbar interbody fusion on biomechanics of neighboring unfused segments. *Spine (Phila Pa 1976)* 1996;21(5):549-555.

42. Nagata H, Schendel MJ, Transfeldt EE, Lewis JL: The effects of immobilization of long segments of the spine on the adjacent and distal facet force and lumbosacral motion. *Spine (Phila Pa 1976)* 1993;18(16):2471-2479.

43. Chen CS, Cheng CK, Liu CL, Lo WH: Stress analysis of the disc adjacent to interbody fusion in lumbar spine. *Med Eng Phys* 2001;23(7):483-491.

44. Cole CD, McCall TD, Schmidt MH, Dailey AT: Comparison of low back fusion techniques: Transforaminal lumbar interbody fusion (TLIF) or posterior lumbar interbody fusion (PLIF) approaches. *Curr Rev Musculoskelet Med* 2009;2(2):118-126.

45. Gottschalk MB, Premkumar A, Sweeney K, et al: Posterolateral lumbar arthrodesis with and without interbody arthrodesis for L4-L5 degenerative spondylolisthesis: A comparative value analysis. *Spine (Phila Pa 1976)* 2015;40(12):917-925.

    This study on the surgical management of L4-L5 degenerative spondylolisthesis determined that the addition of interbody arthrodesis to a posterolateral arthrodesis resulted in equivalent fusion rates, Oswestry Disability Index scores, and Medical Outcomes Study 36-Item Short Form scores compared with posterolateral fusion alone. Level of evidence: III.

46. Imagama S, Kawakami N, Kanemura T, et al: Radiographic adjacent segment degeneration at five years after L4-5 posterior lumbar interbody fusion with pedicle screw instrumentation: Evaluation by computed tomography and annual screening with magnetic resonance imaging. *Clin Spine Surg* 2016.

    Radiographic adjacent-segment degeneration is more frequently detected by CT and MRI than plain radiography. Conserving the posterior connective components is recommended to prevent adjacent-segment degeneration seen on radiographs.

47. Takahashi Y, Sato T, Hyodo H, et al: Incidental durotomy during lumbar spine surgery: Risk factors and anatomic locations. Clinical article. *J Neurosurg Spine* 2013;18(2):165-169.

    Identified risk factors for unintended durotomy are female sex, old age, the presence of degenerative spondylolisthesis, and juxtafacet cysts. High-risk anatomic zones for incidental durotomy are the caudal margin of cranial lamina, cranial margin of caudal lamina, the herniated disk level, and the medial aspect of the facet joint adjacent to the insertion of hypertrophic ligamentum flavum.

48. Grannum S, Patel MS, Attar F, Newey M: Dural tears in primary decompressive lumbar surgery: Is primary repair necessary for a good outcome? *Eur Spine J* 2014;23(4):904-908.

    The evaluation of 14 patients with dural tears after primary decompressive lumbar surgery found that the patients can be successfully managed without primary suture repair without adverse effects on long-term surgical outcomes.

49. Saxler G, Krämer J, Barden B, Kurt A, Pförtner J, Bernsmann K: The long-term clinical sequelae of incidental durotomy in lumbar disc surgery. *Spine (Phila Pa 1976)* 2005;30(20):2298-2302.

50. Ulrich NH, Burgstaller JM, Brunner F, et al; LSOS Study Group: The impact of incidental durotomy on the outcome of decompression surgery in degenerative lumbar spinal canal stenosis: Analysis of the Lumbar Spinal Outcome Study (LSOS) data. A Swiss prospective multi-center cohort study. *BMC Musculoskelet Disord* 2016;17:170.

    A study of 167 patients in the multicenter Lumbar Stenosis Outcome Study found that patients with degenerative lumbar spinal stenosis who underwent primary decompression without fusion had an incidental durotomy rate of 9%. In the patients with incidental durotomy, there were no negative effects on long-term outcome and quality of life.

51. Sato S, Yagi M, Machida M, et al: Reoperation rate and risk factors of elective spinal surgery for degenerative spondylolisthesis: Minimum 5-year follow-up. *Spine J* 2015;15(7):1536-1544.

    Body mass index and disk height were identified as independent risk factors for same-segment degeneration, whereas male sex and facet degeneration were identified as independent risk factors for adjacent-segment degeneration.

52. Kim JY, Ryu DS, Paik HK, et al: Paraspinal muscle, facet joint, and disc problems: Risk factors for adjacent segment degeneration after lumbar fusion. *Spine J* 2016;16(7):867-875.

   The multifactorial occurrence of radiographic evidence of adjacent-segment degeneration is associated with a higher body mass index, preexisting facet and disk degeneration on preoperative examination, and a smaller preoperative relative cross-sectional area of the paraspinal muscles seen on MRI.

53. Yamasaki K, Hoshino M, Omori K, et al: Risk factors of adjacent segment disease after transforaminal inter-body fusion for degenerative lumbar disease. *Spine (Phila Pa 1976)* 2017;42(2):E86-E92.

   A retrospective study of 263 patients concluded that patients with preoperative sagittal imbalance have a statistically significant increased risk of adjacent-segment degeneration. The risk of adjacent-segment degeneration is 5.1 times greater in patients with preoperative pelvic tilt of more than 22.5°.

54. Zhang C, Berven SH, Fortin M, Weber MH: Adjacent segment degeneration versus disease after lumbar spine fusion for degenerative pathology: A systematic review with meta-analysis of the literature. *Clin Spine Surg* 2016;29(1):21-29.

   This systematic review, which included 4,206 patients, concluded that limiting the number of levels fused may have greater effect on avoiding adjacent-segment pathology than changes in fusion strategies.

55. Johans SJ, Amin BY, Mummaneni PV: Minimally invasive lumbar decompression for lumbar stenosis: Review of clinical outcomes and cost effectiveness. *J Neurosurg Sci* 2015;59(1):37-45.

   The benefits of minimally invasive lumbar decompression for lumbar stenosis versus an open approach were a shorter hospital stay, faster return to work, lower rate of infection, and less estimated blood loss. These benefits may make the minimally invasive approach more cost-effective than an open approach.

56. Nerland US, Jakola AS, Solheim O, et al: Minimally invasive decompression versus open laminectomy for central stenosis of the lumbar spine: Pragmatic comparative effectiveness study. *BMJ* 2015;350:h1603.

   Prospective data from the Norwegian Registry for Spine Surgery, which included 885 patients with lumbar central spinal stenosis, are presented. Patients treated with microdecompression or laminectomy were found to have equivalent favorable outcomes at 1-year follow-up.

57. Lee KH, Yeo W, Soeharno H, Yue WM: Learning curve of a complex surgical technique: Minimally invasive transforaminal lumbar interbody fusion (MIS TLIF). *J Spinal Disord Tech* 2014;27(7):E234-E240.

   There is a learning curve for MIS-TLIF. Technical proficiency was obtained after a mean of 44 surgeries.

   MIS-TLIF resulted in shorter surgical times, greater relief of symptoms, and improved pain reduction.

58. Nandyala SV, Fineberg SJ, Pelton M, Singh K: Minimally invasive transforaminal lumbar interbody fusion: One surgeon's learning curve. *Spine J* 2014;14(8):1460-1465.

   Obtaining proficiency and understanding of MIS-TLIF will lead to a reduction in surgical time, estimated blood loss, amount of administered intravenous fluid, and duration of anesthesia.

59. Seng C, Siddiqui MA, Wong KP, et al: Five-year outcomes of minimally invasive versus open transforaminal lumbar interbody fusion: A matched-pair comparison study. *Spine (Phila Pa 1976)* 2013;38(23):2049-2055.

   Retrospective analysis of prospectively collected data comparing clinical and radiographic outcomes of MIS versus open TLIF showed similar fusion rates and clinical outcomes such as Oswestry Disability Index scores, Medical Outcomes Study 36-Item Short Form Health Survey scores, and visual analog scale score for up to 5 years postoperatively.

60. Djurasovic M, Rouben DP, Glassman SD, Casnellie MT, Carreon LY: Clinical outcomes of minimally invasive versus open TLIF: A propensity-matched cohort study. *Am J Orthop (Belle Mead NJ)* 2016;45(3):E77-E82.

   Sixty-four patients either underwent a single- or two-level MIS-TLIF procedure. The patients continued to have the benefits of less muscle dissection and faster recovery at 1 to 2 years after surgery. Similar clinical outcomes were reported to those treated with open TLIF.

61. Goldstein CL, Macwan K, Sundararajan K, Rampersaud YR: Comparative outcomes of minimally invasive surgery for posterior lumbar fusion: A systematic review. *Clin Orthop Relat Res* 2014;472(6):1727-1737.

   This systematic review of MIS versus open TLIF suggested a balance in surgical and clinical outcomes, with comparable rates of intraoperative surgical complications. A slight decrease in perioperative medical complications was reported in the MIS-TLIF cohort.

62. Singh K, Nandyala SV, Marquez-Lara A, et al: A perioperative cost analysis comparing single-level minimally invasive and open transforaminal lumbar interbody fusion. *Spine J* 2014;14(8):1694-1701.

   The authors present the results of a nonrandomized, nonblinded prospective review of 66 consecutive patients who underwent single-level TLIF (33 MIS-TLIF and 33 open TLIF procedures). Patients treated with MIS-TLIF had shorter surgical times, length of hospital stays, average anesthesia time, and mean estimated blood loss. Although hospital reimbursements appear higher in open versus MIS groups, it is the shorter surgical time and length of hospital stay that allows the MIS technique to reduce utilization of resources and increase surgical case volume.

63. Phan K, Mobbs RJ: Minimally invasive versus open laminectomy for lumbar stenosis: A systematic review and meta-analysis. *Spine (Phila Pa 1976)* 2016;41(2):E91-E100.

This systematic review with a meta-analysis compared minimally invasive laminectomy versus open laminectomy for stenosis. Although minimally invasive laminectomy had a similar complication profile with that of the open approach, minimally invasive laminectomy was associated with a shorter length of stay and less estimated blood loss. Level of evidence: I.

64. Hofstetter CP, Hofer AS, Wang MY: Economic impact of minimally invasive lumbar surgery. *World J Orthop* 2015;6(2):190-201.

Although minimally invasive lumbar surgery appears to have the potential to be a cost-effective intervention, more studies are needed to further delineate the indications for MIS spine procedures.

Chapter 19

Axial Pain and Lumbar Degenerative Disk Disease

Richard D. Guyer, MD   Clifton W. Hancock, MD, MS, MBA

Abstract

The surgical treatment of axial back pain historically has been controversial because the diagnosis of the etiology of the pain can be challenging and, as a result, outcomes are variable. However, increasing evidence suggests that the etiology of axial back pain is discoverable and, in the case of discogenic back pain, may be amenable to surgical intervention when nonsurgical management is unsuccessful. Several options exist for surgically treating a symptomatic disk, including two broad categories of surgical options: fusion and arthroplasty. Fusion can be accomplished by a variety of approaches and methods. Many investigational devices are being used in disk arthroplasty, but only two devices have been approved by the FDA. Both fusion and arthroplasty have been demonstrated to improve outcome measures and are increasingly being considered as acceptable options for recalcitrant disk pain. Some evidence suggests that arthroplasty may offer better outcomes when compared with the currently preferred option of fusion and may potentially avoid adjacent-level degeneration.

Dr. Guyer or an immediate family member has received royalties from Alphatec Spine and Nanovis; is a member of a speakers' bureau or has made paid presentations on behalf of Carevature, DePuy Synthes, K2M, and Medtronic; and has stock or stock options held in Lattice Biologics and Spinal Kinetics. Neither Dr. Hancock nor any immediate family member has received anything of value from or has stock or stock options held in a commercial company or institution related directly or indirectly to the subject of this chapter.

Keywords: 360° fusion; anterior lumbar interbody fusion; artificial disk replacement; axial back pain; hybrid fusion; low back pain; lumbar degenerative disk disease; lumbar discogenic pain; posterior fusion

Introduction

Axial back pain resulting from degenerative, painful disks is a common but controversial indication for spine surgery. Several factors complicate the diagnosis of symptomatic degenerative disk disease and fuel debate regarding appropriate surgical management of disk-mediated axial pain. Nonsurgical management and physical therapy result in improved symptoms in most patients. However, if a minimum of 6 months of nonsurgical management is unsuccessful, then fusion or disk replacement surgery may be beneficial in select patients.[1] In appropriately selected patients, surgical treatment has resulted in reduced patient-reported pain and improved patient-reported outcomes; however, meta-analysis data indicate that such improvements may not result in significant changes in functional outcomes.[2,3] Deciding whether to surgically manage axial back pain is further complicated by the difficulty of making a diagnosis of discogenic pain. Currently, no objective pathology test, laboratory value, or radiographic imaging finding exists for diagnosing a symptomatic disk. Rather, the diagnosis is made based on a combination of variables, including a patient history of mechanically induced pain, physical examination, and radiographic evidence of disk degeneration and, in some patients, reproduction of pain on provocative diskography.[4]

Although diskography has been shown to have a high negative predictive value and a moderately high positive predictive value for disk-mediated pain at the level tested, the positive predictive value can change dramatically based on the stringency of the diagnostic criteria applied. Reproduction of pain is the most basic diagnostic criterion for a so-called positive study. More stringent criteria include thresholds for pain intensity, standards for the pressure of the injection, evidence of abnormal disk morphology seen on an imaging study, and a requirement for negative diskography at an adjacent unaffected level. However, one study suggests that performing a negative control during diskography, that is, injection of a normal/adjacent level, can induce degeneration.[5] Thus, although diskography may be the best single objective measure of discogenic pain, it is rarely used, and many surgeons make the diagnosis based on patient history, physical examination findings, and MRI findings, which may be less reliable in establishing a clear diagnosis. In addition to the diagnostic challenges surrounding discogenic back pain, the risks of surgery also are problematic. Complication rates as high as 46% have been reported.[6-8] Although surgical management of discogenic pain resulting from degenerative disk disease is controversial, such treatment can provide improvement in appropriately selected patients.[9]

Epidemiologic Data

Low back pain is one of the most common medical diagnoses in the developed world. It is estimated that more than 80% of adults experience low back pain at some point.[1,4] Structurally visible causes of low back pain such as fracture, substantial instability, and tumor are obvious pain generators, but many other abnormalities, such as degenerative and age-related changes, are more variable in their provocation of pain. A large proportion of the adult population has visible arthritis, osteophytosis, disk space narrowing, facet hypertrophy, and even disk herniation on imaging but remains asymptomatic. Because so many patients are asymptomatic, the cause of low back pain was historically believed to be either multifactorial or undiscoverable unless the pain was accompanied by radicular symptoms. This belief has since been challenged, and although not all axial low back pain is amenable to intervention, it can have an identifiable cause.[4] Systematic application of anesthetic blocks as well as provocative procedures can establish the diagnosis. In 170 patients with axial back pain, a cause of pain was established for all patients.[10-12] Disk degeneration was the most commonly reported cause of pain, accounting for 41.8% of back pain.[10]

Discogenic pain is the most common cause of axial back pain in adults, and it demonstrates an association with age. Degenerative disk disease is a more likely source of axial back pain in younger patients, whereas the prevalence of facet pain and sacroiliac pain increases with increasing age. In studies of more than 350 patients with back pain in which the etiology of pain was evaluated, the mean age of patients with discogenic pain was 43 years, whereas other etiologies for back pain had a mean age greater than 59 years.[10-12] Typically, discogenic pain manifests as a deep ache, as opposed to the sharp or burning pain of radiculopathy. Although discogenic pain can refer to the legs, the distribution is often nondermatomal and not well localized. In the same series of 3,578 patients with back pain, sacroiliac and facet joint pain were more common in females, whereas males were more likely to have discogenic pain.[10-12]

Causes of Discogenic Back Pain

Historically, vertebral disks were thought to be relatively avascular and aneural; however, they do have a neural supply, particularly to the outer one-third of the anulus fibrosus of the intervertebral disk. Although the nucleus pulposus is aneural, the outer anulus fibrosus contains nociceptive fibers from the ventral ramus and sinuvertebral nerve as well as the gray ramus communicans. Injured or inflamed disks also can acquire additional pain fibers; nonmyelinated fibers can grow into annular defects in a granulomatous repair process. Substance P; prostaglandin E$_2$; interleukin-2, -6, and -8; and tumor necrosis factor-alpha, along with other inflammatory cytokines listed in **Table 1**, have been found in abnormal and painful disks. When these cytokines are released into the anulus fibrosus of a deranged intervertebral disk, they may increase pathologic nociception.[4] Not all abnormal disks are painful, however.

It appears as though there is a difference between normal age-related degenerative changes and painful symptomatic disks. The multifactorial changes that occur in disk morphology with aging include mechanical, traumatic, and nutritional accumulated changes resulting in loss of disk height, osteophyte formation, and changes in the anulus fibrosus. This age-related, typically painless degeneration is termed spondylosis deformans. Intervertebral osteochondrosis is the preferred but less commonly used term for the more painful and symptomatic degenerative disk. Intervertebral osteochondrosis in degenerative disk disease is believed to result from the failure of the nucleus pulposus to effectively disperse load and the accompanying annular fissuring and bone marrow changes in the end plate. This annular fissuring and pathomechanical dispersion of load in a disk that is chemically predisposed by cytokines toward pathologic nociception is believed to be the main cause of disk pain. This theory fits well with many of the diagnostic hallmarks of discogenic pain, such as the tendency for pain provocation under load or with disk pressurization (as occurs

Table 1

Chemical Mediators of Spine Pain

Nonneurogenic

Acetylcholine

Adenosine triphosphate

Bradykinin

Dihydroxyeicosatetraenoic acid

Histamine

Interleukin-6

Interleukin-8

Leukotrienes

Prostaglandin E_2

Serotonin

Tumor necrosis factor-alpha

Neurogenic

Angiotensin II

Calcitonin gene-related peptide

Cholecystokinin-like substance

Dynorphin

Enkephalin

Gastrin-releasing peptide

Galanin

Neuropeptide Y

Neurotensin

Somatostatin

Substance P

Vasoactive intestinal peptide

Reproduced from Kang JD, Sowa G, Woods BI: The pathophysiology of axial neck and low back pain, in Rao RD, Smuck M, eds: *Orthopaedic Knowledge Update: Spine 4*. Rosemont, IL, American Academy of Orthopaedic Surgeons, 2012, pp 33-42.

Table 2

Options for the Surgical Management of Recalcitrant Disk Pain

Fusion Procedures

Single-sided

    ALIF

    PSIF

    Direct lateral interbody fusion

Multiple-sided

    360° (ALIF with PSIF)

    PSIF with TLIF or PLIF

    PSIF with lateral interbody

Motion-Preserving Procedures

    Disk replacement

    Multilevel disk replacement

    Hybrid fusion/disk replacement

ALIF = anterior lumbar interbody fusion, PLIF = posterolateral lumbar interbody fusion, PSIF= posterior spinal instrumented fusion, TLIF = transforaminal lumbar interbody fusion.

under diskography). The understanding of pain mediation via a chemically and neurally sensitized disk may also explain why no perfect correlation exists between pain and the presence of structural abnormalities in the disk; the pain response is mediated by the interaction of structural abnormalities with cytokines and free nerve endings and is not intrinsic to the structural abnormalities themselves.[4,9]

Surgical Fusion

Fusion is considered the standard of care for the surgical management of degenerative disk disease. Removal of the nociceptive fibers within the affected disk and restoration of stability can result in substantial improvement in pain. Good results have been achieved with arthrodesis in appropriately selected patients.[13,14]

Many techniques and myriad devices are available for achieving bony union of a spinal motion segment. These methods can be grouped into three general approaches: anterior fusion, which can be performed via an anterior or a lateral approach; posterior fusion; and 360° fusion, which consists of anterior and posterior fusion. Devices used in fusion techniques include rod-and-screw posterior constructs, anterior interbody spacers, and anterior devices that are inserted via a posterior approach such as posterior lumbar interbody fusion (PLIF) and transforaminal lumbar interbody fusion (TLIF). Several different approaches have been described, such as the midline posterior approach or the Wiltse approach. More recently, interbody devices that are inserted via lateral lumbar interbody approaches have been used. Each device has relative advantages and disadvantages. Bone graft options include local or iliac autograft, allograft, or graft substitute. For the anterior portion of the surgery, transperitoneal and retroperitoneal approaches via a variety of incisions have been described.[15] Types of fusion procedures and motion-preserving procedures for the management of recalcitrant disk pain are listed in **Table 2.**

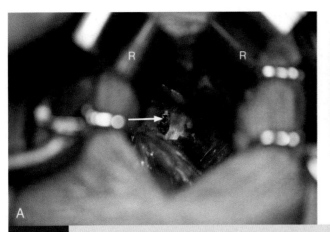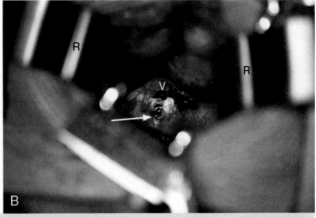

Figure 1 Intraoperative photographs show the retroperitoneal approach at the L4-5 (**A**) and L5-S1 (**B**) levels. In both photographs, the screw (arrow) marks the middle of the disk as visualized intraoperatively and confirmed on fluoroscopy. **A**, The retractor on the left side of the photograph protects the vena cava, aorta, and ureter. **B**, The vascular clips (V) ligate a segmental vessel and aid in mobilizing the iliac veins. Each retractor protects the iliac vessel on that side of the disk. R = retractor, S = screw, V = vascular clips.

Anterior Lumbar Interbody Fusion

Anterior lumbar interbody fusion (ALIF) accesses the disk space using either a transperitoneal or retroperitoneal approach. The vena cava and iliac vessels must be mobilized, and the assistance of an approach surgeon may be warranted. The bifurcation of the iliac vessels typically occurs at the L4 vertebra. Below this level, particularly at L5-S1, access to the spine is achieved through the axilla of the great vessels. An example of the anterior retroperitoneal approach is shown in **Figure 1**. The midline can be clearly visualized via a retroperitoneal approach.

Because the inferior vena cava lies on the right side of the patient's spine and is more friable than the aorta, the retroperitoneal approach typically is performed from the patient's left side. A right-sided approach could be used instead, particularly if the surgeon is working at a level below the bifurcation of the vena cava. For example, a right-sided approach might be desired when addressing a single level in a young patient, because this allows preservation of a clean plane on the patient's left side in the event an adjacent-level procedure is undertaken in the future.

The retroperitoneal approach has several drawbacks. Because the approach is lateral rather than directly on the midline, visualization may be more difficult and exact midline placement of implants can be more challenging. However, with the use of a midline abdominal incision, sufficient retraction, and a combination of direct visualization and fluoroscopy, midline placement of components is usually not problematic. Advantages of the retroperitoneal approach are substantial, particularly regarding the preservation of the sympathetic nerves and the prevention of complications of retrograde ejaculation and sexual dysfunction. According to a study published in 2003, injury

to the sympathetic nerve may result in sexual dysfunction in 13% of patients treated via a transperitoneal approach compared with less than 2% of patients treated via a retroperitoneal approach.[16] Even so, the transperitoneal approach has been well described, is safely used by many surgeons, and may provide a direct anterior approach and visualization of the vertebral column, particularly in patients undergoing revision.

After the vertebral column and disk at the desired level are visualized, a mark is made on the midline of the disk and end plates, and a complete diskectomy is performed. Blunt retractors are used to keep the vena cava or iliac vessels clear of the surgical field. Either handheld or table-based retractors may be used, but the authors of this chapter prefer handheld retractors. A collapsed or compressed inferior vena cava can be difficult to visualize and can have an appearance similar to normal areolar tissue. For this reason, the annulotomy is made with the blade of the knife facing away from the great vessels and curettage of the end plates is performed in a side-to-side manner, restricting any sharp curet to the disk space itself. Violation of the end plate must be avoided because of the risk for implant subsidence as well as increased bleeding, which obscures visualization. Vascular injury and retroperitoneal bleeding are serious complications, with a reported incidence rate of 1% to 7%.[17,18]

After the disk space is cleared, trial implants are placed to determine correct interbody sizing and then the final implant is placed. The surgeon may opt to perforate the middle of the end plate with a curet or burr to allow pluripotent cells and blood from within the vertebral body to aid in fusion. The surgeon must not violate a weight-bearing area of the end plate, however, because doing so can

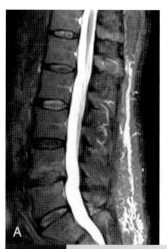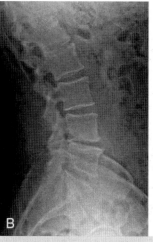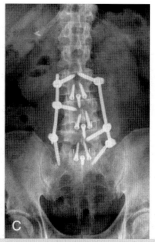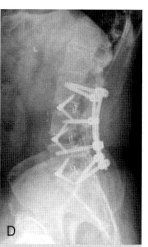

Figure 2 Images of the spine of a 61-year-old man with chronic axial back pain that did not improve after a course of nonsurgical management. Sagittal T2-weighted magnetic resonance image (**A**) and lateral radiograph (**B**) demonstrate mild listhesis of L4-5 and L5-S1. The patient's multilevel disease and instability made him a poor candidate for disk replacement, so 360° fusion was performed. AP (**C**) and lateral (**D**) radiographs obtained after three-level 360° fusion was performed to manage the instability and the painful degenerative level at L3-4.

contribute to subsidence. Performing disk replacement uses an identical approach, and end plate violation is more serious because the ensuing subsidence negates the possible benefits of a motion-preservation device.

Outcomes of ALIF are good and, historically, stand-alone ALIF or ALIF reinforced with posterior instrumented fusion (that is, 360° fusion) has been the standard against which new devices such as artificial disk replacement have been compared. A 2012 study reported a 22.3% rate of reduction in the Oswestry Disability Index (ODI) score at 5-year follow-up after stand-alone ALIF.[14] Likewise, the visual analog scale (VAS) score was improved by 40.6 points. Perhaps the main drawback of ALIF in isolation is the nonunion rate, which historically was reported at 28% to 44%.[19,20] In a more recent 2012 study, using Bagby and Kuslich (BAK) cages and autograft, the rate of pseudarthrosis was 16%.[14] However, the use of newer cage designs has resulted in improved rates of fusion.[21] The use of newer biologics as well as newer ALIF designs that incorporate bioactive surfaces such as porous titanium and fixation screws may have ameliorated the incidence of nonunion. One study demonstrated no difference in fusion rate between the stand-alone SynFix device (a polyetheretherketone cage with integrated plate and screws; DePuy Synthes) and anteroposterior fusion at 2-year follow-up.[21] Fusion rates exceeded 90% in both treatment groups. ALIF is also a good technique for maintaining or improving sagittal alignment.

360° Fusion

Posterior instrumentation with posterolateral fusion, or 360° fusion, may be performed to further stabilize

ALIFs in an effort to promote union (**Figure 2**). Fusion rates are highest after interbody fusion reinforced with transpedicular posterior instrumented fusion.[21,22] However, an increased rate of fusion is associated with the need for a longer surgical time, a second incision and the accompanying risk for infection, as well as the increased pain and morbidity resulting from dissection through the paraspinal musculature. Although in one study the addition of posterior instrumented fusion to ALIF increased the 2-year fusion rate to as high as 94%, this improvement was not significant compared with fusion rates associated with newer ALIF designs.[21] The addition of a posterior approach and pedicle instrumentation increases morbidity, and VAS and ODI scores at 2-year follow-up were lower after anteroposterior lumbar fusion compared with ALIF alone. Satisfaction rates were good or excellent after 78% of 360° fusions and 91% of ALIFs alone.

Although the addition of posterior fixation has drawbacks, it can help achieve fusion in patients in whom host conditions are suboptimal, such as those with osteopenic bone or diabetes, smokers, or in patients in whom posterior decompression is needed. Posterior fixation can also be useful for patients in whom some degree of instability, such as spondylolisthesis or other compromise to posterior structures, exists. However, some authors have suggested a trend toward higher levels of adjacent-segment degeneration with the addition of posterior fusion.[23]

Stand-alone Posterior Approach

Posterior instrumentation with posterolateral fusion for the management of degenerative disk disease can be especially useful in patients in whom an anterior procedure is contraindicated or in patients with radicular and axial symptoms in whom posterior decompression may be planned. Although some concern exists that the use of a posterior approach may contribute to adjacent-segment degeneration, many surgeons maintain that this problem can be ameliorated with preservation of the facets and careful screw placement (the latter to avoid damaging the facets).

In a study in which 72 patients were randomized to undergo posterolateral fusion with instrumentation, only 15% were pain-free at 5-year follow-up.[24] However, 66.7% of patients reported improvement in pain. The average VAS score improved to 30, and the ODI score improved an average of 18 points. In addition, by 5-year follow-up, pain medication was discontinued in 38% of patients who underwent posterior fusion. Fusion rates after posterior-only procedures also compared favorably with historical ALIF values and were comparable to those of 360° fusion, with only 7% of patients undergoing secondary surgery for pseudarthrosis.

Cages designed for posterior insertion during PLIF and TLIF have been developed in an effort to improve the fusion rate; however, use of these cages necessitates the relatively greater insult to the paraspinal musculature of a posterior approach. Minimally invasive techniques such as percutaneous screw placement may somewhat ameliorate this muscular insult, but the authors of this chapter are unaware of any studies evaluating minimally invasive posterior fusion to manage degenerative disk disease. Some surgeons have suggested that TLIF contributes to postoperative adjacent-segment degeneration. Both TLIF and PLIF require at least some nerve root mobilization for insertion, and both techniques have been associated with postoperative radiculopathy. Restoration of sagittal lordosis is more consistently achieved with ALIF than with either TLIF or PLIF.

Lateral Lumbar Interbody Fusion

The lateral approach to the spine to manage disk pain is a relatively new technique. In a study of 28 lateral interbody fusions via a lateral transpsoas approach, a 70.1% improvement in VAS score and a 52% improvement in ODI score were reported at 2-year follow-up.[25] Statistical significance was not reported. Of the 23 patients treated, 3 underwent additional posterior reinforcement similar to that of 360° fusion. The subsidence rate was 14%, but the high fusion rate of 96% was comparable to ALIF or 360° fusion. The average hospital stay was 21 hours.

The lateral approach cannot typically be used to access L5-S1 because of anatomic constraints related to the ilium. Not only are few studies available to support the use of a lateral approach to manage disk pain, but lateral transpsoas interbody fusion also is associated with a relatively high risk of postoperative thigh pain and risk of injury to the lumbar plexus, including the genitofemoral and femoral nerves.[26] A systematic review published in 2015 reported that postoperative thigh pain occurs in up to 61% of patients after lateral transpsoas interbody fusion, with motor deficit occurring in 9% of patients with more severe neurologic injury.[27]

Surgical Reconstruction

Devices

The success of joint arthroplasty in the appendicular skeleton has spurred substantial enthusiasm for joint arthroplasty in the spine. Theoretically, arthroplasty could be performed to remove a painful disk while maintaining segmental motion, which might result in a reduced incidence of adjacent-level degeneration and reduced need for revision at adjacent levels. The use of arthroplasty would also eliminate the fusion-related risk of pseudarthrosis. However, artificial disk replacement (ADR) in the lumbar spine has not had the wide success and acceptance of arthroplasty elsewhere in the body. This is likely the result of a combination of factors. First, the biomechanics of the spine, which is composed of multiple levels, each with three axes of rotation and three articulating surfaces, is biomechanically more complex than many other joints that are amenable to replacement. ADR addresses the disk but not the facet joints. Second, the proximity of the disk to vascular and neurologic structures makes disk arthroplasty somewhat more risky than knee or hip arthroplasty. Third, whereas fusion in the extremities is not desired, fusion in the spine provides a reasonable result. Although patient-reported outcomes data demonstrate equivalence or superiority of disk replacement compared with fusion, disk replacement in the lumbar spine remains controversial.[8,14,28,29]

The ideal disk implant would restore height, mimic normal biomechanics, demonstrate favorable and lasting wear properties, provide stable fixation to bone, and exhibit biocompatibility in terms of its composition and wear particles. Hydraulic, elastic, composite, and mechanical designs have been described.

In hydraulic implants, also known as nucleus replacement implants, the degenerative nucleus pulposus is replaced by a gel prosthesis.[30] Although this approach has potential in theory, such implants can only be used in patients with an intact anulus fibrosus and there is a risk of extrusion of the artificial nuclear material. No hydraulic implant has been approved for use.

An elastic model attempts to mimic normal biomechanics by replacing the disk with a polymer that is

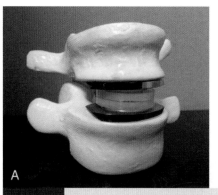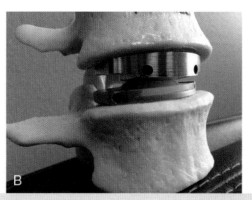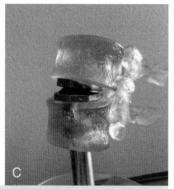

Figure 3 Photographs of formerly and currently available artificial disk replacement implants. **A,** The Charité implant, which is no longer on the market. The ProDisc-L (**B**) and activL disk (**C**) are the two FDA-approved implants currently available for use in the United States.

intended to mimic the normal anulus fibrosus. A test of an elastic model in a small number of patients resulted in shearing of the polymer.[30]

A composite prosthesis is similar to an elastic prosthesis, with the goal of creating a viscoelastic composite that mimics the properties of a normal disk.[30] No such disk replacement has been approved for use in the United States. However, the M6-L artificial lumbar disk (Spinal Kinetics), which is used outside the United States, consists of a conventional keeled two-plate design, with a polycarbonate core wrapped in polyethylene fibers sandwiched between the plates. A clinical trial of this device demonstrated results similar to those of so-called mechanical implants (such as those approved by the FDA) and indicates that the M6-L may offer the advantage of more normal biomechanics and biokinetics.[31]

The FDA-approved mechanical implants have a ball-and-socket articulation with varied degrees of freedom. Several different methods are used to integrate the metal end plates with native bone. As with many hip and knee arthroplasty options, the implants have metal-on-polyethylene articulations. The Charité Artifical Disc (DePuy Spine) was the first FDA-approved artificial disk, but it is no longer on the market. However, its design is similar to that of currently marketed implants and is discussed in this chapter because it is often encountered radiographically. The devices currently on the market are the ProDisc-L (Synthes Spine) and the activL disk (Aesculap Implant Systems; **Figure 3**).

The Charité disk was indicated for skeletally mature patients with degenerative disk disease at one level from L4 to S1, but the implant was reportedly used at higher and multiple levels.[7,14] This mechanical disk replacement has a mobile polyethylene core design consisting of a sliding plastic core between two cobalt-chromium plates. The device is nonconstrained. The end plates affix to

the end plates of the vertebrae with small spikes and titanium spray with hydroxyapatite coating to prevent displacement.[7,14]

The ProDisc-L implant was approved in 2006 for single-level use from L3 to S1.[32] It has a fixed-core design consisting of two cobalt-chromium end plates and a polyethylene spacer. The polyethylene core is domed only on the superior aspect; the inferior aspect is flat and locks into the inferior baseplate. The semiconstrained implant was designed to offer many of the advantages of the Charité implant while addressing concerns regarding potential polyethylene disk extrusion. The chrome plates affix to the end plates via keels and titanium plasma coating.[7,14]

The activL was approved by the FDA in 2015 for single-level use at L4-5 or L5-S1. Similar to the other two devices discussed previously, the activL implant uses polyethylene between two metal end plates. Unlike the ProDisc-L, the activL does not require a keel to achieve fixation to the vertebral end plates (although this option is available); instead, similar to the Charité implant, the activL has small tines or spikes that help prevent displacement. The titanium coating and anatomic shape also aid in fixation. The polyethylene spacer is locked into the lower end plate, which allows a small amount of gliding. This motion mimics the natural axis of rotation.

Several other similar devices have been evaluated in larger series and trials, but are either not FDA-approved or not available in North America. The FlexiCore (Stryker Spine), Kineflex (SpinalMotion), and Maverick lumbar disk (Medtronic) are new arthroplasty designs that have not been approved by the FDA. A recent injunction filed against Medtronic over patent infringement will bar Maverick from the US market for the foreseeable future. Maverick has a metal-on-metal–keeled design with a hyaluronic acid–coated keel

4: Surgical Management of Degenerative Spine Disorders

design to promote osseointegration, and it has a center of rotation at the posterior third of the implant.[8] The FlexiCore is similar in that it has a metal-on-metal bearing center of rotation in the middle of the implant and keelless titanium integration to the end plates. The Kineflex implant, which has a metal-on-metal keeled ball-and-socket design, was scheduled to be presented to the FDA for approval during the summer of 2016 but was voluntarily withdrawn by the company because of concerns about metal-on-metal wear.

Surgical Technique

Similar to ALIF, disk arthroplasty is performed via an anterior abdominal approach. Unlike ALIF, precise placement of the disk in the midline is critical to success. To help locate the midline, a short screw can be placed within the disk at the suspected midline, after which the midline is confirmed on a true AP fluoroscopic image of the screw. After the true midline is confirmed, a complete diskectomy is performed. Many implant systems require release of the posterior longitudinal ligament to prevent uneven tethering of disk motion. Violation of the end plate must be avoided, because such violation can cause implant subsidence and unwanted fusion. Placement of retractors is critical during the annulotomy and resection of the disk, as well as when placing the final implants, because visualization of the midline is important; retractors protect the vasculature from the passage of instruments, trial implants, and the final implant.[28,29] A lumbar disk replacement performed via a retroperitoneal approach is shown in **Figure 4.**

After the disk space is cleared, implant sizing is performed. It is important to place the trial implant toward the posterior aspect of the end plate to ensure that the center of rotation of the disk replacement is similar to the anatomic center of rotation. Anterior placement of the artificial disk can generate increased stress on the posterior facets.

It is critical to observe the edges of the trial implant and final implant as instruments are passed into and out of the disk space because these maneuvers could potentially catch and injure the iliac vein, vena cava, or a segmental branch vein. Vascular injury and retroperitoneal hematoma are serious complications that occur in 1.9% to 2.9% of patients.[28] Because of the relative risk of this step, it is suggested that any surgeon who is unfamiliar with vascular repair techniques enlist the help of an approach surgeon.

Outcomes

Outcomes after arthroplasty appear to be at least comparable with those of fusion in appropriately selected patients. Early studies were often intended to show equivalence between ADR implants and fusion and to report on the complications or safety issues associated with these devices. Recent studies with 2- to 10-year follow-up suggest arthroplasty has some advantages.[8,14,28,29,33,34]

Results of ADR are most impressive at short-term (6-week) follow-up. A retrospective study of 104 patients followed for a mean of 20 months reported a mean 5.8-point decrease in VAS score and a mean 55-point decrease in ODI score, with improvement occurring in the first 6 weeks postoperatively in most patients.[28] Unlike several previous studies, this study demonstrated improved symptoms and favorable results in 17 of 21 patients who also had radicular symptoms. Outcomes are favorable in longer-term studies as well.

In a multicenter prospective trial of 134 implanted Maverick artificial disks, the mean ODI and VAS scores decreased by 25 and 4 points, respectively, at 2-year follow-up.[8] Continued motion of more than 3° at the arthroplasty segment was noted 2 years postoperatively, and improved Medical Outcomes Study 36-Item Short Form (SF-36) and mental component summaries of the SF-36 values were noted. Perhaps most notable in this study are the positive results obtained in return to work and discontinuation of pain medication. At baseline, 43% of patients were not working and more than 90% of them attributed that status to the presence of back pain. At 24 months after disk replacement, 36% of patients were not working, and only 55% cited back pain as the primary reason for being unemployed. Whereas 87% of patients used medication to control pain preoperatively, at 2 years postoperatively, only 45% used medication to control pain. Patient satisfaction was high. This study[8] differed from an earlier study[34] in that it was international in scope, was more inclusive in that it required an institution to perform only 10 disk replacement surgeries per year to meet the eligibility requirements for study participation, and left the decision to implant an ADR up to the individual surgeon, rather than basing it on more strictly constraining inclusion criteria. These parameters address criticisms of earlier studies not being generalizable to broader practice outside of highly specialized centers. Outcomes of disk arthroplasty in the study with these broader inclusion criteria were comparable to those of previous investigations with more narrow inclusion criteria.[8,34]

Similar results were reported in a noninferiority study with a hypothesis that the composite effectiveness outcome of the investigational activL device would be noninferior to the outcome in control patients (patients treated with either of the two FDA-approved implants, the ProDisc-L or Charité).[6] For all three disks, outcomes

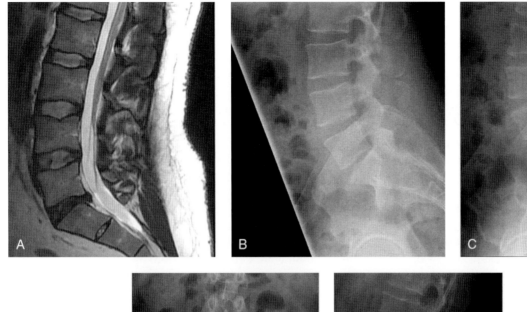

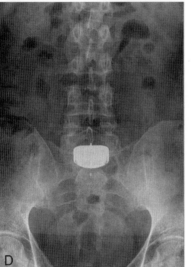

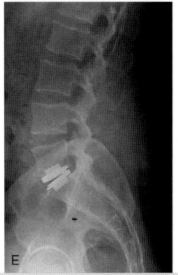

Figure 4	Images of the spine of a 37-year-old man who was an ideal candidate for lumbar artificial disk replacement based on several years of unsuccessful nonsurgical management of his symptomatic degenerative disk disease, relatively minimal degenerative changes at adjacent levels, and his high activity level. **A,** Sagittal T3-weighted MRI demonstrates the symptomatic disk at L5-S1 and minimal degenerative changes at adjacent levels. No instability is evident on flexion (**B**) and extension (**C**) radiographs. Based on the patient's age and activity level, fusion was less desirable than arthroplasty because of the risk of adjacent-level degeneration. AP (**D**) and lateral (**E**) radiographs obtained after the artificial disk was inserted.

measures were better than preoperative values, with 90% of patients treated with the activL implant and 88% of patients treated with either the Charité or ProDisc-L implant achieving at least 15% reduction in ODI scores.

Positive results have been reported 5 and 10 years after arthroplasty as well. A 2012 study reported that arthroplasty demonstrated superiority over ALIF arthrodesis regarding the return to work rate at 5-year follow-up (66% and 47%, respectively).[14] In addition, the rate of secondary surgery was lower after arthroplasty. ODI, VAS, and SF-36 scores were not significantly different

between control and arthroplasty groups when comparing stand-alone ALIF with arthroplasty.[14] In a different study, results after insertion of Charité implants and Kineflex implants were comparable to results of other artificial disks after insertion, with lower ODI scores and improved VAS scores.[7]

In a study of 32 patients treated with 33 Charité implants, long-term improvement in VAS and ODI scores were maintained at a mean follow-up of 11.8 years (7 and 28 points, respectively).[29] Patient satisfaction remained high, with 25 patients (78%) reporting that they would "certainly" undergo disk replacement surgery again under the same circumstances. The mean motion of the arthroplasty was 5.4°, which indicated continued motion in most patients. However, 7 patients (21%) progressed to fibrous or osseous fusion with less than 2° of motion; these patients did not require revision surgery.

Similar results were achieved at 10-year follow-up after insertion of ProDisc II implants.[32] Five of the 54 patients who were available for follow-up required revision surgery, but satisfaction remained high, with a success rate of 77%. When patients with negative preoperative predictors such as facet degeneration, spondylolisthesis, or lateral recess stenosis were excluded, the success rate rose to 87.2%.

Although disk replacement has been touted as theoretically superior to arthrodesis in achieving more normal kinematics and reduced adjacent-segment disease, data supporting a reduction in the rate of adjacent-segment degeneration only recently have been published.[35-38] In a 2012 study evaluating the outcomes of 1,000 consecutive disk replacements at a single center, the revision rate for adjacent-segment disease was only 1.9%.[36] This compared favorably to the results of a systematic review published in 2008 reporting the development of adjacent-segment disease in 14% of patients treated with arthrodesis.[38] Furthermore, in this series the incidence of new degeneration in previously normal adjacent levels was only 6.7% in patients who underwent disk replacement, compared with 23.8% in patients who underwent fusion.

Multiple prospective FDA trials have demonstrated ADR to be equivalent or superior to anterior, posterior, and 360° fusion techniques. Although fusion remains the standard of treatment, with improvements in technique, arthroplasty is becoming an increasingly accepted method for managing back pain resulting from single-level disk derangement between L4 and S1. Whether to expand the indications to include either multilevel arthroplasty or arthroplasty above or below fusion remains controversial. Per the International Society for the Advancement of Spine Surgery Policy Statement on lumbar artificial disks, "Based on a thorough review of the best available evidence-based scientific literature the International Society for the Advancement of Spine Surgery concludes that lumbar ADR is not new, experimental, or investigational. It is a well-tested technology which should predictably lead to better outcomes and less complications than fusion surgery, as well as a protective effect on adjacent levels."[39] However, not all professional organizations or spine surgeons agree, and, because of failures in early attempts at lumbar arthroplasty as well as economic concerns, many still view the procedure with skepticism.

Complications

Complications of ADR are similar to those of anterior fusion procedures. In a retrospective study of registry data, reported complications included retroperitoneal bleeding, abdominal wall bleeding, subsidence, retrograde ejaculation, vaginal dryness, urethral injury, and prosthesis dislocation.[8] Of the complications listed, only dislocation, which occurred in 1% of patients, is exclusive to arthroplasty. The overall complication rate after ADR is 10% to 42%; this rate varies depending on length of follow-up and what constitutes a complication.[6-8,32] In a prospective multicenter study of 134 patients who underwent disk replacement with a Maverick implant, 42% of patients experienced an early adverse event within 6 months postoperatively.[8] These events ranged from abdominal wall complications such as hernia or dehiscence to more serious complications such as vascular injury. Even relatively routine negative outcomes such as early nonspecific back pain were reported as adverse events in this study. Despite this fairly high rate of adverse events, patient satisfaction was relatively high, with 75% of patients experiencing a greater than 15% improvement in ODI score at 6-month follow-up.

Somewhat lower adverse event rates have been reported in other studies. A recent 2016 study reported an adverse event rate of 9% for two different arthroplasty options; most of the data were collected from an institution at which a high volume of lumbar disk replacements are conducted.[7] A 2013 study reported that ADR compared favorably with fusion.[24] In this study, 80 patients were randomized to undergo ADR and 72 to undergo fusion. At 5-year follow-up, complications were reported in 13 patients in the ADR group and in 9 patients in the fusion group. Complications included infection, hematoma, pseudarthrosis, hernia, nerve entrapment, donor site pain, dural tear, meralgia paresthetica, and subsidence. Suspected facet pain was listed as a complication for six patients in the ADR group; if this category is excluded, the complication rate after ADR is less than 5%, which compares favorably with fusion. Whereas 10% of patients who underwent fusion required disk replacement to manage adjacent-level degeneration within 5 years postoperatively, fusion of the ADR level was the most common revision procedure in patients who had previously undergone arthroplasty. The overall revision rate for all reasons was higher after fusion procedures than after arthroplasty (41% and 20%, respectively).

In general, complication rates appear to be similar between fusion and disk replacement. Advantages of ADR appear to include avoidance of nonunion or delayed union and a reduced incidence of adjacent-level disease requiring revision surgery.[35,37] As would be expected, the incidence of facet pain is higher after arthroplasty than after fusion.

Special Considerations and Patient Selection

Patient selection for ADR is paramount in attaining satisfactory results. The selection criteria for ADR include those for fusion to manage axial back pain, but with some additional concerns. ADR is primarily indicated for younger or physiologically younger adults. Patients must be skeletally mature, must not have substantial axial deformity, and must be young enough to expect benefit from motion preservation and to avoid subsidence resulting from decreased bone mineral density. The patients' low back pain should be attributed to a degenerative disk at L4-L5 or L5-S1 (or L3-S1 if using the ProDisc-L), and the patients should have undergone at least 6 months of unsuccessful nonsurgical treatment. In addition, the facets at the treatment level should be relatively healthy.[32]

Absolute contraindications to ADR include systemic infection, osteoporosis or osteopenia (T-score of less than –1.0 on dual-energy x-ray absorptiometry), metal allergy, substantial spinal deformity (greater than 11°), uncontrolled inflammatory disease, and instability. Relative contraindications include radicular leg pain, stenosis, herniated nucleus pulposus, anterolisthesis of grade 1 or higher (grade 1 retrolisthesis might be acceptable), and severe loss of disk height preventing implant insertion. Previous abdominal surgery and multiple level disk degeneration have been noted to be soft contraindications.

Special Concerns

Similar to arthroplasty in other joints, concerns exist regarding the biocompatibility of disk replacement implants, particularly regarding the generation of wear particles. Implant longevity is a concern, but wear particles are of particular concern because they can induce a local immune reaction resulting in osteolysis, which could cause implant subsidence and instability. Furthermore, an aseptic lymphocyte-dominated vasculitis-associated lesion, which has occurred in patients who have metal-on-metal hip prostheses, could result in substantial morbidity were it to occur in close proximity to important vascular and neural elements. However, clinically significant osteolysis appears to be rare in patients who have undergone lumbar disk replacement.[40,41] In a 2015 study on ProDisc-L implant retrieval, osteolysis developed in two of eight patients.[42] One instance occurred after on-label use of the implant. Examination of the implant suggested the occurrence of abnormal abrasion and impingement, which may have resulted in excess particle generation. The second reported case was in a patient who underwent hybrid fusion (disk replacement above a fused segment).

The implant may have been subject to increased forces and shear at this level because of the bridged segment below. A review of retrospective and prospective outcomes studies on several brands of disk replacement did not reveal osteolysis as a common cause of failure, although subsidence has been described as occurring in 1% to 2% of patients in several series.[6-8,14,24,28,29,32,34] The study did not indicate whether subsidence in these cases could have been the result of osteolysis.

Metal-on-metal reactions are potentially more concerning than subsidence from osteolysis. Although aseptic lymphocyte-dominated vasculitis-associated lesions are apparently rare, the condition has occurred in four patients treated at three institutions.[41] Three patients had been treated with the Kineflex metal-on-metal prosthesis, and one had been treated with a metal-on-polyethylene implant. As a result of the metal reactions, cystic masses developed in these patients, generating compression of the thecal sac. In one patient, the mass was sufficiently large to cause renal failure resulting from mass effect on the ureter and vessels.

Multilevel Artificial Disk Replacement

Lumbar disk replacement is an effective treatment for single-level disk disease in appropriately selected patients, with outcomes that are at least equivalent to those of more traditional fusion techniques. Two-level lumbar ADR is more controversial, however. Concerns regarding multilevel ADR include risk of coronal imbalance; hypermobility of the construct, resulting in accelerated facet degeneration and instability; and inability to attain the intended motion at both levels. Vertebral body fracture is also a concern, because the middle segment in a multilevel construct is sandwiched between two prostheses. Depending on the brand and design of the implants, keels may be cut into the middle vertebral body, which may further weaken it biomechanically, thereby predisposing it to fracture.[31,43-45] In the United States, multilevel lumbar disk replacement remains an off-label use. The French National Authority for Health recommended against multilevel lumbar disk replacement[43]

Several recent studies have reported encouraging results for multilevel lumbar disk arthroplasty.[43,44] In addition, the idea of preserving motion over longer segments remains attractive. Functional outcome scores demonstrate continued surgical benefit up to 10 years after multilevel ADR. However, the literature is limited by small sample sizes and low-quality study design.

A 2015 study reported the results of two-level arthroplasty in a retrospective review of 108 patients.[43] Most surgeries were performed at L4-L5 and L5-S1, but 15 patients underwent surgery at L3-L4 and L4-L5. A significant improvement in functional outcome on the ODI and VAS was reported, with a 13-point decrease in ODI as well as a 2.8-point improvement in radicular pain and a 4.3-point improvement in lumbar pain. Bending radiographs demonstrated continued motion at both levels in 74% of patients. Constructs from L4-L5 to L5-S1 seemed to perform best, with 87% of patients having continued bilevel motion at 4-year follow-up. The complication rate of 18% is similar to that of historical ALIF data.

A smaller study published in 2014 reported long-term follow-up data on the subset of patients from the original ProDisc-L clinical trial who underwent multilevel surgery.[44] Twelve of the 13 patients who were available for follow-up at a mean of 9.6 years postoperatively reported satisfaction with the procedure, and the mean ODI score improved significantly, from 70 points preoperatively to 12.9 at final follow-up ($P = 0.002$).

Data are mixed regarding whether results of two-level ADR are superior to those of single-level ADR. Early studies from the mid 2000s found two-level ADR to be approximately equivalent in outcomes to one-level ADR, but surgeons remained less optimistic about the use of ADR in multiple levels because bisegmental surgery was associated with more complications and was more technically demanding.[45] In contrast, a 2015 study of 121 implants in 83 patients reported a 21-point mean improvement in the ODI score after two-level ADR at 24-month follow-up.[31] Patients treated with single-level ADR had a mean 21-point improvement in the ODI score. Reduction in VAS score was similar between the two treatment groups as well. Sixty-eight percent of patients treated with single-level ADR and 87% of patients treated with multilevel ADR reported that their condition was "markedly improved." This difference in patient satisfaction may reflect the relatively greater initial disability after two-level surgery; additionally, this study used a disk replacement design that is not currently on the market. Multilevel ADR did result in a greater number of complications compared with single-level ADR.

In a large prospective FDA trial, 237 patients with two-level degenerative disk disease were randomized to either ADR with the ProDisc-L implant or fusion (165 and 72 patients, respectively).[46] Results at 24-month follow-up were promising regarding outcome measures and the incidence of adjacent-segment degeneration. Of the 148 patients from the arthroplasty group who were evaluated at 2 years postoperatively, 58.8% had a successful outcome and 73.3% had an improvement in ODI score of at least 15 points. This difference was statistically superior to the 47.8% success rate after multilevel fusion, after which only 59.7% of patients achieved an improvement of at least 15 points in the ODI score. The fusion rates are based on the 67 patients from that group who were available for follow-up 2 years postoperatively. Patient satisfaction, SF-36 scores, and narcotic usage at 2 years also improved in the arthroplasty group. However, the manufacturer decided not to apply for FDA approval for multilevel use.

The indications and contraindications for two-level ADR are less well defined than for single-level ADR, but the inclusion and exclusion criteria are similar for both types of ADR. Surgeons who elect to perform multilevel ADR should only do so in patients in whom disk degeneration is present at consecutive levels, preferably at L4-L5 and L5-S1.[31,43-45]

Hybrid Disk Replacement

Even though fusion results in improved ODI and VAS pain scores, concern for the development of adjacent-level degeneration has led to the gradual acceptance of motion-preserving surgery. Although single-level ADR is an accepted alternative to single-level fusion, multilevel ADR remains more controversial than multilevel fusion, even though it seems that a greater propensity for adjacent-level degeneration would result from longer-segment fusions compared with single-level fusions. Proponents of motion-preservation surgery cite suboptimal sagittal balance and longer bridged segments as possible reasons for adjacent-segment degeneration. Proponents of fusion suggest that suboptimal surgical technique such as facet violation and excessive posterior muscle trauma can result in adjacent-segment degeneration. A hybrid approach that combines the benefits of fusion with the benefits of ADR may be indicated for patients in whom concern exists for adjacent-level degeneration after multilevel fusion and/or who are not good candidates for multilevel disk replacement.[47] Several studies with short-term results of hybrid constructs have been published. To date, hybrid constructs appear to be equivalent or superior to both multilevel fusions and multilevel ADRs in terms of ODI and VAS scores[47,48] (Figure 5).

In a randomized clinical trial comparing the use of hybrid constructs with posterior-based fusion to manage two-level degenerative disk disease at L4-L5 and L5-S1, ODI and VAS scores were lower after ALIF with ADR compared with posterior instrumented fusion with the addition of TLIF (mean follow-up, 37 months).[47] Surgical approach may have had an effect on outcomes. All hybrid surgeries were performed via anterior approaches, and all the fusions were performed via posterior approaches. The anterior hybrid approach using ADR and ALIF was found to be a viable alternative to fusion in select patients.

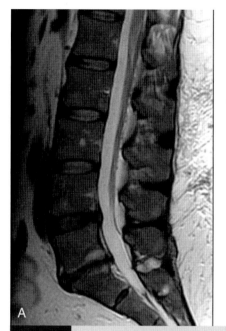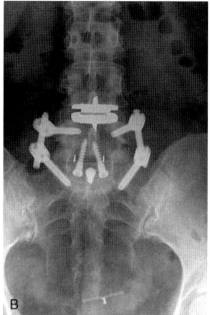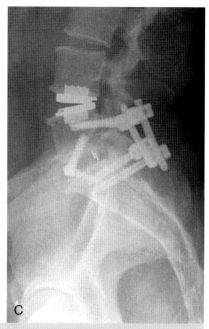

Figure 5 Images from a 43-year-old woman who experienced chronic low back pain and right radicular leg pain resulting from disk herniation at L5-S1. She had previously undergone laminotomy and diskectomy at that level but experienced re-herniation. She also had pain and degeneration at level L4-L5. **A,** Preoperative sagittal T2-weighted MRI. AP (**B**) and lateral (**C**) radiographs obtained after a hybrid approach consisting of anterior lumbar interbody fusion at L5-S1 and disk replacement at L4-L5 with the ProDisc-L to manage the stenosis and herniation as well as the painful L4-L5 diskography level while preserving motion and possibly delaying symptomatic degeneration at more superior levels.

Two-level hybrid constructs also seem to be at least equivalent if not superior to multilevel disk replacement. A hybrid approach may be an option for a greater number of patients, because it does not necessitate the presence of healthy facet joints at the lowest level. In addition, hybrid constructs are associated with lower ODI and VAS scores postoperatively and at 2-year follow-up. In a prospective study of 42 patients undergoing a hybrid technique, ODI scores had improved 53% by 2-year follow up.[48]

There are no clear indications for hybrid fixation. Possible indications include degenerative disk disease of at least two levels, failure of at least 1 year of nonsurgical management, and abnormal imaging findings as well as good posterior musculature. Contraindications are similar to those mentioned previously.[48]

Summary

The etiology of low back pain is often discoverable through examination, imaging, history, and diagnostic injection. A substantial number of patients with low back pain have pain attributable to degenerative disks. Discogenic back pain management is primarily nonsurgical, and modalities such as physical therapy, anti-inflammatory drugs, injections, and activity modification are the first-line interventions. However, in patients who have continued pain that is recalcitrant to nonsurgical management, surgical options exist and have been shown to improve functional and outcome measures in multiple studies. Diskectomy and fusion are the preferred surgical methods for managing discogenic pain and can be accomplished by methods such as posterior spinal instrumented fusion, ALIF, TLIF, PLIF, and lateral interbody fusion, or a combination of these methods. More recently, lumbar disk arthroplasty has been used to address discogenic pain. Unlike fusion, arthroplasty is touted to preserve motion at the surgical segment, thus reducing transferred/abnormal forces on the adjacent levels. This may reduce adjacent-level degeneration and reduce revision rates. Measures such as ODI and VAS suggest slightly better outcomes with arthroplasty than fusion in patients with single-level discogenic pain, although fusion still remains the preferred method of surgical intervention. Multilevel and hybrid use of lumbar arthroplasty also has been described with encouraging results but remains a new and unapproved use of these devices and is considered controversial.

Key Study Points

- Contrary to classic teaching, most axial back pain has a discoverable etiology.

- Surgery for discogenic pain remains controversial. Multiple studies have reported convincing positive results in pain reduction, high patient satisfaction, and improvement in quality of life. However, a well-publicized meta-analysis suggested that patient functional outcomes may remain unchanged compared with nonsurgical treatment.

- The preferred method for surgical treatment of a painful disk is diskectomy and fusion, but lumbar disk replacement is becoming increasingly common and has outcomes that compare favorably with fusion.

- Use of arthroplasty at multiple levels or as part of a hybrid construct has been described with favorable results, but remains an off-label use of lumbar disk replacement.

Annotated References

1. Baliga S, Treon K, Craig NJ: Low back pain: Current surgical approaches. *Asian Spine J* 2015;9(4):645-657.

   This article provides a broad overview of the etiologies and diagnosis of axial back pain along with surgical approaches. The authors discuss ALIF, 360° fusion, lateral fusion, and disk replacement along with some of the difficulties and controversies surrounding each technique.

2. Ibrahim T, Tleyjeh IM, Gabbar O: Surgical versus non-surgical treatment of chronic low back pain: A meta-analysis of randomised trials. *Int Orthop* 2008;32(1):107-113.

3. Bydon M, De la Garza-Ramos R, Macki M, Baker A, Gokaslan AK, Bydon A: Lumbar fusion versus non-operative management for treatment of discogenic low back pain: A systematic review and meta-analysis of randomized controlled trials. *J Spinal Disord Tech* 2014;27(5):297-304.

   A systematic review and meta-analysis of five randomized controlled trials on treating axial back pain is presented. In three studies, analysis showed a statistically significant improvement in the ODI score in the group treated with lumbar fusion, but pooled data revealed no significant difference when compared with the group treated nonsurgically. An overall 7.39-point improvement was reported in the ODI score favoring lumbar fusion, but the authors suggested that this might not be a clinically significant difference. They concluded that either surgical intervention or nonsurgical management is an acceptable treatment.

4. Maus TP, Aprill CN: Lumbar diskogenic pain, provocation diskography, and imaging correlates. *Radiol Clin North Am* 2012;50(4):681-704.

   This article reviews the concept of discogenic pain as one etiology of axial back pain and discusses the role of diskography in the diagnosis of lumbar discogenic pain. It also discusses the literature describing the noninvasive diagnosis of discogenic pain along with less invasive modalities.

5. Carragee EJ, Don AS, Hurwitz EL, Cuellar JM, Carrino JA, Herzog R: Does discography cause accelerated progression of degeneration changes in the lumbar disc: A ten-year matched cohort study. *Spine (Phila Pa 1976)* 2009;34(21):2338-2345.

6. Garcia R Jr, Yue JJ, Blumenthal S, et al: Lumbar total disc replacement for discogenic low back pain: Two-year outcomes of the activL multicenter randomized controlled IDE clinical trial. *Spine (Phila Pa 1976)* 2015;40(24):1873-1881.

   This prospective, multicenter, randomized controlled noninferiority trial reported on lumbar ADRs in patients with symptomatic degenerative disk disease at a single level. This study compared the investigational activL disk replacement with two FDA-approved control devices (ProDisc-L and Charite). The activL disk was found noninferior to the control devices (*P* <0.001). Level of evidence: II.

7. Guyer RD, Pettine K, Roh JS, et al: Five-year follow-up of a prospective, randomized trial comparing two lumbar total disc replacements. *Spine (Phila Pa 1976)* 2016;41(1):3-8.

   This prospective, randomized controlled, multicenter study compared outcomes of the Charité Artificial Disc and the Kineflex-L artificial disk at a follow-up of 5 years. Also reported are data on serum ion levels in the subgroup of patients receiving metal-on-metal implants. Level of evidence: I.

8. Assaker R, Ritter-Lang K, Vardon D, et al: Maverick total disc replacement in a real-world patient population: A prospective, multicentre, observational study. *Eur Spine J* 2015;24(9):2047-2055.

   This prospective international study collected outcomes data on the Maverick ADR for 2 years postoperatively. Statistically significant improvements in mean disability (–25.4) and low back pain intensity (–4.0) scores were observed at 6 months postoperatively (*P* <0.0001). The complication rate was reported to be 42%. The outcome and complication rates in this study may be more applicable to ADRs performed outside of large, high-volume centers because the minimum number of ADRs performed per year at the participating sites was only 10.

9. Mirza SK, Deyo RA, Heagerty PJ, Turner JA, Martin BI, Comstock BA: One-year outcomes of surgical versus nonsurgical treatments for discogenic back pain: A community-based prospective cohort study. *Spine J* 2013;13(11):1421-1433.

This prospective cohort study reported on patients with axial back pain seeking surgical consultation. Outcomes data are reported on patients presenting with discogenic axial back pain, and surgically and nonsurgically treated groups are compared. After controlling for baseline differences between groups, surgical treatment showed some benefit over nonsurgical treatment.

10. DePalma MJ, Ketchum JM, Saullo T: What is the source of chronic low back pain and does age play a role? *Pain Med* 2011;12(2):224-233.

In 358 consecutive patients with back pain, 153 underwent definitive diagnostic injections to determine the source of the pain. In all patients, the cause of pain was determined. This study investigated the association between age and etiology of back pain. The authors found that, the younger the patient, the more likely that low back pain is discogenic pain. Facet or sacroiliac joint pain is more likely in older adults.

11. DePalma MJ, Ketchum JM, Saullo TR: Multivariable analyses of the relationships between age, gender, and body mass index and the source of chronic low back pain. *Pain Med* 2012;13(4):498-506.

The authors of this study report on the same group of patients that they described in a 2011 study. One hundred fifty-three patients underwent definitive diagnostic injections to determine the source of their back pain, which was determined in all the patients. Associations were found between low back pain and age, body mass index, and sex. Younger males were more likely to have degenerative disk disease as an etiology for low back pain, whereas females were more likely to have facet joint or sacroiliac joint pain. Older age was associated with an increasing likelihood of having a nondiscogenic source of pain.

12. DePalma MJ, Ketchum JM, Trussell BS, Saullo TR, Slipman CW: Does the location of low back pain predict its source? *PM R* 2011;3(1):33-39.

In 156 patients with low back pain, each patient was queried as to the exact location of the pain. The presence of midline low back pain was found to be suggestive of pain from the anulus fibrosus of a deranged intervertebral disk. Paramidline low back pain was associated with facet or sacroiliac joint pain. Diagnostic injections were successfully used to determine the etiology of pain in all of the patients.

13. McGrory JE, Guyer RD: Lumbar fusion: A defensible option for discogenic low back pain? *Semin Spine Surg* 2011;23(4):227-234.

A discussion of the difficulty and controversy surrounding the surgical treatment of axial discogenic back pain is presented. The use of diskography as well as the outcomes and fusion rates of several fusion methods are discussed.

14. Guyer RD, Thongtrangan I, Ohnmeiss DD: Outcomes of CHARITE lumbar artificial disk versus fusion: 5-year data. *Semin Spine Surg* 2012;24(1):32-36.

The 5-year results of ADR using the Charité disk were compared against results in a control group treated with ALIF with iliac crest autograft. Useful outcomes data for both ALIF and ADR are reported, including VAS and ODI scores. In this study, the ADR group had improved functional outcomes based on the ODI, VAS, and some components of the SF-36. The incidence of adjacent-level degeneration was lower for ADR than for that of the fusion group.

15. Mobbs RJ, Phan K, Malham G, Seex K, Rao PJ: Lumbar interbody fusion: Techniques, indications and comparison of interbody fusion options including PLIF, TLIF, MI-TLIF, OLIF/ATP, LLIF and ALIF. *J Spine Surg* 2015;1(1):2-18.

The authors discuss surgical options for interbody fusion of the lumbar spine, including PLIF, ALIF, TLIF, minimally invasive TLIF, oblique fusion approaches, and lateral lumbar interbody fusion. Basic technical descriptions of each approach as well as associated risks are discussed.

16. Sasso RC, Burkus JK, LeHuec JC: Retrograde ejaculation after anterior lumbar interbody fusion: Transperitoneal versus retroperitoneal exposure. *Spine (Phila Pa 1976)* 2003;28(10):1023-1026.

17. Mobbs RJ, Phan K, Daly D, Rao PJ, Lennox A: Approach-related complications of anterior lumbar interbody fusion: Results of a combined spine and vascular surgical team. *Global Spine J* 2016;6(2):147-154.

A retrospective analysis of prospectively collected cohort data on complications and outcomes of patients undergoing ALIF for lumbar fusion is presented. Complications included intraoperative vascular injury, retroperitoneal hematoma, and retrograde ejaculation. Importantly, this article also evaluated ALIF with the use of an approach surgeon. The inclusion of a vascular surgeon is recommended to reduce complications and length of hospital stay.

18. Bateman DK, Millhouse PW, Shahi N, et al: Anterior lumbar spine surgery: A systematic review and meta-analysis of associated complications. *Spine J* 2015;15(5):1118-1132.

This systematic review of the literature investigated complications associated with anterior lumbar spine surgery. The overall complication rate was 14.1%. Complications included venous injury (3.2%) and retrograde ejaculation (2.7%). The possible use of an access surgeon is discussed.

19. Stauffer RN, Coventry MB: Anterior interbody lumbar spine fusion: Analysis of Mayo Clinic series. *J Bone Joint Surg Am* 1972;54(4):756-768.

20. Penta M, Fraser RD: Anterior lumbar interbody fusion. A minimum 10-year follow-up. *Spine (Phila Pa 1976)* 1997;22(20):2429-2434.

21. Strube P, Hoff E, Hartwig T, Perka CF, Gross C, Putzier M: Stand-alone anterior versus anteroposterior lumbar interbody single-level fusion after a mean follow-up of 41 months. *J Spinal Disord Tech* 2012;25(7):362-369.

Fusion rates have been reported to be higher after ALIF with transpedicular fixation than those of ALIF alone.

4: Surgical Management of Degenerative Spine Disorders

However, some new ALIF devices using integrated screws are now available and may not require posterior instrumentation to achieve similar fusion rates. This study investigates one such device. VAS and ODI scores, complication rates for traditional 360° ALIF, and integrated devices are discussed.

22. Christensen FB: Lumbar spinal fusion. Outcome in relation to surgical methods, choice of implant and postoperative rehabilitation. *Acta Orthop Scand Suppl* 2004;75(313):2-43.

23. Park P, Garton HJ, Gala VC, Hoff JT, McGillicuddy JE: Adjacent segment disease after lumbar or lumbosacral fusion: Review of the literature. *Spine (Phila Pa 1976)* 2004;29(17):1938-1944.

24. Sköld C, Tropp H, Berg S: Five-year follow-up of total disc replacement compared to fusion: A randomized controlled trial. *Eur Spine J* 2013;22(10):2288-2295.

   In this prospective randomized controlled trial, 152 patients underwent treatment with either ADR or fusion. ODI and SF-36 measures were collected at 1, 2, and 5 years. Both groups showed clinical improvement at 5-year follow-up, but ODI improvement was greater in the ADR group. Important to this study is its unusually high 99% follow-up rate at 5 years.

25. Marchi L, Oliveira L, Amaral R, et al: Lateral interbody fusion for treatment of discogenic low back pain: Minimally invasive surgical techniques. *Adv Orthop* 2012;2012:282068.

   Outcomes of lateral interbody fusion performed for discogenic back pain in a small group of 22 patients are reported along with radiographic data. Good descriptions of the lateral approach and interbody technique are provided. Fusion was achieved in 93% of the patients and, at the 24-month follow-up, improvement was reported in the mean ODI score.

26. Mandelli C, Colombo EV, Sicuri GM, Mortini P: Lumbar plexus nervous distortion in XLIF® approach: An anatomic study. *Eur Spine J* 2016;25(12):4155-4163.

   This anatomic cadaver study describes proximity of the lumbar plexus during the lateral interbody approach at the L2-L3 and L4-L5 levels. Distortion of the femoral nerve or genitofemoral nerve while docking or opening the retractor was analyzed.

27. Gammal ID, Spivak JM, Bendo JA: Systematic review of thigh symptoms after lateral transpsoas interbody fusion for adult patients with degenerative lumbar spine disease. *Int J Spine Surg* 2015;9:62.

   This systematic review of the literature evaluating postoperative thigh symptoms in patients treated with lateral interbody fusion showed that the incidence of thigh symptoms varied in the studies reported. The incidence was as high as 60.7% overall, and as many as 9.3% of patients sustained a nerve injury that resulted in a motor deficit.

28. Mostofi K: Total disc arthroplasty for treating lumbar degenerative disc disease. *Asian Spine J* 2015;9(1):59-64.

   This retrospective study of 104 patients treated with ADR reported improvements in outcomes data. Of importance, 92 of 104 patients returned to work after surgery. The complications rate of 9.6% compared favorably with rates reported in the literature.

29. Lu SB, Hai Y, Kong C, et al: An 11-year minimum follow-up of the Charite III lumbar disc replacement for the treatment of symptomatic degenerative disc disease. *Eur Spine J* 2015;24(9):2056-2064.

   This study reports the 11-year outcomes of the Charité III ADR in 35 patients. A successful outcome was reported in 87.5 % of the patients. Revision surgery was performed in two patients for adjacent-segment degeneration and pedicle fracture. Implant motion and radiographic appearance also were evaluated.

30. Sakalkale DP, Bhagia SA, Slipman CW: A historical review and current perspective on the intervertebral disc prosthesis. *Pain Physician* 2003;6(2):195-198.

31. Schätz C, Ritter-Lang K, Gössel L, Dreßler N: Comparison of single-level and multiple-level outcomes of total disc arthroplasty: 24-month results. *Int J Spine Surg* 2015;9:14.

   A multicenter, prospective study of the implantation of the M6-L artificial lumbar disk in 83 patients with discogenic back pain found that patients treated with single- or double-level ADR, showed improvement in both ODI and VAS scores at 24 months. Importantly, the M6-L represents a viscoelastic, rather than purely mechanical implant.

32. Park SJ, Lee CS, Chung SS, Lee KH, Kim WS, Lee JY: Long-term outcomes following lumbar total disc replacement using ProDisc-II: Average 10-year follow-up at a single institute. *Spine (Phila Pa 1976)* 2016;41(11):971-977.

   Patients treated using the ProDisc-II implant were analyzed at 1, 2, 5, 7, and 10 years after surgery. Interestingly, patients were grouped into "good" and "bad" groups; "good" patients underwent surgery for degenerative disk disease, whereas "bad" patients underwent ADR for mixed pathologies. ODI scores were improved at all time points. Success rates and patient satisfaction were higher in patients who were "good" candidates than in patients with broader indications for treatment. A strict patient selection process is mandatory for successful outcomes in ADR. Level of evidence: IV.

33. Gornet MF, Schranck F, Wharton ND, et al: Optimizing success with lumbar disc arthroplasty. *Eur Spine J* 2014;23(10):2127-2135.

   Using data from a prospective study on ADR, the imaging studies of 99 patients treated with single-level lumbar disk arthroplasty were evaluated to identify variables that were significantly associated with good or bad outcomes at the 5-year follow-up. Factors associated with poor results included preoperative disk height less than 8 mm, Modic type 2 changes elsewhere (multilevel disease), low lordosis, misshapen end plates (flat or convex), low levels of fatty replacement in the paraspinal musculature, and substantial facet joint or disk degeneration. Better patient outcomes were associated with a larger percentage of the end plate covered with the implant, larger implant heights, greater increases in disk space heights, and near-normal lumbar lordosis.

34. Gornet MF, Burkus JK, Dryer RF, Peloza JH: Lumbar disc arthroplasty with Maverick disc versus stand-alone interbody fusion: A prospective, randomized, controlled, multicenter investigational device exemption trial. *Spine (Phila Pa 1976)* 2011;36(25):E1600-E1611.

The results of trial use of the Maverick ADR for single-level discogenic pain in 577 patients is reported. This study compared the Maverick ADR with stand-alone ALIF. Importantly, the results of ADR are more impressive because differences in outcomes should not be attributable to any posterior approach and instrumentation in the control group. The ADR group had significantly better improvement in outcome measures and patient satisfaction.

35. Blumenthal SL, Zigler JE, Guyer RD, Ohnmeiss DD: Abstract 523: Long-term evaluation of re-operation rates for lumbar total disc replacement and fusion: Analysis of 1,237 patients. International Society for the Advancement of Spine Surgery 2013 Annual Conference. Scottsdale, Arizona, International Society for the Study of the Lumbar Spine, 2013, Available at http://www.isass.org/abstracts/isass13_oral_posters/isass13-523-Long-term-Evaluation-of-Re-operation-Rates-for-Lumbar-Total-Disc-Repla.html, Accessed January 25, 2017.

Analysis was conducted on a database of all ADRs performed at a large spine center with a high volume of ADRs (1,237 patients from 5 different investigational studies, including 67 control patients treated with fusion). Patients were treated with single-level, multilevel, or hybrid ADRs. The longest follow-up was 134 months. Revision rates were 10.4% for ADRs, 11.6% for hybrid ADRs, and 20.9% for fusions.

36. Zigler JE, Glenn J, Delamarter RB: Five-year adjacent-level degenerative changes in patients with single-level disease treated using lumbar total disc replacement with Pro-Disc-L versus circumferential fusion. *J Neurosurg Spine* 2012;17(6):504-511.

This study reported 5-year results of adjacent-level degenerative changes in patients treated with ADR versus fusion. No changes in adjacent levels occurred at 5 years in 90.8% of ADR patients. This rate compares favorably with results of fusion in which 71.4% of patients did not have progression of adjacent-level degeneration.

37. Rainey S, Blumenthal SL, Zigler JE, Guyer RD, Ohnmeiss DD: Analysis of adjacent segment reoperation after lumbar total disc replacement. *Int J Spine Surg* 2012;6:140-144.

This retrospective review of charts and radiographs from 1,000 patients who underwent ADR reported a revision rate of 2.0% for adjacent-level degeneration. Preoperative MRI data for adjacent-level pathology were reported for this group.

38. Harrop JS, Youssef JA, Maltenfort M, et al: Lumbar adjacent segment degeneration and disease after arthrodesis and total disc arthroplasty. *Spine (Phila Pa 1976)* 2008;33(15):1701-1707.

39. Zigler J, Garcia R: ISASS Policy Statement: Lumbar artificial disc. *Int J Spine Surg* 2015;9:7.

This policy statement from the International Society for the Advancement of Spine Surgery is intended to educate providers (and insurance companies) about recent evidence on ADR. The current devices available are discussed and suggested indications for ADR are reviewed along with an overview of recent outcomes studies. Universal insurance coverage was recommended for single-level lumbar ADR in patients meeting established selection criteria.

40. Veruva SY, Lanman TH, Isaza JE, MacDonald DW, Kurtz SM, Steinbeck MJ: UHMWPE wear debris and tissue reactions are reduced for contemporary designs of lumbar total disc replacements. *Clin Orthop Relat Res* 2015;473(3):987-998.

A histologic analysis was performed on tissue samples obtained from 11 ADR explantations. Seven samples were from mobile-bearing ADRs and four were from fixed-bearing ADRs. No significant differences were attributed to the type of implant. Particle-induced reactions in ADR and the relative rarity of significant osteolysis are discussed.

41. Guyer RD, Shellock J, MacLennan B, et al: Early failure of metal-on-metal artificial disc prostheses associated with lymphocytic reaction: Diagnosis and treatment experience in four cases. *Spine (Phila Pa 1976)* 2011;36(7):E492-E497.

In this case report, four ADRs were revised because of metal-on-metal reactions. Cystic masses developed in these patients, which caused compression of the thecal sac. In one patient, the mass was sufficiently large to cause renal failure resulting from the mass' effect on the ureter and vessels. Three patients received a metal-on-metal prosthesis, and one received a metal-on-polyethylene implant.

42. Veruva SY, Lanman TH, Hanzlik JA, Kurtz SM, Steinbeck MJ: Rare complications of osteolysis and periprosthetic tissue reactions after hybrid and non-hybrid total disc replacement. *Eur Spine J* 2015;24(suppl 4):S494-S501.

The authors discuss two cases of particle-induced tissue reactions after ADR. Symptomatic osteolysis, which is a relatively rare complication in ADR, occurred.

43. Trincat S, Edgard-Rosa G, Geneste G, Marnay T: Two-level lumbar total disc replacement: Functional outcomes and segmental motion after 4 years. *Orthop Traumatol Surg Res* 2015;101(1):17-21.

This study reports on outcomes after 4 years of two-level lumbar disk replacement in 108 patients. Two-level arthroplasty demonstrated improvement in outcome measures. This study also discusses some of the controversy surrounding multilevel disk replacement, including the French

Health Authority recommendation against multilevel arthroplasty

44. Balderston JR, Gertz ZM, McIntosh T, Balderston RA: Long-term outcomes of 2-level total disc replacement using ProDisc-L: Nine- to 10-year follow-up. *Spine* 2014;39(11):906-910.

    Fifteen patients who underwent two-level lumbar ADR were assessed preoperatively and at 2, 5, and 9 years postoperatively. Substantial improvement in ODI was reported at the 2-year follow-up and was maintained at the 9-year follow-up.

45. Di Silvestre M, Bakaloudis G, Lolli F, Vommaro F, Parisini P: Two-level total lumbar disc replacement. *Eur Spine J* 2009;18(suppl 1):64-70.

46. Delamarter R, Zigler JE, Balderston RA, Cammisa FP, Goldstein JA, Spivak JM: Prospective, randomized, multicenter Food and Drug Administration investigational device exemption study of the ProDisc-L total disc replacement compared with circumferential arthrodesis for the treatment of two-level lumbar degenerative disc disease: Results at twenty-four months. *J Bone Joint Surg Am* 2011;93(8):705-715.

    This randomized controlled trial compared 237 patients treated with ADR or circumferential arthrodesis. At 2 years, 58.8% of ADR patients met criteria that allowed classification of treatment success compared with 47.8% in the arthrodesis group. In addition, ODI and SF-36 measures were significantly better in the ADR group than the fusion group. This study used ALIF with posterior spinal interbody fusion rather than stand-alone ALIF. As such, it is uncertain if the improvements in outcomes are attributable to motion preservation or avoidance of posterior approaches. Level of evidence: I.

47. Hoff EK, Strube P, Pumberger M, Zahn RK, Putzier M: ALIF and total disc replacement versus 2-level circumferential fusion with TLIF: A prospective, randomized, clinical and radiological trial. *Eur Spine J* 2016;25(5):1558-1566.

    Outcomes data from hybrid fusions (ADR with an adjacent-level fusion) are compared with two-level TLIF with posterior pedicle screw stabilization at L4-S1 in 64 patients. At a mean follow-up of 37 months, patients treated with hybrid fusion had significantly lower VAS scores immediately postoperatively and at follow-up compared with the TLIF patients.

48. Le Huec JC, Aunoble S, Meyrat R, Al Sawad Y: Hybrid surgery: Fusion and disc arthroplasty is superior to two disc arthroplasties in the lumbar spine. Randomized controlled trial. *World Spinal Column J* 2010;1:2-10.

Chapter 20

Sacroiliac Joint Dysfunction

John Glaser, MD

Abstract

Sacroiliac joint dysfunction as a cause of sacroiliac joint pain can be difficult to discern. Evaluation should consist of a thorough history, physical examination, and diagnostic imaging, which can include diagnostic injections. Although nonsurgical measures often are effective, surgical treatment can be considered in the appropriate candidate, if necessary. Percutaneous surgical techniques have recently become common for the treatment of sacroiliac joint pain.

Keywords: diagnostic injection; percutaneous; sacroiliac joint

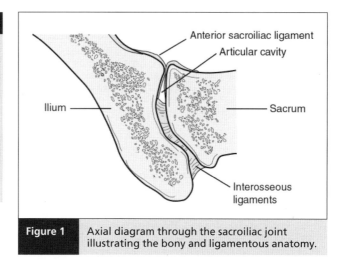

Figure 1 Axial diagram through the sacroiliac joint illustrating the bony and ligamentous anatomy.

Introduction

The sacroiliac joint has been recognized as a potential source of pain and disability for more than 100 years. The first available report of sacroiliac surgery was published in 1908, establishing a history of publication approximately as long as that of spine fusion.[1] Before the understanding of lumbar disk pathology advanced in the middle third of the 20th century, the sacroiliac joint was also considered a source of sciatic pain. Surgical treatment of painful sacroiliac joints in the absence of infection, major trauma, or other source of instability has historically been controversial, possibly because of the well-known difficulties encountered when trying to identify specific anatomic structures responsible for back pain. Earlier techniques involved open procedures with bone grafting and, in some reports, fixation.[2] In the past decade, techniques for percutaneous fixation and fusion have become common and more than a dozen implant systems are currently available.

Dr. Glaser or an immediate family member serves as a board member, owner, officer, or committee member of the American Orthopaedic Association and the North American Spine Society.

Anatomy, Biomechanics, and Innervation

The sacroiliac joint is the articulation of the ilium with the S1 and S2 sacral segments (and occasionally S3, especially in males).[3] The joint shape varies greatly and changes with skeletal growth. Six percent of US adults also have sacralization of the fifth lumbar vertebra.[4] The sacroiliac joint is considered amphiarthrodial, although it also can be considered diarthrodial because it has articular cartilage on its ventral aspect and intra-articular ligaments dorsally. The mean cartilaginous surface area is almost 1,000 mm^2 for women and 1,140 mm^2 for men[5] (**Figure 1**).

The sacroiliac joint transfers load from the lower extremities to the spine and facilitates childbirth. Stability is provided by the bony anatomy and ligamentous support. The sacrum is wider on its cranial and anterior surfaces, which creates a keystone effect in the pelvic ring during weight bearing. The dorsal ligamentous complex is thick and strong; the ventral ligaments are much thinner and often incomplete. Ventral leakage of injected contrast material has been reported to occur in more than one-half of injections.[6] The joint also has a higher coefficient of friction than any diarthrodial joint because of the interdigitating ridges and grooves.[7]

The sacral roots exit at each sacral level via foramina on both the dorsal and ventral surfaces bilaterally. The

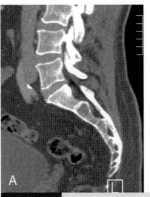 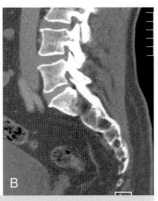

Figure 2 **A,** Sagittal CT obtained at the medial edge of the sacral foramina shows the position of the medial foramen slightly cephalad to the disk remnant. **B,** Sagittal CT scan obtained slightly more lateral shows the position of the foramen at the level of the disk remnant.

medial aspect of the foramen is often slightly cephalad to the disk remnant on a lateral radiograph or sagittal CT scan. Moving laterally, the foramen extends caudally, where it often overlies the disk remnant (**Figure 2**).

Sacroiliac joint motion is described as nutation, which primarily is ventral rotation of the sacrum on the ilium around its transverse axis at S2.[8] Various methods have been used to evaluate the amount of sacroiliac joint motion. Although results have varied, a few degrees of nutation are generally noted. Females are slightly more mobile than males. No quantifiable difference in nutation exists between symptomatic and asymptomatic joints,[9] although this finding has been debated. Doppler imaging of vibrations is an uncommon and controversial test that seems to show differences in laxity between symptomatic and asymptomatic joints.[10] Alternatively, sacroiliac joint pain can arise from counternutation.[3]

Innervation of the sacroiliac joint is still not completely defined. Studies have provided evidence for innervation from L5 to S4.[11,12] Axons associated with nociception also have been found in the articular cartilage of the sacroiliac joint and periarticular ligaments.[13]

Epidemiology

The incidence of sacroiliac pain in patients with chronic low back pain has been estimated to be between 10% and 30%; comparative local anesthetic blocks have been used to predict pain response.[14,15] The incidence of sacroiliac pain following lumbar fusion in patients who are symptomatic for low back pain has been reported to be between 32% and 43%.[16,17] Although lumbar fusions that extend to the pelvis are more frequently implicated than those that do not, lumbar fusions that do not extend to the pelvis are also reported as a predisposing factor.[18]

Evaluation

History

Most patients with sacroiliac joint symptoms will report pain with activity, such as while ascending and descending stairs.[19] In patients who have not undergone previous lumbar fusion, a history of trauma is common but not universal. A common complaint also seems to be pain while rolling over in bed. The pain is generally in the region of the posterior superior iliac spine, but also has been noted to radiate to the groin and down the leg to a varied extent.[20] However, sacroiliac pain has no cardinal symptoms.[21]

Physical Examination

In addition to a standard physical examination for spine problems, sacroiliac tests should also be used to establish a diagnosis of sacroiliac joint pain. No single maneuver is diagnostic for sacroiliac pain, but when three or more tests have positive results, the likelihood of sacroiliac pain increases. In some cases, at least 50% of pain relief following repeated, fluoroscopically guided injections is considered diagnostic for sacroiliac pain.[20-23]

With the Fortin finger test, the patient is asked to place his or her finger on the area of greatest pain; placement around the posterior superior iliac spine is considered a positive result. The remaining tests are performed in the supine position; reproduction of the patient's pain is considered a positive result for the tests listed in **Table 1**.

Imaging

The incidence of radiographic degeneration is high in asymptomatic individuals. Imaging alone cannot be used to diagnose or screen for degenerative causes of sacroiliac joint pain.[24] Imaging can help diagnose infectious problems, fracture, or tumor. Three-dimensional imaging such as CT or MRI also is important in defining anatomy for surgical planning.

Diagnostic Injection

Diagnostic injection is the best test to confirm that pain originates in the sacroiliac joint. Studies have reported differences in injection techniques, amounts of contrast material and/or anesthetic used, and levels of pain relief required for a response to be considered positive. The use of contrast material to verify intra-articular needle position, a relatively small amount of anesthetic injected (approximately 2 mL), and at least 50% pain relief are generally accepted criteria.[23] Repeated injections are often

Table 1

Physical Examination Maneuvers for Sacroiliac Pain

Examination Test	Description
Thigh thrust test	Directed pressure is placed on the knee with the hip and knee flexed to 90°
Pelvic compression test	Medially directed pressure is applied to the iliac crests
Pelvic distraction test	Laterally directed pressure is applied at the anterior superior iliac spine
Patrick or flexion, abduction, external rotation test	The heel of the foot is placed on the symptomatic side on the contralateral patella. The examiner places one hand on the contralateral anterior superior iliac spine to stabilize the pelvis. Posteriorly directed pressure is applied to the medial knee of the symptomatic side.
Gaenslen test	The buttock of the symptomatic side lies over the edge of the examination table to allow the hip to extend. The hip and knee of the contralateral side are held in flexion with the thigh against the abdomen. The hip on the symptomatic side is extended. Posteriorly directed pressure is applied to the anterior thigh if needed.

recommended because high false-positive rates have been reported for a single injection.[22]

Nonsurgical Treatment

Medication

Although no study specifically examines the use of medication for sacroiliac pain in patients without spondyloarthropathy, an attempted trial of judicious medication use seems prudent. As with many benign musculoskeletal pain problems, NSAIDs or muscle relaxants can provide enough benefit to avoid more aggressive interventions.[21]

Exercise

Exercise for back pain is well established. Although studies examining the role of exercise specifically in patients with sacroiliac pain are limited, exercise is a commonly used modality.[25]

Bracing

Evidence supporting sacroiliac bracing is limited to anecdote and smaller studies. Cadaver studies have shown reduced sagittal rotation of the sacroiliac joint with the application of a pelvic belt.[26]

Manual Therapy

Although it has been shown that manipulation does not actually change the position of the sacroiliac joint, some patients report therapeutic benefit. Major complications seem to be rare.[27,28]

Prolotherapy

Prolotherapy (also called proliferation therapy or regenerative injection therapy) is the injection, generally into soft tissues, of an irritant solution such as a combination of dextrose, glycerin, and phenol. Two studies have been performed on patients with chronic low back pain, but not necessarily sacroiliac pain.[29,30] Patients received double-blind injections in the lumbar and sacroiliac regions. Patients in one of the studies also underwent spine manipulation.[30] Both studies reported moderate benefit at 6 months for both groups, with significant improvement in the prolotherapy groups compared with those who received sham injections.

Injection and Neurotomy

Intra-articular steroid injections and radiofrequency neurotomy of the sacroiliac joint both have been studied.[12,14,31,32] The most recent systematic review analyzed results for patients with pain lasting for more than 3 months who had not been successfully treated with nonsurgical measures.[14] Some patients experienced substantial benefit from each of the treatment modalities, although the evidence was considered limited for both.

Surgical Measures

When nonsurgical measures have been ineffective in a patient who is considered an appropriate surgical candidate, sacroiliac surgery can be considered. The first case of sacroiliac fusion was reported in 1908.[1] Infectious disease was likely the most common reason for surgery early in the 20th century. From the later 20th century until recently, sacroiliac joint fusion was most commonly performed in the setting of high-energy trauma and pelvic instability.

Earlier surgical techniques involved various forms of open exposure, decortication, and grafting without fixation. Multiple approaches have been described, including anteromedial and posterior approaches to the joint for posterior superior iliac spine osteotomy (**Figure 3**). As internal fixation techniques evolved, use of the sacroiliac joint included screw fixation across the joint, posterior plating, transiliac rod fixation, and use of pedicle screw fixation systems.[2,33-37] Most instrumented techniques use posterior approaches, but anterior fixation and fusion also has been performed.[38] Postoperative immobilization and rehabilitation also have varied greatly.

The results of open sacroiliac fusion have been mixed. A recent systematic review of six studies concluded that sacroiliac fusion appeared to be satisfactory as treatment to alleviate pain in the pelvic girdle.[39] Most series showed moderate improvement; one study noted unsatisfactory results of bilateral fusion with fixation.[36] One long-term study reported minimal differences at 23-year follow-up between patients who underwent fusion and patients treated nonsurgically.[40] Rates of complications and pseudarthrosis have varied among studies.

Over the past decade, percutaneous fixation and/or fusion has become much more common.[41] Multiple percutaneous systems are available with varied techniques. Some systems use implants inserted into the joint along its axis.[42] Other systems cross the joint from lateral to medial.[43-45] Some systems involve decortication and grafting; others rely on bony ingrowth on the implants.[43,44,46] No study has compared the different percutaneous techniques. The best-studied technique involves plasma-coated titanium implants inserted from lateral to medial:[19,44,45] Smooth pins are placed across the joint with radiographic guidance, followed by preparation with a drill and broach. The implants are then tapped into place (**Figure 4**). Good-quality imaging and thorough

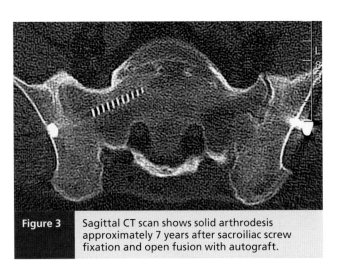

Figure 3   Sagittal CT scan shows solid arthrodesis approximately 7 years after sacroiliac screw fixation and open fusion with autograft.

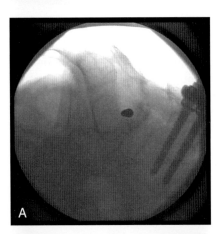

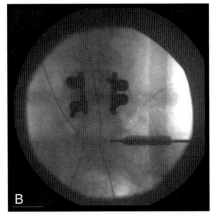

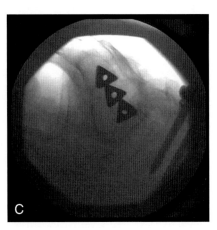

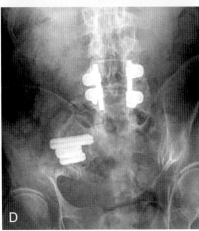

Figure 4   Images demonstrate percutaneous fixation and fusion. **A,** Lateral fluoroscopic image shows initial pin placement. **B,** AP fluoroscopic image obtained after bone preparation shows cage being advanced over the guidewire. **C,** Lateral fluoroscopic image shows three cages after implantation. **D,** Postoperative AP pelvic radiograph.

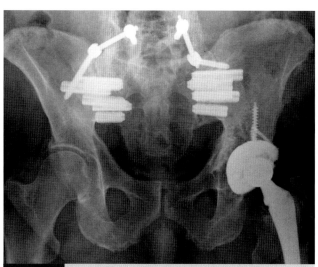

Figure 5   AP pelvic radiograph shows symptomatic implant loosening after bilateral implantation. The patient underwent implantation of additional components as well as supplemental lumbopelvic fixation.

knowledge of the anatomy is critical.[47,48] Structures at risk include the sacral nerve roots within the foramina, the L5 roots anterior to the sacral ala, and the contents of the sacral spinal canal. Electromyographic stimulation of the implants can be performed but its value is unclear. Postoperative management varies but protected ambulation is usually allowed, followed by rehabilitation at the discretion of the treating physician.

Both prospective studies of this technique were industry sponsored; one study compared surgical with nonsurgical management,[19] the other prospectively followed patients treated surgically.[45] Both studies showed significant improvements in pain and function at 2 years. Adverse events included a small number of device-related complications and revision surgeries. A postmarket analysis noted a 3.8% rate of complaints related to the device.[49] A review of complications from a large health insurer's database noted a somewhat higher complication rate (16.4%), especially for infection (4.1%).[41]

One small study compared minimally invasive and open techniques.[38] The findings favored percutaneous technique for length of hospital stay, length of surgery, and blood loss. Clinical improvement was seen in both groups but was greater in the minimally invasive group.

Evaluation of continued or recurrent pain can be difficult. CT can help assess implant position and may be able to help diagnose pseudarthrosis. Indications and outcomes for revision surgery have not been published. Revision surgery can involve multiple techniques including

removal and/or replacement of implants, open bone grafting, or additional forms of fixation (**Figures 5**).

Summary

The treatment of sacroiliac dysfunction can be challenging. No technique provides a universal benefit. Nonsurgical measures can be effective and should be attempted before surgery is considered. In the appropriate candidate, surgery can be performed with an acceptable complication rate. Percutaneous techniques have the potential to improve quality of life but long-term studies are lacking.

Key Study Points

- Pain from the sacroiliac joint is best diagnosed by using diagnostic intra-articular injections.
- Physical examination maneuvers directed toward the sacroiliac joint are helpful but not diagnostic for sacroiliac dysfunction.
- Nonsurgical measures can be effective and should generally be tried before considering surgical intervention.
- Surgical intervention can improve pain and function for recalcitrant sacroiliac pain in appropriately selected patients.

Annotated References

1. Painter CF: Excision of the os innominatum: Arthrodesis of the sacroiliac synchondrosis. *Boston Med Surg Jrnl* 1908;207.

2. Buchowski JM, Kebaish KM, Sinkov V, Cohen DB, Sieber AN, Kostuik JP: Functional and radiographic outcome of sacroiliac arthrodesis for the disorders of the sacroiliac joint. *Spine J* 2005;5(5):520-528, discussion 529.

3. Vleeming A, Schuenke MD, Masi AT, Carreiro JE, Danneels L, Willard FH: The sacroiliac joint: An overview of its anatomy, function and potential clinical implications. *J Anat* 2012;221(6):537-567.

   The authors present an extensive review of the current state of knowledge regarding the structure and function of the sacroiliac joint.

4. Tague RG: High assimilation of the sacrum in a sample of American skeletons: Prevalence, pelvic size, and obstetrical and evolutionary implications. *Am J Phys Anthropol* 2009;138(4):429-438.

5. Ebraheim NA, Madsen TD, Xu R, Mehalik J, Yeasting RA: Dynamic changes in the contact area of the sacroiliac joint. *Orthopedics* 2003;26(7):711-714.

6. Fortin JD, Dwyer AP, West S, Pier J: Sacroiliac joint: pain referral maps upon applying a new injection/arthrography technique: Part I. Asymptomatic volunteers. *Spine (Phila Pa 1976)* 1994;19(13):1475-1482.

7. Vleeming A, Volkers AC, Snijders CJ, Stoeckart R: Relation between form and function in the sacroiliac joint. Part II: Biomechanical aspects. *Spine (Phila Pa 1976)* 1990;15(2):133-136.

8. Sturesson B, Selvik G, Udén A: Movements of the sacroiliac joints: A roentgen stereophotogrammetric analysis. *Spine (Phila Pa 1976)* 1989;14(2):162-165.

9. Sturesson B, Uden A, Vleeming A: A radiostereometric analysis of movements of the sacroiliac joints during the standing hip flexion test. *Spine (Phila Pa 1976)* 2000;25(3):364-368.

10. Damen L, Buyruk HM, Güler-Uysal F, Lotgering FK, Snijders CJ, Stam HJ: The prognostic value of asymmetric laxity of the sacroiliac joints in pregnancy-related pelvic pain. *Spine (Phila Pa 1976)* 2002;27(24):2820-2824.

11. Grob KR, Neuhuber WL, Kissling RO: Innervation of the sacroiliac joint of the human [German]. *Z Rheumatol* 1995;54(2):117-122.

12. Patel N, Gross A, Brown L, Gekht G: A randomized, placebo-controlled study to assess the efficacy of lateral branch neurotomy for chronic sacroiliac joint pain. *Pain Med* 2012;13(3):383-398.

    In this study, 51 subjects with sacroiliac joint pain were randomized 2:1 to lateral branch neurotomy with cooled radiofrequency electrodes versus a sham procedure. Multiple quality-of-life instruments showed substantial benefit to neurotomy versus the sham procedure for up to 9 months after treatment. Level of evidence: II.

13. Szadek KM, Hoogland PV, Zuurmond WW, De Lange JJ, Perez RS: Possible nociceptive structures in the sacroiliac joint cartilage: An immunohistochemical study. *Clin Anat* 2010;23(2):192-198.

14. Hansen HC, McKenzie-Brown AM, Cohen SP, Swicegood JR, Colson JD, Manchikanti L: Sacroiliac joint interventions: A systematic review. *Pain Physician* 2007;10(1):165-184.

15. Schwarzer AC, Aprill CN, Bogduk N: The sacroiliac joint in chronic low back pain. *Spine (Phila Pa 1976)* 1995;20(1):31-37.

16. DePalma MJ, Ketchum JM, Saullo TR: Etiology of chronic low back pain in patients having undergone lumbar fusion. *Pain Med* 2011;12(5):732-739.

    In this review of 170 patients with low back pain, 28 had been treated with fusion. All patients underwent multiple diagnostic blockades to attempt to identify the source of pain. The sacroiliac joint was considered to be the pain source in 12 of the 28 patients. Level of evidence: IV.

17. Liliang PC, Lu K, Liang CL, Tsai YD, Wang KW, Chen HJ: Sacroiliac joint pain after lumbar and lumbosacral fusion: Findings using dual sacroiliac joint blocks. *Pain Med* 2011;12(4):565-570.

    Of 130 patients with pain lasting more than 3 months and a history of fusion, 52 had three or more provocative findings positive for sacroiliac joint pain and underwent dual diagnostic blocks. Of these, 21 had greater than 75% relief with both blocks and were considered to have sacroiliac joint pain. Level of evidence: IV.

18. Ha KY, Lee JS, Kim KW: Degeneration of sacroiliac joint after instrumented lumbar or lumbosacral fusion: A prospective cohort study over five-year follow-up. *Spine (Phila Pa 1976)* 2008;33(11):1192-1198.

19. Polly DW, Swofford J, Whang PG, et al; INSITE Study Group: Two-year outcomes from a randomized controlled trial of minimally invasive sacroiliac joint fusion vs. non-surgical management for sacroiliac joint dysfunction. *Int J Spine Surg* 2016;10:28.

    In this randomized prospective study, 148 patients received either porous-coated implants or were treated nonsurgically. At the 6-month follow-up, patients in the surgical treatment group had a success rate three times greater than that of control patients. The satisfaction rate in the surgical group was 78% at 12 months and 70% at 24 months. Level of evidence: II.

20. Fortin JD, Falco FJ: The Fortin finger test: An indicator of sacroiliac pain. *Am J Orthop (Belle Mead NJ)* 1997;26(7):477-480.

21. Dreyfuss P, Dreyer SJ, Cole A, Mayo K: Sacroiliac joint pain. *J Am Acad Orthop Surg* 2004;12(4):255-265.

22. Simopoulos TT, Manchikanti L, Singh V, et al: A systematic evaluation of prevalence and diagnostic accuracy of sacroiliac joint interventions. *Pain Physician* 2012;15(3):E305-E344.

    In this systematic review of diagnostic techniques for sacroiliac joint pain, improvement of 50% or better was considered a positive result. Most studies suggested point prevalence at approximately 25%. Evidence was good for diagnostic accuracy of injections, fair for provocation maneuvers, and limited for imaging studies. Level of evidence: III.

23. Szadek KM, van der Wurff P, van Tulder MW, Zuurmond WW, Perez RS: Diagnostic validity of criteria for sacroiliac joint pain: A systematic review. *J Pain* 2009;10(4):354-368.

24. Eno JJ, Boone CR, Bellino MJ, Bishop JA: The prevalence of sacroiliac joint degeneration in asymptomatic adults. *J Bone Joint Surg Am* 2015;97(11):932-936.

In this study, 500 pelvic CT scans obtained for patients with no back pain or trauma were retrospectively reviewed for evidence of sacroiliac joint degeneration. The prevalence of degeneration was 65.1%; 30.5% was considered to be significant degeneration. Level of evidence: IV.

25. Mooney V, Pozos R, Vleeming A, Gulick J, Swenski D: Exercise treatment for sacroiliac pain. *Orthopedics* 2001;24(1):29-32.

26. Vleeming A, Buyruk HM, Stoeckart R, Karamursel S, Snijders CJ: An integrated therapy for peripartum pelvic instability: A study of the biomechanical effects of pelvic belts. *Am J Obstet Gynecol* 1992;166(4):1243-1247.

27. Guo X, Zhao Y: Treating subluxation of sacroiliac joint by manipulation: A report of 100 cases. *J Tradit Chin Med* 1994;14(3):192-194.

28. Tullberg T, Blomberg S, Branth B, Johnsson R: Manipulation does not alter the position of the sacroiliac joint: A roentgen stereophotogrammetric analysis. *Spine (Phila Pa 1976)* 1998;23(10):1124-1128, discussion 1129.

29. Klein RG, Eek BC, DeLong WB, Mooney V: A randomized double-blind trial of dextrose-glycerine-phenol injections for chronic, low back pain. *J Spinal Disord* 1993;6(1):23-33.

30. Ongley MJ, Klein RG, Dorman TA, Eek BC, Hubert LJ: A new approach to the treatment of chronic low back pain. *Lancet* 1987;330(8551):143-146.

31. Luukkainen RK, Wennerstrand PV, Kautiainen HH, Sanila MT, Asikainen EL: Efficacy of periarticular corticosteroid treatment of the sacroiliac joint in non-spondylarthropathic patients with chronic low back pain in the region of the sacroiliac joint. *Clin Exp Rheumatol* 2002;20(1):52-54.

32. Slipman CW, Lipetz JS, Plastaras CT, et al: Fluoroscopically guided therapeutic sacroiliac joint injections for sacroiliac joint syndrome. *Am J Phys Med Rehabil* 2001;80(6):425-432.

33. Belanger TA, Dall BE: Sacroiliac arthrodesis using a posterior midline fascial splitting approach and pedicle screw instrumentation: A new technique. *J Spinal Disord* 2001;14(2):118-124.

34. Giannikas KA, Khan AM, Karski MT, Maxwell HA: Sacroiliac joint fusion for chronic pain: A simple technique avoiding the use of metalwork. *Eur Spine J* 2004;13(3):253-256.

35. Smith-Petersen MNR, Rogers WA: End-result study of arthrodesis of the sacro-iliac joint for arthritis: Traumatic and non-traumatic. *J Bone Joint Surg* 1926;8(1):118-136.

36. Schütz U, Grob D: Poor outcome following bilateral sacroiliac joint fusion for degenerative sacroiliac joint syndrome. *Acta Orthop Belg* 2006;72(3):296-308.

37. Waisbrod H, Krainick JU, Gerbershagen HU: Sacroiliac joint arthrodesis for chronic lower back pain. *Arch Orthop Trauma Surg* 1987;106(4):238-240.

38. Ledonio CG, Polly DW Jr, Swiontkowski MF: Minimally invasive versus open sacroiliac joint fusion: Are they similarly safe and effective? *Clin Orthop Relat Res* 2014;472(6):1831-1838.

Forty-nine patients from two institutions were treated with sacroiliac joint fusion between 2006 and 2012. Ten patients were excluded from the retrospective review because of incomplete data. Of the 39 patients reviewed, 22 underwent open fusion and 17 underwent minimally invasive sacroiliac joint fusion. Both groups had improvement in the Oswestry Disability Index scores, but patients in the minimally invasive group had significantly greater improvement and shorter surgical time and length of hospital stay. Level of evidence: III.

39. Lingutla KK, Pollock R, Ahuja S: Sacroiliac joint fusion for low back pain: A systematic review and meta-analysis. *Eur Spine J* 2016;25(6):1924-1931.

This systematic review of six observational studies showed statistical and clinical improvement in patients with pelvic girdle pain who underwent sacroiliac joint fusion. Level of evidence: III.

40. Kibsgård TJ, Røise O, Sudmann E, Stuge B: Pelvic joint fusions in patients with chronic pelvic girdle pain: A 23-year follow-up. *Eur Spine J* 2013;22(4):871-877.

In this long-term study, 50 patients who underwent fusion were compared with 28 control patients. Oswestry Disability Index and Medical Outcomes Study 36-Item Short Form showed moderately high pain and disability scores, although 65% of patients thought that surgery had been beneficial. Level of evidence: IV.

41. Schoell K, Buser Z, Jakoi A, et al: Postoperative complications in patients undergoing minimally invasive sacroiliac fusion. *Spine J* 2016;16(11):1324-1332.

The Pearl Diver patient record database of Humana-identified patients who underwent sacroiliac fusion from 2007 to 2014 reported an overall complication rate of 16.4% at 6 months, The rate of infection was 4.1% and the rate of nervous system complications was 6.2% Level of evidence: II.

42. Wise CL, Dall BE: Minimally invasive sacroiliac arthrodesis: Outcomes of a new technique. *J Spinal Disord Tech* 2008;21(8):579-584.

43. Mason LW, Chopra I, Mohanty K: The percutaneous stabilisation of the sacroiliac joint with hollow modular anchorage screws: A prospective outcome study. *Eur Spine J* 2013;22(10):2325-2331.

In this study, 55 patients were followed for a mean of 36 months after sacroiliac joint fusion using a plasma-coated hollow modular anchorage screw filled with demineralized bone matrix. Mean Medical Outcomes Study 36-Item Short Form and visual analog scale scores showed significant improvements. Level of evidence: IV.

44. Rudolf L, Capobianco R: Five-year clinical and radiographic outcomes after minimally invasive sacroiliac joint fusion using triangular implants. *Open Orthop J* 2014;8:375-383.

In this retrospective review of patients who underwent minimally invasive sacroiliac joint fusion, 88% of the patients had substantial clinical improvement and the mean visual analog scale score decreased from 8.3 to 2.4 at a mean follow-up of 5 years. Level of evidence: IV.

45. Duhon BS, Bitan F, Lockstadt H, Kovalsky D, Cher D, Hillen T; SIFI Study Group: Triangular titanium implants for minimally invasive sacroiliac joint fusion: 2-year follow-up from a prospective multicenter trial. *Int J Spine Surg* 2016;10:13.

In this prospective multicenter study of 172 patients who underwent minimally invasive sacroiliac joint fusion with 2-year follow-up, visual analog scale scores decreased from 79.8 to 26 and Oswestry Disability Index decreased from 55 to 31. The number of patients using opioids decreased from 76.2% to 55.0%. Seven adverse events and eight revisions were reported. Level of evidence: II.

46. Al-Khayer A, Hegarty J, Hahn D, Grevitt MP: Percutaneous sacroiliac joint arthrodesis: A novel technique. *J Spinal Disord Tech* 2008;21(5):359-363.

47. Ebraheim NA, Xu R, Challgren E, Heck B: Location of the sacral pedicle, foramina, and ala on the lateral aspect of the sacrum: A radiographic study. *Orthopedics* 1998;21(6):703-706.

48. Wolinsky P, Lee M: The effect of C-arm malrotation on iliosacral screw placement. *J Orthop Trauma* 2007;21(7):427-434.

49. Miller LE, Reckling WC, Block JE: Analysis of postmarket complaints database for the iFuse SI Joint Fusion System®: A minimally invasive treatment for degenerative sacroiliitis and sacroiliac joint disruption. *Med Devices (Auckl)* 2013;6:77-84.

In 5,319 patients treated with a specific sacroiliac joint fusion system, 204 complaints were reported. Nerve impingement was noted in 4 patients and recurrent pain in 43; 72 implants were placed improperly. Of 96 patients who underwent revision surgery, 56 occurred in the early postoperative period and 40 in the late postoperative period. Postmarket surveillance may underreport the true incidence of problems. Level of evidence: III.

Section 5

Spine Deformity

SECTION EDITOR:

Ronald A. Lehman Jr, MD

Chapter 21

Early-Onset Scoliosis and Congenital Spine Anomalies

Brian J. Kelley, MD, PhD   Michael G. Vitale, MD, MPH

Abstract

Early-onset scoliosis is the development of any spinal curvature before age 10 years. This disorder has congenital, structural, thoracogenic, neuromuscular, syndromic, and idiopathic etiologies. The Classification of Early-Onset Scoliosis has been developed to stratify these heterogeneous entities, improve clinical acumen, and foster research. Pulmonary problems, which are linked to progressive thoracic cavity development and lung volume, are frequent comorbidities in patients with early-onset scoliosis. Treatment goals are to correct and/or control spinal deformity and preserve skeletal growth until skeletal maturity, at which time definitive correction may take place. Treatment options for patients with early-onset scoliosis range from observation to definitive surgical correction. Observation may be appropriate for nonprogressive, balanced curves. If a curve is progressing, bracing and/or casting may be used to improve spinal alignment and balance. If curve progression continues despite nonsurgical management, surgical curve control measures are instituted. The best surgical option is dictated by the overall clinical condition of the individual patient.

Keywords: Classification of Early-Onset Scoliosis; congenital scoliosis; etiology; idiopathic scoliosis; thoracogenic scoliosis

Introduction

Early-onset scoliosis (EOS) is broadly defined as any spinal curvature that develops before the patient is 10 years old. Infantile scoliosis occurs in infants and children younger than 4 years, and juvenile scoliosis occurs in children age 4 to 10 years. Many children with EOS have a significant comorbid condition. The Classification of Early-Onset Scoliosis (C-EOS) has been well validated, is reliable, and has excellent prognostic value.[1-3] The C-EOS evaluates patients based on age, curve etiology, major Cobb angle, kyphosis, and an optional progression modifier. Use of the C-EOS allows targeted treatment decisions (**Figure 1**). Proper diagnosis and classification are critical because each scoliosis etiology has a unique pathophysiology that dictates specific treatment options.

Pulmonary Pathophysiology

The etiology of EOS is inextricably linked to lung development and physiology. Lung compliance is greatest at birth, when the thoracic cage primarily is composed of cartilage, and lung musculature is at its weakest. Compliance decreases with age as bone replaces cartilage within the thoracic framework, and lung muscles begin to strengthen. Because the ribs and their corresponding muscular attachments articulate with the thoracic spine, alterations in spine shape or trajectory can have

Dr. Vitale or an immediate family member has received royalties from Biomet; serves as a paid consultant to Biomet and Stryker; serves as an unpaid consultant to Wellinks; has received research or institutional support from Biomet, Children's Spine Foundation, Orthopaedic Research and Education Foundation, Scoliosis Research Society, Pediatric Orthopaedic Society of North America, and Orthopaedic Scientific Research Foundation; has received non-income support (such as equipment or services), commercially derived honoraria, or other non–research-related funding (such as paid travel) from Biomet, DePuy, FOX Family Foundation, Children's Spine Foundation, Medtronic, OMEGA Medical Grants Association, and Synthes; and serves as a board member, owner, officer, or committee member of the Children's Spine Foundation, International Pediatric Orthopaedic Symposium, and Pediatric Orthopaedic Society of North America. Neither Dr. Kelley nor any immediate family member has received anything of value from or has stock or stock options held in a commercial company or institution related directly or indirectly to the subject of this chapter.

5: Spine Deformity

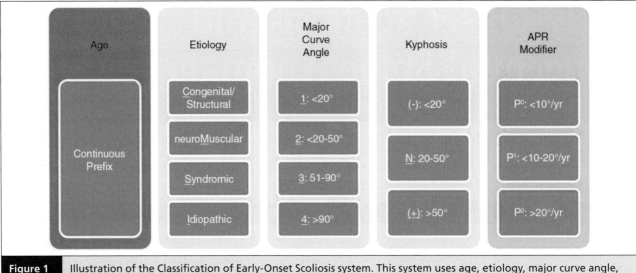

Age	Etiology	Major Curve Angle	Kyphosis	APR Modifier
Continuous Prefix	Congenital/Structural	1: <20°	(-): <20°	P⁰: <10°/yr
	neuroMuscular	2: <20-50°	N: 20-50°	P¹: <10-20°/yr
	Syndromic	3: 51-90°	(+): >50°	P²: >20°/yr
	Idiopathic	4: >90°		

Figure 1 Illustration of the Classification of Early-Onset Scoliosis system. This system uses age, etiology, major curve angle, kyphosis, and an optional progression modifier. APR = annual progression rate. (Reproduced with permission from Williams BA, Matsumoto H, McCalla DJ, et al: Development and initial validation of the Classification of Early-Onset Scoliosis (C-EOS). *J Bone Joint Surg Am* 2014;96[16]:1359-1367.)

a profound effect on respiratory function. Some spine deformities may not appear with clinically relevant respiratory findings, but a substantial deformity can diminish total lung volume. Decreased total lung volume lowers tidal volumes and leads to increased work of breathing and/or an elevated respiratory rate.[4] This constellation of deformity-related musculoskeletal and pulmonary findings along with related clinical symptoms is called thoracic insufficiency syndrome.[5] Treatment strategies for EOS-related respiratory issues must be based on a multidisciplinary approach, with a particular emphasis on pulmonary expertise.[6] Alveolar growth and development continue through adolescence, and the timing of surgery often is affected by pulmonary considerations.

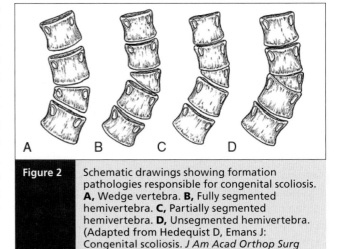

Figure 2 Schematic drawings showing formation pathologies responsible for congenital scoliosis. **A,** Wedge vertebra. **B,** Fully segmented hemivertebra. **C,** Partially segmented hemivertebra. **D,** Unsegmented hemivertebra. (Adapted from Hedequist D, Emans J: Congenital scoliosis. *J Am Acad Orthop Surg* 2004;12[4]:266-275.)

Etiology and Natural History

Congenital, Structural, and Thoracogenic Scoliosis

Most incidences of congenital scoliosis are sporadic and lack a clear genetic component. The incidence of congenital scoliosis is unknown but is estimated at 1 in 1,000 live births.[7,8] Large epidemiologic studies indicate that more girls than boys are affected. Congenital scoliosis may result from fetal exposure to an insult during embryonic spinal development between the fourth and sixth weeks of gestation. Preclinical studies have suggested carbon monoxide and hypoxia as possible causes of congenital vertebral malformations.[9,10] Although no clear genetic factors have been identified, several candidate genes in animal models and humans were found to have a strong association with vertebral body dysgenesis.[7,8]

Congenital scoliosis is recognized as a failure of vertebral body formation and/or segmentation resulting in spine deformity during embryonic development[11] (**Figures 2 and 3**). Formation defects include hemivertebrae and wedge vertebrae. A hemivertebra, which results from a complete unilateral formation failure, is classified as fully segmented, partially segmented, or unsegmented depending on whether a normal disk space is present; or is classified as incarcerated or nonincarcerated depending on whether the pedicle is in line with adjacent pedicles. In a wedge vertebra, a partial formation failure on one side of the vertebra results in diminished vertebral body height. Bony and intervertebral disk architecture is otherwise

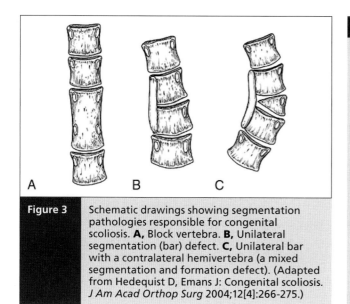

Figure 3 Schematic drawings showing segmentation pathologies responsible for congenital scoliosis. **A,** Block vertebra. **B,** Unilateral segmentation (bar) defect. **C,** Unilateral bar with a contralateral hemivertebra (a mixed segmentation and formation defect). (Adapted from Hedequist D, Emans J: Congenital scoliosis. *J Am Acad Orthop Surg* 2004;12[4]:266-275.)

Table 1

Representative Neuromuscular Conditions Leading to Early-Onset Scoliosis

Arthrogryposis

Cerebral palsy

Congenital myotonia

Hereditary motor sensory neuropathy (Charcot-Marie-Tooth disease)

Muscular dystrophies
  Becker
  Duchenne
  Limb girdle
  Myotonic (Steinert)

Myelomeningocele

Poliomyelitis

Spinal cord injury

Spinal muscular atrophy
  Acute infantile (type 1)
  Werdnig-Hoffmann (types 2 and 3)

Spinocerebellar dysfunction (Friedreich ataxia)

normal. Segmentation defects include block vertebrae, unilateral bars, and unilateral bars with a contralateral hemivertebra (a mixed defect). A block vertebra results from a bilateral segmentation failure, which causes the absence of the disk space between adjacent vertebral bodies. A unilateral bar is a bony structure that fuses the disks and facets on one side of the vertebral column. Deformity progression depends on the anomaly type and location.[12] Reported rates of progression (as measured by the per-year increase in curve degrees) are less than 2° for a block or wedge vertebra, 2° to 5° for a hemivertebra, and 5° to 10° for a unilateral bar with a contralateral hemivertebra. The most significant deformity occurs with a thoracolumbar location. The most rapid progression occurs during the rapid growth phases during the first 5 years of life and puberty.

Congenital scoliosis often is accompanied by spinal dysraphism or an intraspinal anomaly such as diastematomyelia, syringomyelia, or tethered cord.[13-15] The mesodermal layer responsible for vertebral body formation also is responsible for urogenital, cardiac, and pulmonary systems. Abnormalities of vertebral body embryology may be linked to maldevelopment within these systems, and concomitant cardiac and renal abnormalities are common. Children with congenital scoliosis should be screened for urogenital, cardiac, and pulmonary pathologies, especially if surgery is being considered. In addition to a comprehensive clinical history, physical examination and plain radiographs, advanced imaging and additional testing should be used to evaluate for associated conditions.

Thoracogenic scoliosis is found in patients with multiple congenital rib fusions (ie, spondylocostal-spondylothoracic dysostosis). Vertebral anomalies also may be present as well as changes in the chest wall following thoracic surgery, which may function as a unilateral spinal tether.[16]

Neuromuscular Scoliosis

The term neuromuscular scoliosis encompasses a variety of conditions that can appear at any time in life as a mild to severe deformity (**Table 1**). The highly variable natural history of these neuromuscular deformities often is linked to progressive pulmonary complications. Most patients have curve progression independent of the neuromuscular diagnosis. Muscle weakness has been assumed to be a cause of scoliosis development, but the pathophysiology remains unclear; there is no association among the etiology, pattern of weakness, and curve pattern.[17] The factors associated with scoliosis development include age of onset of neuromuscular disease, ambulatory status, and the severity or rapidity of muscle weakness progression.[18] Many patients have a kyphoscoliotic deformity secondary to loss of trunk stability. A long, collapsing C-shaped curve is typical, but any other curve morphology also is possible (**Figure 4**). Pelvic obliquity should be considered in an evaluation of neuromuscular scoliosis. The combination of pelvic obliquity and neuromuscular scoliosis leads to spinal imbalance with corresponding dermal pressure points.[17] Like congenital scoliosis, neuromuscular scoliosis often is accompanied by associated

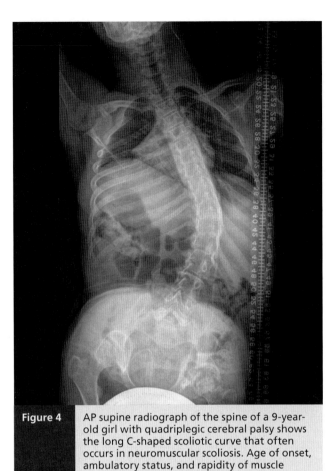

Figure 4 AP supine radiograph of the spine of a 9-year-old girl with quadriplegic cerebral palsy shows the long C-shaped scoliotic curve that often occurs in neuromuscular scoliosis. Age of onset, ambulatory status, and rapidity of muscle weakness are the most important factors associated with curve progression in patients with neuromuscular scoliosis.

Table 2	
Scoliosis Research Society Classification of Neuromuscular Scoliosis	
Type	**Associated Conditions**
Neuropathic	Upper motor neuron disease
	Lower motor neuron disease
	Mixed upper and lower motor neuron disease
	Spinocerebellar dysfunction
	Hereditary motor sensory neuropathy
Myopathic	Muscular dystrophy
	Arthrogryposis
	Congenital myopathies

and previously underappreciated intraspinal anomalies.[19-21] The course of idiopathic scoliosis is quite different from that of other scoliosis deformities. In some patients, infantile- or juvenile-onset idiopathic scoliosis is resolved without surgical or nonsurgical treatment.[22] Idiopathic curves often are more flexible than curves in other EOS conditions and therefore are more amenable to nonsurgical interventions before the optimal time for definitive surgical treatment. The patient's age at the time of diagnosis distinguishes infantile idiopathic scoliosis (age 0 to 3 years) from juvenile idiopathic scoliosis (age 4 to 10 years) or the more common adolescent idiopathic scoliosis (age older than 10 years to 18 years).

pathologies requiring a multidisciplinary treatment approach. The Scoliosis Research Society classifies neuromuscular scoliosis as neuropathic or myopathic (**Table 2**).

Syndromic Scoliosis

Syndromic scoliosis typically has an underlying hereditary component. Scoliosis is a component of the patient's phenotype in numerous pathologic conditions with highly variable natural histories (**Table 3**). Most types of syndromic scoliosis require intervention to control curve progression. Any potential intervention must be considered as part of a comprehensive treatment plan that often involves multiple clinical disciplines. If intervention is indicated, its goals often are dictated by the clinical severity of the scoliotic curvature and/or patient prognosis.

Idiopathic Infantile and Juvenile Scoliosis

The causes of idiopathic scoliosis are unknown as the name suggests, although there may be a familial etiology (**Figure 5**). Research suggests links to genetic factors

Evaluation

A detailed patient history and physical examination are essential, with emphasis on spine and neurologic evaluations, review of radiographic findings, and screening for associated anomalies. Careful testing of abdominal reflexes sometimes indicates an underlying spinal dysraphism. If the child can participate in pulmonary function testing, any restrictive lung disease can be detected, along with its potential for progression. Full-length radiographs are evaluated for spinal alignment and balance. In younger children who unable to stand, radiographs are taken in the position of maximum gravity. The deformity is measured in the sagittal and coronal planes, and pelvic and shoulder balance are documented. Associated rib cage abnormalities also are noted. CT is reserved for evaluating structural abnormalities such as congenital scoliosis or rib fusions. To minimize radiation exposure, CT often is deferred until the patient is scheduled for surgery. The risks of sedation for children who are at least 1 year old approach those for considerably older children,

Table 3

Representative Syndromic Conditions Leading to Early-Onset Scoliosis

Alagille syndrome

Down syndrome

Ehlers-Danlos syndrome

Goldenhar syndrome

Klippel-Feil syndrome

Marfan syndrome

Neurofibromatosis

Osteogenesis imperfecta

Prader-Willi syndrome

Spondylothoracic dysplasia–Jarcho-Levin syndrome (associated with mesoderm posterior protein 2 [*MESP2*] gene) and spondylocostal dysplasia (associated with mutations in delta-like 3 [*DLL3*]), *MESP2*, lunatic fringe [*LFNG*], and hairy/enhancer of split 7 [*HES7*] genes)

Trisomy 18

VACTERL (vertebral, anorectal, cardiovascular, tracheoesophageal, renal, limb) associations

and therefore MRI can be used in these patients to rule out spinal dysraphism.

Treatment

Treatment strategies for a patient with EOS must consider the patient's age at the time of diagnosis as well as the future growth potential of the spine. Given the heterogeneity of scoliotic findings, treatment options must be tailored to the patient's clinical condition. Treatments range from observation and nonsurgical management to definitive surgical correction, and often as the child grows they involve a multimodal continuum of therapies.[23] Ideally the treatment plan is designed to preserve growth until the patient reaches skeletal maturity, when definitive correction can take place. Nonsurgical strategies often are preferred to more invasive treatments. The treatment goals include minimizing the spinal deformity and the extent of the final spinal fusion while maximizing thoracic volume and function as well as the child's overall development.[16] The emphasis is on curve progression rather than the absolute magnitude of the curve as highlighted by the C-EOS system.

Nonsurgical Management

Nonsurgical management options include observation and bracing or casting. Observation is reserved for a

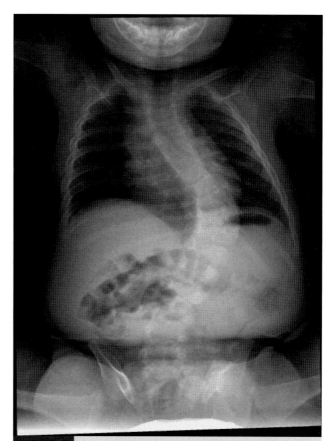

Figure 5 AP seated radiograph shows idiopathic scoliosis in a 2-year-old boy being treated with serial casting. The spinal deformity cannot be attributed to any discernable structural lesion or underlying diagnosis. Early-onset idiopathic curves typically are flexible and therefore amenable to longitudinal nonsurgical treatment strategies.

nonprogressive, balanced curve, especially if it is unlikely to deteriorate. Examples of this type of curve are those resulting from a block vertebra or a hemimetameric shift, in which two contralateral hemivertebrae are separated by at least one normal vertebra. The suggested follow-up protocol includes obtaining plain radiographs every 6 to 12 months with serial assessments of spinal balance and Cobb angle measurements. The deformity may be relatively stable during middle childhood, which occurs between periods of more rapid progression during infancy and early adolescence. Because of concern about cumulative radiation over the course of the patient's childhood, a reference plain radiograph of the chest may serve for the initial diagnosis and management. Supine radiographs may be sufficient for an infant. When the child is able to stand and walk, weight-bearing full-length PA and lateral radiographs should be obtained.[8] Positional changes often are associated with changes in Cobb angle measurements.

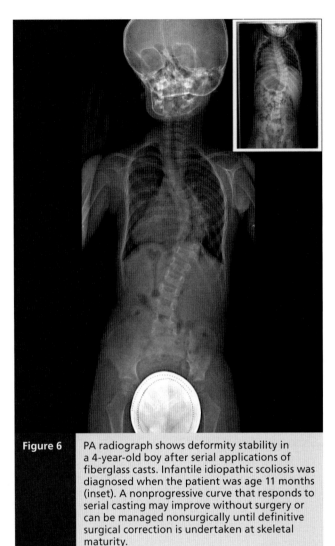

Figure 6 PA radiograph shows deformity stability in a 4-year-old boy after serial applications of fiberglass casts. Infantile idiopathic scoliosis was diagnosed when the patient was age 11 months (inset). A nonprogressive curve that responds to serial casting may improve without surgery or can be managed nonsurgically until definitive surgical correction is undertaken at skeletal maturity.

Consistency in measuring the curve is paramount for identifying progression. Additional imaging studies to identify spinal dysraphism also may be needed during early childhood.

The curve typically is monitored until the Cobb angle exceeds 25° with more than 10° of documented progression.[23] If the Cobb angle exceeds this threshold, bracing or casting can allow skeletal growth to continue while improving spinal balance (**Figure 6**). In patients with EOS, bracing or casting is most appropriate for a long flexible curve or a compensatory curve. For example, progressive infantile idiopathic EOS may respond to a Mehta casting regimen, which is based on the measurement of the rib–vertebral angle difference (a measure of the difference in each of the angles of the ribs attached to the apical vertebra, with 20° or less associated with a nonprogressive or resolving curve).[24] However, several types of EOS deformities include a short, rigid curve that

does not respond to bracing. Even if the curve does not appear to respond to serial casting and bracing, these strategies may succeed in controlling curve progression and allow surgery to be delayed.[25] Bracing or casting also can be used as an adjunct treatment strategy after surgical correction by providing supplementary support and protecting the instrumentation.

Exercise regimens such as the Schroth method can be used alone or in combination with bracing to improve the spinal deformity by increasing muscle strength and promoting trunk elongation. This treatment is designed only for flexible curves and is limited by the necessity for patient participation. Little evidence supports the use of scoliosis-specific physical therapy in patients with EOS.

Surgical Intervention

The guiding principles for early surgical correction in patients with EOS are to improve the spinal deformity and balance while preserving spine growth until definitive correction can take place at skeletal maturity. Earlier surgery is indicated if the patient has progressive respiratory or neurologic symptoms. Collectively, growth-friendly surgical strategies are intended to control the patient's continuing spine and chest development.[26,27] The three types of surgery designed to preserve spine growth are distraction based, guided growth, and compression based.[28]

Posterior distraction-based techniques apply forces across a deformed spinal segment. Distraction maneuvers recontour the spine using temporary rods positioned along the spinal axis by screw or hook constructs anchored to the spine, ribs, and/or pelvis. Over time, the patient undergoes a series of smaller surgical procedures to lengthen the rod and thus promote improved spinal alignment. Types of rods include traditional growing rods, which provide scoliosis control; the Vertical Expandable Prosthetic Titanium Rib (DePuy Synthes) device, which provides thoracic expansion; and hybrid rods[23,26,29] (**Figure 7**). Thoracic expansion is reserved for patients with a primary deformity involving the thoracic cage, such as rib fusions or thoracic insufficiency syndrome. The strategy for using magnetically manipulated growing rods is similar but does not require additional surgery because the rods can be lengthened using an external magnetic device[30-32] (**Figure 8**). With a guided-growth implant strategy such as the Shilla technique, screws are placed to create a short apical fusion, and additional proximal and distal screws not rigidly attached to rods slide over the rod as the spine grows, thereby directing growth along the rod trajectory[33,34] (**Figure 9**). The formerly used Luque trolley system technique was based on similar principles. Compression-based techniques use compressive implants to halt growth on the convex

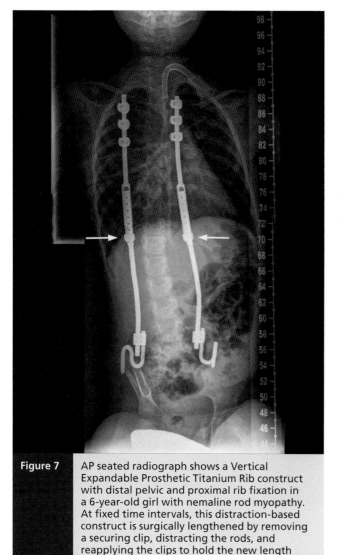

Figure 7   AP seated radiograph shows a Vertical Expandable Prosthetic Titanium Rib construct with distal pelvic and proximal rib fixation in a 6-year-old girl with nemaline rod myopathy. At fixed time intervals, this distraction-based construct is surgically lengthened by removing a securing clip, distracting the rods, and reapplying the clips to hold the new length (arrows).

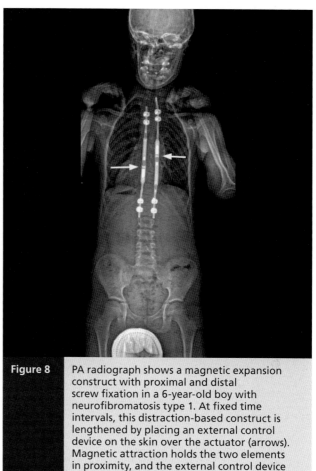

Figure 8   PA radiograph shows a magnetic expansion construct with proximal and distal screw fixation in a 6-year-old boy with neurofibromatosis type 1. At fixed time intervals, this distraction-based construct is lengthened by placing an external control device on the skin over the actuator (arrows). Magnetic attraction holds the two elements in proximity, and the external control device elongates the actuator by a predetermined length without additional surgery.

side of the curve. Often this technique uses an anterior approach without fusion[35,36] (**Figure 10**). Staples or tethers are placed across the growth plates, and concave growth proceeds with the goal of curve balance. In practice, spinal growth after a compression-based procedure can be unpredictable.[37] The initial research provided proof of concept, with many incidences of curve diminution; however, the determination of appropriate indications and optimal implants continues to evolve. In contrast to a posterior technique, the use of an anterior compression-based technique may eliminate the requirement for definitive fusion when a child reaches skeletal maturity. Distraction-based and guided-growth strategies currently are more often used than compression-based strategies because they are more familiar to surgeons and involve less surgical morbidity.

Definitive surgical correction often combines spinal fusion with techniques intended to improve spinal alignment and balance. Conversion of a growth-friendly construct can be difficult. Obtaining axial plane correction often requires osteotomies because the spine has become stiff from the relative immobilization induced by the initial implants. Fusion surgery seeks to halt the progress of the deformity by locking the spine into its current shape. Before fusion, spinal alignment can be improved in multiple planes by compression, distraction, and/or derotation of spinal implants combined with Smith-Petersen or pedicle subtraction spinal osteotomies. These techniques can be especially effective when used asymmetrically or in combination. The possible long-term consequences of definitive fusion before skeletal maturity include the crankshaft phenomenon, in which postfusion posterior growth inhibition combined with continued anterior growth causes a new or worsening deformity.

Although delaying definitive surgical correction until the patient reaches skeletal maturity always is preferred, earlier surgical intervention may be necessary. The patient

5: Spine Deformity

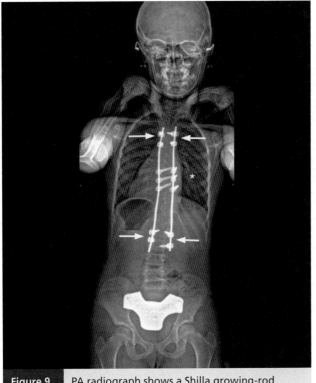

Figure 9 PA radiograph shows a Shilla growing-rod construct (a guided-growth construct) with proximal and distal screws in a 5-year-old girl with idiopathic scoliosis whose curve had progressed despite nonsurgical treatment. A short-segment apical screw-rod construct (asterisk) is complemented by proximal and distal screws that accommodate the rod but do not lock it into place. Spinal growth occurs in a guided fashion as the proximal and distal screws move along the tracks created by the rods (arrows).

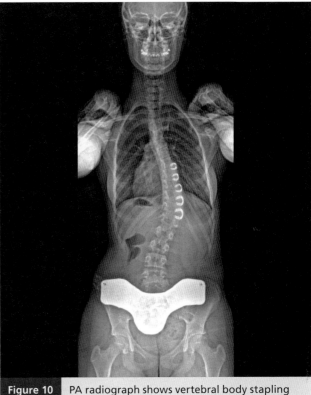

Figure 10 PA radiograph shows vertebral body stapling in a 10-year-old girl with idiopathic scoliosis. In this compression-based surgical intervention, the staples tether the spinal column along the curve convexity while allowing concave growth to balance the deformity. Unpredictable spinal growth and long-term durability have limited the use of staple correction in deformity correction.

may require complex spinal reconstruction involving abnormal skeletal elements in isolation, as in a hemivertebrectomy, or in combination, as in vertebral column resection. In hemivertebra resection, the bony element most often is removed through a posterior-only approach (**Figure 11**). Complete excision followed by limited spinal fusion can correct the deformity, but the patient's family should be counseled that there is a substantial risk that further surgery will be required. Resection ideally is undertaken before a secondary compensatory curve develops so that the potential fusion length can be limited.[38] It is preferable to wait until progression is obvious and the patient is at least 24 to 30 months old. The contraindications to resection include evidence of spinal dysraphism at the same level, inability to use internal or external bracing after resection, the presence of rigid deformities above or below the level, and vascular anomalies that may not be correctible.[8] If the spinal malalignment is too severe

to correct, vertebral column resection may be required. This elimination of the abnormal elements will shorten the spine and is thus reserved for the most severe spinal deformities. The removed spinal segment often is replaced with a synthetic cage augmented by autograft or allograft bone in addition to spinal instrumentation (**Figure 12**). Complex reconstruction surgeries have a greater risk of bleeding and neurologic injury when compared with other spinal fusion procedures. It is recommended that these procedures be performed by experienced surgeons with appropriate ancillary providers.[39,40]

Outcomes

The heterogeneity of EOS pathology limits the validity of any overall assessment of outcomes. EOS with an idiopathic etiology may be resolved spontaneously or with the use of early casting. Similar strategies often are ineffective for treating congenital scoliosis, which is more likely than idiopathic EOS to require definitive surgical

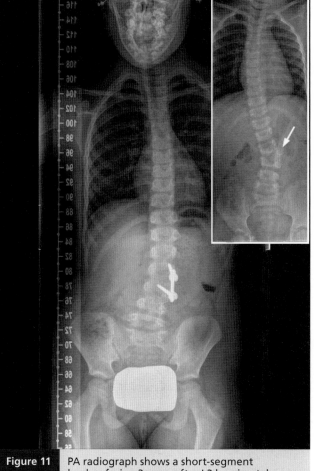

Figure 11 PA radiograph shows a short-segment lumbar fusion 3 years after L3 hemivertebra resection (inset arrow) in a 7-year-old girl whose condition initially appeared as spinal asymmetry. A congenital curve secondary to a hemivertebra typically does not respond to nonsurgical therapies, and early surgical intervention leads to the best deformity correction and long-term outcome. Complete removal of the hemivertebra followed by a short-segment fusion allows curve correction and growth preservation in the remaining spinal column.

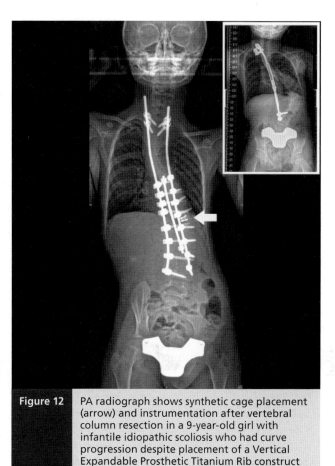

Figure 12 PA radiograph shows synthetic cage placement (arrow) and instrumentation after vertebral column resection in a 9-year-old girl with infantile idiopathic scoliosis who had curve progression despite placement of a Vertical Expandable Prosthetic Titanium Rib construct 3 years earlier (inset). This surgical option typically is reserved for a complex and/or rigid deformity that cannot be corrected by a less invasive surgical strategy.

correction. Patients with a neuromuscular or syndromic deformity often undergo surgical correction at a relatively early age because their disease is likely to rapidly progress. These patients also have the greatest risk of postoperative morbidity because of related medical conditions. It is important to remember that although general guidelines are useful for directing therapeutic strategies, the treatment must be tailored to the individual patient's needs and overall health.

Numerous recent studies have evaluated casting and bracing protocols and surgical interventions in patients with EOS.[27,41,42] Some of the earliest studies of outcomes after spinal fusion in young patients found that deformity progression was stabilized but that persistent or worsening restrictive lung disease and occasional deformity recurrence led to a poor quality of life.[43-45] These analyses resulted in the development of delayed treatment strategies that promote nonsurgical therapy and then to growth-friendly surgical options that allow continued bony growth through childhood.[23,26,46] The heterogeneity of the patient population presents a substantial challenge to clinical research, which will greatly benefit from multicenter collaboration.

It is well understood that patients with EOS can have substantial perturbations in health-related quality of life. A questionnaire developed to provide a disease-specific measure of quality of life and outcomes in patients with EOS has been well validated within the past few years.[1,47] A related classification system for reporting surgical complications involving the growing spine also has been developed.[48]

Summary

EOS remains a challenging condition because of the relatively young age of patients at diagnosis as well as the numerous accompanying comorbidities. It is important to correctly diagnose EOS and understand its etiology. The treatment strategies are directed by etiology and natural history. Concomitant pulmonary pathophysiology necessitates the treatment of the spinal deformity with simultaneous preservation of the chest wall and lung growth. Unless the curve regresses or progression ceases, initial treatment is designed to preserve bony growth until skeletal maturity, when definitive correction can take place. Several therapeutic options are available to treat EOS, ranging from nonsurgical strategies to complex spinal column reconstruction. Overall treatment strategies involve a multimodal approach that must be tailored over time to the individual patient's needs.

Key Study Points

- EOS is defined as the development of any curvature of the spine in a patient younger than 10 years. The C-EOS has been developed to stratify diagnoses based on age, etiology, major Cobb angle, degree of kyphosis, and an optional progression modifier. Concomitant pulmonary comorbidities often contribute to the overall pathologic condition.

- The etiologies of EOS can be congenital, neuromuscular, syndromic, or idiopathic. Each etiology has unique pathologic characteristics and clinical findings that dictate the potential progression of the disease and management options.

- The goals of treatment are to correct and/or control the deformity and preserve skeletal growth potential until the patient reaches skeletal maturity, at which time definitive correction can be undertaken, if necessary.

- Distraction-based, guided-growth, or compression-based growth-friendly surgical strategies can be used before definitive correction. Each strategy has strengths and weaknesses and must be tailored to the patient's clinical condition.

- The outcomes of intervention are difficult to compare among groups of patients because of the heterogeneity of the pathologies.

Annotated References

1. Williams BA, Matsumoto H, McCalla DJ, et al: Development and initial validation of the Classification of Early-Onset Scoliosis (C-EOS). *J Bone Joint Surg Am* 2014;96(16):1359-1367.

   The authors discuss the development and validation of a novel classification system to stratify EOS into categories that document age, etiology, major Cobb angle, and kyphosis and have an optional progression modifier.

2. Cyr M, Hilaire TS, Pan Z, Thompson GH, Vitale MG, Garg S; Children's Spine Study Group, Growing Spine Study Group: Classification of Early Onset Scoliosis has excellent interobserver and intraobserver reliability. *J Pediatr Orthop* 2017;37(1):e1-e3.

   The C-EOS demonstrated high levels of interobserver and intraobserver agreement, which confirmed it as a reliable tool for clinical communication and research. Level of evidence: II.

3. Park HY, Matsumoto H, Feinberg N, et al: The Classification for Early-Onset Scoliosis (C-EOS) correlates with the speed of vertical expandable prosthetic titanium rib (VEPTR) proximal anchor failure. *J Pediatr Orthop* 2015;Nov 13 [Epub ahead of print].

   The C-EOS was applied to failure rates for the proximal Vertical Expandable Prosthetic Titanium Rib. The C-EOS demonstrated the ability to discriminate the speeds of failure, which suggests that it may have potential value in guided decision making. Level of evidence: III.

4. Fletcher ND, Bruce RW: Early onset scoliosis: Current concepts and controversies. *Curr Rev Musculoskelet Med* 2012;5(2):102-110.

   The authors discuss the diagnosis, evaluation, and treatment of EOS.

5. Campbell RM Jr, Smith MD, Mayes TC, et al: The characteristics of thoracic insufficiency syndrome associated with fused ribs and congenital scoliosis. *J Bone Joint Surg Am* 2003;85(3):399-408.

6. Herring MJ, Putney LF, Wyatt G, Finkbeiner WE, Hyde DM: Growth of alveoli during postnatal development in humans based on stereological estimation. *Am J Physiol Lung Cell Mol Physiol* 2014;307(4):L338-L344.

   This study of human alveolar development reported exponential growth within the first 2 years of life followed by continued growth at a reduced rate in adolescence.

7. Giampietro PF, Dunwoodie SL, Kusumi K, et al: Progress in the understanding of the genetic etiology of vertebral segmentation disorders in humans. *Ann N Y Acad Sci* 2009;1151:38-67.

8. Shah SA, Song K: Congenital scoliosis, in Weinstein SL, Flynn JM, eds: *Lovell and Winter's Pediatric Orthopedics,*

ed 7. Philadelphia, PA, Lippincott Williams and Wilkins, 2014, pp 698-738.

The authors discuss the multiple aspects of congenital scoliosis.

9. Loder RT, Hernandez MJ, Lerner AL, et al: The induction of congenital spinal deformities in mice by maternal carbon monoxide exposure. *J Pediatr Orthop* 2000;20(5):662-666.

10. Alexander PG, Tuan RS: Carbon monoxide-induced axial skeletal dysmorphogenesis in the chick embryo. *Birth Defects Res A Clin Mol Teratol* 2003;67(4):219-230.

11. Winter RB, Moe JH, Eilers VE: Congenital scoliosis: A study of 234 patients treated and untreated: Part I. Natural history. *J Bone Joint Surg Am* 1968;50(1):1-15.

12. McMaster MJ, Ohtsuka K: The natural history of congenital scoliosis: A study of two hundred and fifty-one patients. *J Bone Joint Surg Am* 1982;64(8):1128-1147.

13. McMaster MJ: Occult intraspinal anomalies and congenital scoliosis. *J Bone Joint Surg Am* 1984;66(4):588-601.

14. Ghandhari H, Tari HV, Ameri E, Safari MB, Fouladi DF: Vertebral, rib, and intraspinal anomalies in congenital scoliosis: A study on 202 Caucasians. *Eur Spine J* 2015;24(7):1510-1521.

    This observational study of 202 Caucasian patients revealed diastematomyelia as the most common intraspinal anomaly associated with congenital scoliosis.

15. Gupta N, Rajasekaran S, Balamurali G, Shetty A: Vertebral and intraspinal anomalies in Indian population with congenital scoliosis: A study of 119 consecutive patients. *Asian Spine J* 2016;10(2):276-281.

    This study of an Indian population reported that tethered cord was the most common intraspinal anomaly associated with congenital scoliosis.

16. Skaggs DL, Guillaume T, El-Hawary R, Emans J, Mendelow M, Smith J; Scoliosis Research Society Growing Spine Committee: Early onset scoliosis consensus statement. *Spine Deform* 2015;3(2):107.

    A consensus statement by the SRS committee classifies EOS etiologies and provides definitions.

17. Ouellet JA, Arlet V: Neuromuscular scoliosis, in Boos N, Aebi M, eds, *Spinal Disorders: Fundamentals of Diagnosis and Treatment*. Berlin, Germany, Springer-Verlag, 2008, pp 663-692.

18. Berven S, Bradford DS: Neuromuscular scoliosis: Causes of deformity and principles for evaluation and management. *Semin Neurol* 2002;22(2):167-178.

19. Grauers A, Danielsson A, Karlsson M, Ohlin A, Gerdhem P: Family history and its association to curve size and treatment in 1,463 patients with idiopathic scoliosis. *Eur Spine J* 2013;22(11):2421-2426.

    Based on the self-assessment questionnaire responses of 1,463 patients with idiopathic scoliosis, the authors found larger curve sizes in patients with a positive family history of scoliosis, but no relationship between family history and sex or age of onset.

20. Grauers A, Wang J, Einarsdottir E, et al: Candidate gene analysis and exome sequencing confirm LBX1 as a susceptibility gene for idiopathic scoliosis. *Spine J* 2015;15(10):2239-2246.

    A case-control study of a Scandinavian cohort using exome sequencing found a highly significant association between an intergenic variant downstream of the *LBX1* gene and idiopathic scoliosis.

21. Zhang W, Sha S, Xu L, Liu Z, Qiu Y, Zhu Z: The prevalence of intraspinal anomalies in infantile and juvenile patients with "presumed idiopathic" scoliosis: A MRI-based analysis of 504 patients. *BMC Musculoskelet Disord* 2016;17:189.

    This MRI evaluation of patients with infantile or juvenile idiopathic scoliosis revealed an approximate 20% incidence of neural abnormality. This finding suggests the need for the increased use of advanced imaging for all patients with scoliosis who are younger than 10 years.

22. Thompson SK, Bentley G: Prognosis in infantile idiopathic scoliosis. *J Bone Joint Surg Br* 1980;62(2):151-154.

23. Yang S, Andras LM, Redding GJ, Skaggs DL: Early-onset scoliosis: A review of history, current treatment, and future directions. *Pediatrics* 2016;137(1):e20150709.

    This review article discusses EOS along with nonsurgical and surgical treatment options, including growth-friendly techniques.

24. Mehta MH: The rib-vertebra angle in the early diagnosis between resolving and progressive infantile scoliosis. *J Bone Joint Surg Br* 1972;54(2):230-243.

25. Baulesh DM, Huh J, Judkins T, Garg S, Miller NH, Erickson MA: The role of serial casting in early-onset scoliosis (EOS). *J Pediatr Orthop* 2012;32(7):658-663.

    Casting regimens for patients with idiopathic and nonidiopathic EOS are compared. A trend toward improved deformity correction in patients with idiopathic pathology was found, along with normal longitudinal thoracic growth in all patients. Level of evidence: III.

26. Gomez JA, Lee JK, Kim PD, Roye DP, Vitale MG: "Growth friendly" spine surgery: Management options for the young child with scoliosis. *J Am Acad Orthop Surg* 2011;19(12):722-727.

    The authors review growth-friendly surgical treatment options for children with scoliosis, including distraction-based, guided-growth, and compression-based strategies. These treatments are aimed at curve control and maintenance of spinal and thorax growth.

5: Spine Deformity

27. Wessell NM, Martus JE, Halanski MA, Snyder B, Truong W: What's new in pediatric spine growth modulation and implant technology for early-onset scoliosis? *J Pediatr Orthop* 2016; Jul 11 [Epub ahead of print].

A literature review of recent articles discussing growth-friendly surgical treatment options for EOS is presented.

28. Skaggs DL, Akbarnia BA, Flynn JM, Myung KS, Sponseller PD, Vitale MG; Chest Wall and Spine Deformity Study Group; Growing Spine Study Group; Pediatric Orthopaedic Society of North America; Scoliosis Research Society Growing Spine Study Committee: A classification of growth friendly spine implants. *J Pediatr Orthop* 2014;34(3):260-274.

Growth-friendly spine implant systems are classified into three categories (distraction-based, compression-based, and guided-growth) to improve communication and facilitate comparative studies.

29. Campbell RM Jr, Smith MD, Hell-Vocke AK: Expansion thoracoplasty: The surgical technique of opening-wedge thoracostomy. *J Bone Joint Surg Am* 2004;86(suppl 1):51-64.

30. Akbarnia BA, Mundis GM Jr, Salari P, Yaszay B, Pawelek JB: Innovation in growing rod technique: A study of safety and efficacy of a magnetically controlled growing rod in a porcine model. *Spine (Phila Pa 1976)* 2012;37(13):1109-1114.

This in vivo randomized study of magnetically controlled growing rod technology within a porcine model indicated attainment of 80% of predicted spinal height using remote distraction and an accelerated increase in spinal height after implant removal.

31. Akbarnia BA, Cheung K, Noordeen H, et al: Next generation of growth-sparing techniques: Preliminary clinical results of a magnetically controlled growing rod in 14 patients with early-onset scoliosis. *Spine (Phila Pa 1976)* 2013;38(8):665-670.

This prospective nonrandomized study of the use of a magnetically controlled growing rod technique in patients with progressive EOS reported comparable safety and distraction efficacy compared with standard growing rod therapy.

32. Dannawi Z, Altaf F, Harshavardhana NS, El Sebaie H, Noordeen H: Early results of a remotely-operated magnetic growth rod in early-onset scoliosis. *Bone Joint J* 2013;95(1):75-80.

This single institutional study discusses outcomes and complications of magnetic growing rod placement in a small cohort of patients with EOS.

33. McCarthy RE, Sucato D, Turner JL, Zhang H, Henson MA, McCarthy K: Shilla growing rods in a caprine animal model: A pilot study. *Clin Orthop Relat Res* 2010;468(3):705-710.

34. McCarthy RE, McCullough FL: Shilla growth guidance for early-onset scoliosis: Results after a minimum of five years of follow-up. *J Bone Joint Surg Am* 2015;97(19):1578-1584.

This study of patients treated with Shilla growth guidance surgery reported a relatively high complication rate but the ability to achieve reasonable curve control until definitive surgical correction.

35. Betz RR, Ranade A, Samdani AF, et al: Vertebral body stapling: A fusionless treatment option for a growing child with moderate idiopathic scoliosis. *Spine (Phila Pa 1976)* 2010;35(2):169-176.

36. Trobisch PD, Samdani A, Cahill P, Betz RR: Vertebral body stapling as an alternative in the treatment of idiopathic scoliosis. *Oper Orthop Traumatol* 2011;23(3):227-231.

Vertebral body stapling as an effective treatment in skeletally immature patients with idiopathic scoliosis was demonstrated in this study from a single institution.

37. Uzumcugil A, Cil A, Yazici M, et al: Convex growth arrest in the treatment of congenital spinal deformities, revisited. *J Pediatr Orthop* 2004;24(6):658-666.

38. Yaszay B, O'Brien M, Shufflebarger HL, et al: Efficacy of hemivertebra resection for congenital scoliosis: A multicenter retrospective comparison of three surgical techniques. *Spine (Phila Pa 1976)* 2011;36(24):2052-2060.

This multicenter retrospective study compared the following three surgical treatments for congenital scoliosis: hemiepiphysiodesis, instrumented fusion without hemivertebra excision, and instrumented hemivertebra resection. A higher percentage of deformity correction was found with hemivertebra resection than with hemiepiphysiodesis or instrumented fusion without resection.

39. Jeszenszky D, Haschtmann D, Kleinstück FS, et al: Posterior vertebral column resection in early onset spinal deformities. *Eur Spine J* 2014;23(1):198-208.

The effectiveness of vertebral column resection in EOS was demonstrated in this small case series.

40. Chang DG, Yang JH, Lee JH, et al: Pediatric posterior vertebral column resection (PVCR): Before and after ten years of age: Greater than 10-year follow-up. *Spine (Phila Pa 1976)* 2016;41(21):E1271-E1278.

Long-term follow-up of patients with congenital scoliosis treated with vertebral column resection showed improvement in the Cobb angle when surgery was performed before the patient was 10 years of age. Level of evidence: IV.

41. Thorsness RJ, Faust JR, Behrend CJ, Sanders JO: Nonsurgical management of early-onset scoliosis. *J Am Acad Orthop Surg* 2015;23(9):519-528.

The potential effect of serial casting on idiopathic and smaller magnitude curves is discussed.

42. Dede O, Sturm PF: A brief history and review of modern casting techniques in early onset scoliosis. *J Child Orthop* 2016;10(5):405-411.

   The authors discuss casting history, indications, and techniques for patients with EOS.

43. Goldberg CJ, Gillic I, Connaughton O, et al: Respiratory function and cosmesis at maturity in infantile-onset scoliosis. *Spine (Phila Pa 1976)* 2003;28(20):2397-2406.

44. Vitale MG, Matsumoto H, Bye MR, et al: A retrospective cohort study of pulmonary function, radiographic measures, and quality of life in children with congenital scoliosis: An evaluation of patient outcomes after early spinal fusion. *Spine (Phila Pa 1976)* 2008;33(11):1242-1249.

45. Karol LA: Early definitive spinal fusion in young children: What we have learned. *Clin Orthop Relat Res* 2011;469(5):1323-1329.

   A review of the literature revealed Chiari malformation as the most common intraspinal anomaly in patients with infantile and juvenile idiopathic scoliosis.

46. Sturm PF, Anadio JM, Dede O: Recent advances in the management of early onset scoliosis. *Orthop Clin North Am* 2014;45(4):501-514.

   Growth-friendly surgical options for EOS are discussed.

47. Matsumoto H, Williams B, Park HY, et al: The final 24-item Early Onset Scoliosis Questionnaires (EOSQ-24): Validity, reliability and responsiveness. *J Pediatr Orthop* 2016.

   Assessment of the 24-item Early Onset Scoliosis Questionnaire indicated that it is a valid and reliable measurement tool to evaluate outcomes.

48. Smith JT, Johnston C, Skaggs D, Flynn J, Vitale M: A new classification system to report complications in growing spine surgery: A multicenter consensus study. *J Pediatr Orthop* 2015;35(8):798-803.

   A classification system was developed to report complications from growth-friendly spine surgery so that comparisons can be made between different treatment techniques.

5: Spine Deformity

Chapter 22

Juvenile and Adolescent Idiopathic Scoliosis

Daniel Bouton, MD   Daniel J. Sucato, MD, MS

Abstract

Idiopathic scoliosis is the most common structural deformity of the spine in the juvenile and adolescent populations. It is a complex, three-dimensional torsional change of the spinal column for which no definitive etiology can be determined. The focus of orthopaedic treatment is to prevent curve progression through bracing and/or surgery. Although the efficacy of bracing has been proved in recent years, much research has been focused on predicting which patients will have curve progression despite appropriate brace management. In the juvenile population, treatment strategies are aimed at preventing curve progression while allowing the spinal column and thorax to grow to an appropriate size. In adolescents with a progressive curve, surgical intervention may prevent progression while obtaining appropriate spinal balance in the coronal and sagittal planes. Complications in the treatment of idiopathic scoliosis can be categorized as postoperative infection, pseudarthrosis, and the very rarely occurring neurologic deficits. Important advances in standardizing patient care have markedly diminished the frequency of these complications. Current research is focused on improving the quality of care and minimizing the risks of complications.

Keywords: adolescent; idiopathic; juvenile; scoliosis

Introduction

Scoliosis has been described since ancient times and is defined as a lateral deviation of at least 10° from the normal coronal alignment of the spine. However, scoliosis is well understood to be a complex, three-dimensional torsion of the spinal column. Idiopathic scoliosis, a structural curvature of the spine for which no definitive etiology can be determined, is the most common type of structural scoliosis, accounting for almost 80% of incidences. Idiopathic scoliosis is classified based on the age of the patient at initial diagnosis. Infantile idiopathic scoliosis is diagnosed in children younger than 3 years, and juvenile idiopathic scoliosis (JIS) is diagnosed in children age 4 to 9 years. Together, these two conditions often are called early-onset scoliosis. Adolescent idiopathic scoliosis (AIS) is diagnosed in patients older than 10 years and up to 18 years of age.

Clinical Evaluation

Scoliosis in a child or adolescent often is detected during a school screening program, and the patient subsequently is referred to an orthopaedic surgeon. The clinical evaluation should begin with a thorough history and physical examination. Similar conditions such as spondylolysis, spondylolisthesis, and Scheuermann kyphosis should be ruled out. Back pain occurs in approximately 32% of adolescents with idiopathic scoliosis, but its cause is identified in only 10% of patients, despite appropriate imaging.[1] It is of value to obtain a girl's menstrual history for estimating future growth potential.

Patients typically have one of several noticeable physical characteristics, including a high shoulder, a scapular

Dr. Bouton or an immediate family member has received nonincome support (such as equipment or services), commercially derived honoraria, or other non–research-related funding (such as paid travel) from OrthoPediatrics. Dr. Sucato or an immediate family member has received royalties from Globus Medical and serves as a board member, owner, officer, or committee member of the Pediatric Orthopaedic Society of North America and the Scoliosis Research Society.

5: Spine Deformity

prominence, or an asymmetry of the trunk or flank. The physical examination is critical to rule out any underlying neurologic causes of the deformity. Attention should be focused on cutaneous manifestations of spinal dysraphism such as midline hemangiomas, hairy tufts, and dimpling. A thorough neurologic examination of motor strength, sensation, and lower extremity reflexes is important. The umbilical or abdominal reflexes are most predictive of a neural axis abnormality. A subtle cavovarus or pes cavus foot deformity sometimes is the only clue to an underlying neurologic condition.

Radiographic Evaluation

The radiographic evaluation is similar for patients with JIS or AIS. Standing PA and lateral long-cassette radiographs of the entire spine and pelvis are required. Bending and supine radiographs usually are reserved for preoperative guidance. Measurement of the Cobb angle from the most tilted caudal and cephalic vertebrae toward the concavity is useful for quantifying the deformity, although this measurement has an interobserver variability of 6° to 7°.[2] Radiographs should be scrutinized for any evidence of congenital vertebral anomalies, absent posterior elements, or rib abnormalities. Particular attention should be given to the sagittal profile—thoracic hypokyphosis at the apex is characteristic of idiopathic scoliosis—and junctional kyphosis, which indicates that both curves may be structural. The rib–vertebral angle difference is less valuable for predicting the progression of the curve in patients with JIS than in those with infantile idiopathic scoliosis, and it is not routinely used in the evaluation of patients with JIS.[3]

MRI should be considered for every patient with JIS. Intraspinal abnormalities exist in 18% to 20% of patients in whom a diagnosis of JIS is made before age 10 years.[4] Male sex and left thoracic or right lumbar curve patterns were positively associated with a neural lesion on MRI.[5,6] MRI should be considered for a patient with AIS if the patient has an abnormal curve pattern (especially a left thoracic curve), rapid curve progression, an abnormal neurologic examination, apical thoracic kyphosis, or persistent neck pain and headache.

Juvenile Idiopathic Scoliosis

Epidemiology and Natural History

JIS comprises 13% to 16% of all cases of idiopathic scoliosis diagnosed in the United States.[7,8] Girls are affected more often than boys, and the female-to-male ratio increases with age. The average age at diagnosis is almost 7 years, although a diagnosis tends to be made earlier in boys than in girls.[9] JIS is more likely to progress, more likely to require surgical intervention, and less likely to respond to bracing than AIS.[10]

JIS most often appears during a relatively quiescent time between periods of rapid spinal column growth in infancy and adolescence. As a result, the initial curve progression may be slow or moderate, and patients, families, and the surgeon may not be aware of the potential for future problems. Ultimately, however, 70% of patients with JIS have deformity progression requiring treatment.[11] Untreated patients were found to have a higher mortality rate beginning at age 40 to 50 years, which mainly resulted from pulmonary compromise, than either the general population or patients with AIS.[12]

Classification

The Lenke classification of AIS can be applied to JIS; the six curve types, three lumbar coronal modifiers, and three thoracic sagittal modifiers are the same.[13] The most common patterns in both JIS and AIS are right thoracic and double major curves. Several noteworthy modifications of the Lenke classification apply to JIS, however. The curve having the largest Cobb angle is determined to be the major curve and is considered structural. Side-bending radiographs are not used in JIS to determine whether a minor curve is structural. A main thoracic curve is considered structural if its apical vertebra or disk space fails to touch the C7 plumb line. Similarly, a thoracolumbar or lumbar curve is considered structural if its apex fails to touch the center sacral vertical line. A proximal thoracic curve is considered structural if the contralateral first rib is elevated with respect to the ipsilateral first rib.

Treatment

Curve progression is more likely in JIS than AIS, but observation is appropriate for a patient with JIS who has a curve of less than 20° to 25°. Depending on the patient's age, the curve magnitude, and the severity of clinical deformity, surveillance-interval radiographs should be obtained every 4 to 12 months.[10] As the adolescent growth spurt approaches, the patient must be followed more closely because a minimally progressive curve can quickly worsen.[14]

Nonsurgical management of JIS varies depending on the age and size of the patient. The two most common nonsurgical modalities are casting and bracing. In infantile-onset scoliosis, cast or brace treatment can lead to curve resolution, but in JIS the goal is to prevent curve progression. Bracing most often is chosen over casting because of ease of use and patient and family acceptance. For patients with a rigid curve who are younger than 5 years, the choice may be serial casting with a Risser cast that is changed every 6 to 12 weeks. The goal of casting is to stabilize the curve so that the patient can continue to further treatment with bracing.[10] In most patients with JIS, bracing is indicated for curves larger than 20° to 25° but smaller than 50°. Patients with JIS have more remaining years of growth until skeletal maturity than patients with AIS, and the task of controlling the curve, therefore, is more challenging. Multiple braces often are needed as the child continues to grow. Maintaining compliance throughout these years can be difficult. Nonetheless, brace treatment of patients with JIS can be successful, particularly for those with curves less than 30°.[15]

Several different types of braces can be used to treat JIS or AIS. In general, the two categories are full-time braces and nighttime overcorrection braces. The most commonly used full-time brace is the underarm thoracolumbosacral orthosis, which uses corrective molds fabricated into a plastic brace.[16] It is important to be aware that a brace-induced rib deformity can result from pressure on the soft rib cage of a relatively young patient who must undergo a long period of treatment with the thoracolumbosacral orthosis.[13]

Nighttime overcorrection braces, such as the Charleston and Providence braces, are advantageous because they need to be worn only at night; this factor theoretically improves patient compliance. The success rates of nighttime bracing vary but are correlated with the best in-brace correction. On average, patients with successfully treated curves were found to have an in-brace correction of 102%; those who eventually required surgical intervention had an in-brace correction of only 73%.[17]

A comparison of JIS and AIS curves requiring surgical treatment found that the JIS curves were larger, more kyphotic, and less well compensated and that their apex and stable vertebra were more caudal.[18] No one surgical treatment has been universally successful for treating JIS. Each of the many different surgical options has its own set of complications and shortcomings. In general, surgical treatments are categorized as growth-friendly options or definitive fusion. Interest in growth-friendly procedures has increased with findings about the long-term complications associated with early thoracic fusion. Posterior-only fusion at a young age carries the risk of continued anterior growth and crankshaft deformity as well as pulmonary complications.[19] Patients at the greatest risk for the development of crankshaft deformity are younger than 10 years, with open triradiate cartilage and Risser grade 0 skeletal maturity. In the past, anterior fusion would have been strongly considered in addition to posterior fusion for these patients, but all-pedicle-screw constructs may obviate the need for anterior fusion in some patients.[20,21] The Sanders hand classification is gaining

popularity because of its seemingly good interobserver and intraobserver reliability and its ability to provide more detailed information with respect to the timing of peak height velocity in patients with AIS.[22,23]

The goal of treatment in patients with JIS is to halt curve progression with nonsurgical methods while allowing time for additional spinal column growth in an attempt to avoid surgical treatment until the patient is at an appropriate age for definitive spinal fusion. Many growth-friendly technologies have been developed to lessen the burden of traditional growing-rod constructs. Although there are no definitive indications, a survey of expert surgeons concluded that growing-rod posterior constructs should be considered for patients who are younger than 8 to 10 years, have a curve larger than 60°, and either have documented curve progression despite compliant brace wear or cannot tolerate brace wear.[24] Growing-rod constructs were introduced in 1978 and were improved by the advent of dual-rod submuscular constructs intended to improve the amount of growth obtained at each lengthening while minimizing the risk of complications.[25] In comparison with single-rod techniques, dual-rod techniques were found to provide better initial correction and maintenance of correction, with a lower complication rate.[26]

A currently used technique involves fusing the end vertebra to an adjacent vertebra using double-level pedicle screws for distal and proximal fixation. A proximal level as cranial as T1 or T2 often is chosen to avoid the risk of junctional kyphosis. Two rods are placed proximally and distally and are connected at some point in between, usually in an area of neutral sagittal alignment such as the thoracolumbar junction. Rod overlap allows for future lengthening. To achieve maximal growth, lengthening is done at intervals of less than 6 months. Anterior or posterior apical fusion sometimes is done simultaneously with the initial rod implantation, but the combination of apical fusion and growing-rod constructs can lead to curve stiffening and crankshaft deformity as well as other complications. The use of dual growing rod placement without apical fusion resulted in better initial correction and better maintenance of correction at 2-year follow-up.[27]

Although growing-rod constructs have several advantages over early spine fusion, every lengthening procedure carries risks from anesthesia and infection. Magnetically controlled growing rods have been enthusiastically received as a means of limiting risks. These devices can be gradually distracted by using a remote device in an outpatient setting (**Figure 1**). The rods are implanted in a fashion similar to that used for traditional growing rods, with anchor points placed proximally and distally.

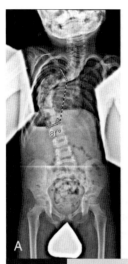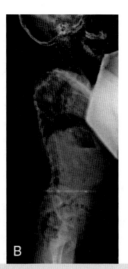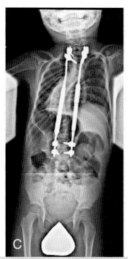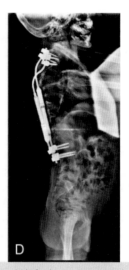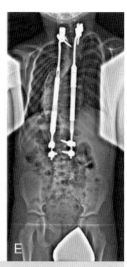

Figure 1 AP **(A)** and lateral **(B)** standing radiographs showing a hyperkyphotic left thoracic curve measuring 81° in the coronal plane in a 6-year-old patient with early-onset idiopathic scoliosis. Postoperative AP **(C)** and lateral **(D)** standing radiographs showing a magnetically controlled growing-rod construct inserted from T1 to L3, with posterior spinal fusion at T1-T2 and L2-L3. **E,** AP standing radiograph showing improvement in the coronal plane 10 months after surgery. Both growing rods had been magnetically lengthened in the clinic at 4-month intervals. The two lengthening procedures achieved a total 10 mm of lengthening.

The rod contains an internal magnet that can be rotated through an external device to lengthen or shorten the construct. Although these devices are still in development, their use is increasing. Small case studies reported good results.[28-30] At a follow-up of approximately 2 years, a 43% to 56% Cobb angle correction was achieved with an average T1-T12 height increase of 0.8 mm per month.[30] However, a complication was reported in as many as 38.8% of patients, and 27.8% required at least one revision surgery (not including the definitive fusion).[31] The most common complications were screw pullout, rod breakage, and decreased effectiveness of successive lengthenings. Larger prospective studies are warranted to further investigate this new technology.

Spinal growth modulation in the form of vertebral body staples or flexible tethers has been proposed for treating young patients with either JIS or AIS. In theory, this method would improve the coronal curve by halting growth on the convex side of the curve, in accordance with the Heuter-Volkmann principle, and allowing growth on the concave side. Multiple techniques have been used for spinal growth modulation, none of which have yet been approved by the FDA. A retrospective study of nitinol staples placed from end vertebra to end vertebra found that success depended on the curve having a relatively small preoperative magnitude; 78% of thoracic curves smaller than 35° remained static or improved, compared with 25% of thoracic curves larger than 35°.[32] The complications included pneumothorax, staple displacement, and overcorrection. Anterior spinal tethering is a growth-modulation technique suggested for use in hypokyphotic thoracic curves larger than 40° in patients with substantial growth remaining.[33] Bicortical screws are placed in the vertebral bodies from end vertebra to end vertebra and connected with a tether. This technique often is performed thoracoscopically, and it requires the lung to be deflated for adequate visualization. A retrospective study of 11 patients at 2-year follow-up found an average Cobb angle correction of 70% as well as axial rotational improvement.[33] Two patients required tether loosening to prevent overcorrection. The procedure carries all of the risks of anterior thoracolumbar spinal surgery. The long-term motion of the instrumented segment and disks is unknown, and further study is needed to determine the ultimate role of this technique in the treatment of JIS.

Adolescent Idiopathic Scoliosis

Epidemiology, Etiology, and Natural History

AIS is defined as a structural curvature of the spine in the coronal plane in patients older than 10 years up to 18 years of age. The estimated prevalence of AIS is approximately 3%.[34] Curves of increasing severity are less common in AIS than in JIS. Almost equal numbers of girls and boys have a relatively small curve, but the ratio of girls to boys increases with curve severity; the ratio is 7.2:1 for patients with a curve requiring orthopaedic treatment.[35]

The exact cause of AIS is unknown but probably is multifactorial. Investigation into a possible genetic component is promising. A candidate gene has been identified. A recent gene-targeting study reported that the removal of G protein-coupled receptor 126 (*GPR126*) from mouse chondrocytes resulted in an idiopathic scoliosis deformity.[36]

The natural history of AIS is variable and depends on skeletal maturity and curve magnitude at diagnosis. In a skeletally immature patient (Risser grade 0 or 1) a curve larger than 20° is at a high risk for progression.[37] Much depends on whether the patient has reached peak height velocity, which can be difficult to estimate until it has passed. After skeletal maturity, curves progress less quickly than before skeletal maturity. Thoracic curves larger than 50° tend to progress at a rate of approximately 1° per year into adulthood.[38] The mortality rate among patients with AIS is similar to that of the general population. Chronic back pain, lumbar osteoarthritis, and slight dissatisfaction with body image have been associated with AIS.[39]

Classification

The Lenke classification was developed to describe AIS curve patterns and guide surgical planning.[40] This comprehensive classification system takes into account both the coronal and sagittal planes. In patients with AIS, unlike those with JIS, side-bending radiographs are obtained to determine whether a minor curve should be considered surgically structural. A minor curve that corrects to less than 25° is not categorized as a structural curve and is not included in the definitive fusion. As in JIS, care must be taken to evaluate the sagittal contour, specifically at the junctional zones (T2-T5 and T10-L2) because kyphosis larger than 20° in these areas can render a curve structural regardless of its characteristics in the coronal plane.

Treatment

In general, three types of treatments are used for patients with AIS: observation, bracing, and surgical intervention. Most adolescents can be simply observed because of the low probability that their curve will progress.[37] An algorithm developed to provide guidance to the surgeon specifies that patients with a curve magnitude of less than 25° can be observed regardless of skeletal maturity as defined by the Risser sign. If the patient's skeletal maturity is at Risser grade 1 or 2, a curve as large as 30° can be observed with radiographic follow-up at regular intervals until skeletal maturity is reached. If the patient has less growth remaining (Risser grade 3, 4, or 5), a curve as large as 40° to 45° can be treated with observation. These guidelines are general, however, and treatment must be tailored to the individual patient. The

iliac apophysis often does not ossify until an average of 18 months after the curve acceleration phase. Because of this finding, attempts have been made to better stratify patients in the Risser 0 stage regarding the likelihood of curve progression. The Tanner-Whitehouse method, which uses radiographs of the hand to assess skeletal maturity, has been more closely correlated with the timing of peak growth velocity and may better predict which patients in the Risser 0 stage would likely benefit from brace treatment.[41] Attempts have been made to predict curve progression using a DNA-based test (ScoliScore; Axial Biotech). Despite promising initial results, a recent independent evaluation found no difference in the scores of patients with and without curve progression.[42] Currently, this expensive test is not indicated in the management of AIS.

Brace treatment has had resurgent popularity in recent years. Several well-designed studies found a clear benefit to brace treatment for some patients in comparison with observation (**Figure 2**). The indications for brace treatment in patients with AIS include a primary curve of 25° to 40° and skeletal immaturity (Risser grade 0, 1, or 2). Girls should be premenarchal or less than 1 year postmenarchal. Brace wear was clearly acknowledged as a viable treatment option after a National Institutes of Health–funded randomized prospective study was ended earlier than scheduled because the efficacy of bracing had been established.[43] The curve did not progress to surgical magnitude in 75% of patients who underwent bracing compared with 42% of patients in the observation group. Brace treatment was found to be dosage dependent; at least 16 hours of daily wear generally is recommended.[44] The Charleston nighttime overcorrection brace, which is worn only for 8 to 10 hours per day, is an alternative to a full-time brace. The Charleston brace has been found to be as effective as the Milwaukee and Boston full-time braces, but a comparison study concluded that the Charleston brace should be reserved for use in patients with a single lumbar or thoracolumbar curve smaller than 35°.[45] Although brace treatment allows many patients to avoid surgery, it is not universally successful. The risk that brace treatment will be unsuccessful is greatest in a patient who is not compliant with treatment, is at Risser grade 0, has open triradiate cartilage, or has a curve of 30° or larger.[46] Compliance was improved and the amount of curve progression was decreased when temperature sensors in the brace were used to provide the patient with feedback about compliance.[47]

A desire to avoid surgical intervention has incentivized patients and their families to seek alternative nonsurgical modalities. Physical therapy and scoliosis-specific exercises have become increasingly popular. In theory, a dedicated physical therapy program aimed at conditioning the muscles in an asymmetric torso and back might improve spinal alignment. Modest improvement in scoliosis control has been reported, but a systematic review

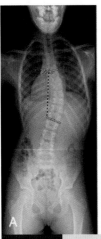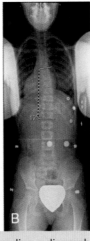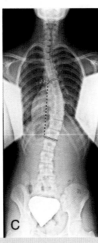

Figure 2 **A,** PA standing radiograph showing a 36° right thoracic curve in a girl age 10 years, 4 months. Open triradiate cartilages and Risser grade 0 iliac apophysis can be seen. The patient was premenarchal. **B,** PA standing radiograph showing the patient wearing a thoracolumbosacral orthosis, with correction of the curve to 12° in the coronal plane. **C,** PA standing radiograph showing a stable curve with no progression achieved by age 17 years. Closed triradiate cartilages and Risser grade 4 iliac apophysis can be seen. The patient's height increased 26.1 cm throughout the course of treatment.

determined that a lack of high-quality evidence precluded recommending the use of scoliosis-specific exercises.[48]

Recent reports suggest that patients treated with the Schroth exercise method have improvement in Scoliosis Research Society (SRS)-22r scores and self-image, with a trend toward less risk for curve progression in skeletally immature patients.[49,50] *Programs using scoliosis-specific exercises are labor intensive, the therapist must be certified, and results have been mixed.

Surgery is a reasonable option for patients with a thoracic curve exceeding 50° at skeletal maturity because continuing progression would be expected.[51] Lumbar curves of smaller magnitude (40° to 45°) also can be surgically treated because these curves have a propensity to worsen over time, and the clinical deformity may be unacceptable. Posterior spinal fusion with segmental pedicle screw instrumentation has become the mainstay of treatment, although anterior fusion remains a viable option for certain curve patterns. Pedicle screws offer better three-column correctional power than older hook-and-rod constructs (**Figure 3**).

The Lenke classification system has been useful for standardizing the selection of curves to be treated with posterior spinal fusion.[40] It is important to determine whether each curve is structural and to include all structural curves in the fusion construct. In general, the upper instrumented vertebra is the proximal end vertebra for a thoracic or thoracolumbar-lumbar curve. If the proximal thoracic curve is structural, T2 is often selected as the upper instrumented vertebra. Clinical shoulder balance

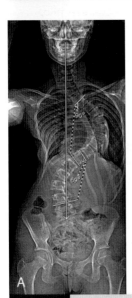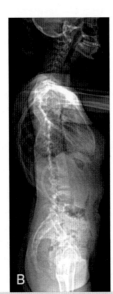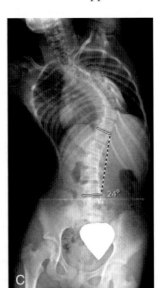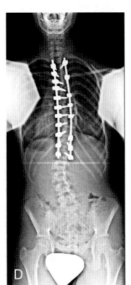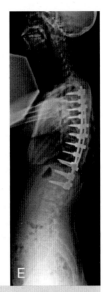

Figure 3 PA (**A**) and lateral (**B**) radiographs from a 14-year-old girl demonstrate thoracic and lumbar curves measuring 96° and 69°, respectively, in the coronal plane, and a hypokyphotic sagittal contour. **C,** Supine left-bending radiograph demonstrates improvement of the left lumbar curve to 24° in the coronal plane. A T3-L1 posterior instrumented spinal fusion was performed. Standing radiographs obtain at the 2-year follow-up show substantial improvement in the coronal (**D**) and sagittal (**E**) planes.

Table 1

Fusion Level Guidelines for Adolescent Idiopathic Scoliosis Curve Patterns

Lenke Primary Curve Type	Upper Instrumented Vertebra	Lowest Instrumented Vertebra
1	Proximal end vertebra[a]	Most distal vertebra touched by center sacral vertical line or neutral vertebra[b]
2	Proximal end vertebra	Most distal vertebra touched by center sacral vertical line or neutral vertebra[b]
3	Proximal end vertebra[a]	Distal end vertebra[c]
4	Proximal end vertebra	Distal end vertebra[c]
5	Proximal end vertebra	Distal end vertebra[c]
6	Proximal end vertebra[a]	Distal end vertebra[c]

[a]T2 if the left shoulder is elevated, T3 if the shoulders are level, T4 if the right shoulder is elevated.

[b]If the preoperative neutral and distal end vertebrae are the same or have a one-level difference. If the neutral vertebra is two or three levels caudal to the end vertebra, the lowest instrumented vertebra should be one level cephalad to the neutral vertebra.

[c]One level cephalad to the distal end vertebra if it crosses the midline and adequately derotates on a convex bending radiograph.

should be considered in determining whether the proximal thoracic curve is structural. Deciding on the lowest instrumented vertebra often is more controversial. Coronal and sagittal balance should be considered. Often the lowest instrumented vertebra is the lowest vertebra that last touches the center sacral vertical line, especially for a thoracic curve. Guidelines have been proposed based on the relationship of the distal end vertebra to the neutral vertebra, which is the most cephalad vertebra with a neutral axial plane rotation.[52] In patients with single or double thoracic curves, the following rules apply. When the preoperative end and neutral vertebrae are the same or have a one-level gap, the lowest instrumented vertebra should be the neutral vertebra. If the neutral vertebra is two or three levels distal to the end vertebra, the fusion should end one level proximal to the neutral vertebra. In a double major curve or a thoracolumbar-lumbar curve, it is generally accepted to use the lowest end vertebra as the lowest instrumented vertebra. Bending radiographs can be useful for refining the selection of the lowest instrumented vertebra and determining the fusion level. For example, if L3 is the end vertebra and the L3 vertebral body crosses the center sacral vertical line in right-bending radiographs, fusion can stop at L3. Otherwise, fusion should be extended to L4 (**Figure 3**) and (**Table 1**).

Anterior spinal fusion has been used less often since the advent of thoracic pedicle screws but still is a viable option and was found to achieve excellent three-dimensional correction in single thoracolumbar-lumbar curve patterns. A prospective study comparing anterior and posterior spinal fusion for Lenke type 5 curves found shorter fusions and lower costs with anterior fusion, with no difference in safety or efficacy.[53] Proponents of an all-posterior approach, however, suggest that fusion levels are similar, correction is the same, and surgical time is shorter with a posterior fusion than an anterior fusion. In addition, an all-posterior approach obviates the need for chest tube placement and most likely contributes to less time in the hospital.

Important advances have been made in the care of patients with AIS after posterior fusion. Multimodal pain control regimens and early mobilization have resulted in a decrease in hospital length of stay and complications. The use of an accelerated discharge pathway was found to decrease length of stay by almost 50% without an increase in readmissions or early complications.[54] Further research is being undertaken to improve the efficiency and quality of care while controlling costs in an increasingly cost-sensitive healthcare environment.

Surgical Complications

Like any surgical intervention, posterior spinal fusion carries substantial risks that must be discussed preoperatively with the patient and family. Neurologic injury and surgical site infection are uncommon but must be considered. Spinal cord monitoring is critical to the safety of any surgery for spinal deformity. Intraoperative neurologic monitoring has become the standard of care. The combination of somatosensory-evoked potentials and transcranial motor-evoked potentials decreases the risk of an unrecognized injury to the spinal cord. A large multicenter study found that 3.4% of patients undergoing posterior spinal fusion for AIS had a critical change on

5: Spine Deformity

monitoring with combined somatosensory-evoked and transcranial motor-evoked potentials, and the surgeon responded intraoperatively. Intraoperative neurologic monitoring detected all transient motor or sensory deficits.[55] The wake-up test has limited use in a patient with idiopathic scoliosis when advanced monitoring is used.

Surgical site infection can be associated with substantial morbidity, increased costs, and poor long-term outcomes. Rates of delayed surgical site infection as high as 6.9% were reported in patients with AIS,[56] although other studies reported much lower percentages.[57,58]

Surgical site infection has been associated with medical comorbidities, blood transfusions, and not having used a postoperative drain.[59] A recent retrospective analysis showed that two doses of postoperative antibiotic prophylaxis were as effective as continued dosing until drain removal.[60] Routine use of prophylactic vancomycin and ceftazidime as well as pulsatile lavage has been promoted to minimize the infection risk.[61] Further research is needed to establish clear practice guidelines for minimizing the risk of surgical site infection in patients with AIS.

Summary

Idiopathic scoliosis is common in children and adolescents. Many advances have been made in nonsurgical and surgical treatment of JIS and AIS. Treatment with a brace is now widely accepted as an effective strategy for controlling curve progression in many patients. Surgical treatment can prevent curve progression into adulthood and achieve appropriate spinal balance in the coronal and sagittal planes. Surgical complications are uncommon but can be devastating. Ongoing clinical research can be expected to lead to improved outcomes and quality of care with a minimal risk of complications.

Key Study Points

- Idiopathic scoliosis, a three-dimensional deformity of the spinal column, is the most common type of scoliosis in children and adolescents.
- Brace treatment is effective for preventing progression of a curve to a surgical magnitude in certain adolescents with remaining spine growth. Its efficacy is dosage dependent.
- Posterior instrumented spinal fusion is the mainstay of treatment for adolescent patients with a curve larger than 50°. Much of the current research is focused on improving clinical outcomes while minimizing the risk of complications.

Annotated References

1. Ramirez N, Johnston CE, Browne RH: The prevalence of back pain in children who have idiopathic scoliosis. *J Bone Joint Surg Am* 1997;79(3):364-368.

2. Morrissy RT, Goldsmith GS, Hall EC, Kehl D, Cowie GH: Measurement of the Cobb angle on radiographs of patients who have scoliosis: Evaluation of intrinsic error. *J Bone Joint Surg Am* 1990;72(3):320-327.

3. Mehta MH: The rib-vertebra angle in the early diagnosis between resolving and progressive infantile scoliosis. *J Bone Joint Surg Br* 1972;54(2):230-243.

4. Dobbs MB, Lenke LG, Szymanski DA, et al: Prevalence of neural axis abnormalities in patients with infantile idiopathic scoliosis. *J Bone Joint Surg Am* 2002;84(12):2230-2234.

5. Evans SC, Edgar MA, Hall-Craggs MA, Powell MP, Taylor BA, Noordeen HH: MRI of 'idiopathic' juvenile scoliosis: A prospective study. *J Bone Joint Surg Br* 1996;78(2):314-317.

6. Zhang W, Sha S, Xu L, Liu Z, Qiu Y, Zhu Z: The prevalence of intraspinal anomalies in infantile and juvenile patients with "presumed idiopathic" scoliosis: A MRI-based analysis of 504 patients. *BMC Musculoskelet Disord* 2016;17:18. Medline

On MRI, 94 of 504 patients (18.7%) with scoliosis were found to have a neural axis abnormality. Male sex as well as left thoracic and right lumbar curve patterns were found to be associated with the presence of a neural axis abnormality. Level of evidence: IV.

7. Ponseti IV, Friedman B: Prognosis in idiopathic scoliosis. *J Bone Joint Surg Am* 1950;32(2):381-395.

8. Keiser RP, Shufflebarger HL: The Milwaukee brace in idiopathic scoliosis: Evaluation of 123 completed cases. *Clin Orthop Relat Res* 1976;118:19-24.

9. Robinson CM, McMaster MJ: Juvenile idiopathic scoliosis: Curve patterns and prognosis in one hundred and nine patients. *J Bone Joint Surg Am* 1996;78(8):1140-1148.

10. Dobbs MB, Weinstein SL: Infantile and juvenile scoliosis. *Orthop Clin North Am* 1999;30(3):331-341, vii.

11. Tolo VT, Gillespie R: The characteristics of juvenile idiopathic scoliosis and results of its treatment. *J Bone Joint Surg Br* 1978;60(2):181-188.

12. Pehrsson K, Larsson S, Oden A, Nachemson A: Long-term follow-up of patients with untreated scoliosis: A study of mortality, causes of death, and symptoms. *Spine (Phila Pa 1976)* 1992;17(9):1091-1096.

13. Lenke LG, Dobbs MB: Management of juvenile idiopathic scoliosis. *J Bone Joint Surg Am* 2007;89(suppl 1):55-63.

14. Charles YP, Daures JP, de Rosa V, Diméglio A: Progression risk of idiopathic juvenile scoliosis during pubertal growth. *Spine (Phila Pa 1976)* 2006;31(17):1933-1942.

15. Aulisa AG, Guzzanti V, Marzetti E, Giordano M, Falciglia F, Aulisa L: Brace treatment in juvenile idiopathic scoliosis: A prospective study in accordance with the SRS criteria for bracing studies. *Scoliosis* 2014;9:3.

    In a prospective study of 113 patients with JIS treated with a brace, 106 (93.8%) had curve correction or stabilization and only 7 (6.2%) had progression at 2-year follow-up. Brace wear was more effective for curves smaller than 30°. Level of evidence: II.

16. Schiller JR, Thakur NA, Eberson CP: Brace management in adolescent idiopathic scoliosis. *Clin Orthop Relat Res* 2010;468(3):670-678.

17. Jarvis J, Garbedian S, Swamy G: Juvenile idiopathic scoliosis: The effectiveness of part-time bracing. *Spine (Phila Pa 1976)* 2008;33(10):1074-1078.

18. McElroy MJ, Sponseller PD, Fuhrhop SK, et al; Harms Study Group; Growing Spine Study Group: Clinically significant differences exist between curves in operative idiopathic early-onset scoliosis and adolescent idiopathic scoliosis. *Spine (Phila Pa 1976)* 2013;38(16):1368-1374.

    Compared with surgically treated AIS curves, surgically treated early-onset scoliosis curves were larger, more kyphotic, and less well compensated, and they had a more caudal apex and stable vertebra. Level of evidence: III.

19. Dubousset J, Herring JA, Shufflebarger H: The crankshaft phenomenon. *J Pediatr Orthop* 1989;9(5):541-550.

20. Burton DC, Asher MA, Lai SM: Scoliosis correction maintenance in skeletally immature patients with idiopathic scoliosis: Is anterior fusion really necessary? *Spine (Phila Pa 1976)* 2000;25(1):61-68.

21. Tao F, Zhao Y, Wu Y, et al: The effect of differing spinal fusion instrumentation on the occurrence of postoperative crankshaft phenomenon in adolescent idiopathic scoliosis. *J Spinal Disord Tech* 2010;23(8):e75-e80.

22. Nicholson AD, Sanders JO, Liu RW, Cooperman DR: The relationship of calcaneal apophyseal ossification and Sanders hand scores to the timing of peak height velocity in adolescents. *Bone Joint J* 2015;97-B(12):1710-1717.

    Radiographs of the calcaneus and hand, along with height measurements, were obtained yearly in 94 patients between the ages of 3 and 18 years. The objective of the study was to determine the utility of these two studies in determining the time of peak height velocity. The calcaneal staging demonstrated four of six stages prior to the time of peak height velocity, whereas the Sanders method demonstrated two of eight stages. These data provide good information for clinicians when evaluating young children with idiopathic scoliosis to best determine the risk of curve progression based on the timing of peak height velocity.

23. Vira S, Husain Q, Jalai C, et al: The interobserver and intraobserver reliability of the Sanders classification versus the Risser stage. *J Pediatr Orthop* 2017;37(4):e246-e249.

    Interobserver and intraobserver reliability were compared using the Sanders classification and the Risser staging methods for determining peak height velocity in patients with idiopathic scoliosis. Twenty scoliosis radiographs and 20 hand radiographs from 11th-grade students were evaluated by four groups–orthopaedic residents, spine fellows, spine surgeons, and radiologists. The findings demonstrated better interobserver and intraobserver reliability for the Sanders classification compared with the Risser staging method; attending surgeons had good reliability using the Sanders classification. Level of evidence: III.

24. Yang JS, McElroy MJ, Akbarnia BA, et al: Growing rods for spinal deformity: Characterizing consensus and variation in current use. *J Pediatr Orthop* 2010;30(3):264-270.

25. Moe JH, Kharrat K, Winter RB, Cummine JL: Harrington instrumentation without fusion plus external orthotic support for the treatment of difficult curvature problems in young children. *Clin Orthop Relat Res* 1984;185:35-45.

26. Thompson GH, Akbarnia BA, Kostial P, et al: Comparison of single and dual growing rod techniques followed through definitive surgery: A preliminary study. *Spine (Phila Pa 1976)* 2005;30(18):2039-2044.

27. Akbarnia BA, Breakwell LM, Marks DS, et al; Growing Spine Study Group: Dual growing rod technique followed for three to eleven years until final fusion: The effect of frequency of lengthening. *Spine (Phila Pa 1976)* 2008;33(9):984-990.

28. Cheung KM, Cheung JP, Samartzis D, et al: Magnetically controlled growing rods for severe spinal curvature in young children: A prospective case series. *Lancet* 2012;379(9830):1967-1974.

    A prospective case study of two patients with JIS who were treated with magnetically controlled growing rods found improvement in the Cobb angle from 67° to 29° at 24-month follow-up. The length of the instrumented segment increased by a mean 1.9 mm with each distraction. No complications were noted.

29. Hickey BA, Towriss C, Baxter G, et al: Early experience of MAGEC magnetic growing rods in the treatment of early onset scoliosis. *Eur Spine J* 2014;23(suppl 1):S61-S65.

    At a minimum 23-month follow-up, eight patients had a mean 43% correction in the Cobb angle after magnetic growing-rod placement. The complications included screw pullout, rod breakage, and loss of distraction. Level of evidence: IV.

30. La Rosa G, Oggiano L, Ruzzini L: Magnetically controlled growing rods for the management of early-onset scoliosis: A preliminary report. *J Pediatr Orthop* 2017;37(2):79-85.

    At an average 27-month follow-up, 10 patients had a mean Cobb angle correction from 64.7° to 28.5°. The

5: Spine Deformity

T1-T12 height increased an average 0.8 mm per month. Three patients had complications. Level of evidence: IV.

31. Choi E, Yazsay B, Mundis G, et al: Implant complications after magnetically controlled growing rods for early onset scoliosis: A multicenter retrospective review. *J Pediatr Orthop* 2016; Epub ahead of print.

   Twenty-one of 54 patients (38.9%) had at least one complication at a mean 19.4-month follow-up after implantation of magnetically controlled growing rods. Fifteen patients (27.8%) had at least one revision surgery. Proximal or distal fixation-related complications were most common. Level of evidence: IV.

32. Lavelle WF, Samdani AF, Cahill PJ, Betz RR: Clinical outcomes of nitinol staples for preventing curve progression in idiopathic scoliosis. *J Pediatr Orthop* 2011;31(1suppl):S107-S113.

   A retrospective review of 28 patients (mean age, 9.4 years) treated with vertebral body stapling found no change or a decrease in Cobb angle in 78% if the original thoracic curve was smaller than 35°. Level of evidence: III.

33. Samdani AF, Ames RJ, Kimball JS, et al: Anterior vertebral body tethering for idiopathic scoliosis: Two-year results. *Spine (Phila Pa 1976)* 2014;39(20):1688-1693.

   A retrospective review of 11 consecutive patients who underwent anterior vertebral body tethering found an average Cobb angle correction of 70% at 2-year follow-up. Two patients required the tether to be loosened to prevent overcorrection. Level of evidence: IV.

34. Nachemson AL, Lonstein JE, Weinstein SL: *Report of the Prevalence and Natural History Committee of the Scoliosis Research Society.* Denver, CO, Scoliosis Research Society, 1982.

35. Rogala EJ, Drummond DS, Gurr J: Scoliosis: Incidence and natural history. A prospective epidemiological study. *J Bone Joint Surg Am* 1978;60(2):173-176.

36. Karner CM, Long F, Solnica-Krezel L, Monk KR, Gray RS: Gpr126/Adgrg6 deletion in cartilage models idiopathic scoliosis and pectus excavatum in mice. *Hum Mol Genet* 2015;24(15):4365-4373.

   A knockout mice model was used to provide genetic evidence that loss of *GPR126* in osteochondroprogenitor cells alters spinal column development. Microtomographic and radiographic studies revealed several hallmarks of AIS.

37. Lonstein JE, Carlson JM: The prediction of curve progression in untreated idiopathic scoliosis during growth. *J Bone Joint Surg Am* 1984;66(7):1061-1071.

38. Weinstein SL, Ponseti IV: Curve progression in idiopathic scoliosis. *J Bone Joint Surg Am* 1983;65(4):447-455.

39. Weinstein SL, Zavala DC, Ponseti IV: Idiopathic scoliosis: Long-term follow-up and prognosis in untreated patients. *J Bone Joint Surg Am* 1981;63(5):702-712.

40. Lenke LG, Betz RR, Harms J, et al: Adolescent idiopathic scoliosis: A new classification to determine extent of spinal arthrodesis. *J Bone Joint Surg Am* 2001;83(8):1169-1181.

41. Sanders JO, Browne RH, McConnell SJ, Margraf SA, Cooney TE, Finegold DN: Maturity assessment and curve progression in girls with idiopathic scoliosis. *J Bone Joint Surg Am* 2007;89(1):64-73.

42. Roye BD, Wright ML, Matsumoto H, et al: An independent evaluation of the validity of a DNA-based prognostic test for adolescent idiopathic scoliosis. *J Bone Joint Surg Am* 2015;97(24):1994-1998.

   Results of the ScoliScore test did not differ based on whether patients had curve progression. The positive predictive value (0.27) and negative predictive value (0.87) were lower in previously published reports by the test developers. Level of evidence: III.

43. Weinstein SL, Dolan LA, Wright JG, Dobbs MB: Effects of bracing in adolescents with idiopathic scoliosis. *N Engl J Med* 2013;369(16):1512-1521.

   A prospective study was ended before its scheduled completion date because the efficacy of bracing had been established. Brace wear was successful in preventing progression to a surgical-magnitude curve in 75% of patients compared with 42% of patients in the observation group. Level of evidence: I.

44. Katz DE, Herring JA, Browne RH, Kelly DM, Birch JG: Brace wear control of curve progression in adolescent idiopathic scoliosis. *J Bone Joint Surg Am* 2010;92(6):1343-1352.

45. Katz DE, Richards BS, Browne RH, Herring JA: A comparison between the Boston brace and the Charleston bending brace in adolescent idiopathic scoliosis. *Spine (Phila Pa 1976)* 1997;22(12):1302-1312.

46. Karol LA, Virostek D, Felton K, Jo C, Butler L: The effect of the Risser stage on bracing outcome in adolescent idiopathic scoliosis. *J Bone Joint Surg Am* 2016;98(15):1253-1259.

   Patients who were at Risser stage 0 were found to be at risk for requiring surgery despite compliant brace wear. Other risk factors in brace treatment were the presence of open triradiate cartilage and a curve of at least 30°. Level of evidence: II.

47. Karol LA, Virostek D, Felton K, Wheeler L: Effect of compliance counseling on brace use and success in patients with adolescent idiopathic scoliosis. *J Bone Joint Surg Am* 2016;98(1):9-14.

   Feedback about brace wear compliance led to an improved level of compliance and decreased curve progression in patients undergoing bracing for AIS. Level of evidence: II.

48. Romano M, Minozzi S, Zaina F, et al: Exercises for adolescent idiopathic scoliosis: A Cochrane systematic review. *Spine (Phila Pa 1976)* 2013;38(14):E883-E893.

A systematic review found only two randomized controlled studies of scoliosis-specific exercises for the treatment of AIS. A lack of high-quality evidence precluded a recommendation for using scoliosis-specific exercises. Level of evidence: II.

49. Schreiber S, Parent EC, Moez EK, et al: The effect of Schroth exercises added to the standard of care on the quality of life and muscle endurance in adolescents with idiopathic scoliosis: An assessor and statistician blinded randomized controlled trial. *Scoliosis* 2015;10:24.

Fifty patients with AIS were randomly assigned to two treatment groups—standard of care or standard of care plus supervised Schroth exercises. The exercises were taught over five sessions in the first 2 weeks of the study. Patients were evaluated with the Biering-Sorensen and SRS-22r outcome instruments at 3 and 6 months. Patients in the Schroth exercise group had greater improvement in the Biering-Sorensen score than the patients receiving standard care alone (32.3 versus 4.8, respectively). At 6 months, the self-image and pain domains improved in the Schroth group and declined in the standard care group. There were some ceiling effects with the SRS-22r scores that may require the development of a new outcome scoring system to assess patients receiving nonsurgical care.

50. Schreiber S, Parent EC, Khodayari Moez E, et al: Schroth physiotherapeutic scoliosis-specific exercises added to the standard of care lead to better Cobb angle outcomes in adolescents with idiopathic scoliosis: An assessor and statistician blinded randomized controlled trial. *PLoS One* 2016;11(12):e0168746.

This study analyzed the effect of a 6-month Schroth exercise program and standard care intervention on the overall Cobb angle in patients with AIS compared with standard care alone. They found that, in a patient with a 51.2° curve at baseline, the addition of Schroth exercises would result in a 6-month curve of 49° compared with a curve of 55° in patients who did not perform the Schroth exercises.

51. Weinstein SL, Dolan LA, Cheng JC, Danielsson A, Morcuende JA: Adolescent idiopathic scoliosis. *Lancet* 2008;371(9623):1527-1537.

52. Suk SI, Kim JH, Kim SS, Lim DJ: Pedicle screw instrumentation in adolescent idiopathic scoliosis (AIS). *Eur Spine J* 2012;21(1):13-22.

Fusion levels for AIS were evaluated, and a classification system was proposed based on vertebral body rotation. Proposed guidelines for distal fusion levels were based on the location of the neutral vertebra.

53. Wang Y, Fei Q, Qiu G, et al: Anterior spinal fusion versus posterior spinal fusion for moderate lumbar/thoracolumbar adolescent idiopathic scoliosis: A prospective study. *Spine (Phila Pa 1976)* 2008;33(20):2166-2172.

54. Fletcher ND, Andras LM, Lazarus DE, et al: Use of a novel pathway for early discharge was associated with a 48% shorter length of stay after posterior spinal fusion for adolescent idiopathic scoliosis. *J Pediatr Orthop* 2017;37(2):92-97.

A case-control study compared patients after surgery for AIS when an accelerated discharge pathway or a traditional discharge pathway was used. Patients in the accelerated pathway group had a 48% shorter length of stay than those in the traditional pathway group. There were no differences in rates of readmission or wound complications. Level of evidence: III.

55. Schwartz DM, Auerbach JD, Dormans JP, et al: Neurophysiological detection of impending spinal cord injury during scoliosis surgery. *J Bone Joint Surg Am* 2007;89(11):2440-2449.

56. Hahn F, Zbinden R, Min K: Late implant infections caused by Propionibacterium acnes in scoliosis surgery. *Eur Spine J* 2005;14(8):783-788.

57. Smith JS, Shaffrey CI, Sansur CA, et al; Scoliosis Research Society Morbidity and Mortality Committee: Rates of infection after spine surgery based on 108,419 procedures: A report from the Scoliosis Research Society Morbidity and Mortality Committee. *Spine (Phila Pa 1976)* 2011;36(7):556-563.

This review of the SRS's morbidity and mortality database of more than 100,000 patients assessed the rates of postoperative wound infection associated with spine surgery. The incidence of wound infection for pediatric patients ranged from 0.9% for degenerative disease to 5.4% for kyphosis. The risk factors for infection were revision surgery, performance of spinal fusion, and the use of spine implants.

58. Cahill PJ, Warnick DE, Lee MJ, et al: Infection after spinal fusion for pediatric spinal deformity: Thirty years of experience at a single institution. *Spine (Phila Pa 1976)* 2010;35(12):1211-1217.

59. Ho C, Sucato DJ, Richards BS: Risk factors for the development of delayed infections following posterior spinal fusion and instrumentation in adolescent idiopathic scoliosis patients. *Spine (Phila Pa 1976)* 2007;32(20):2272-2277.

60. Kamath VH, Cheung JP, Mak KC, et al: Antimicrobial prophylaxis to prevent surgical site infection in adolescent idiopathic scoliosis patients undergoing posterior spinal fusion: 2 doses versus antibiotics till drain removal. *Eur Spine J* 2016;25(10):3242-3248.

A retrospective comparative analysis of 226 patients who underwent posterior spinal fusion for AIS found that two doses of postoperative antibiotic were as effective as continued use until drain removal. Level of evidence: III.

61. Myung KS, Glassman DM, Tolo VT, Skaggs DL: Simple steps to minimize spine infections in adolescent idiopathic scoliosis. *J Pediatr Orthop* 2014;34(1):29-33.

A retrospective review found significantly decreased infection rates after posterior spinal fusion for AIS when vancomycin and ceftazidime were routinely used as chemoprophylaxis with intraoperative pulsatile lavage. Level of evidence: III.

Chapter 23
Neuromuscular Spine Deformity

Paul Sponseller, MD, MBA   Oussama Abousamra, MD

Abstract

Scoliosis is common in children with neuromuscular disorders. Impaired trunk balance and the strength of trunk muscles are important factors in the pathomechanism of scoliosis. The specific characteristics of each neuromuscular disorder determine the efficacy of nonsurgical management, the indications for surgery, the time of intervention, and the expected postoperative complications. Segmental posterior spinal fusion has been an effective definitive treatment for neuromuscular scoliosis, and the role of growth-modulating devices in younger children has been recently reported. In general, the complication rate is higher in patients with neuromuscular conditions than in children and adolescents who have scoliosis and no comorbidities. Treatment techniques and the postoperative course differ in each disorder. Despite advances in scoliosis surgery and an improved understanding of underlying neuromuscular mechanisms in many disorders, further research is needed to provide optimal orthopaedic care for children with neuromuscular disorders and scoliosis.

Keywords: cerebral palsy; Duchenne muscular dystrophy; neuromuscular scoliosis; Rett syndrome; spinal muscular atrophy

Introduction

Neuromuscular scoliosis describes a heterogeneous group of disorders.[1,2] Upper or lower motor neuron disorders

Dr. Sponseller or an immediate family member has received royalties from Globus Medical and DePuy; serves as a paid consultant to DePuy; has received research or institutional support from DePuy; and serves as a board member, owner, officer, or committee member of the Scoliosis Research Society. Neither Dr. Abousamra nor any immediate family member has received anything of value from or has stock or stock options held in a commercial company or institution related directly or indirectly to the subject of this chapter.

may be seen with a deficit in the brain, such as cerebral palsy and Rett syndrome; the spinal cord, such as myelomeningocele and spinal muscular atrophy (SMA); or the peripheral muscles, such as Duchenne muscular dystrophy.[3] It is important to review the recent literature regarding spinal deformity in these disorders and discuss prevalence and nonsurgical and perioperative management.

Cerebral Palsy

Prevalence

Cerebral palsy is the most common cause of neuromuscular scoliosis.[3] A recent study showed that the patient's function, as described by the Gross Motor Function Classification System (GMFCS), is a major factor in scoliosis development.[4] The highest risk of scoliosis (approximately 50%) has been noted in children younger than 18 years with a GMFCS level of IV or V.[4] Therefore, scoliosis surveillance in children with cerebral palsy is recommended based on age and the GMFCS level.[4]

Clinical assessment, by visual examination of the patient in the sitting position, has been shown to be a valid screening method for scoliosis in children with cerebral palsy and should be performed regularly in at-risk patients.[5]

Nonsurgical Treatment

Bracing has not been effective for the treatment of scoliosis in children with cerebral palsy.[4,6] No evidence exists that brace treatment affects the natural history of the condition;[3] however, a brace may be more effective in achieving clinical improvement of sitting ability in patients with long C-shaped curves than in those with short curves.[6]

Surgical Treatment

Indications and Preoperative Risk Factors

It has been suggested that curves greater than 50° are an indication for surgery.[7] The most common corrective surgery for scoliosis in patients with cerebral palsy is posterior spinal fusion with instrumentation from T2 to the pelvis.[8] Because this procedure may represent extensive elective surgery for children with cerebral palsy, a multi-disciplinary approach has been recommended during the perioperative period.[8] Multiple preoperative comorbidities associated with cerebral palsy recently have been evaluated to identify risk factors for postoperative complications.[9-12] Gastroesophageal reflux has been shown to be a risk factor for infection, and feeding difficulties with dependence on gastrostomy and jejunostomy tubes have been associated with the increased risk of deep wound infections and postoperative pancreatitis.[9-11]

Considerations

Intraoperative traction is a valuable adjunct. Posterior fusion is performed with anchors consisting of pedicle screws, tapes, or wires at key levels, including the apex. The spine is made flexible enough to achieve balance. Correction may be produced by distraction, compression, and cantilever bending of the spine.

Intraoperative monitoring of somatosensory-evoked potentials and transcranial electric motor-evoked potentials has been recommended, even for patients with severe motor deficits, to ensure that movement, sensation, and bladder function remain intact.[13] Hydrocephalus and cortical atrophy are predictive factors of signal limitations, and cervical electrodes to stimulate descending neurogenic-evoked potentials should be used if transcranial motor signals cannot be obtained after multiple arrays are tried.[14] Descending neurogenic motor potentials are antidromic stimuli from cervical laminar or epidural electrodes, and they are recorded at the popliteal nerves, which traverse multiple pathways. Descending neurogenic motor potentials may provide motor data in patients whose motor cortex is difficult to stimulate.[14] Intraoperative blood loss has been shown to be substantially greater in patients with cerebral palsy undergoing scoliosis surgery compared with patients with other neuromuscular and nonneuromuscular conditions treated with scoliosis correction procedures.[15] Tranexamic acid has been effective in reducing blood loss and the need for cell-salvage transfusions.[16]

A recent study reported comparable radiographic results in patients treated with posterior-only instrumentation and those treated with combined surgery.[17] The use of posterior-only instrumentation also resulted in shorter surgical times and decreases in the hospital length of stay. The Luque-Galveston procedure as well as pedicle screw instrumentation have been effective in correcting scoliosis deformity with a low complication rate.[18-20] In a matched patient study comparing a technique using unit rod instrumentation with a pedicle screw construct, better correction of the Cobb angle, less blood loss, and a shorter hospital length of stay were reported with the

pedicle screw construct.[20] No differences, however, were found in correction of pelvic obliquity, complications, or the need for revision surgery.

Correction of pelvic obliquity also was found to be similar in patients treated using unit rod instrumentation, iliac screws, or sacral alar iliac screws.[21] Sacral pedicle screw augmentation and placing bilateral pedicle screws in L5 and S1 have been recommended for strengthening the spinopelvic fixation construct[22,23] (**Figure 1**). Pedicle screw density consisting of more than 50% of the fixation construct is superior to a low density construct (consisting of <50% of the pedicle screw construct).[24] Sacral alar iliac screws have a lower failure rate than that of iliac screws, and failure of rod-to-screw connectors is the major factor in creating this difference between the two implants.[25] However, these studies included different neuromuscular pathologies in addition to cerebral palsy. Studies have acknowledged the increased cost of pedicle screw constructs compared with unit rod instrumentation.[9,20,24] Further research with long-term follow-up is needed to detect any differences in late complications and revision surgeries between different instrumentation methods. Anterior and posterior approaches are reserved for the most severe curves (greater than approximately 110° with associated lordosis; **Figure 2**).

Growth-modulating techniques have been effective in correcting scoliosis and pelvic obliquity and delaying definitive fusion in young children with cerebral palsy and severe scoliosis; however, deep wound infections have been a common surgical complications with a rate of approximately 30%.[26]

Outcomes

A high complication rate, with a major complication rate of approximately 40%, has been reported after spinal fusion in patients with cerebral palsy.[9,27] Pulmonary complications such as atelectasis, pleural effusion, and pneumonia are the most common complications. When indicated, preoperative training with noninvasive positive-pressure ventilation has been shown to be effective in improving respiratory outcomes and reducing the incidence of respiratory complications.[28] Gastrointestinal complications also are common (19% to 50%).[9,27] Deep wound infection occurs in approximately 5% of patients.[9,27] A multilayered wound closure technique performed by a plastic surgeon has been proposed recently, and the rate of postoperative wound complications has significantly changed from 19% with routine closure to zero with plastic multilayered closure.[29]

The addition of central neuromotor impairment categories allow the GMFCS levels to be subclassified. The inability to swallow well (requiring a G-tube), to speak, to

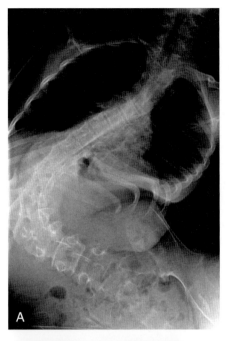
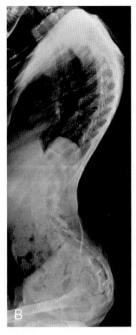
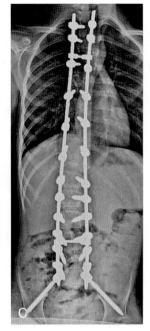
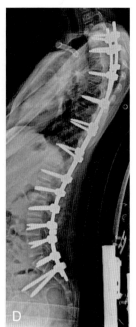

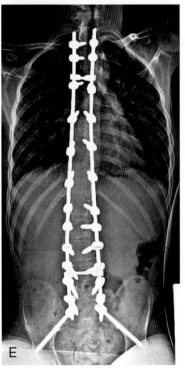
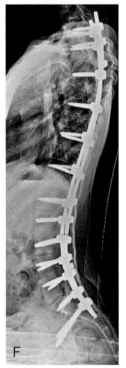

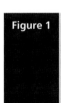

Figure 1 Preoperative AP (**A**) and lateral (**B**) radiographs of the spine of a 14-year-old boy with cerebral palsy show severe scoliosis and pelvic obliquity. Postoperative AP (**C**) and lateral (**D**) radiographs after posterior spinal fusion and spinopelvic fixation. AP (**E**) and lateral (**F**) radiographs 5 years after surgery show maintenance of correction.

control the airway (requiring tracheostomy), and cortical excitability (seizures) allow GMFCS level V to be subclassified as levels 5.0 through 5.3, depending on the number of additional impairments.[12] Patients at GMFCS level 5.0 do not have any of these impairments, whereas patients at GMFCS level 5.3 have three or four of these functional impairments. This subclassification has been associated with increased risk of postoperative complications as well as a decreased health-related quality of life.[9,10,12,27,30] Intraoperative factors such as estimated blood loss and the level of training of the first surgical assistant also have been proposed as factors affecting complication rates.[27,31] Optimizing the medical condition of patients preoperatively and controlling intraoperative factors should be part of the routine approach in spinal fusion surgery for patients with cerebral palsy to achieve the best possible outcomes.

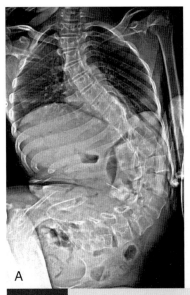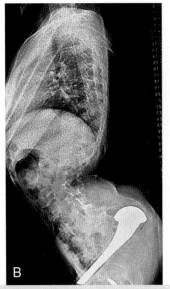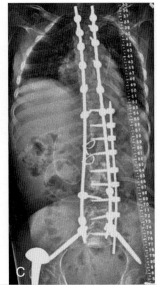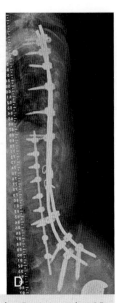

Figure 2 Preoperative AP (**A**) and lateral (**B**) radiographs the spine of a 17-year-old girl with cerebral palsy. Postoperative AP (**C**) and lateral (**D**) radiographs shows anterior and posterior fusion with instrumentation.

Rett Syndrome

Prevalence and Nonsurgical Treatment
Scoliosis is the most common orthopaedic condition seen in children with Rett syndrome.[32] It has been reported that scoliosis will develop in 75% of children with Rett syndrome by 13 years of age.[32] C- or S-shaped curves can be seen, with poorer function and walking ability associated with C-shaped curves.[33] There is no consensus that bracing is beneficial in reducing the progression of scoliosis in children with Rett syndrome.[32]

Surgical Treatment
Indications
Spinal fusion is considered when a curve reaches 40° to 50°.[32] The survival of children with Rett syndrome who undergo spinal fusion for severe scoliosis has been shown to be better than that of children treated nonsurgically.[34] This observation was more marked for children with early-onset scoliosis in whom surgery could have a protective effect on respiratory function.[34]

Considerations
Posterior spinal fusion has been the most commonly reported method of fixation.[35-37] Pelvic fixation is usually needed to correct pelvic obliquity and restore sitting balance[35] (**Figure 3**). In addition, because progression of pelvic obliquity and spinopelvic imbalance is expected in Rett syndrome, pelvic fixation obviates the need for revision surgery as the patient's condition deteriorates.[35]

Outcomes
A length of hospital stay of approximately 3 weeks has been reported in patients with Rett syndrome who undergo scoliosis surgery.[36,37] Respiratory problems remain the most common major complication after spinal fusion in children with Rett syndrome.[35-37] Despite the poor bone quality of these patients, implant failure has not been a reported complication.[35-37] However, a 2015 study reported multiple vertebral dislocation events in one patient that occurred proximal to T3-ilium fixation.[38] In this patient, a recurrent proximal junctional failure with spondyloptosis and grade IV spondylolisthesis was reported after index and revision spinal fusions.

Myelomeningocele

Prevalence and Nonsurgical Treatment
Scoliosis has been reported in up to 80% of children with myelomeningocele and increases in frequency in patients with higher spinal lesions.[39] Many children with myelomeningocele have difficulty maintaining their sitting balance because of paralysis of their abdominal, thoracic, and lumbar extensor muscles.[39] Bracing has been reported to lower the rate of progression in myelomeningocele.[40]

Surgical Treatment
Indications
The complexity of factors involved in myelomeningocele has made it difficult to identify a single factor as the cause of sitting imbalance and functional limitations. Scoliosis magnitude, as defined by the Cobb angle,

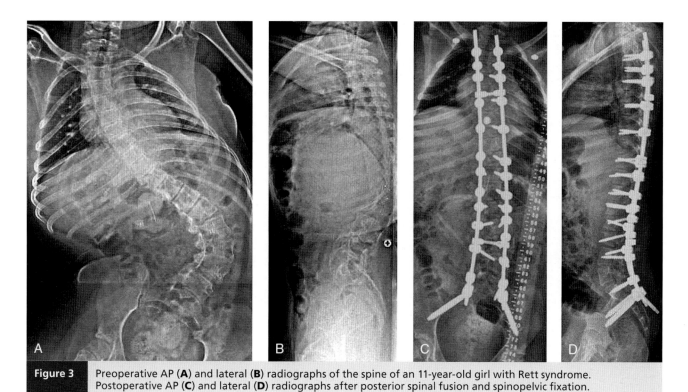

Figure 3   Preoperative AP (**A**) and lateral (**B**) radiographs of the spine of an 11-year-old girl with Rett syndrome. Postoperative AP (**C**) and lateral (**D**) radiographs after posterior spinal fusion and spinopelvic fixation.

is not considered a good indicator of sitting imbalance, has been weakly related to restrictive lung function in children with myelomeningocele, and has no established relationship with physical function or self-perception.[39-41]

Sitting balance by itself has been related to better overall quality of life and physical function, and ambulatory status has not been related to quality of life and self-perception.[41,42] However, having mobility independence appears to contribute more to health-related quality of life than being independent in self-care or being wheelchair dependent.[43] A negative effect of surgery on walking ability has been reported.[44] A recent study with long-term follow-up did not find a difference in sitting balance between children who were treated with surgery and those who were not treated surgically.[45] Variable results and an array of complicated factors have prevented the establishment of clear surgical indications and have made surgical planning for patients with scoliosis and myelomeningocele especially difficult. Individual assessment by an experienced surgeon is needed. Correction of congenital anomalies represent opportunities for focal improvement (**Figure 4**). MRI is helpful in detecting Chiari deformity, syrinx, and tethering, and it should be performed prior to surgery. If a ventriculoperitoneal shunt is in place, shunt function should be assessed prior to surgery.

Considerations

Recent efforts have been made to decrease the high rate of pseudarthrosis and implant failure, reported after spinal fusion in patients with myelomeningocele.[46] Minimally invasive lateral interbody fusion has been reported for four patients (minimum 2-year follow-up) and has been proposed as a method providing acceptable fusion rates with maintenance of correction through midterm follow-up.[46] Anterior-only fusion is another option to avoid the scarred posterior region. The orthopaedic surgeon should consider the need for a plastic surgery consultation if muscle and skin coverage pose problems.[47]

Outcomes

A complication rate as high as 80% has been reported after spinal fusion in patients with myelomeningocele.[44] A 2014 study reported infection in approximately 33% of patients and pseudarthrosis in 18% of patients over long-term follow-up.[45] Revision surgery was needed for many patients during the follow-up period.

In addition to careful preoperative planning, these findings have led to the recent conclusions that although spinal fusion in patients with myelomeningocele corrects the coronal deformity and halts scoliosis progression, it has a high complication rate and no clear effect on health-related quality of life.[45] The decision for surgery should be made on a case-by-case basis, with consideration

5: Spine Deformity

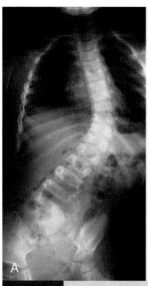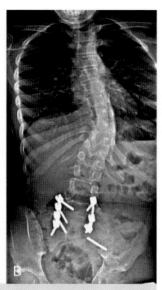

Figure 4 **A,** Preoperative AP spine radiograph of a 3.5-year-old girl with lipomeningocele. **B,** AP radiograph of the spine 10 years after hemivertebra excision and posterior fusion.

of the effect of the curve on the individual's pain and function.

Myelokyphosis is a focal gibbus with a high lumbar apex. Because it frequently leads to nonhealing skin erosions, surgical correction is indicated. Options include gradual distraction using the Vertical Expandable Prosthetic Titanium Rib (DePuy Synthes) if the curve is flexible, or resection of a more rigid gibbus with growing rods or trolley instrumentation (termed a sagittal Shilla technique because the apical control involves the sagittal plane)[48](**Figure 5**).

Spinal Muscular Atrophy

Prevalence and Nonsurgical Treatment
Scoliosis in children with SMA contributes to sitting instability and respiratory compromise.[49] Scoliosis develops in nearly all children with SMA.[50,51] The functional profile of the patient, as described by the disease type, has been reported as a predictor of scoliosis progression.[49] Scoliosis develops earlier in life in children who have type II SMA and no walking ability, and their curves tend to be more progressive with lung function degradations than those of children with type III SMA who can ambulate.[49] The differences between SMA types have been important in assessing the prognosis for the development of scoliosis, pelvic obliquity, and pulmonary insufficiency.[49] Newer treatments for SMA, such as intrathecal nusinersen, have recently shown promising results in changing the course of the disease.[52,53]

Nonsurgical treatment using braces has been suggested as a temporary solution for SMA patients between the ages of 4 and 10 years.[54] The aim of the brace is to improve trunk stability and seated position and to temporarily delay the progression of scoliosis.[54] For ambulatory children who require free trunk movement for gait stabilization, braces are rarely indicated because of the possible loss of walking ability caused by limiting trunk mobility.[51,54]

Surgical Treatment
Indications
Surgical correction has been considered the method of choice for nonambulatory patients when a curve becomes greater than 50°.[51] The best age for spinal fusion is 10 to 12 years, if possible, because surgical stabilization at a younger age is associated with a high risk of dorsal fusion and the crankshaft phenomenon[51,55] (**Figure 6**).

Considerations
Posterior spinal fusion with segmental instrumentation has become the standard for scoliosis correction in SMA.[55] The use of growing rods have been described for young children approximately 6 to 8 years of age.[56,57] Rods are effective in controlling curves and pelvic obliquity and have demonstrated a means to promote thoracic growth and seating height.[56-58]

Outcomes
Respiratory complications have been most frequently encountered in the postoperative period.[55,56,59] However, lower complication rates than those of Duchenne muscular dystrophy and infantile and juvenile idiopathic scoliosis have been reported in some studies.[26,59]

Duchenne Muscular Dystrophy

Prevalence and Nonsurgical Treatment
It has been reported that scoliosis develops in almost all patients with Duchenne muscular dystrophy who are wheelchair dependent and are not receiving steroid treatment.[60] However, glucocorticoid administration has shown a long-term protective effect against the development of spinal deformity in children with Duchenne muscular dystrophy.[61]

Surgical Treatment
Indications
Early surgical treatment of scoliosis in patients with Duchenne muscular dystrophy has been recommended, before the curve reaches 40°.[62,63] Deterioration of respiratory function is slowed after surgical correction of the scoliotic curve.[64,65]

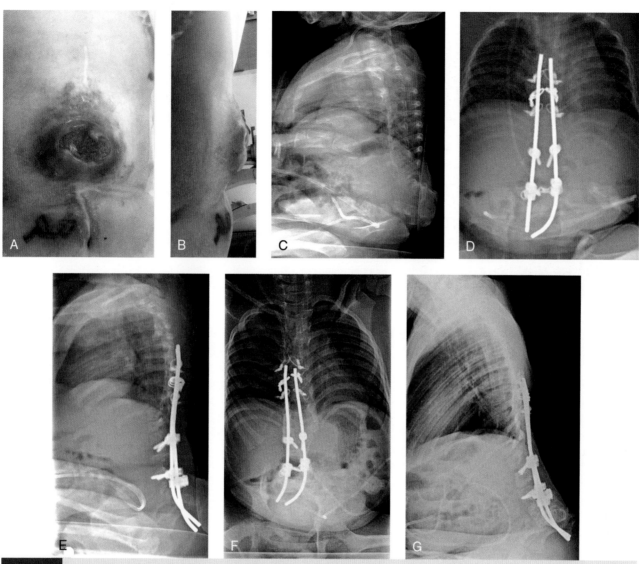

Figure 5 **A** and **B,** Preoperative clinical photographs show a posterior skin defect in an 11-month-old boy with myelomeningocele. **C,** Preoperative AP spine radiograph at 1.6 years of age shows severe kyphosis. Surgery was performed after more than 6 months of wound care. Postoperative AP (**D**) and lateral (**E**) spine radiographs after kyphectomy and a sagittal Shilla technique (limited apical fusion with growth allowed proximally and distally). AP (**F**) and lateral (**G**) radiographs at 3.5 years after surgery showing maintenance of correction.

Considerations

Segmental instrumentation using sublaminar wires or pedicle screws has been effective in providing good correction and stability.[66-68] Fusion from T2 to the pelvis can be performed. The aim is to avoid progression of pelvic obliquity and the possible need for further surgery, especially in a patient with a deteriorating medical condition[66] (**Figure 7**). Osteoporosis and increased blood loss should be anticipated.

Outcomes

A high rate of postoperative complications has been reported for patients with Duchenne muscular dystrophy.[66,69] Implant-related complications are more common when sublaminar wires are used.[66] Wound infection also is a common complication.[59,66,69] In one study, patients with Duchenne muscular dystrophy had a higher overall complication rate and a higher wound infection rate than patients with other neuromuscular disorders.[69] Hepatotoxicity has recently been described as a unique postoperative complication in patients with Duchenne muscular dystrophy and was not seen in patients with other neuromuscular disorders.[69]

Despite the high complication rate, children with Duchenne muscular dystrophy who undergo scoliosis correction have improved sitting balance, slower

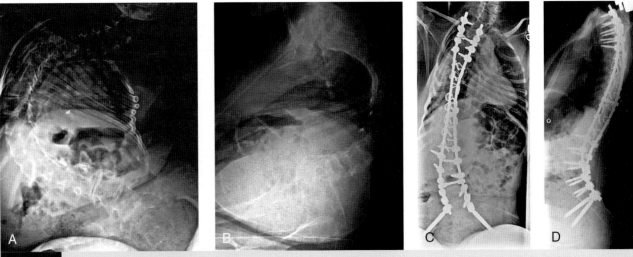

Figure 6 Preoperative AP (**A**) and lateral (**B**) spine radiographs of a 16-year-old girl with spinal muscular atrophy. Postoperative AP (**C**) and lateral (**D**) radiographs 1 year after posterior spinal fusion.

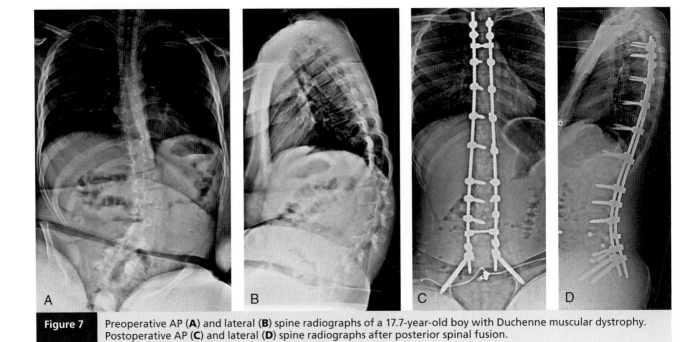

Figure 7 Preoperative AP (**A**) and lateral (**B**) spine radiographs of a 17.7-year-old boy with Duchenne muscular dystrophy. Postoperative AP (**C**) and lateral (**D**) spine radiographs after posterior spinal fusion.

deterioration of respiratory function, and improvement of performance of the activities of daily living compared with children who are treated nonsurgically.[64]

Summary

Scoliosis is a common orthopaedic deformity in children with neuromuscular disorders. The differences in pathophysiology between these disorders and the variations in the neurologic level of involvement impose different risk factors that play an important role in guiding treatment. Although many children need surgery and spinal fusion as a definitive treatment for scoliosis, a specific multidisciplinary management approach in the context of each disorder would likely lead to improved postoperative outcomes. Further research in this field is needed to determine optimal orthopaedic care for children with neuromuscular disorders and scoliosis.

Key Study Points

- Posterior spinal fusion with segmental instrumentation is the most appropriate method of fixation for most children with neuromuscular scoliosis.

- A high postoperative complication rate is seen after spinal fusion in patients with neuromuscular scoliosis. Respiratory and wound problems are the most common complications.

- Growth-modulating techniques have been recently investigated and are effective for managing severe neuromuscular scoliosis that develops in the first decade of life.

- Steroid therapy is effective in decreasing the need for scoliosis surgery in children with Duchenne muscular dystrophy.

- Spinal fusion is helpful in decreasing the rate of deterioration of pulmonary function in children with Duchenne muscular dystrophy or SMA.

Annotated References

1. Brooks JT, Sponseller PD: What's new in the management of neuromuscular scoliosis. *J Pediatr Orthop* 2016;36(6):627-633.

   This literature review of neuromuscular scoliosis showed that growing rods are effective in correcting scoliosis for this population. Intraoperative neuromonitoring, although variable, seems to be safe. Blood loss is higher compared with other scoliosis categories. Patients with neuromuscular disorders have a high rate of surgical site infection. Level of evidence: IV.

2. Canavese F, Rousset M, Le Gledic B, Samba A, Dimeglio A: Surgical advances in the treatment of neuromuscular scoliosis. *World J Orthop* 2014;5(2):124-133.

   This literature review of neuromuscular scoliosis reported that the likelihood and severity of scoliosis increases with the degree of neuromuscular involvement. Although neuromuscular scoliosis can be well corrected with different constructs, there is a high rate of associated complications.

3. Williamson BJ: Surgical management of neuromuscular scoliosis, in Bentley G, ed: *European Surgical Orthopaedics and Traumatology.* Berlin, Germany, Springer, 2014, pp 499-519.

   The author of this book chapter reported that spinal deformity in neuromuscular disorders results from a lack of muscular control and muscular weakness. Although there are similarities between neuromuscular disorders, each disorder is unique, and looking at neuromuscular scoliosis as a single condition underestimates the consideration needed to establish a treatment plan.

4. Persson-Bunke M, Hägglund G, Lauge-Pedersen H, Wagner P, Westbom L: Scoliosis in a total population of children with cerebral palsy. *Spine (Phila Pa 1976)* 2012;37(12):E708-E713.

   A population of 666 children with cerebral palsy was followed with annual examinations. Analysis showed that the incidence of scoliosis increased with the GMFCS level and age. The study authors concluded that follow-up programs for early detection of scoliosis should be based on the child's GMFCS level and age.

5. Persson-Bunke M, Czuba T, Hägglund G, Rodby-Bousquet E: Psychometric evaluation of spinal assessment methods to screen for scoliosis in children and adolescents with cerebral palsy. *BMC Musculoskelet Disord* 2015;16:351.

   Data from 28 children with cerebral palsy were studied. There was excellent interrater reliability for both clinical examination and scoliometer measurements. A high concurrent validity of the psychometric evaluation was found compared with the Cobb angle. Clinical spinal examinations seem appropriate as a screening tool to identify scoliosis in children with cerebral palsy.

6. Nakamura N, Uesugi M, Inaba Y, Machida J, Okuzumi S, Saito T: Use of dynamic spinal brace in the management of neuromuscular scoliosis: A preliminary report. *J Pediatr Orthop B* 2014;23(3):291-298.

   Fifty-two patients with neuromuscular disorders were treated using a dynamic spinal brace. Preliminary findings showed that dynamic spinal braces may be effective for early-stage scoliosis. The brace also improved sitting stability and caregiver satisfaction.

7. Sewell MD, Wallace C, Malagelada F, et al: Does spinal fusion and scoliosis correction improve activity and participation for children with GMFCS level 4 and 5 cerebral palsy? *Medicine (Baltimore)* 2015;94(49):e1907.

   A retrospective data review of 70 children with GMFCS level IV/V and scoliosis is presented. Thirty-six children underwent observation or brace treatment, and 34 underwent surgical treatment. Questionnaire and radiographic data were reviewed over a 2-year period. Spinal fusion was associated with an improvement in activity and participation, whereas nonsurgical treatment was associated with a small reduction in activity and participation.

8. Theroux MC, DiCindio S: Major surgical procedures in children with cerebral palsy. *Anesthesiol Clin* 2014;32(1):63-81.

   The authors describe the most common major procedures used to treat children with cerebral palsy. Spine fusion is the most extensive surgery in this population. Children with cerebral palsy have many comorbid conditions that can result in increased morbidity and even mortality in the perioperative period.

9. Nishnianidze T, Bayhan IA, Abousamra O, et al: Factors predicting postoperative complications following spinal fusions in children with cerebral palsy scoliosis. *Eur Spine J* 2016;25(2):627-634.

5: Spine Deformity

This retrospective review included 303 children with cerebral palsy who underwent posterior spinal fusion. Preoperative risk scores and postoperative complication scores were recorded. G-tube dependence is a predictive risk factor for complications after posterior spinal fusion in patients with cerebral palsy.

10. Abousamra O, Nishnianidze T, Rogers KJ, et al: Risk factors for pancreatitis after posterior spinal fusion in children with cerebral palsy. *J Pediatr Orthop B* 2016;Aug 6 [Epub ahead of print].

A retrospective data review included 300 children with cerebral palsy who underwent posterior spinal fusion. Results showed that acute chemical pancreatitis, as measured by elevated pancreatic enzymes, developed in 55% of the children. Gastrostomy dependence increased the risk of postoperative pancreatitis. Although no mortality was reported, the hospital stay was longer for children who had pancreatitis.

11. Chidambaran V, Gentry C, Ajuba-Iwuji C, et al: A retrospective identification of gastroesophageal reflux disease as a new risk factor for surgical site infection in cerebral palsy patients after spine surgery. *Anesth Analg* 2013;117(1):162-168.

A retrospective data analysis of 30 children with cerebral palsy in whom infection developed after spinal fusion showed that 70% had an incisional surgical site infection. Although many of the infections were polymicrobial, the most common pathogens identified were gram-negative bacilli. Gastroesophageal reflux disease increases the risk of infection in children with cerebral palsy after spinal fusion.

12. Jain A, Sponseller PD, Shah SA, et al; Harms Study Group: Subclassification of GMFCS level-5 cerebral palsy as a predictor of complications and health-related quality of life after spinal arthrodesis. *J Bone Joint Surg Am* 2016;98(21):1821-1828.

From a prospective cerebral palsy registry, 199 patients at GMFCS level V were identified. Subgroups were assigned based on the presence of a gastrostomy tube, tracheostomy, seizures, and nonverbal status. Major complications increased substantially in patients with higher GMFCS level V subtypes. Level of evidence: III.

13. Pastorelli F, Di Silvestre M, Vommaro F, et al: Intraoperative monitoring of somatosensory (SSEPs) and transcranial electric motor-evoked potentials (tce-MEPs) during surgical correction of neuromuscular scoliosis in patients with central or peripheral nervous system diseases. *Eur Spine J* 2015;24(suppl 7):931-936.

Intraoperative neuromonitoring records of 40 patients with neuromuscular scoliosis were reviewed. No false-negative results were found. A relatively high incidence of false-positive results was noted in patients with central nervous system disorders. Although multimodality neuromonitoring is safe and effective to detect spinal cord and peripheral nerve dysfunction in neuromuscular scoliosis surgery, the interpretation of neurophysiologic data may be challenging in this population.

14. Mo AZ, Asemota AO, Venkatesan A, Ritzl EK, Njoku DB, Sponseller PD: Why no signals? Cerebral anatomy predicts success of intraoperative neuromonitoring during correction of scoliosis secondary to cerebral palsy. *J Pediatr Orthop* 2015;Dec 17 [Epub ahead of print].

The intraoperative neuromonitoring records of 206 children with cerebral palsy who underwent scoliosis surgery were reviewed. There was a significant association of periventricular leukomalacia, hydrocephalus, and encephalomalacia with lack of meaningful and interpretable signals, especially transcranial motor-evoked potentials. Level of evidence: IV.

15. Jain A, Njoku DB, Sponseller PD: Does patient diagnosis predict blood loss during posterior spinal fusion in children? *Spine (Phila Pa 1976)* 2012;37(19):1683-1687.

The authors present a retrospective review of 617 patients with 37 different diagnoses who underwent spinal fusion surgery. Patients with cerebral palsy had more blood loss than patients with other diagnoses. Patients with neuromuscular and syndromic disorders had more blood loss than patients with idiopathic scoliosis and Scheuermann kyphosis.

16. Dhawale AA, Shah SA, Sponseller PD, et al: Are antifibrinolytics helpful in decreasing blood loss and transfusions during spinal fusion surgery in children with cerebral palsy scoliosis? *Spine (Phila Pa 1976)* 2012;37(9):E549-E555.

A multicenter retrospective review of prospectively collected data included 84 patients with cerebral palsy who underwent spinal fusion. Estimated blood loss was substantially reduced with the use of antifibrinolytic agents. Tranexamic acid was more effective than epsilon-aminocaproic acid in decreasing blood loss and cell salvage transfusion.

17. Beckmann K, Lange T, Gosheger G, et al: Surgical correction of scoliosis in patients with severe cerebral palsy. *Eur Spine J* 2016;25(2):506-516.

A retrospective review of 57 patients with cerebral palsy compared the radiographic and clinical results between posterior surgery and combined posterior and anterior surgery. Posterior-only surgery appears to lead to comparable radiographic results with shorter surgical times and shorter intensive care unit and hospital stays than combined surgery. The duration of surgery was a relevant predictor of complications.

18. Lonstein JE, Koop SE, Novachek TF, Perra JH: Results and complications after spinal fusion for neuromuscular scoliosis in cerebral palsy and static encephalopathy using Luque Galveston instrumentation: Experience in 93 patients. *Spine (Phila Pa 1976)* 2012;37(7):583-591.

This retrospective cohort analysis included 93 patients with cerebral palsy who underwent spinal fusion using Luque-Galveston instrumentation. The study concluded that this technique is a safe and effective procedure. Pseudarthroses were detected late and were the main reason for additional surgery.

19. Tsirikos AI, Mains E: Surgical correction of spinal deformity in patients with cerebral palsy using pedicle screw instrumentation. *J Spinal Disord Tech* 2012;25(7):401-408.

   A retrospective review of prospectively collected data included 45 patients with cerebral palsy who underwent spinal fusion. The authors reported that pedicle screw instrumentation can achieve excellent correction of spinal deformity in quadriplegic patients with cerebral palsy along with low complication and revision rates and high parent satisfaction.

20. Fuhrhop SK, Keeler KA, Oto M, et al: Surgical treatment of scoliosis in non-ambulatory spastic quadriplegic cerebral palsy patients: A matched cohort comparison of unit rod technique and all-pedicle screw constructs. *Spine Deform* 2013;1(5):389-394.

   A matched cohort study compared unit rod and pedicle screw constructs for scoliosis correction. Pedicle screws achieved better correction of the coronal Cobb angle and resulted in less blood loss and a shorter hospital length of stay. No differences were found in the correction of pelvic obliquity, complications, or the need for revision surgery.

21. Abousamra O, Nishnianidze T, Rogers KJ, Bayhan IA, Yorgova P, Shah SA: Correction of pelvic obliquity after spinopelvic fixation in children with cerebral palsy: A comparison study with minimum two-year follow-up. *Spine Deform* 2016;4(3):217-224.

   A retrospective review of prospectively collected, single-institution data included 77 patients and compared pelvic obliquity correction among three spinopelvic fixation techniques. Iliac screws and sacral alar iliac screws were similar to the unit rod in comparative effectiveness and implant safety profile. Level of evidence: III.

22. Dubory A, Bachy M, Bouloussa H, Courvoisier A, Morel B, Vialle R: Screw augmentation for spinopelvic fixation in neuromuscular spine deformities: Technical note. *Eur Spine J* 2015;24(11):2580-2587.

   The authors report on 10 patients who underwent spinopelvic fixation for neuromuscular spine deformity. It was concluded that sacral pedicle screw augmentation enhances the pelvic obliquity correction obtained using a posterior procedure.

23. Myung KS, Lee C, Skaggs DL: Early pelvic fixation failure in neuromuscular scoliosis. *J Pediatr Orthop* 2015;35(3):258-265.

   A retrospective review of posterior spinal fusion with pelvic fixation included 41 patients with neuromuscular disorders. The authors found that not placing bilateral pedicle screws at L5 and S1, in addition to two iliac screws, was associated with a 35% early failure rate of pelvic fixation. Level of evidence: IV.

24. Funk S, Lovejoy S, Mencio G, Martus J: Rigid instrumentation for neuromuscular scoliosis improves deformity correction without increasing complications. *Spine (Phila Pa 1976)* 2016;41(1):46-52.

   A retrospective review included data from 80 patients who had surgery for neuromuscular scoliosis and spinopelvic fixation. Constructs were defined as nonrigid (>50% sublaminar wires) and rigid (≥50% pedicle screws). The greater cost of rigid spinal implants may be justified when considering improved deformity correction, the lower rate of pseudarthrosis, and avoidance of open anterior release with its associated additional surgical time, cost, and morbidity.

25. Shabtai L, Andras LM, Portman M, et al: Sacral alar iliac (SAI) screws fail 75% less frequently than iliac screws in neuromuscular scoliosis. *J Pediatr Orthop* 2016.

   A review of 101 children with neuromuscular scoliosis treated with spinal fusion and pelvic fixation showed that sacral alar iliac screws had a lower rate of implant failure and revision surgery compared with iliac screws. The most important advantage of the sacral alar iliac screws may be obviation of the need for a screw-to-rod connector. Level of evidence: III.

26. McElroy MJ, Sponseller PD, Dattilo JR, et al; Growing Spine Study Group: Growing rods for the treatment of scoliosis in children with cerebral palsy: A critical assessment. *Spine (Phila Pa 1976)* 2012;37(24):E1504-E1510.

   A multicenter retrospective review of 27 children with cerebral palsy who underwent growing rod treatment for scoliosis is presented. The study concluded growing rods via a posterior-only approach are effective, and constructs extending to the pelvis control pelvic obliquity more effectively. The most common complications were deep wound infection (30%).

27. Samdani AF, Belin EJ, Bennett JT, et al: Major perioperative complications after spine surgery in patients with cerebral palsy: Assessment of risk factors. *Eur Spine J* 2016;25(3):795-800.

   The authors present a prospective longitudinal cohort study of 127 patients with cerebral palsy treated with spine surgery. A major complication occurred in 39.4% of the patients, with pulmonary problems being the most common type of complication. Risk factors included greater preoperative kyphosis, staged procedures, a lack of antifibrinolytic use, and increased blood loss. Level of evidence: II.

28. Khirani S, Bersanini C, Aubertin G, Bachy M, Vialle R, Fauroux B: Non-invasive positive pressure ventilation to facilitate the post-operative respiratory outcome of spine surgery in neuromuscular children. *Eur Spine J* 2014;23(suppl 4):S406-S411.

   Thirteen patients with nonidiopathic scoliosis who underwent posterior spinal fusion were trained to use noninvasive positive pressure ventilation and a mechanical insufflator exsufflator device to decrease postoperative respiratory complications. No respiratory complications were observed after scoliosis surgery with preoperative and postoperative respiratory training, which emphasizes the interest in this type of management for high-risk patients.

5: Spine Deformity

29. Ward JP, Feldman DS, Paul J, et al: Wound closure in nonidiopathic scoliosis: Does closure matter? *J Pediatr Orthop* 2015; Jul 24 [Epub ahead of print].

Two groups of patients with neuromuscular scoliosis were compared in terms of wound complication rates in this retrospective review that included a total of 76 patients. The wound complication rate was significantly reduced from 19% in the nonstandardized closure group to zero in the group treated with plastic multilayered closure. This finding suggests that the wound closure method plays a major role in lowering the incidence of wound complications. Level of evidence: III.

30. Basques BA, Chung SH, Lukasiewicz AM, et al: Predicting short-term morbidity in patients undergoing posterior spinal fusion for neuromuscular scoliosis. *Spine (Phila Pa 1976)* 2015;40(24):1910-1917.

A retrospective cohort study of 940 patients with neuromuscular scoliosis who underwent spinal fusion reported that 133 patients had an adverse event and 99 had a severe adverse event. An American Society of Anesthesiologists Classification of 3 or greater was found to be the only independent risk factor for any adverse event and severe adverse events. Body mass index for age in the 95th percentile or greater was the only risk factor for hospital readmission. Level of evidence: III.

31. Shrader M, Falk M, Segal L, Wood W, Boan C, White G: Minimizing complications in scoliosis surgery in children with cerebral palsy. *Dev Med Child Neurol* 2015;1(57):44-45.

A prospective, matched cohort analysis with a consecutive series of patients with cerebral palsy who underwent posterior spinal fusion compared procedures performed by two attending surgeons and procedures performed by a team led by a single surgeon. The authors concluded that the use of a second attending surgeon decreased surgical time, blood loss, the complication rate, and the length of the hospital stay.

32. Downs J, Bergman A, Carter P, et al: Guidelines for management of scoliosis in Rett syndrome patients based on expert consensus and clinical evidence. *Spine (Phila Pa 1976)* 2009;34(17):E607-E617.

A draft of scoliosis guidelines was created based on a literature review and open-ended questions. A version of the draft was sent to an international multidisciplinary panel of clinicians to reach consensus agreement. A comprehensive life span approach to the management of scoliosis in patients with Rett syndrome was recommended. Surgery should be considered when the Cobb angle is approximately 40° to 50° and must be supported by specialist management of anesthesia, pain control, seizures, and early mobilization.

33. Riise R, Brox JI, Sorensen R, Skjeldal OH: Spinal deformity and disability in patients with Rett syndrome. *Dev Med Child Neurol* 2011;53(7):653-657.

The authors report on 25 patients with Rett syndrome and radiographically confirmed scoliosis. Functional level in females with Rett syndrome measured according to the Barthel Index showed significant correlation with the scoliosis curve type. A low score was associated with a C-shaped curve involving all the spine and pelvis.

34. Downs J, Torode I, Wong K, et al; Rett syndrome spinal fusion group: Surgical fusion of early onset severe scoliosis increases survival in Rett syndrome: A cohort study. *Dev Med Child Neurol* 2016;58(6):632-638.

This study estimated the effects of spinal surgery on survival in 140 females with Rett syndrome and severe scoliosis. After adjusting for mutation type and age of scoliosis onset, the rate of death was lower in patients treated with surgery than in patients who were not surgically treated.

35. Gabos PG, Inan M, Thacker M, Borkhu B: Spinal fusion for scoliosis in Rett syndrome with an emphasis on early postoperative complications. *Spine (Phila Pa 1976)* 2012;37(2):E90-E94.

The findings of a retrospective study of 16 patients with Rett syndrome treated with posterior spinal fusion and unit rod instrumentation is presented. Spinal fusion can achieve a satisfactory technical result. Major complications included respiratory problems (61%) and gastrointestinal problems (21%).

36. Hammett T, Harris A, Boreham B, Mehdian SM: Surgical correction of scoliosis in Rett syndrome: Cord monitoring and complications. *Eur Spine J* 2014;23(suppl 1):S72-S75.

A retrospective review of 11 children with Rett syndrome showed that scoliosis surgery in Rett syndrome carries a very high rate of complications and is associated with an average hospital stay of 3 weeks. Both caregivers and surgeons should be aware of these findings when planning an intervention. The authors suggest aggressive physical optimization of these patients prior to surgery, with an emphasis on nutrition.

37. Karmaniolou I, Krishnan R, Galtrey E, Cleland S, Vijayaraghavan R: Perioperative management and outcome of patients with Rett syndrome undergoing scoliosis surgery: A retrospective review. *J Anesth* 2015;29(4):492-498.

A retrospective review of 24 children with Rett syndrome who underwent spinal fusion showed a high incidence of postoperative complications in this population. Extreme postoperative vigilance is required, and recovery in a high-dependency unit is recommended.

38. Pisano AJ, Wagner SC, Helgeson MD, Jex JW: Multiple vertebral dislocation events after fusion for scoliosis in Rett syndrome. *Spine J* 2015;15(12):e61-e62.

The authors present a case report of a female patient with Rett syndrome who underwent posterior spinal fusion. Two weeks later, spondyloptosis was found at T3-T4. Open reduction and extension of fusion to T1 was performed. Eight months later, grade IV anterolisthesis was found at C4-C5, with compression of the central canal.

39. Patel J, Walker JL, Talwalkar VR, Iwinski HJ, Milbrandt TA: Correlation of spine deformity, lung function, and

seat pressure in spina bifida. *Clin Orthop Relat Res* 2011;469(5):1302-1307.

Thirty-two patients with myelodysplasia and scoliosis were retrospectively reviewed. All patients displayed a reduction in forced vital capacity, which was not related to increasing scoliosis. A history of pressure ulcers did not correlate with spinal deformity or measures of seated pressure.

40. Wai EK, Young NL, Feldman BM, Badley EM, Wright JG: The relationship between function, self-perception, and spinal deformity: Implications for treatment of scoliosis in children with spina bifida. *J Pediatr Orthop* 2005;25(1):64-69.

41. Bartnicki B, Synder M, Kujawa J, Stańczak K, Sibiński M: Siting stability in skeletally mature patients with scoliosis and myelomeningocele. *Ortop Traumatol Rehabil* 2012;14(4):383-389.

A prospective study enrolled 19 patients with myelomeningocele and scoliosis, and showed that the value of the Cobb angle was not a good indicator of sitting balance in patients with scoliosis and myelomeningocele. Stable sitting was related to better overall quality of life and physical function.

42. Schmidt G, Synder M, Pieszyński I, Kujawa J, Sibiński M: Walking patterns of skeletally mature patients with scoliosis and myelomeningocele [Polish]. *Chir Narzadow Ruchu Ortop Pol* 2011;76(6):319-323.

This prospective study of 19 patients with myelomeningocele and scoliosis reported that walking ability may deteriorate with age. Patients' general physical function, quality of life, self-perception, and motivation are not related to ambulatory status.

43. Schoenmakers MA, Uiterwaal CS, Gulmans VA, Gooskens RH, Helders PJ: Determinants of functional independence and quality of life in children with spina bifida. *Clin Rehabil* 2005;19(6):677-685.

44. Schoenmakers MA, Gulmans VA, Gooskens RH, Pruijs JE, Helders PJ: Spinal fusion in children with spina bifida: Influence on ambulation level and functional abilities. *Eur Spine J* 2005;14(4):415-422.

45. Khoshbin A, Vivas L, Law PW, et al: The long-term outcome of patients treated operatively and non-operatively for scoliosis deformity secondary to spina bifida. *Bone Joint J* 2014;96-B(9):1244-1251.

The authors present a retrospective review of 45 patients with scoliosis secondary to spina bifida; 34 patients were treated surgically and 11 were treated nonsurgically. At a mean follow-up of 14.1 years, both groups were statistically similar with respect to walking capacity, sitting balance, and health-related quality of life.

46. Iorio JA, Jakoi AM, Steiner CD, et al: Minimally invasive lateral interbody fusion in the treatment of scoliosis associated with myelomeningocele. *Surg Technol Int* 2015;26:371-375.

A retrospective review is presented of four patients with myelomeningocele and severe scoliosis who underwent posterior spinal fusion and staged minimally invasive lateral interbody fusion. At a minimum follow-up of 2 years, fusion was achieved in all the patients.

47. Sponseller PD, Young AT, Sarwark JF, Lim R: Anterior only fusion for scoliosis in patients with myelomeningocele. *Clin Orthop Relat Res* 1999;364:117-124.

48. Margalit A, Sponseller PD: Myelokyphectomy in spina bifida: The modified Fackler or sagittal Shilla technique. *Op Tech Orthop* 2016;26(4):222-228. Available at: http://www.sciencedirect.com/science/article/pii/S1048666616300386. Accessed January 12, 2017.

The authors describe the modified Fackler (sagittal Shilla) technique. This technique is used to address severe focal kyphosis in a child 9 years of age or younger with myelomeningocele. This procedure is associated with good long-term outcomes, including increased and sustained curve correction, a decrease in the number of surgeries, and gains in height.

49. Fujak A, Raab W, Schuh A, Richter S, Forst R, Forst J: Natural course of scoliosis in proximal spinal muscular atrophy type II and IIIa: Descriptive clinical study with retrospective data collection of 126 patients. *BMC Musculoskelet Disord* 2013;14:283.

Data on scoliosis, pelvic obliquity, and inspiratory vital capacity were evaluated for 126 patients. Differences between type II and type IIIA SMA should be taken into consideration in managing scoliosis in children.

50. Garg S: Management of scoliosis in patients with Duchenne muscular dystrophy and spinal muscular atrophy: A literature review. *J Pediatr Rehabil Med* 2016;9(1):23-29.

The author presents a literature review of scoliosis in patients with SMA and Duchenne muscular dystrophy. Nonsurgical treatment has not been effective at scoliosis prevention. The main goal of surgical treatment is to improve sitting balance and prevent scoliosis progression. Comprehensive and multidisciplinary preoperative evaluations are vital to reduce the risk of surgical treatment.

51. Haaker G, Fujak A: Proximal spinal muscular atrophy: Current orthopedic perspective. *Appl Clin Genet* 2013;6(11):113-120.

This literature review focused on the orthopaedic management of SMA. Surgical spine stabilization using multisegmental dorsal stabilization is the method of choice for treating scoliosis in nonambulatory patients no younger than 10 to 12 years of age. Satisfactory solutions of surgical therapy for severe scoliosis in very young children are lacking.

52. Chiriboga CA, Swoboda KJ, Darras BT, et al: Results from a phase 1 study of nusinersen (ISIS-SMN(Rx)) in children with spinal muscular atrophy. *Neurology* 2016;86(10):890-897.

A total of 28 patients with SMA enrolled in this open-label phase 1 study. The goal of the study was to examine safety, tolerability, pharmacokinetics, and preliminary clinical efficacy of intrathecal nusinersen. Results from this study support continued development of nusinersen for treatment of SMA. Level of evidence: IV.

53. Haché M, Swoboda KJ, Sethna N, et al: Intrathecal injections in children with spinal muscular atrophy: Nusinersen clinical trial experience. *J Child Neurol* 2016;31(7):899-906.

This study summarizes the lumbar puncture experience in children with SMA in a phase 1 open-label study of nusinersen and its extension. Seventy-three lumbar punctures were performed in 28 children. The most common adverse events were headache, back pain, and postlumbar puncture syndrome. Lumbar punctures were successfully performed in children with SMA. The frequency of adverse events related to lumbar puncture was similar to that previously reported in children undergoing this procedure.

54. Fujak A, Kopschina C, Forst R, Mueller LA, Forst J: Use of orthoses and orthopaedic technical devices in proximal spinal muscular atrophy: Results of survey in 194 SMA patients. *Disabil Rehabil Assist Technol* 2011;6(4):305-311.

The purpose of this study was to determine the use of orthopaedic and assistive devices by patients with SMA based on a survey of 194 patients. The survey results may help formulate a strategy for providing assistive devices to patients with SMA that will be better adapted to the needs of the individual patient.

55. Fujak A, Raab W, Schuh A, Kreß A, Forst R, Forst J: Operative treatment of scoliosis in proximal spinal muscular atrophy: Results of 41 patients. *Arch Orthop Trauma Surg* 2012;132(12):1697-1706.

Scoliosis in 24 patients with SMA was treated using the ISOLA system (DePuy Spine), and 17 patients were treated with telescopic rods. Unsatisfactory results were reported with telescopic rods because of the crankshaft phenomenon. For nonambulatory patients, definitive stabilization is recommended beginning at approximately 10 to 12 years of age.

56. McElroy MJ, Shaner AC, Crawford TO, et al: Growing rods for scoliosis in spinal muscular atrophy: Structural effects, complications, and hospital stays. *Spine (Phila Pa 1976)* 2011;36(16):1305-1311.

The authors present a retrospective analysis of 15 patients with SMA treated with growing rods. Although growing rods improved trunk height and the space available for lung ratio and controlled curve progression and pelvic obliquity, they did not alter rib collapse.

57. Chandran S, McCarthy J, Noonan K, Mann D, Nemeth B, Guiliani T: Early treatment of scoliosis with growing rods in children with severe spinal muscular atrophy: A preliminary report. *J Pediatr Orthop* 2011;31(4):450-454.

A retrospective review of 11 patients with SMA and scoliosis who were treated with growing rod constructs showed substantial correction of the Cobb angle postoperatively, with no surgical complications identified. The study concluded that a growing rod construct is an effective option in the treatment of scoliosis in SMA. Level of evidence: IV.

58. Long WD III, Smith BG: A review: The use of growing rods to treat scoliosis in patients with spinal muscular atrophy. *Semin Spine Surg* 2012;24(3):164-168.

The authors present a literature review of the use of growing rods in the treatment of scoliosis in children with SMA. It was concluded that the growing rod technique demonstrated a means to enable children with severe scoliosis secondary to SMA to grow in terms of sitting height and chest and lung development.

59. Burow M, Forst R, Forst J, Hofner B, Fujak A: Perioperative complications of scoliosis surgery in patients with Duchenne muscular dystrophy and spinal muscular atrophy: Focusing on wound healing disorders. *Int J Neurosci* 2016;21:1-7.

A retrospective study of 180 patients (142 with Duchenne muscular dystrophy and 38 with SMA) showed that the most common complications after scoliosis surgery are respiratory and cardiac problems. Wound healing disorder is a severe complication and is associated with prolonged therapy.

60. Shapiro F, Zurakowski D, Bui T, Darras BT: Progression of spinal deformity in wheelchair-dependent patients with Duchenne muscular dystrophy who are not treated with steroids: Coronal plane (scoliosis) and sagittal plane (kyphosis, lordosis) deformity. *Bone Joint J* 2014;96-B(1):100-105.

The extent of scoliosis was assessed on sitting AP spine radiographs in 88 consecutive nonambulatory patients with Duchenne muscular dystrophy who were not receiving steroid treatment. Scoliosis developed in nearly all patients with Duchenne muscular dystrophy who were not receiving steroids after they become wheelchair dependent. The degree of deformity progressed over time.

61. Lebel DE, Corston JA, McAdam LC, Biggar WD, Alman BA: Glucocorticoid treatment for the prevention of scoliosis in children with Duchenne muscular dystrophy: Long-term follow-up. *J Bone Joint Surg Am* 2013;95(12):1057-1061.

Fifty-four ambulatory boys with Duchenne muscular dystrophy were enrolled in a nonrandomized comparative study of glucocorticoid deflazacort. The long-term use of deflazacort resulted in a substantial decrease in the need for spinal surgery. Level of evidence: II.

62. Hsu JD, Quinlivan R: Scoliosis in Duchenne muscular dystrophy (DMD). *Neuromuscul Disord* 2013;23(8):611-617.

This literature review of scoliosis in patients with Duchenne muscular dystrophy concluded that regular monitoring for scoliosis should be performed in a nonambulatory child. If scoliosis is present, surgical treatment should be undertaken at an early stage. Careful multidisciplinary preoperative assessment and perioperative care are required.

63. Cawley DT, Carmody O, Dodds MK, McCormack D: Early limited instrumentation of scoliosis in Duchenne muscular dystrophy: Is a single-rod construct sufficient? *Spine J* 2015;15(10):2166-2171.

A retrospective study of 41 patients with Duchenne muscular dystrophy was performed to assess outcomes after posterior single-rod instrumentation and bilateral spinal fusion for neuromuscular scoliosis. The authors advocate early surgical intervention using a limited instrumentation technique to maintain sitting balance and minimize perioperative morbidity.

64. Suk KS, Lee BH, Lee HM, et al: Functional outcomes in Duchenne muscular dystrophy scoliosis: Comparison of the differences between surgical and nonsurgical treatment. *J Bone Joint Surg Am* 2014;96(5):409-415.

The authors report on 66 patients with Duchenne muscular dystrophy and scoliosis. Surgery improved function and decreased the rate of deterioration of forced vital capacity compared with patients treated nonsurgically. Level of evidence: II.

65. Chua K, Tan CY, Chen Z, et al: Long-term follow-up of pulmonary function and scoliosis in patients with Duchenne's muscular dystrophy and spinal muscular atrophy. *J Pediatr Orthop* 2016;36(1):63-69.

A retrospective study of 40 patients (29 with Duchenne muscular dystrophy and 11 with SMA) showed that scoliosis surgery in these patients results in a long-term decreased rate of decline in pulmonary function over a follow-up period of more than 10 years. The frequency of chest infections was not improved by scoliosis surgery. Level of evidence: III.

66. Scannell BP, Yaszay B, Bartley CE, Newton PO, Mubarak SJ: Surgical correction of scoliosis in patients with Duchenne muscular dystrophy: 30-year experience. *J Pediatr Orthop* 2016; Jan 11 [Epub ahead of print].

A single-center retrospective study of 60 patients with Duchenne muscular dystrophy and scoliosis who were treated over 30 years concluded that both pedicle screws and Luque instrumentation improved the coronal Cobb angle. The pedicle screw group had improved and maintained pelvic obliquity. Both groups had high complication rates. Level of evidence: IV.

67. Mehdian H, Perez-Romera AB, Nasto LA, Kapinas A: Surgical outcome of scoliosis correction in Duchenne muscular dystrophy (DMD) using different instrumentation constructs. Spine J, 2016. Available at: http://www.thespinejournalonline.com/article/S1529-9430(15)01916-6/abstract. Accessed January 5, 2017.

A retrospective case series of 43 patients with Duchenne muscular dystrophy and scoliosis who were treated with sublaminar wire or pedicle screw constructs showed that all constructs were equally effective. Pedicle screw constructs showed better results in terms of reduced surgical time and blood loss, and better maintenance of correction.

68. Mehta SS, Modi HN, Srinivasalu S, et al: Pedicle screw-only constructs with lumbar or pelvic fixation for spinal stabilization in patients with Duchenne muscular dystrophy. *J Spinal Disord Tech* 2009;22(6):428-433.

69. Duckworth AD, Mitchell MJ, Tsirikos AI: Incidence and risk factors for post-operative complications after scoliosis surgery in patients with Duchenne muscular dystrophy: A comparison with other neuromuscular conditions. *Bone Joint J* 2014;96-B(7):943-949.

A retrospective review of 110 patients with neuromuscular scoliosis who underwent spinal fusion was performed to compare the incidence and risk factors for postoperative complications in patients with different neuromuscular disorders. Patients with Duchenne muscular dystrophy had an increased overall complication rate. Hepatotoxicity was unique to patients with Duchenne muscular dystrophy.

5: Spine Deformity

Chapter 24

Adult Spine Deformity

Zeeshan M. Sardar, MD, MSc   Ronald A. Lehman Jr, MD   Lawrence G. Lenke, MD

Abstract

Adult spine deformity represents a spectrum of pathology related to regional deformity, with or without global malalignment. Both coronal and sagittal plane problems can have a negative effect on the patient's quality of life. Nonsurgical treatment should emphasize physical therapy and spinal injections, as needed, for neural issues. Surgical treatment focuses on relieving symptomatic stenosis and realigning the deformed spine into a more normal regional and, especially, global alignment.

Dr. Lehman or an immediate family member is a member of a speakers' bureau or has made paid presentations on behalf of DePuy, Medtronic, and Stryker; serves as a paid consultant to Medtronic; serves as a board member, owner, officer, or committee member of AOSpine, the Cervical Spine Research Society, the North American Spine Society, and the Scoliosis Research Society. Dr. Lenke or an immediate family member has received royalties from Medtronic and Quality Medical Pub; serves as a paid consultant to DePuy, K2M, and Medtronic; has received research or institutional support from AOSpine, DePuy, EOS Imaging, the Scoliosis Research Society, and the Setting Scoliosis Straight Foundation; has received nonincome support (such as equipment or services), commercially derived honoraria, or other non-research–related funding (such as paid travel) from Evans Family Donation (grateful patient philanthropic support), the Fox Family Foundation (philanthropic research funding from grateful patient), and Fox Rothschild, LLC (expert witness in a patent infringement case); and serves as a board member, owner, officer, or committee member of Global Spine Outreach and the Orthopaedic Research and Education Foundation). Neither Dr. Sardar nor any immediate family member has received anything of value from or has stock or stock options held in a commercial company or institution related directly or indirectly to the subject of this chapter.

Keywords: adult deformity; degenerative scoliosis; idiopathic scoliosis; sagittal balance; spine reconstruction

Introduction

Spine deformity in adult patients is increasing in prevalence because of the increasing number of elderly individuals.[1] Depending on the criteria used, the prevalence of scoliosis in adults older than 60 years has been reported to be higher than 60%.[1-4] Most often, scoliosis is defined as curvature of the spine with a Cobb angle greater than 10° in the coronal plane.[5] However, deformity also can exist in the sagittal plane (kyphosis or lordosis), the axial plane (rotation), or multiple planes. Therefore, the term adult spine deformity will be used instead of adult scoliosis.

The evaluation of the sagittal plane of the spine is critical in adults.[4,6-11] Malalignment in the sagittal plane can affect a patient's ability to maintain an upright posture with the head over the pelvis and feet. Studies have shown the importance of sagittal spine alignment and its correlation with health-related quality of life (HRQOL) measures.[2,12,13] Medical professionals treating these patients are becoming increasingly aware of the effects of spine deformity and its associated disability.

Classification of Adult Spine Deformity

The most common form of adult spine deformity is degenerative, although many other types of spine deformities exist. Adult spine deformity has been classified into four major groups[5] (**Table 1**). Type 1 is primary degenerative scoliosis or de novo scoliosis. Type 2 is progressive idiopathic scoliosis, with or without degeneration. Type 3a is secondary adult scoliosis in the context of pelvic obliquity or a secondary curve in idiopathic, congenital, or neuromuscular scoliosis, and type 3b is secondary adult scoliosis in the context of a metabolic bone disease such as osteoporosis, with or without degeneration and/or fractures. Although this classification system describes spine deformity in a large number of adults, it omits several other important groups of patients with spine deformities

Table 1			

Adult Scoliosis Types

Type	Description	Curve Location	Etiology
1	Primary degenerative scoliosis (de novo scoliosis)	Commonly lumbar or thoracolumbar with apex at L2-L3 or L3-L4	Asymmetric disk degeneration and facet joint degeneration
2	Progressive idiopathic scoliosis	Similar to adolescent idiopathic scoliosis	Progression of adolescent form of idiopathic scoliosis because of mechanical reasons or degeneration
3a	Secondary adult scoliosis	Commonly thoracolumbar/lumbosacral	Secondary to: An adjacent thoracic or thoracolumbar curve of idiopathic, neuromuscular, or congenital origin Pelvic obliquity Lumbosacral transitional anomaly
3b	Secondary scoliosis	Variable	Metabolic bone disease, osteoporosis

such as those with iatrogenic sagittal imbalance. This group includes patients who have undergone prior lumbar, lumbosacral, or thoracolumbar surgery; however, in these patients the spine was instrumented in a position of decreased lordosis relative to the pelvic incidence (PI). A second group includes patients with junctional spine deformity, which can be defined as proximal or distal junctional failure resulting in the development of a spine deformity in patients who had undergone prior spine fusion. A third group includes patients with posttraumatic deformity, which can be defined as spine deformity (typically in the sagittal plane) resulting from a high-energy traumatic fracture. This type of deformity presents as an acute or progressive deformity. A fourth group includes patients with a pathologic deformity resulting from an infectious or neoplastic process in the spine. **Table 2** presents a more comprehensive etiologic listing of the types of adult spine deformity.

Although knowing the etiology of the deformity is important in guiding treatment, it does not provide information on location and severity, which is equally important in determining the course of treatment and surgical options. In 2006, the Scoliosis Research Society (SRS) proposed a classification system for adult spine deformity based on radiographic parameters and using concepts from the King-Moe and the Lenke classification systems.[14,15] The SRS classification used the following six coronal and one sagittal curve types: type 1, single thoracic; type 2, double thoracic; type 3, double major; type 4, triple major; type 5, thoracolumbar; type 6, lumbar (idiopathic or de novo); and type 7, single sagittal plane deformity without an associated coronal curve. Although the Lenke classification system for

adolescent idiopathic scoliosis has been widely accepted and used in the selection of fusion levels, the SRS classification lacks a clear application to patient management and clinical relevance.[16] Therefore, it has not been widely used.

The SRS-Schwab Adult Spinal Deformity Classification[2,12] was subsequently developed to incorporate the Schwab classification based on HRQOL measures and radiographic outcomes, including pelvic parameters. While describing the deformity in both the coronal and sagittal planes, this classification places emphasis on the sagittal plane because of its substantial effect on patient outcomes. In the coronal plane, the curve type is based on the Cobb angle measurement of the thoracic and thoracolumbar/lumbar curves. A curve is considered major if it measures more than 30°. Four curve types are defined (**Table 3**). In curve type T, the thoracic curve is the only major curve. In curve type L, the thoracolumbar/lumbar curve is the only major curve. In curve type D, both the thoracic and thoracolumbar/lumbar curves are major curves. In curve type N, there is no major curve in the coronal plane.

Three sagittal modifiers are then assigned to the curve type: the difference in angles between the PI and lumbar lordosis (LL; [PI-LL mismatch]), the pelvic tilt (PT), and the sagittal vertical axis (SVA). Each of these modifiers is assigned a grade of 0, +, or ++, depending on the severity of the condition as outlined in **Table 3**. These modifiers also serve to set the goal for alignment after surgical correction of the spine deformity. In a 2013 multicenter review of 341 patients with adult spine deformities, patients who had improvement in the SRS-Schwab sagittal modifiers were significantly more likely to achieve

Table 2

Comprehensive Etiology-Based Adult Spine Deformity Classification

Type	Description	Subtype
1	Adult degenerative spine deformity	Not applicable
2	Adult idiopathic spine deformity	A: Progressive idiopathic scoliosis without previous surgical treatment B: Development of spine deformity adjacent to previous surgical fusion
3	Iatrogenic sagittal imbalance	A: Previous fusion for idiopathic scoliosis (eg, flat back deformity related to Harrington rods instrumentation) B: Previous fusion, commonly for degenerative condition with lack of adequate lordosis
4	Junctional spine deformity	A: Deformity related to proximal junctional failure after a previous fusion surgery B: Deformity related to distal junctional failure after a previous fusion surgery
5	Posttraumatic spine deformity	A: Acute deformity after trauma B: Chronic progressive deformity after trauma
6	Pathologic spine deformity	A: Neoplastic B: Infectious
7	Metabolic-related spine deformity	Osteoporosis, other metabolic bone disorder
8	Other spine deformity	Congenital, neuromuscular, syndromic

Table 3

The Scoliosis Research Society—Schwab Adult Spine Deformity Classification

Coronal Curve Types	Sagittal Modifiers
T: Thoracic only Lumbar curve <30°	PI – LL Grade 0: PI – LL <10° Grade +: 10° <PI – LL <20° Grade ++: PI – LL >20°
L: Thoracolumbar/lumbar only Thoracic curve <30°	Global alignment Grade 0: SVA <4 cm Grade +: 4 cm <SVA <9.5 cm Grade ++: SVA >9.5 cm
D: Double curve Thoracic and thoracolumbar/lumbar >30°	PT Grade 0: PT <20° Grade +: 20° <PT <30° Grade ++: PT >30°
N: No major coronal deformity All coronal curves <30°	Not applicable

LL = lumbar lordosis, PI = pelvic incidence, PT = pelvic tilt, SVA = sagittal vertical axis.

a minimal clinically important difference (MCID) for HRQOL measures.[12]

Natural History

Because of the many types of adult spine deformities, this section will focus on patients with a degenerative spine deformity. These patients typically seek treatment in the sixth or seventh decade of life (male to female ratio, 1:1).[1] Radiographic features of curves prone to progression include increasing intervertebral disk degeneration, lateral olisthesis of 6 mm or more, an intercrestal line through L5 instead of L4, apical vertebral rotation of grade II or higher, and a Cobb angle greater than 30°.[1,17,18]

In a review of the radiographs of 24 patients with degenerative scoliosis less than 30°, 11 of the patients (46%) had a lateral olisthesis of more than 5 mm at L3-L4.[17] Interestingly, the mean progression of left-sided curves was 3° per year, whereas right-sided curves progressed at a mean of 1.5° per year.

Clinical Presentation

Adult patients with spine deformity most commonly seek an evaluation because of new or progressive pain.[1] Individuals with degeneration of the lumbar/lumbosacral spine have varying amounts of back and/or leg pain. The back pain can be focally located at the apex of the curve or at the lumbosacral fractional curve. More diffuse back pain and muscle fatigue is reported by patients who have substantial sagittal and/or coronal imbalance (Figure 1). Back pain that occurs mainly when the patient is upright and improves on lying down portends a good prognostic sign for relief with surgical stabilization and is probably indicative of mechanical instability.

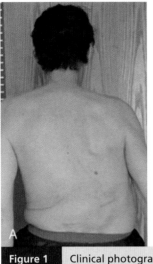
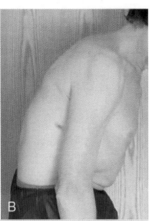

Figure 1 Clinical photographs of 67-year-old man with degenerative scoliosis. **A,** Posterior view of the patient's back shows coronal imbalance toward the left side. **B,** The lateral view shows the stooped forward posture associated with sagittal imbalance.

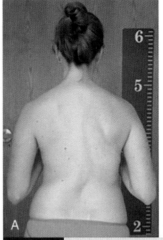
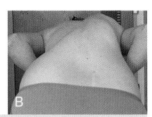

Figure 2 Clinical photographs of a 30-year-old woman with idiopathic scoliosis and a progressive deformity. **A,** The posterior view shows thoracolumbar scoliosis and scapular asymmetry. **B,** A rib prominence is seen on a forward-bending view of the patient's back.

Patients with degenerative spine deformity often have varying degrees of accompanying spine stenosis. Symptoms depend on the location of the stenosis. Patients have radicular symptoms from compression of nerve roots in the foramina on the concavity of the spine curves. This is especially common in the lumbosacral fractional curve. Patients with more central stenosis have neurogenic claudication when standing and walking.

Although older adults tend to seek medical attention because of pain or disability, younger adults often present because of worsening deformity with a changing trunk position (**Figure 2**). Dissatisfaction with appearance is another reason patients seek medical attention.

The preoperative evaluation of a patient with an adult spine deformity begins with a thorough history and physical examination. Patients are asked about the existence of back pain, leg pain, and symptoms of neurogenic claudication. It is important to quantify the intensity of the pain and related disability caused by both leg and back pain. Information about alleviating and aggravating factors also should be elicited.

A patient's medical and surgical history can be used to determine the etiology of a spine deformity as outlined in **Table 2**. It is important to determine if a diagnosis of scoliosis was made in adolescence or childhood; if prior spine surgeries were performed; and if spine infection, tumor, or traumatic injury has occurred. The medical history also is useful in documenting the general health of a patient and comorbidities that can affect the risks associated with complex procedures to correct deformity.

It is especially important to determine if a patient has a history of smoking or if a diagnosis of osteoporosis has been made.

Patients are asked about the presence of extremity weakness and sensory changes as well as bowel and/or bladder dysfunction. Difficulties with gait and balance can be related to lumbar stenosis but are more often caused by coexistent cervical myelopathy, which has been reported in up to 28% of patients.[1] A history of declining functional status or the use of walking aids should be elicited. It is important to note which nonsurgical treatment measures have been tried and which have been successful.

Physical Examination

The physical examination is of prime importance. The patient should be appropriately disrobed to allow for evaluation of the spine deformity. The examination should begin with inspection of the patient in the standing position, with his or her hips and knees extended. Overall coronal and sagittal balance should be observed, along with the patient's ability to bend laterally. Patients with a sagittal plane deformity often use various compensation methods such as retroversion of the pelvis, which is noted by flattening of the buttocks. Patients with more severe deformities also attempt to compensate with hip and knee flexion. To better understanding the amount of sagittal plane deformity, it is important to examine the patient with his or her hips and knees extended if that position can be tolerated. A patient also should be assessed for leg-length inequality. Other important observations are the presence of shoulder inequality, rib prominence, waist-line asymmetry, and truncal shift.

For a younger adult patient with an idiopathic spine deformity, the scoliometer angle is measured with the patient in the forward-bending position and then in the prone position. These measurements provide information about the magnitude of rotation and flexibility of the spine.

The patient's gait should be carefully analyzed for abnormal patterns, including antalgic, high-stepping (sign of footdrop), scissoring, wide-based, Trendelenburg, unsteady, and slow gaits. The patient's ability to heel walk, toe walk, tandem walk, and perform a one-leg stand also are evaluated. These tests can indicate signs of subtle weakness and myelopathy.

A complete neurologic examination of the upper and lower extremities is performed. This examination includes testing motor strength and sensation in the extremities. Deep tendon reflexes and abdominal reflexes are tested to look for hyperreflexia or asymmetry. To look for signs of myelopathy, the patient is examined for the presence of the Hoffman sign, inverted radial reflex, Babinski reflex, and ankle clonus.

The patient is examined in the prone and supine positions to assess for flexibility of the spine. This is particularly helpful in those with kyphosis or sagittal imbalance. The peripheral pulses of the lower extremities are palpated, and the skin is inspected for signs of peripheral vascular disease. The hips and knees are examined, and range of motion is checked to ensure that the pain is not related to hip or knee pathology instead of spine pathology. This examination also allows the physician to check for hip or knee flexion contractures, which can complicate patient positioning in the operating room.

Radiography and Advanced Diagnostics

EOS System

Full-length standing PA and lateral radiographs should be obtained for all patients. The EOS system (EOS Imaging) can be used to obtain standing radiographs, with a patient's hips and knees extended, elbows flexed, and fingertips on the clavicles[19-21] (**Figure 3**). The EOS imaging system is a slot-scanning device that allows simultaneous acquisition of two orthogonal radiographs (PA and lateral views).[19-21] The device has two coupled pairs of radiation sources and detectors that capture the radiographic image using a synchronized vertical movement.[20] Because of the slot-scanning nature of the machine, the radiographs appear in a 1:1 scale for size and volume for the entire radiograph as opposed to standard radiographs in which

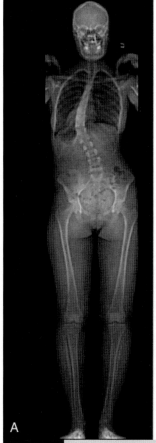
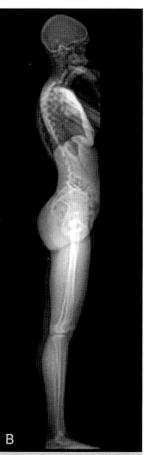

Figure 3 Simultaneously obtained PA (**A**) and lateral (**B**) standing full-length radiographs of a patient with the hips and knees extended, elbows flexed, and fingertips on the clavicles.

magnification varies because of the distance of the body part from the x-ray beam.[20] Because the images are taken simultaneously, EOS software also can be used to reconstruct a three-dimensional model of the bony structure from the radiographs.[19-21]

The EOS device reduces the radiation dose by six to nine times in the thoracolumbar region compared with the dose from a standard radiography system.[19] EOS system image quality is substantially better for all structures in coronal and lateral views than those obtained with a standard radiography system, with the exception of visualization of the spinous processes, which are better seen with a standard system.[19] The substantial reduction in radiation dose and improved image quality benefits young adults, especially females, who may require frequent follow-up radiography because they have an increased risk for deformity progression.

Weight-bearing radiographic images can be acquired with the EOS system. These full-length radiographs allow for global and regional deformity assessments.

The radiographs must include adequate visualization of the auditory meatus proximally and the femoral heads distally. In addition, the head-to-toe radiographs obtained using the EOS system can show the patient's use of compensatory measures such as hip and knee flexion. The radiographs should be carefully evaluated for evidence of degeneration, disk collapse, vertebral osteophytes, scoliosis, kyphosis, and anterior or lateral olisthesis.

Deformity Assessment
Coronal Plane
PA radiographs are used to measure the Cobb angles of the thoracic, thoracolumbar, lumbar, and the lumbosacral fractional curves in the coronal plane. PA radiographs are viewed with the heart on the left side, and alignment is measured. To determine coronal balance, a vertical line (called the C7 plumb line [C7PL]) is drawn from the middle of the C7 vertebral body.[1] Another vertical line, called the central sacral vertical line (CSVL), is drawn from the center of the sacrum. The distance between the C7PL and CSVL is defined as the coronal balance (**Figure 4**). If the CSVL and C7PL match, the coronal balance is described as neutral. If the C7PL lies to the right of the CSVL, the coronal balance is described as positive, and if the C7PL lies to the left of the CSVL, the coronal balance is described as negative. PA radiographs also can be used to look for leg-length inequality and pelvic obliquity. Repeat radiography with a shoe lift may be obtained to limit the effect of such external factors on coronal balance.

EOS imaging allows assessment of global alignment from head to toe (**Figure 5**). To assess global coronal alignment, a vertical line is drawn from the center of gravity of the head at the midpoint of both infraorbital margins (the head coronal vertical axis). In a patient with neutral global coronal alignment, the head coronal vertical axis should fall in the center of the sacrum and the midpoint of the center of the hips, knees, and ankles.

PA radiographs also are used to assess for scoliosis by measuring the Cobb angles of the curves. The Cobb angle of a curve is the angle between the proximal and distal end vertebrae of a curve (**Figure 6**). The end vertebra is defined as the most tilted vertebra in the horizontal plane. The location of the curve is based on the location of the apical vertebra, which is the vertebra that is the most displaced from the midline, the most horizontal, and the most rotated. The SRS defines a curve as thoracic if the apex is between the T2 vertebra and the T11-T12 disk; a curve is thoracolumbar if the apex is between the T12 and the L1 vertebrae, and lumbar if the apex is at or below the L1-L2 disk.

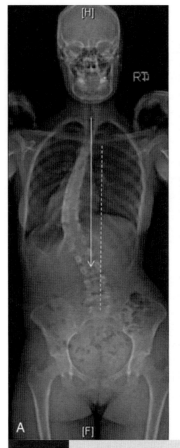
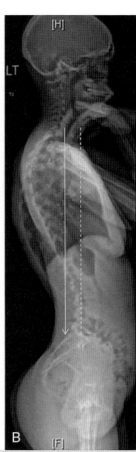

Figure 4   **A,** The dashed line on this PA radiograph represents the central sacral vertical line (CSVL) and the solid line with the arrow represents the C7 plumb line (C7PL). The horizontal distance between these two lines is the coronal vertical axis or coronal balance. Because the C7PL is to the left of the CSVL in this patient, the coronal balance would be described as negative. **B,** Lateral radiograph of the spine. The dashed line represents the posterior sacral vertical line (PSVL) drawn from the superior-posterior corner of S1. The solid line with the arrow represents the C7PL. The horizontal distance between these two lines is the sagittal vertical axis (SVA) or sagittal balance. Because the C7PL is posterior to the PSVL, the SVA would be described as negative.

Certain types of radiographs can provide valuable information about the flexibility of a deformity. These radiographs include PA side-bending and supine views to assess the flexibility of the scoliotic curves in the coronal plane and to sort structural from nonstructural curves.

Sagittal Plane
Lateral radiographs, which are generally viewed with the patient facing toward the right, are used to measure the pelvic parameters and the sagittal profile of the patient. Supine cross-table lateral radiographs can help in the

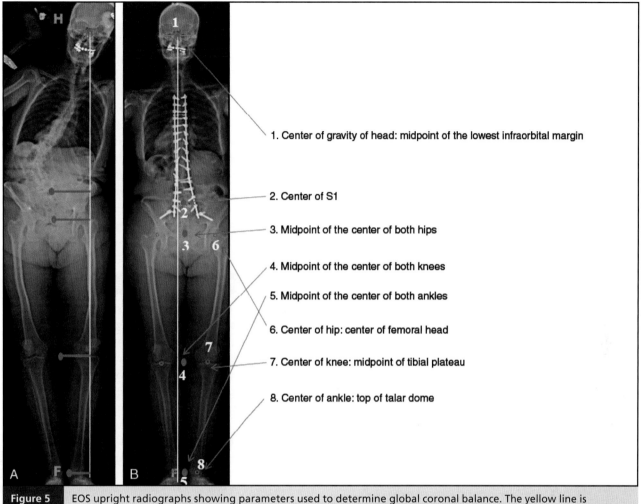

1. Center of gravity of head: midpoint of the lowest infraorbital margin

2. Center of S1

3. Midpoint of the center of both hips

4. Midpoint of the center of both knees

5. Midpoint of the center of both ankles

6. Center of hip: center of femoral head

7. Center of knee: midpoint of tibial plateau

8. Center of ankle: top of talar dome

Figure 5 EOS upright radiographs showing parameters used to determine global coronal balance. The yellow line is dropped from the center of the gravity of the head, showing its position in relationship to the shown landmarks (red dots/lines). **A,** PA radiograph shows a significantly positive (to the right) head coronal vertical axis as shown by the deviation of the line from the vertical axis in relationship to the sacrum, hips, knees, and ankles. **B,** Postoperative PA radiograph of the same patient after spine deformity correction surgery shows almost neutral global coronal balance.

assessment of the rigidity of kyphotic deformities. For example, a spine may have markedly positive sagittal imbalance, but supine radiographs showing flexibility can obviate the need for a three-column osteotomy (**Figure 7**). Most physicians routinely obtain flexibility radiographs during surgical planning for adult spine deformity correction.

Magnetic Resonance Imaging

An MRI scan is obtained for all patients preoperatively to assess for stenosis of the spinal canal and neuroforamina. MRI can be used to assess the degree of stenosis and identify the structures causing the stenosis (ligamentum flavum, disk, osteophytes, facets, or cysts). T2-weighted sagittal and axial images are best used to identify and assess spine stenosis. In addition, T2-weighted images are

used to look for effusions in the facet joints that could suggest instability. T1-weighted images can be used to look for a lack of fat in the neuroforamina, which suggests foraminal stenosis.

Computed Tomography

A CT scan is almost always obtained for surgical planning. For patients who had prior surgeries, pseudarthrosis sites and laminectomy defects may be identified. The position of any preexisting spine instrumentation is assessed to ensure that the pedicle screws are of appropriate length and not causing a harmful violation of the pedicles. CT also is used to analyze the width, length, location, and rotation of the pedicles that will undergo instrumentation during surgery. In addition, CT can be used to look for preexisting anterior and posterior fusion between spine

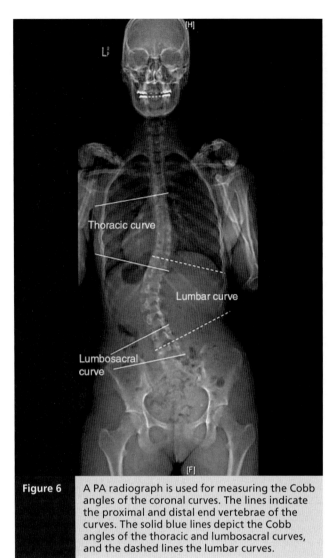

Figure 6 A PA radiograph is used for measuring the Cobb angles of the coronal curves. The lines indicate the proximal and distal end vertebrae of the curves. The solid blue lines depict the Cobb angles of the thoracic and lumbosacral curves, and the dashed lines the lumbar curves.

Dual-Energy X-ray Absorptiometry

Females and elderly patients undergoing reconstructive spine surgery should undergo dual-energy x-ray absorptiometry. Patients with severe osteopenia or osteoporosis (femoral neck T-score ≤ –2.5) may benefit from medical management of bone loss.[22] Supplemental vitamin D and calcium are recommended for most of these patients. The 2016 American Association of Clinical Endocrinologists guidelines recommend that patients with osteoporosis and a moderate fracture risk without previous fragility fractures be treated with alendronate, denosumab, risedronate, or zoledronic acid. For patients with high fracture risk or those with a prior fragility fracture, treatment with denosumab, teriparatide, or zoledronic acid is recommended.[23]

Adult Spine Deformity and Disability

Adult spine deformity can lead to substantial disability and adversely affect quality of life. A retrospective analysis of 497 patients with symptomatic adult spine deformity compared their Medical Outcomes Study 36-Item Short Form physical and mental component summary scores with reported US normative and chronic disease scores.[7] The mean physical component summary for adult patients with a spine deformity was found to be significantly lower than that of the total US population. The disability caused by symptomatic adult spine deformity increased with age and worsened more rapidly than that of US age-generational norms. In addition, the authors reported that the physical component summary score was worse with an increasing SVA and decreasing LL. Disability caused by thoracic scoliosis was less severe than that caused by lumbar scoliosis and was similar to that of individuals with chronic low back pain. The patients who had the worse physical component summary scores were those with lumbar scoliosis combined with an SVA greater than +10 cm. The scores of these patients were worse than those of patients with limited vision and limited upper and lower extremity use. The mean physical component summary score for patients with symptomatic adult spine deformity was worse than that of patients with chronic back pain and hypertension and was similar to that of patients with medical conditions such as cancer, diabetes, and heart disease.

Many studies have confirmed the importance of sagittal balance and its effect on HRQOL.[4,6-11,24] Restoring sagittal balance by improving the SVA and PT and creating proportionate LL have been shown to improve patient outcomes.[9-11] One study reported that the T1 spinopelvic inclination had the strongest correlation with each

segments, even in cases in which spine surgeries have not been performed previously, because spontaneous fusion of spine segments can occur in conditions such as infection, ankylosing spondylitis, and severe idiopathic or degenerative deformity.

CT used in conjunction with MRI can help differentiate stenosis caused by bone from that caused by soft tissues. CT myelography may be required in patients who are unable to undergo MRI or if metal artifact degradation is present.

For complex primary or revision cases, a three-dimensional CT reconstruction can provide useful information. In patients with abnormal anatomy or if a complex osteotomy is planned, a three-dimensional printed spine model can be obtained to help in the placement of pedicle screws and osteotomy planning (**Figure 8**). The ability to reference a life-size model in the operating room is helpful in difficult surgeries.

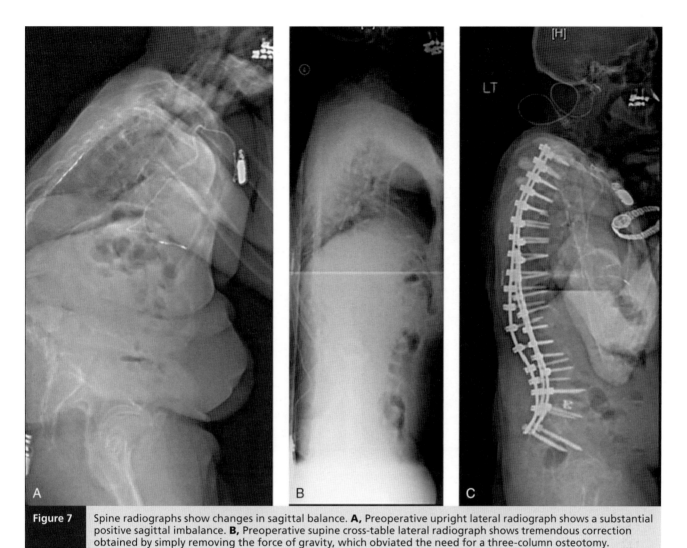

Figure 7 Spine radiographs show changes in sagittal balance. **A,** Preoperative upright lateral radiograph shows a substantial positive sagittal imbalance. **B,** Preoperative supine cross-table lateral radiograph shows tremendous correction obtained by simply removing the force of gravity, which obviated the need for a three-column osteotomy. **C,** Postoperative upright lateral radiograph of the same patient shows good sagittal balance after surgery.

HRQOL measure, followed by the SVA and PT.[10] The goals for optimal sagittal alignment include a T1 spinopelvic inclination less than 0°, an SVA less than 5 mm, PT less than 20°, and PI-LL mismatch less than ±9°.[9,11]

Coronal balance is important in patients with deformity because an imbalance of greater than 4 cm has been associated with moderate disability.[25] Other factors that substantially correlate with pain include lateral vertebral olisthesis, L3 and L4 end plate obliquity angles (degrees from horizontal), LL, and thoracic kyphosis.[8] The magnitude, but not the location of the lateral olisthesis, has been shown to affect pain.[8]

Many radiographic measurements affect the HRQOL. The goal of deformity correction surgery is to obtain a spine that is globally balanced in the coronal and sagittal planes using these parameters to define the amount of correction required.

Nonsurgical Treatment

The benefit of nonsurgical treatment in patients with adult spine deformity has not been established; however, for patients with moderate symptoms without evidence of substantial instability or neurologic deficits, nonsurgical treatment can be initiated.[26-28] Nonsurgical treatment includes physical therapy that focuses on core strengthening and endurance.[1] Patients also can be referred to physicians for spine injections and medical management of pain. In general, bracing is not recommended for adult patients because it has the potential to cause further deconditioning and is unable to halt curve progression.[1]

Multimodal medical pain management includes NSAIDs, muscle relaxants, and medications such as pregabalin and gabapentin for nerve pain. Narcotic medications are avoided for nonsurgical management, especially

5: Spine Deformity

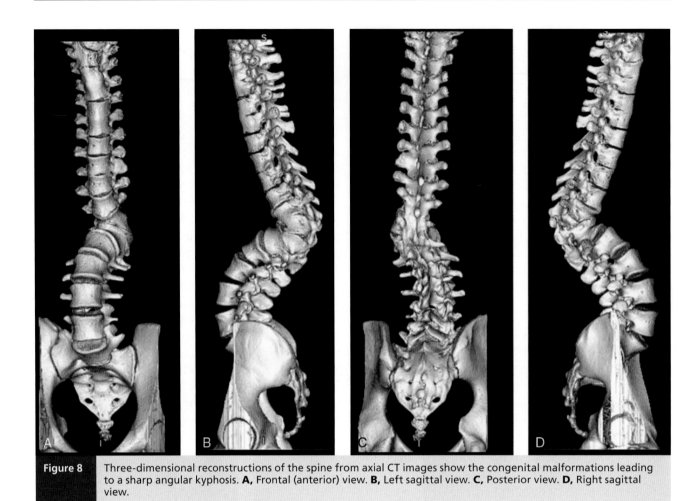

Figure 8 Three-dimensional reconstructions of the spine from axial CT images show the congenital malformations leading to a sharp angular kyphosis. **A,** Frontal (anterior) view. **B,** Left sagittal view. **C,** Posterior view. **D,** Right sagittal view.

in elderly patients. Nonnarcotic pain medications also should be used judiciously in elderly patients. NSAIDs can cause complications such as gastric ulcers, renal problems, cardiovascular issues, and increased bleeding, whereas muscle relaxants can cause oversedation.

A systematic review of nonsurgical treatment in patients with adult deformity revealed indeterminate support for physical therapy, chiropractic care, and bracing based on level IV evidence. Level III evidence for the use of injections also showed an indeterminate effect.[26] It was concluded that no single nonsurgical treatment option for adult spine deformity was supported in the literature. In a comparative review of patients with adult lumbar scoliosis who were treated with surgical and nonsurgical measures and followed for 2 years, no improvement was seen in the nonsurgical cohort over the 2-year period and there was a trend toward a decline in HRQOL scores.[27]

Nevertheless, nonsurgical treatment can be used in patients with stable curves without substantial neurologic deficits. However, these patients should be reevaluated at defined intervals to evaluate the efficacy of nonsurgical treatment and assess the need for referral for surgical consideration. The cost of ongoing nonsurgical treatment without improvement in a patient's symptoms must be considered. The mean cost of nonsurgical treatment in these patients was estimated to be $10,815 over a 2-year period, ranging from $9,704 for patients with mild symptoms to $14,022 for patients with more severe symptoms.[28] Patients who are not good surgical candidates because of medical comorbidities and are not improving with nonsurgical measures may have to accept an altered lifestyle.

Surgical Treatment

Indications

Patients who do not improve after a trial of nonsurgical treatment can be considered for surgical treatment if back and/or leg pain continue and their quality of life is substantially affected. Other indications for surgical treatment include the presence of severe deformity, decompensation in the sagittal or coronal plane, progression of deformity, the presence of instability, and/or the presence of neurologic deficit. The presence of progressive neurologic deficits is rare in patients with primary spine deformity, but it is common in patients with junctional failure after a prior surgery and may warrant urgent surgical treatment.

If surgery is considered appropriate, the details of the proposed surgery should be discussed with the patient, including the benefits, potential risks, and possible complications. Poor medical health, advanced cardiopulmonary disease, or other organ failures are contraindications for surgery. In addition, patients with mental conditions that would prevent active participation in perioperative education and rehabilitation programs are not considered good candidates for surgery. The presence of severe osteoporosis is a relative contraindication to elective spine reconstruction.

Intraoperative Neuromonitoring

The use of intraoperative neuromonitoring is recommended during any spine deformity surgery. Neurologic complications can occur in deformity correction procedures, especially in those involving large deformities, angular deformities, or correction of kyphosis. The purpose of using intraoperative neuromonitoring is to allow rapid intraoperative detection of neurologic complications so that they can be investigated and corrected immediately to avoid long-term neurologic deficits. The common modalities used for intraoperative neuromonitoring include continuous passive electromyography, somatosensory-evoked potentials (SSEPs), and transcranial motor-evoked potentials (MEPs).[29] SSEPs alone have low sensitivity but a high specificity for detecting true neurologic changes.[29] The combined use of the three modalities showed a sensitivity of 100% and a specificity of 84.3% in 102 patients undergoing spine deformity correction without a major osteotomy.[29] Warning criteria were a 50% decrease in the amplitude of SSEPs from baseline or complete loss of MEPs in the limb of interest. However, the sensitivity changed to 67%, with the specificity increasing to 98%, in cases that involved a major osteotomy.

A 2014 study reported on 1,162 patients who had intraoperative monitoring with MEPs during their spine deformity correction procedures.[30] The warning criterion used by the authors was an amplitude decrease of greater than 80% that was synchronously and logically associated with a high-risk surgical maneuver (such as pedicle screw insertion, osteotomy, or deformity correction) and was not caused by systemic and anesthetic factors. The authors reported 100% sensitivity and 99.7% specificity in their cohort with the use of MEPs. All patients who

demonstrated some neurologic deficit postoperatively were identified during surgery with the use of MEPs. Another series of 354 patients reported a sensitivity of 100% and a specificity of 99.3% in deformity correction cases with the use of multimodal intraoperative neuromonitoring.[31]

The use of multimodal intraoperative neuromonitoring is imperative during spine deformity correction surgeries and has a high sensitivity and specificity for identifying a true neurologic event. A 2014 study described a consensus-based checklist and guidelines for the use of intraoperative neuromonitoring during spine deformity surgery.[32] The following guidelines were recommended for practices in the United States. (1) A team approach should be used. A surgeon, an anesthesiologist, and qualified neuromonitoring personnel should be involved in the identification and communication of neuromonitoring changes. (2) SSEP monitoring should be used. (3) Transcranial MEPs and/or descending neurogenic-evoked potentials should be used. (4) A 50% degradation in SSEP signal amplitude from baseline, and/or a sustained decrease in transcranial MEP signal amplitude, and/or a decrease in descending neurogenic-evoked potential signal of more than 60% are "significant warning criteria." (5) A wake-up test should always be considered for patients undergoing surgery for spine deformity if there is persistent signal degradation or if the patient cannot be monitored.

If a neuromonitoring alert occurs, it is recommended that a checklist of items be followed for addressing the issue in a systematic fashion[32] (**Figure 9**). For centers at which spine deformity surgery is performed, the checklist should be placed in the operating room so it can immediately be followed by all team members in the event of an intraoperative neuromonitoring alert.

Intraoperative Hemostasis

Spine deformity correction surgery can be very complex with long surgical times and extensive blood loss. Procedures involving major osteotomies can require massive intraoperative transfusions.[33] The potential for massive blood loss has increased interest in the use of tranexamic acid (TXA).[33] TXA binds to plasminogen and plasmin and inhibits fibrinolysis in the surgical area. Aprotinin and epsilon-aminocaproic acid also have been used, although aprotinin is rarely used because of its association with renal failure and cerebrovascular and cardiac events.[33] Fifty-nine patients who underwent spine deformity correction surgery were divided into two groups; one group received TXA, and a control group did not receive TXA.[33] An intravenous TXA loading dose of 100 mg/kg over a 20-minute period was used before skin incision,

Checklist for the Response to Intraoperative Neuromonitoring Changes in Patients with a Stable Spine

GAIN CONTROL OF ROOM	ANESTHETIC/SYSTEMIC	TECHNICAL/NEUROPHYSIOLOGIC	SURGICAL
❑ Intraoperative pause: stop case and announce to the room	❑ Optimize mean arterial pressure (MAP)	❑ Discuss status of anesthetic agents	❑ Discuss events and actions just prior to signal loss and consider reversing actions:
❑ Eliminate extraneous stimuli (e.g. music, conversations, etc.)	❑ Optimize hematocrit	❑ Check extent of neuromuscular blockade and degree of paralysis	❑ Remove traction (if applicable)
❑ Summon ATTENDING anesthesiologist, SENIOR neurologist or neurophysiologist, and EXPERIENCED nurse	❑ Optimize blood pH and pCO$_2$	❑ Check electrodes and connections	❑ Decrease/remove distraction or other corrective forces
	❑ Seek normothermia	❑ Determine pattern and timing of signal changes	❑ Remove rods
			❑ Remove screws and probe for breach
❑ Anticipate need for intraoperative and/or perioperative imaging if not readily available	❑ Discuss POTENTIAL need for wake-up test with ATTENDING anesthesiologist	❑ Check neck and limb positioning; check limb position on table especially if unilateral loss	❑ Evaluate for spinal cord compression, examine osteotomy and laminotomy sites

ONGOING CONSIDERATIONS	
❑ REVISIT anesthetic/systemic considerations and confirm that they are optimized	❑ Intraoperative and/or perioperative imaging (e.g. O-arm, fluoroscopy, x-ray) to evaluate implant placement
❑ Wake-up test	
❑ Consultation with a colleague	
❑ Continue surgical procedure versus staging procedure	
❑ IV steroid protocol: Methylprednisolone 30 mg/kg in first hr, then 5.4 mg/kg/hr for next 23 hrs	

Figure 9 Checklist for response to intraoperative neuromonitoring changes. (Reproduced with permission from Vitale MG, Skaggs DL, Pace GI, et al: Best practices in intraoperative neuromonitoring in spine deformity surgery: Development of an intraoperative checklist to optimize response. *Spine Deform* 2014;2[5]:333-339.)

followed by a maintenance infusion of 10 mg/kg/hr until skin closure. An approximate 50% reduction in blood loss and a significantly lower transfusion rate was reported for the TXA group compared with the non-TXA group. No thromboembolic events or renal failures occurred in the TXA group.

A much lower bolus dose of 10 mg/kg TXA followed by a maintenance dose of 1 mg/kg/hr was used in a randomized double-blinded trial.[34] Perioperative blood loss was 25% to 30% lower in patients who received TXA. Interestingly, the postoperative coagulation profiles (prothrombin time, international normalized ratio, and platelet counts) for patients in the TXA and control groups were similar.

A 2015 meta-analysis investigating the efficacy of TXA in reducing blood loss in spine surgery found that TXA significantly reduced intraoperative, postoperative, and total blood loss and led to a reduction in the percentage of patients requiring transfusion.[33] One patient in the TXA group had a myocardial infarction, and deep vein thrombosis developed in one patient in the placebo group. Blood loss was lower with a higher dose of TXA. A low dose of TXA was defined as a bolus dose of less than 10 mg/kg followed by a maintenance dose of less than 10 mg/kg/hr, whereas a high dose of TXA was defined as a bolus dose of 10 to 100 mg/kg followed by a maintenance dose of greater than 10 mg/kg/hr.

Further trials are currently underway to evaluate the efficacy of TXA use in adult spine deformity surgery and patients with spine trauma. A loading dose of 50 mg/kg followed by a maintenance dose of 5 mg/kg/hr for spine deformity surgery is used by some surgeons.

Surgical Options

Selecting the optimal surgical approach is a complex process aided by focusing on the reason the patient is seeking treatment. Reasons may include leg pain, back pain, neurologic deficit, substantial imbalance, or progressive deformity.

Decompression Alone

Older patients with medical comorbidities and symptoms of radiculopathy or neurogenic claudication without substantial back pain may be candidates for limited decompression alone.[1] Although this option may appear attractive for elderly patients, this procedure has a high revision rate because the degree of spine instability may increase after laminectomy in a patient with spine deformity. This is especially likely if the decompression is performed at the apex of the curve, at an olisthetic segment, or at the bottom of a rigid curve.[1] However, decompression alone can be considered in patients with small stable curves who are not candidates for spine reconstruction.

Decompression With Limited Fusion

In contrast with decompression alone, frail patients may be better served with decompression and limited fusion. A 2012 study evaluated patients older than 65 years with mild degenerative scoliosis greater than 30° and spine stenosis.[35] Seventy-five percent of the patients who underwent decompression alone had recurrence of symptoms within 5 years compared with 36% of the patients in the group who underwent decompression with limited fusion. Thirty-one percent of patients who underwent decompression alone had recurrence of symptoms within 6 months.

Minimally invasive surgical decompression for patients with spine deformity and stenosis also has resulted in a high revision rate, particularly when lateral olisthesis is present.[36] In this patient population, a better functional outcome has been reported with decompression and limited fusion compared with decompression alone.[37]

Deformity Correction

The selection of fusion levels can vary based on the type of spine deformity being treated. Patients with degenerative spine deformities usually have lumbar scoliosis and sagittal imbalance. In these patients, the distal and proximal fusion levels should be neutral and stable. Typically, the distal fusion level is either L5 or S1. L5 can be chosen as the distalmost level in adults with good bone quality, a fractional curve less than 15°, and a relatively healthy L5-S1 motion segment (ie, no spondylolisthesis, previous decompression, spinal stenosis, or fixed obliquity). If these conditions are not met, S1 must be chosen

as the distalmost fusion level.[1,38] Stopping the fusion at L5 carries the risk of decompensation of the L5-S1 level and the need for revision surgery and extension of the fusion. However, stopping the fusion at S1 carries the risk of pseudarthrosis at the lumbosacral junction.[1,38] Performing an interbody fusion at L5-S1 along with the addition of pelvic fixation may lower the risk of pseudarthrosis.

The selected proximal fusion level should be both stable and neutral. In addition, the proximal level should not be at the apex of the thoracic kyphosis (T5-T8) and should not be at a vertebra with a kyphotic disk segment below it.

For patients with adult idiopathic deformity, in addition to the aforementioned criteria, structural scoliotic curves also should be included in the fusion. The factors usually considered in selecting the proximal level for adolescent idiopathic scoliosis should be evaluated. However, complete correction of the coronal Cobb angle during surgery is not required. The main goal is to achieve balance in the coronal and sagittal planes.

The all-posterior approach is the most commonly used approach in adult spine deformity surgery. The patient is positioned prone on a surgical frame that allows improved lumbar lordosis and radiographic imaging or a Jackson table with two chest pads, two pelvic pads, and two thigh pads. The abdomen should hang free to aid in decreasing blood loss. The chest pads should be positioned so that there is no pressure on the axillae. The hips are kept in an extended position to allow the lumbar spine to sag and increase LL. The knees are positioned in partial flexion, and the bony prominences around the knees and ankles are well padded. If appropriate LL is lacking on preoperative standing radiographs, substantial LL can be gained with this method in most patients undergoing primary reconstructions, and major osteotomies can be avoided.[39]

Segmental spine fixation is achieved using pedicle screws. Pedicle screw-and-rod constructs also can be used to correct the deformity from the posterior approach. The posterior approach also allows direct decompression of the neural elements. In addition, interbody fusions at L4-L5 and L5-S1 can be performed using the transforaminal lumbar interbody fusion technique (**Figure 7**). The use of this technique in spine deformity surgery has achieved a fusion rate equivalent to that of anterior lumbar interbody fusion, while resulting in shorter surgical times.[40]

Patients with osteoporosis present a special challenge because of the effect of poor bone quality on spinal fixation. Fixation strength can be improved by using multiple fixation points and hydroxyapatite-coated screws, augmenting screw fixation with polymethyl methacrylate bone cement, and providing anterior column support in addition to posterior fixation.

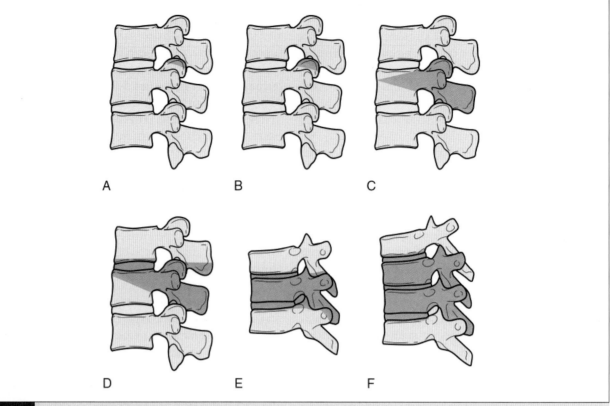

| Figure 10 | Illustration of osteotomy classification grades. **A,** A grade 1 osteotomy involves resection of only the inferior facet at a given level, requires a mobile disk space, and can provide 5° to 10° of correction at each level. **B,** A grade 2 osteotomy is the same as a posterior column osteotomy. **C,** A grade 3 osteotomy is the same as a pedicle subtraction osteotomy and can achieve between 25° to 35° of correction at a level. **D,** A grade 4 osteotomy is similar to the modified pedicle subtraction osteotomy that was previously described. **E,** A grade 5 osteotomy is the same as a vertebral column resection and is a powerful tool in correcting sharp, angular, and rigid deformities. **F,** A grade 6 osteotomy extends the vertebral resection over more than one vertebra. |

Spine Osteotomies

The posterior approach can be used to perform spine osteotomies if further correction in the coronal or sagittal plane is required. There are three main types of spine osteotomies. A posterior column osteotomy involves removal of bilateral facets, interspinous ligament, and the ligamentum flavum. It is a chevron-shaped osteotomy, and it was previously referred to as a Smith-Petersen osteotomy in patients with ankylosed facets and a Ponte osteotomy in patients with Scheuermann kyphosis and unfused facets.[41-43] Careful assessment of preoperative radiographs is required to ensure that a posterior column osteotomy is performed at levels that have mobile disks.

A pedicle subtraction osteotomy is a three-column osteotomy that involves a posterior column osteotomy cephalad and caudad to the level of the pedicle subtraction osteotomy.[41-43] In addition, the pedicles are removed bilaterally, and a wedge-shaped decancellation of the vertebral body is performed along with removal of the posterior vertebral wall that spans the wedge. In a modified or

extended pedicle subtraction osteotomy, the cephalad end plate of the vertebral body is removed along with the overlying disk.

A vertebral column resection starts as a pedicle subtraction osteotomy but both the cephalad and caudad end plates and disks also are removed.[41-43]

A classification system for osteotomies based on six anatomic grades of resection has been proposed[41] (**Figure 10**). The advent of strong segmental pedicle screw instrumentation along with posterior-based osteotomies has allowed surgeons to correct all spine deformities using a posterior-only approach.

Multiple-Rod Constructs

The two main regions of high stress resulting in pseudarthrosis and rod fracture are the lumbosacral junction and the sites of three-column osteotomies (grades 3 to 6). The rate of implant failure has been reported to be as high as 30% after three-column osteotomies.[44] A rod fracture incidence of 5.4% has been reported in adult patients who underwent spine deformity surgery, which increased to 14.9% in patients who also underwent a pedicle subtraction osteotomy.[45] Most rod fractures after a pedicle subtraction osteotomy occurred at a mean of 10 months postoperatively, which suggests that the limitations of implant strength, possibly resulting from excessive rod contouring at the pedicle subtraction osteotomy site, may be a reason for early failure. Using more than two rods at the sites of three-column osteotomies substantially reduces the risk of rod fracture and revision surgery.[44] In a study of 264 patients who underwent pedicle subtraction osteotomy (mean follow-up, 2 years), no failures occurred in those treated with a four-rod construct and interbody fusion caudad and cephalad to the osteotomy site, whereas the highest rate of failure (34%) occurred in patients with two-rod constructs and no interbody fusion caudad and cephalad to the osteotomy site.[46]

The authors of a 2014 study recommended using multiple-rod constructs across three-column osteotomy sites because this technique reduced the risk of rod fracture from approximately 17% to 3%. The revision rate because of pseudarthrosis decreased from 6% to zero because of no complete implant failures in the groups with multiple-rod constructs.[44]

Minimally Invasive and Hybrid Approaches

Minimally invasive surgery for spine deformity correction has been introduced over the past decade. These techniques typically involve anterior, lateral, or transforaminal approaches to the disk space that offer less disruption of the surrounding, normal anatomy. The interbody fusion is typically augmented by minimally invasive posterior pedicle screw instrumentation and fusion.[47-51]

Currently, minimally invasive techniques are primarily applicable to small spine deformities and are not recommended for patients with a preoperative SVA greater than 60 mm, a PI-LL mismatch greater than 30°, or thoracic kyphosis greater than 60°.[52,53] Minimally invasive deformity correction can be used in patients with a standing SVA greater than 60 mm or a flexible deformity that corrects to less than 60 mm in the supine position.[53] This technique is not recommended for rigid deformities with fused segments and for patients with osteoporosis.

The use of hybrid approaches that combine minimally invasive interbody fusion techniques with open posterior approaches have been advocated.[47] A comparison of minimally invasive, hybrid, and open surgeries for adult spine deformity revealed that the mean correction achieved by minimally invasive techniques was 5.5° compared with 10.2° for the open posterior approach and 20.6° for the hybrid approach. The mean SVA correction was 25 mm in the open group compared with minimal SVA correction for the minimally invasive group. However, this study did not evaluate severe spine deformities. The mean preoperative SVA was 33 mm for the minimally invasive group, 56.5 mm for the hybrid group, and 54.4 mm for the group treated with an open approach. The mean postoperative SVA was less than 33 mm for all groups. The only conclusion that can be drawn from these data is that all three options are viable for treating adult patients with small spine deformities and no substantial preoperative sagittal imbalance. The efficacy of minimally invasive approaches for treating severe spine deformities has not been established.

Although minimally invasive approaches may not be appropriate for patients with substantial spine deformity, they may present an option for those with less severe spine deformities. Minimally invasive techniques confer a lower risk of infections, less blood loss, and a lower risk of early revision surgery and hospital readmission compared with traditional open posterior procedures.[47,54,55] Nevertheless, it is important to recognize the unique complications that can occur with minimally invasive procedures. In addition to the typical risks involved with spinal instrumentation, complications introduced by minimally invasive lateral and anterior approaches can include pleural effusions, ureteral injury, iliac vein injury, quadriceps palsy, and abdominal wall herniation.[56]

Proximal Junctional Kyphosis

Segmental pedicle screw instrumentation provides spine surgeons with the ability to achieve rigid fixation. However, this increase in rigidity has led to an increase in the incidence of proximal junctional kyphosis (PJK), which may occur in 10% to 40% of deformity correction procedures.[57] PJK greater than 10° is abnormal, but the magnitude of this angle has not been shown to correlate with poor outcomes.[58] Revision surgery is usually not performed based only on the magnitude of the proximal junctional kyphotic angle. Revision surgery is generally reserved for patients with PJK coexistent with instrumentation failure, traumatic spine injury, neurologic deficit, or substantial pain. Risk factors for the development of PJK include age older than 55 years, a high body mass index, combined anterior-posterior surgery, and distal fusion to the sacrum.[58,59] Patients requiring revision surgery for PJK have been found to have higher postoperative LL and larger SVA corrections than patients without PJK.[57] Rarely, catastrophic failure at the proximal junction can lead to spinal cord injury.

Using a computer-based preoperative model, an 86% accuracy rate was reported in predicting clinically significant PJK greater than 20°.[60] The strongest predictors of PJK were age; the lowermost instrumented vertebra in the sacroiliac region (L5-S1); the use of a pedicle screw as the implant type versus hooks for the upper instrumented vertebra; an upper instrumented vertebra in the thoracolumbar region (T10-L3); and the preoperative SVA, PT, and PI-LL mismatch.

Patients with substantial osteopenia (mean T-score, –1.7) or osteoporosis are at substantial risk for the development of acute fractures at the top of a long construct.[59] The treatment of osteoporosis with teriparatide may improve bone mineral density and reduce the rate of PJK.[61] A threefold reduction in the rate of PJK was reported in patients treated with teriparatide immediately after surgery and continuing for 18 months.[61]

Other suggestions for reducing the risk of PJK include limited dissection proximally using minimally invasive techniques, contouring the proximal part of the rod into kyphosis for a smooth transition into uninstrumented levels, performing interspinous soft-tissue augmentation at the upper instrumented vertebra and the next most cephalad vertebra using braided polyester fiber tape, performing a cement injection at the upper instrumented vertebra and the next cephalad instrumented vertebra, and applying tethers at the proximal junction. However, evidence supporting these techniques remains sparse.

Outcomes and Complications

Adult patients who underwent spine deformity correction surgery were evaluated to identify factors before surgery that would predict reaching (at the least) the MCID.[6] It was found that reaching a MCID was most likely in patients with more substantial deformities as identified by loss of LL, a positive SVA, and intervertebral subluxation. In addition, the achievement of a MCID after surgery was more likely in patients with lower HRQOL scores. Other factors predictive of reaching a MCID were surgical fixation to the sacrum and the need for an osteotomy (factors that indirectly measured the severity of the deformity).

Surgeries for adult spine deformity are associated with a high complication rate that increases in procedures requiring three-column osteotomies.[6,42,43,62,63] Minor complications include urinary tract infection, superficial wound infection, postoperative ileus, transient neurapraxia, deep vein thrombosis, dural tears, minor pulmonary complications, and postoperative delirium. The rate of major complications has been reported to be as high as 40%.[62] Major complications can include substantial neurologic deficit, pulmonary embolism, or a major cardiovascular or cerebrovascular event. Complications requiring revision surgery also are considered major complications and can include deep wound infection, pseudarthrosis, implant failure, implant malposition, and PJK.

Summary

Adult spine deformity encompasses a wide spectrum of etiologies, clinical presentations, and treatment options. Patients may have symptoms of leg pain, back pain, progressive deformity, or neurologic deficits. Complete evaluation of the patient involves a careful clinical history, physical examination, and diagnostic evaluation with full-length radiographs, MRI, and CT.

Treatment is aimed at addressing a patient's symptoms. Because spine deformity can result in substantial disability in an adult patient, physicians involved in the surgical treatment of these patients should be familiar with the realignment goals and techniques of surgery, especially in the sagittal plane.

Treatment decision-making is shared between the physician and the patient. Surgical treatment has a high complication rate and requires a high level of understanding and participation by the patient in the postoperative rehabilitation process. Family/caregiver support is absolutely necessary. Posterior open approaches remain the standard for complex deformity cases, whereas minimally invasive approaches can be considered for patients with small deformities.

Surgical treatment can result in excellent outcomes in properly selected patients, with a reduction in pain and improvement in HRQOL scores.

Key Study Points

- Adult spine deformity encompasses a wide spectrum of etiologies, clinical presentations, and treatment options.

- The disability caused by adult spine deformity is similar to disability related to medical conditions such as cancer, diabetes, and heart disease.

- The goals for optimal sagittal alignment include T1 spinopelvic inclination less than 0°, SVA less than 5 mm, PT less than 20°, and a PI-LL mismatch less than ±9°.

- Risk factors for PJK are age; osteoporosis; lowermost instrumented vertebra in the sacroiliac region; the use pedicle screws as the implant type versus hooks for the upper instrumented vertebra; an upper instrumented vertebra in the thoracolumbar region (T10-L3); and preoperative SVA, PT, and PI-LL mismatch.

- Multimodal intraoperative neuromonitoring using SSEPs, transcranial MEPs, and electromyography provide a high sensitivity and specificity in identifying neurologic deficits intraoperatively.

Annotated References

1. Ailon T, Smith JS, Shaffrey CI, et al: Degenerative spinal deformity. *Neurosurgery* 2015;77(suppl 4):S75-S91.

   This review article on degenerative spine deformity focuses on evaluation, management, and outcomes of patients with adult spinal deformity.

2. Schwab F, Ungar B, Blondel B, et al: Scoliosis Research Society: Schwab adult spinal deformity classification. A validation study. *Spine (Phila Pa 1976)* 2012;37(12):1077-1082.

   Twenty-one adult deformity cases were assessed by nine raters to determine interrater and intrarater variability in applying the SRS-Schwab adult deformity classification. Excellent interrater and intrarater agreement was reported for curve type and each modifier separately.

3. Schwab F, Dubey A, Gamez L, et al: Adult scoliosis: Prevalence, SF-36, and nutritional parameters in an elderly volunteer population. *Spine (Phila Pa 1976)* 2005;30(9):1082-1085.

4. Protopsaltis T, Schwab F, Bronsard N, et al; International Spine Study Group: The T1 pelvic angle, a novel radiographic measure of global sagittal deformity, accounts for both spinal inclination and pelvic tilt and correlates with health-related quality of life. *J Bone Joint Surg Am* 2014;96(19):1631-1640.

   A multicenter study of 559 patients with adult spine deformity was undertaken to investigate a new radiographic measure and its correlation with HRQOL measures. It was found that a T1 pelvic angle of 20° corresponded with the presence of substantial disability. Level of evidence: II.

5. Aebi M: The adult scoliosis. *Eur Spine J* 2005;14(10):925-948.

6. Schwab FJ, Lafage V, Farcy JP, Bridwell KH, Glassman S, Shainline MR: Predicting outcome and complications in the surgical treatment of adult scoliosis. *Spine (Phila Pa 1976)* 2008;33(20):2243-2247.

7. Bess S, Line B, Fu KM, et al; International Spine Study Group: The health impact of symptomatic adult spinal deformity: Comparison of deformity types to United States population norms and chronic diseases. *Spine (Phila Pa 1976)* 2016;41(3):224-233.

   The effect of symptomatic adult spine deformity on Medical Outcomes Study 36-Item Short Form physical and mental component summary scores was compared with the effect on scores of other chronic conditions and US population norms. Level of evidence: III.

8. Schwab FJ, Smith VA, Biserni M, Gamez L, Farcy JP, Pagala M: Adult scoliosis: A quantitative radiographic and clinical analysis. *Spine (Phila Pa 1976)* 2002;27(4):387-392.

9. Schwab F, Lafage V, Patel A, Farcy JP: Sagittal plane considerations and the pelvis in the adult patient. *Spine (Phila Pa 1976)* 2009;34(17):1828-1833.

10. Lafage V, Schwab F, Patel A, Hawkinson N, Farcy JP: Pelvic tilt and truncal inclination: Two key radiographic parameters in the setting of adults with spinal deformity. *Spine (Phila Pa 1976)* 2009;34(17):E599-E606.

11. Schwab F, Patel A, Ungar B, Farcy JP, Lafage V: Adult spinal deformity-postoperative standing imbalance: How much can you tolerate? An overview of key parameters in assessing alignment and planning corrective surgery. *Spine (Phila Pa 1976)* 2010;35(25):2224-2231.

12. Smith JS, Klineberg E, Schwab F, et al; International Spine Study Group: Change in classification grade by the SRS-Schwab Adult Spinal Deformity Classification predicts impact on health-related quality of life measures: Prospective analysis of operative and nonoperative treatment. *Spine (Phila Pa 1976)* 2013;38(19):1663-1671.

   This multicenter study by the International Spine Study Group reported that changes in the sagittal modifiers of the SRS-Schwab classification at 1 year correlated with changes in HRQOL outcomes in patients with adult spine deformity. Level of evidence: III.

13. Schwab F, Farcy JP, Bridwell K, et al: A clinical impact classification of scoliosis in the adult. *Spine (Phila Pa 1976)* 2006;31(18):2109-2114.

14. Lowe T, Berven SH, Schwab FJ, Bridwell KH: The SRS classification for adult spinal deformity: Building on the

5: Spine Deformity

King/Moe and Lenke classification systems. *Spine (Phila Pa 1976)* 2006;31(19 suppl):S119-S125.

15. Berven SH, Lowe T: The Scoliosis Research Society classification for adult spinal deformity. *Neurosurg Clin N Am* 2007;18(2):207-213.

16. Lenke LG, Betz RR, Harms J, et al: Adolescent idiopathic scoliosis: A new classification to determine extent of spinal arthrodesis. *J Bone Joint Surg Am* 2001;83(8):1169-1181.

17. Chin KR, Furey C, Bohlman HH: Risk of progression in de novo low-magnitude degenerative lumbar curves: Natural history and literature review. *Am J Orthop (Belle Mead NJ)* 2009;38(8):404-409.

18. Faraj SS, Holewijn RM, van Hooff ML, de Kleuver M, Pellisé F, Haanstra TM: De novo degenerative lumbar scoliosis: A systematic review of prognostic factors for curve progression. *Eur Spine J* 2016;25(8):2347-2358.

    A systematic review of 12 studies reported that factors for de novo degenerative lumbar scoliosis curve progression included intervertebral disk degeneration, an intercrest line through L5 instead of L4, and lateral vertebral translation 6 mm or greater.

19. Deschênes S, Charron G, Beaudoin G, et al: Diagnostic imaging of spinal deformities: Reducing patients radiation dose with a new slot-scanning X-ray imager. *Spine (Phila Pa 1976)* 2010;35(9):989-994.

20. Illés T, Somoskeöy S: The EOS™ imaging system and its uses in daily orthopaedic practice. *Int Orthop* 2012;36(7):1325-1331.

    The authors review the use of EOS imaging in orthopaedic and spine practices. The principles behind EOS technology are discussed, and its use in reconstructing three-dimensional models is highlighted.

21. Ilharreborde B, Dubousset J, Le Huec JC: Use of EOS imaging for the assessment of scoliosis deformities: Application to postoperative 3D quantitative analysis of the trunk. *Eur Spine J* 2014;23(suppl 4):S397-S405.

    Forty-nine patients with adolescent idiopathic scoliosis were evaluated with three-dimensional reconstructions of the spine and thorax to assess changes in thoracic volume resulting from the surgical correction of scoliosis. All parameters substantially improved after surgery.

22. Pinkerton JV, Thomas S, Dalkin AC: Osteoporosis treatment and prevention for postmenopausal women: Current and future therapeutic options. *Clin Obstet Gynecol* 2013;56(4):711-721.

    Current medical management options for postmenopausal women with osteoporosis are reviewed and novel treatment strategies currently under investigation are discussed.

23. Camacho PM, Petak SM, Binkley N, et al: American Association of Clinical Endocrinologists and American College of Endocrinology Clinical Practice Guidelines for the Diagnosis and Treatment of Postmenopausal Osteoporosis: 2016. Executive summary. *Endocr Pract* 2016;22(9):1111-1118.

    The guidelines published by two national endocrinology organizations concerning the diagnosis and treatment of osteoporosis in postmenopausal women are reviewed.

24. Knott PT, Mardjetko SM, Techy F: The use of the T1 sagittal angle in predicting overall sagittal balance of the spine. *Spine J* 2010;10(11):994-998.

25. Glassman SD, Berven S, Bridwell K, Horton W, Dimar JR: Correlation of radiographic parameters and clinical symptoms in adult scoliosis. *Spine (Phila Pa 1976)* 2005;30(6):682-688.

26. Everett CR, Patel RK: A systematic literature review of nonsurgical treatment in adult scoliosis. *Spine (Phila Pa 1976)* 2007;32(19 suppl):S130-S134.

27. Bridwell KH, Glassman S, Horton W, et al: Does treatment (nonoperative and operative) improve the two-year quality of life in patients with adult symptomatic lumbar scoliosis: A prospective multicenter evidence-based medicine study. *Spine (Phila Pa 1976)* 2009;34(20):2171-2178.

28. Glassman SD, Carreon LY, Shaffrey CI, et al: The costs and benefits of nonoperative management for adult scoliosis. *Spine (Phila Pa 1976)* 2010;35(5):578-582.

29. Quraishi NA, Lewis SJ, Kelleher MO, Sarjeant R, Rampersaud YR, Fehlings MG: Intraoperative multimodality monitoring in adult spinal deformity: Analysis of a prospective series of one hundred two cases with independent evaluation. *Spine (Phila Pa 1976)* 2009;34(14):1504-1512.

30. Zhuang Q, Wang S, Zhang J, et al: How to make the best use of intraoperative motor evoked potential monitoring? Experience in 1162 consecutive spinal deformity surgical procedures. *Spine (Phila Pa 1976)* 2014;39(24):E1425-E1432.

    This retrospective study of 1,162 patients was undertaken to establish a protocol for MEP warning criteria with high sensitivity and specificity in detecting intraoperative spinal cord injury. MEP monitoring based on the authors' protocol achieved good sensitivity and specificity and provided valuable information for intraoperative decision making.

31. Bhagat S, Durst A, Grover H, et al: An evaluation of multimodal spinal cord monitoring in scoliosis surgery: A single centre experience of 354 operations. *Eur Spine J* 2015;24(7):1399-1407.

    In this retrospective series, multimodal monitoring with the combined use of SSEPs and MEPs was shown to be superior to single modality monitoring for the detection of impending spinal cord injury.

32. Vitale MG, Skaggs DL, Pace GI, et al: Best practices in intraoperative neuromonitoring in spine deformity surgery: Development of an intraoperative checklist to optimize response. *Spine Deform* 2014;2(5):333-339.

A group of spine experts discuss the results of their collaboration to create a consensus-based checklist for use in the operating room in the event of change detected by intraoperative neuromonitoring. The roles of the various teams in the operating room are highlighted, and a stepwise approach is outlined for troubleshooting problems.

33. Xie J, Lenke LG, Li T, et al: Preliminary investigation of high-dose tranexamic acid for controlling intraoperative blood loss in patients undergoing spine correction surgery. *Spine J* 2015;15(4):647-654.

    This retrospective study addresses the use of high-dose TXA in spine deformity surgery. The TXA group received an intravenous loading dose of 100 mg/kg, followed by a maintenance infusion of 10 mg/kg/hr. The study demonstrated safety and efficacy of high-dose TXA use, especially in patients undergoing posterior vertebral column resection.

34. Wong J, El Beheiry H, Rampersaud YR, et al: Tranexamic acid reduces perioperative blood loss in adult patients having spinal fusion surgery. *Anesth Analg* 2008;107(5):1479-1486.

35. Daubs MD, Lenke LG, Bridwell KH, Cheh G, Kim YJ, Stobbs G: Decompression alone versus decompression with limited fusion for treatment of degenerative lumbar scoliosis in the elderly patient. *Evid Based Spine Care J* 2012;3(4):27-32.

    The authors present the results of a retrospective analysis of 55 patients older than 65 years with lumbar curves greater than 30° who were treated with either laminectomy alone or laminectomy with limited fusion. Results suggest that decompression with limited fusion may be a better option in preventing the earlier return of symptoms of spinal stenosis.

36. Kelleher MO, Timlin M, Persaud O, Rampersaud YR: Success and failure of minimally invasive decompression for focal lumbar spinal stenosis in patients with and without deformity. *Spine (Phila Pa 1976)* 2010;35(19):E981-E987.

37. Transfeldt EE, Topp R, Mehbod AA, Winter RB: Surgical outcomes of decompression, decompression with limited fusion, and decompression with full curve fusion for degenerative scoliosis with radiculopathy. *Spine (Phila Pa 1976)* 2010;35(20):1872-1875.

38. Sardar ZM, Ouellet JA, Fischer DJ, Skelly AC: Outcomes in adult scoliosis patients who undergo spinal fusion stopping at L5 compared with extension to the sacrum. *Evid Based Spine Care J* 2013;4(2):96-104.

    Controversies related to stopping spinal fusion at L5 versus the sacrum are addressed in this systematic review of patients who underwent surgical correction of spine deformity.

39. Harimaya K, Lenke LG, Mishiro T, Bridwell KH, Koester LA, Sides BA: Increasing lumbar lordosis of adult spinal deformity patients via intraoperative prone positioning. *Spine (Phila Pa 1976)* 2009;34(22):2406-2412.

40. Dorward IG, Lenke LG, Bridwell KH, et al: Transforaminal versus anterior lumbar interbody fusion in long deformity constructs: A matched cohort analysis. *Spine (Phila Pa 1976)* 2013;38(12):E755-E762.

    This retrospective study compared the use of transforaminal lumbar interbody fusion versus anterior lumbar interbody fusion at the lumbosacral region in patients undergoing spinal fusion for deformity. The complications and union rates of the two techniques are compared along with their capacity to achieve focal and global deformity correction.

41. Schwab F, Blondel B, Chay E, et al.: The comprehensive anatomical spinal osteotomy classification. *Neurosurgery* 2015;76(suppl 1):S33-41; discussion S41.

    The authors propose a classification system for spinal osteotomies that details a progressive ranking based on magnitude. In addition, a universal framework is provided to describe spinal osteotomies.

42. Dorward IG, Lenke LG, Stoker GE, Cho W, Koester LA, Sides BA: Radiographic and clinical outcomes of posterior column osteotomies in spinal deformity correction. *Spine (Phila Pa 1976)* 2014.

    The authors analyze data from 128 patients who underwent posterior column osteotomies for primary or revision surgeries. Correction of sagittal and coronal parameters is assessed along with clinical outcomes.

43. Dorward IG, Lenke LG: Osteotomies in the posterior-only treatment of complex adult spinal deformity: A comparative review. *Neurosurg Focus* 2010;28(3):E4.

44. Hyun SJ, Lenke LG, Kim YC, Koester LA, Blanke KM: Comparison of standard 2-rod constructs to multiple-rod constructs for fixation across 3-column spinal osteotomies. *Spine (Phila Pa 1976)* 2014;39(22):1899-1904.

    This retrospective study compared 66 patients treated with two-rod constructs and 66 patients treated multiple-rod constructs for fixation in three-column osteotomies performed for correction of spine deformity. A multiple-rod construct was found to be a safe and effective method of providing increased stability across three-column osteotomy sites. Level of evidence: III.

45. Smith JS, Shaffrey CI, Ames CP, et al: Assessment of symptomatic rod fracture after posterior instrumented fusion for adult spinal deformity. *Neurosurgery* 2012;71(4):862-867.

    The authors used a multicenter database to assess the rate of rod fracture after posterior spinal instrumentation and fusion. A lower rate of rod fracture was found with cobalt-chromium rods than with titanium alloy or stainless steel rods.

46. Gupta M, Henry JK, Schwab F, et al: Reducing rod breakage and pseudarthrosis in pedicle subtraction osteotomy: The importance of rod number and configuration in 264 patients with 2-year follow-up. *Global Spine J* 2016. Available at: https://www.thieme-connect.de/DOI/DOI?10.1055/s-0036-1582911. Accessed March 15, 2017.

5: Spine Deformity

This retrospective review of various rod configurations provides evidence advocating the use of satellite rods over accessory rods for augmentation at pedicle subtraction osteotomy sites.

47. Haque RM, Mundis GM Jr, Ahmed Y, et al; International Spine Study Group: Comparison of radiographic results after minimally invasive, hybrid, and open surgery for adult spinal deformity: A multicenter study of 184 patients. *Neurosurg Focus* 2014;36(5):E13.

The ability to achieve radiographic correction of spine deformity with minimally invasive versus hybrid versus open surgery in adult patients is addressed in this multicenter retrospective study.

48. Anand N, Baron EM, Khandehroo B: Does minimally invasive transsacral fixation provide anterior column support in adult scoliosis? *Clin Orthop Relat Res* 2014;472(6):1769-1775.

This single-center retrospective case series reports on the use of transsacral fixation in conjunction with minimally invasive spinal deformity correction. In carefully selected patients, transsacral fixation may allow safe lumbosacral fusion without iliac fixation when long-segment constructs are used. Level of evidence: IV.

49. Anand N, Baron EM, Khandehroo B, Kahwaty S: Long-term 2- to 5-year clinical and functional outcomes of minimally invasive surgery for adult scoliosis. *Spine (Phila Pa 1976)* 2013;38(18):1566-1575.

This retrospective single-center analysis provides support for minimally invasive surgical correction of adult scoliosis.

50. Anand N, Baron EM: Minimally invasive approaches for the correction of adult spinal deformity. *Eur Spine J* 2013;22(suppl 2):S232-S241.

Various minimally invasive techniques for interbody fusion and percutaneous screw placement for correction of adult spine deformity are reviewed.

51. Bach K, Ahmadian A, Deukmedjian A, Uribe JS: Minimally invasive surgical techniques in adult degenerative spinal deformity: A systematic review. *Clin Orthop Relat Res* 2014;472(6):1749-1761.

The authors present a systematic review of outcomes reported for minimally invasive techniques for correction of adult degenerative spine deformity. All 13 articles reviewed had level IV evidence.

52. Anand N, Baron EM, Khandehroo B: Limitations and ceiling effects with circumferential minimally invasive correction techniques for adult scoliosis: Analysis of radiological outcomes over a 7-year experience. *Neurosurg Focus* 2014;36(5):E14.

The authors report on a single-center retrospective review of the radiographs of 90 patients who underwent scoliosis correction with minimally invasive techniques. Limits are proposed for the magnitude of deformity in the coronal

and sagittal planes that may not be successfully corrected with minimally invasive techniques.

53. Mummaneni PV, Shaffrey CI, Lenke LG, et al; Minimally Invasive Surgery Section of the International Spine Study Group: The minimally invasive spinal deformity surgery algorithm: A reproducible rational framework for decision making in minimally invasive spinal deformity surgery. *Neurosurg Focus* 2014;36(5):E6.

A consensus-based algorithm is presented by a group of experts in spine deformity. The algorithm provides guidelines to determine if a patient with spine deformity should undergo minimally invasive surgery for deformity correction.

54. Anand N, Sardar ZM, Simmonds A, Khandehroo B, Kahwaty S, Baron EM: Thirty-day reoperation and readmission rates after correction of adult spinal deformity via circumferential minimally invasive surgery: Analysis of a 7-year experience. *Spine Deform* 2016;4(1):78-83.

With focus on value-based care, this article provides an argument in support of using minimally invasive techniques for spinal deformity correction to reduce early revision surgery and readmission rates. Level of evidence: IV.

55. Uribe JS, Deukmedjian AR, Mummaneni PV, et al; International Spine Study Group: Complications in adult spinal deformity surgery: An analysis of minimally invasive, hybrid, and open surgical techniques. *Neurosurg Focus* 2014;36(5):E15.

The authors present the results of a multicenter analysis of complications encountered during various surgical techniques used in the correction of adult spine deformities.

56. Anand N, Baron EM: Urological injury as a complication of the transpsoas approach for discectomy and interbody fusion. *J Neurosurg Spine* 2013;18(1):18-23.

The rare complication of injury to the genitourinary system during transpsoas lumbar diskectomy and fusion are presented along with guidance on complication management.

57. Kim HJ, Bridwell KH, Lenke LG, et al: Patients with proximal junctional kyphosis requiring revision surgery have higher postoperative lumbar lordosis and larger sagittal balance corrections. *Spine (Phila Pa 1976)* 2014;39(9):E576-E580.

The unresolved issues of PJK after adult scoliosis surgery is discussed in this case-control study from a single institution. Risk factors for PJK requiring revision are proposed based on the collected data.

58. Bridwell KH, Lenke LG, Cho SK, et al: Proximal junctional kyphosis in primary adult deformity surgery: Evaluation of 20 degrees as a critical angle. *Neurosurgery* 2013;72(6):899-906.

The unsolved problem of PJK is discussed based on retrospective data from a single institution. Older age, obesity, constructs starting in the lower thoracic spine, and fusion to the sacrum are identified as factors associated with PJK of 20° or more.

59. O'Leary PT, Bridwell KH, Lenke LG, et al: Risk factors and outcomes for catastrophic failures at the top of long pedicle screw constructs: A matched cohort analysis performed at a single center. *Spine (Phila Pa 1976)* 2009;34(20):2134-2139.

60. Scheer JK, Osorio JA, Smith JS, et al; and the International Spine Study Group: Development of validated computer based pre-operative predictive model for proximal junction failure (PJF) or clinically significant PJK with 86% accuracy based on 510 ASD patients with 2-year follow-up. *Spine (Phila Pa 1976)* 2016.

To develop and test a computer-based model for predicting PJK in patients undergoing surgical treatment of adult spine deformity, 510 patients were retrospectively studied. Important factors in the development of PJK were patient age, lowest instrumented vertebra, preoperative sagittal balance, type of upper instrumented vertebral implant, upper instrumented vertebra, preoperative PT, and preoperative PI-LL mismatch.

61. Yagi M, Ohne H, Konomi T, et al: Teriparatide improves volumetric bone mineral density and fine bone structure in the UIV+1 vertebra, and reduces bone failure type PJK after surgery for adult spinal deformity. *Osteoporos Int* 2016;27(12):3495-3502.

After spine deformity surgery, the outcomes of 43 patients given teriparatide therapy and 33 control patients who did not receive teriparatide were compared. Patients in the teriparatide group showed a decrease in PJK caused by vertebral failure.

62. Cho SK, Bridwell KH, Lenke LG, et al: Major complications in revision adult deformity surgery: Risk factors and clinical outcomes with 2- to 7-year follow-up. *Spine (Phila Pa 1976)* 2012;37(6):489-500.

The authors report on major long-term complications associated with revision adult spine deformity surgery and their effect on clinical outcomes.

63. O'Neill KR, Lenke LG, Bridwell KH, Neuman BJ, Kim HJ, Archer KR: Factors associated with long-term patient-reported outcomes after three-column osteotomies. *Spine J* 2015;15(11):2312-2318.

Patient-reported outcomes, complication rates, and revision rates are reported for 120 patients who underwent three-column osteotomies for spinal deformity.

Chapter 25

Sagittal Imbalance of the Spine

Serena S. Hu, MD   Kirkham B. Wood, MD

Abstract

The mobile human spine is made up of the cervical, thoracic, and lumbar regions. Each region has characteristic curvatures in the sagittal plane, which together allow an individual to maintain the appropriate vertical posture. Deviations from normal sagittal alignment can result in pain and functional decline. The three basic types of sagittal balance deviations are local, regional, and global.

Keywords: balance; fusion; instrumentation; osteotomy; sagittal balance

Introduction

The normal adult human spine has carefully balanced curvatures in both the coronal (AP) and sagittal (lateral) planes. The spine is said to be in balance when the head is resting in a position directly centered over the distal sacrum and pelvis. Less muscular energy is expended to maintain this stance than any other; therefore, it has been described as the cone of economy.[1,2] Conversely, a loss of specific curvature in a region or the entire spinal column requires increased energy expenditure to gain upright posture, and loading of the motion segments is asymmetric. The resulting degenerative or arthritic changes can cause pain, weakness, and spine deformity. Sagittal plane malalignment can have disabling consequences.[3-6]

Dr. Hu or an immediate family member has received royalties from NuVasive; has stock or stock options held in NuVasive; and serves as a board member, owner, officer, or committee member of the American Orthopaedic Association and the Scoliosis Research Society. Dr. Wood or an immediate family member has received royalties from Globus Medical; is a paid consultant for Alphatec Spine; and has stock or stock options held in TranS1.

A patient with scoliosis has abnormal curvatures in the coronal plane, often leading to arthritis, stenosis, and pain. In recent years, however, significant sagittal plane malalignment has been demonstrated to have an even more dramatic effect on patient functioning than scoliosis.

Definitions

The cervical, thoracic, and lumbar regions of the normal adult spine have inherent curvatures. Together, these three regions maintain a harmonious balance of the head and neck over the sacrum and pelvis[3,7] (**Figure 1**). The normal cervical and lumbar spine curvatures are lordotic. In between, the thoracic spine (T1 through T12) is kyphotic. The normal range of cervical spine lordosis is 31° to 49°.[3] Normal lumbar lordosis (LL) ranges from 40° to more than 80°.[3,8-12] The normal kyphotic range of the thoracic spine is even broader and has been measured from 20° to 70°.[3,8-12] Together, the three curves balance one another so that the base of the cervical spine ideally is centered just over the sacrum and pelvis.

Normal intervertebral alignments within each region of the thoracolumbar spine were described based on large radiographic studies of adults without symptoms[10,11] (**Figure 2**). In the upper and lower aspects of the thoracic spine, there was 1° to 3° of sagittal kyphosis between adjacent vertebrae; the central region from T3 to T9 had 4° to 5° of kyphosis between adjacent vertebrae. The sagittal alignment of the thoracolumbar junction tends to be relatively neutral. In the lumbar spine, the amount of lordosis increases with each segmental level; almost two-thirds of normal LL is found at the lowest two levels (L4-L5 and L5-S1). As a result, small changes in caudal alignment can have a profound effect on the overall alignment of the cervical spine relative to the pelvis.

Sagittal plane abnormalities can be radiographically described in three ways, but all can be primarily understood as an exaggeration or deficiency of normal cervical or LL or thoracolumbar kyphosis.[3,13] A local (focal) sagittal plane abnormality is limited to one or two functional spine units, each of which comprises two vertebral bodies,

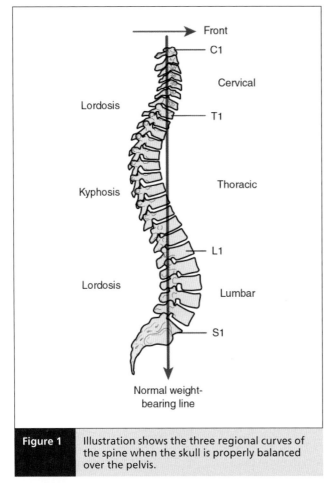

Figure 1 Illustration shows the three regional curves of the spine when the skull is properly balanced over the pelvis.

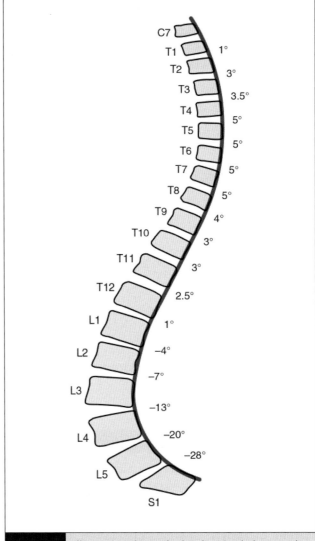

Figure 2 Illustration shows the local sagittal plane angles of the thoracolumbar spine segments.

the intervening disk, and the associated ligaments. The change in sagittal alignment is limited to that area and usually does not affect the alignment of the spinal region or the overall balance of the head and cervical spine over the pelvis. Posttraumatic kyphosis after a burst fracture and lumbar spondylolisthesis with local kyphotic angulation are examples of a local sagittal abnormality.

A regional sagittal plane abnormality encompasses multiple vertebral segments and leads to clear changes in the profile of the spinal region. The cephalad and/or caudad areas are able to compensate so that the overall balance of the head and neck is not substantially changed from its normal position over the sacrum and pelvis. Examples of regional sagittal plane abnormalities are Scheuermann thoracic kyphosis and kyphosis of the cervicothoracic junction, as in postoperative junctional kyphosis (**Figures 3** and **4**).

A global sagittal plane deformity substantially affects the position of the head and neck over the sacrum and pelvis. The abnormality can be in the thoracic, thoracolumbar, or lumbar spine but most commonly is in the caudal aspect of the spine, where the effect on overall alignment can be most profound. Examples of global malalignment are so-called flatback deformity, which can develop idiopathically or iatrogenically after surgery (**Figure 5**), and postlaminectomy kyphosis, especially if the patient is young and the procedure involved the lower lumbar spine. Dramatic sagittal plane abnormalities can accompany ankylosing spondylitis, often resulting from loss of curvature in all three regions of the spine and severe lateral plane imbalance (**Figure 6**).

Spinopelvic Parameters

The important contribution of the pelvis to overall spine sagittal alignment has become clear during the past few

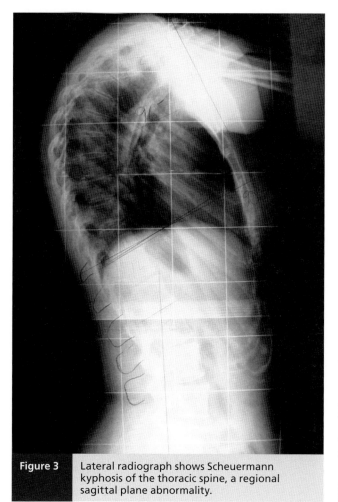

Figure 3 Lateral radiograph shows Scheuermann kyphosis of the thoracic spine, a regional sagittal plane abnormality.

decades. Pelvic incidence (PI) is a sagittal plane measurement of the relationship of the sacrum to the pelvis and the femoral heads; it was first described in adolescents with isthmic spondylolisthesis and adults with a spine deformity[14] (**Figure 7**). This angular measurement combines the sacral slope (the top of S1 relative to the horizontal) and the pelvic tilt (PT; the relationship in the sagittal plane of the femoral heads to the sacrum). In a typical adult without symptoms, the PI is 50° to 55°[3,9,14,15] and is fixed at skeletal maturity. In individuals with greater values of PI, a higher degree of LL is required to maintain balance.[3,14,15]

It has become increasingly apparent in reconstruction surgery for adult spine deformity that the most important predictor of the radiographic and clinical outcome is the restoration of sagittal alignment.[4,16,17] The greatest improvements in health-related quality-of-life measures were seen in patients who had the greatest improvement in C7 plumb line balance,[16] although the sagittal vertical axis (SVA) increases with age. PI, as first described for spondylolisthesis, now is also used in surgical planning

for adult deformity. PI was found to be a strong predictor of the amount of LL a patient requires to maintain the sagittal profile and normal function (preferred value, PI = LL ± 9).[9,14,18-20] Mathematical equations involving total kyphosis, lordosis, and PI have been combined for surgical planning.[14,21] A study of health-related quality-of-life outcomes found that optimal postoperative results were achieved if the SVA was less than 50 mm and the PT was less than 25°.[18] Postoperative lordosis should be within 9° to 10° of the PI measurement.[18,22]

The PT was found to be predictive of a successful surgical outcome and is an important part of surgical planning.[21] The normal PT measurement is approximately 12°, and PT of less than 25° was found to be the measurement most closely related to postoperative clinical satisfaction.[3,13] A larger PT is caused by an increase in pelvic retroversion as the patient attempts to bring the head over the pelvis.[21,23] Global tilt, which is defined as the sum of the PT and the C7 vertical tilt (the angular value of the SVA), was proposed as a method of measuring and predicting sagittal alignment that is more reliable and less sensitive to positional changes than the PT or the SVA alone[24] (**Figure 8**). The T9 tilt, which can be understood as the vertical projection of the center of weight behind the hip joints, must be measured with thoracic kyphosis and the underlying PI to best predict the lordosis needed for an optimal clinical outcome[15] (**Figure 9**).

Clinical Assessment

The symptoms of a sagittal plane abnormality of a local or regional nature typically are restricted to the affected level. The degeneration that can accompany an isthmic spondylolisthesis can be seen at the disk level, the adjacent spine unit, or the foraminal level with root impingement. The pain from posttraumatic kyphosis emanates from degenerated disks above or below the fracture or from facet arthritis posterior to the malalignment. The sagittal plane abnormalities of thoracic kyphosis similarly can lead to pain from disk or facet overload. With a larger deformity, substantial muscular stretching and fatigue can occur, especially when the patient is standing.[25,26] Similar processes occur in junctional kyphosis above or below a previous fusion.

The clinical assessment of a patient with a global sagittal plane deformity becomes increasingly complicated as many regions, segments, and tissues become involved. The symptoms of spine arthritis can depend on the deformity, but with global malalignment, the head and neck fall so far forward that the patient experiences overwhelming muscular ache and fatigue when attempting to remain upright. The patient often has increasing

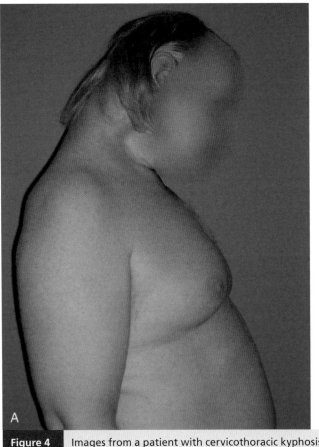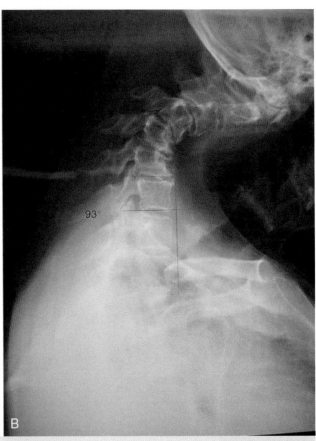

Figure 4 Images from a patient with cervicothoracic kyphosis, a regional sagittal plane abnormality. **A,** Clinical photograph. **B,** Lateral radiograph.

difficulty standing, but minimal symptoms manifest when seated or lying down. It is important to examine the patient in more than one position (especially upright) when the patient is most able to describe the location of symptoms and provocative activities. Spine flexibility should be assessed through flexion and extension maneuvers. Local kyphotic deformities also can be manually assessed for flexibility. In addition, a patient with global malalignment should be examined while supine on the examining table to assess flexibility. Some patients have an apparently severe sagittal plane deformity while standing that is completely corrected with gentle relaxation on the examining table. Conversely, there may be no reduction in this position if the deformity is truly rigid; this condition may require a multicolumn osteotomy or vertebral resection.

The cornerstone radiographic measurement is the C7 plumb line relative to the sacrum (the SVA). In young adults, the C7 plumb line should fall at or posterior to the posterior corner of the sacrum.[3,7] With aging, the normal loss of height from desiccation of the lumbar disks results in loss of LL. In an asymptomatic individual in the eighth decade of life, it is normal for the C7 plumb line to fall a few centimeters anterior to the sacrum.[11,13,27]

All lateral radiographs should permit the spine to be visualized from the base of the skull, where cervical alignment to the hips and upper femurs can be observed. The patient must stand as erect as possible, preferably unsupported, with the hips and knees as fully extended as possible. A false assessment of the overall spine alignment may result if, for example, the hips are flexed (voluntarily or by contracture); therefore, accurate surgical planning may be jeopardized. A fixed flexion contracture of the hip or knee must be measured and factored into preoperative planning.

Current surgical procedures are intended to rebalance the spine so that the C7 plumb line will fall as close to the sacrum as possible. Initially, many surgeons attempted to realign C7 to an optimal position behind the sacrum, but the result was to create junctional issues, kyphosis, and fracture in many older patients. In recent years, surgeons have tempered their zeal for perfect spinal alignment to account for the normal aging process.[3,8]

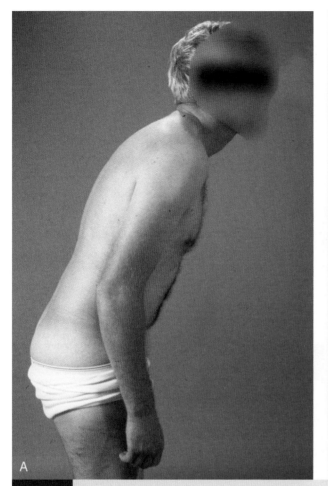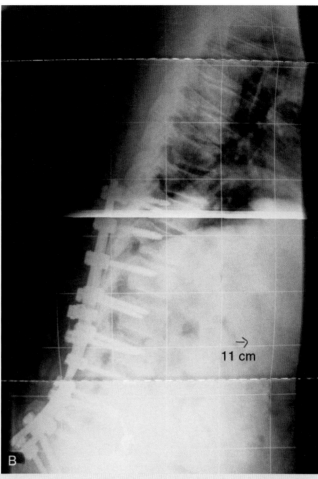

11 cm

| Figure 5 | Images from a patient with iatrogenic flatback deformity, a global sagittal malalignment deformity. **A,** Clinical photograph. **B,** Lateral radiograph. |

The flexibility of the malalignment should be radiographically studied if surgical correction is being considered for a patient with a local or regional deformity in the sagittal plane. A lateral radiograph taken with the patient supine and a semirigid bolster placed under the apex of the deformity can provide information as to the surgical correctability of the deformity. Flexion-extension radiographs can be used to assess the motion characteristics of a local deformity such as spondylolisthesis. In a patient with spondylolisthesis, a simple comparison of the upright lateral radiograph with a supine MRI can provide more information than flexion-extension radiographs.[28]

as well as local modalities such as heat, massage, ice, ultrasound, and electrical stimulation. The judicious use of NSAIDs can be considered, but the use of narcotic medication is not advisable. The patient can be assisted in making an appropriate treatment decision by the provision of information and understanding and conversing with patients who are similarly affected. Simple lifestyle changes sometimes help reduce the inciting stimuli to a satisfactory level. Nonsurgical care was found to have a minimal or guarded effect on improving pain and function, however, and the cumulative costs of such care may be substantial.[29,30]

Treatment

Nonsurgical treatment can be considered if the patient is neurologically intact and the primary considerations are pain relief and functional improvement. Structured physical therapy includes weight training, aerobic and anaerobic conditioning, strengthening, and stretching

Local Sagittal Abnormalities

Posttraumatic Kyphosis

Posttraumatic kyphosis is most closely associated with an ignored or inadequately treated flexion-distraction fracture of the thoracolumbar spine, such as a Chance fracture.[31-33] Nonsurgical treatment of a severe burst fracture

5: Spine Deformity

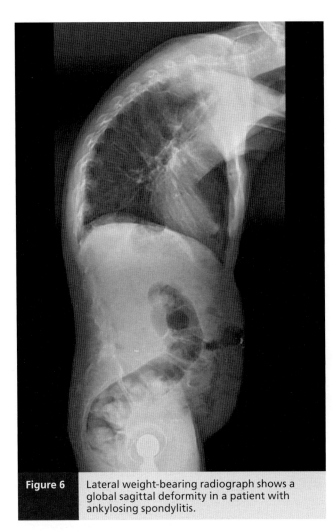

Figure 6 Lateral weight-bearing radiograph shows a global sagittal deformity in a patient with ankylosing spondylitis.

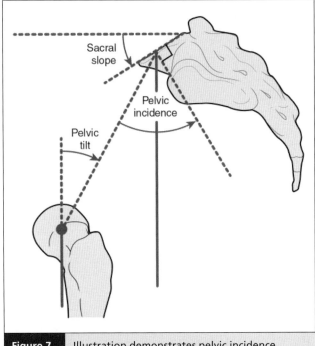

Figure 7 Illustration demonstrates pelvic incidence, which combines the sacral slope and pelvic tilt.

can lead to a similar deformity. The pain probably results from a combination of disk degeneration above or below the fractured bone and posterior ligament laxity. Surgery can be considered after unsuccessful nonsurgical treatment. Surgical reconstruction is intended to stabilize the affected segments while realigning them to the extent possible. The stabilizing fusion was found to be more important for pain relief than sagittal realignment.[34] If the affected segment is flexible and some realignment can be achieved during examination or positioning under anesthesia, only a simple posterior reconstruction of the failed tension band may be necessary. Disk space release, anterior corpectomy with posterior instrumentation, or a posterior three-column osteotomy can be considered for a rigid deformity.

Isthmic Spondylolisthesis

Dozens of surgical procedures have been described for treating adult isthmic spondylolisthesis.[35-37] No one procedure is suitable for all patients because of individual differences in vertebral translation, local kyphosis, rigidity, age, and neural element compression. The typical caudal location of the isthmic slip in the lumbar spine requires the application of sagittal alignment principles, however. Reduction of the sagittal translation is much less critical in spondylolisthesis reconstruction than reduction of any lumbosacral kyphosis. Overly aggressive translation reduction was associated with an increased risk of neural injury.[37-41] It is recommended that the normal horizontal position of L4 be restored to the extent possible (**Figure 10**).

Regional Sagittal Abnormalities

Many adults in late life have thoracic kyphosis that is painful and fatiguing; the condition may have been present from young adulthood but is relatively asymptomatic. Like patients with a global sagittal plane deformity, most patients with a regional malalignment abnormality such as Scheuermann kyphosis experience the most intense symptoms when standing for an extended period of time. Many patients are dissatisfied with the cosmetic appearance of the deformity and seek correction.

The flexibility of the spine should be assessed clinically and radiographically. Full spine imaging from the occiput to the proximal femurs is required.[12] The flexibility analysis often requires a lateral radiograph of the thoracic spine taken with a semirigid bolster placed under the deformity

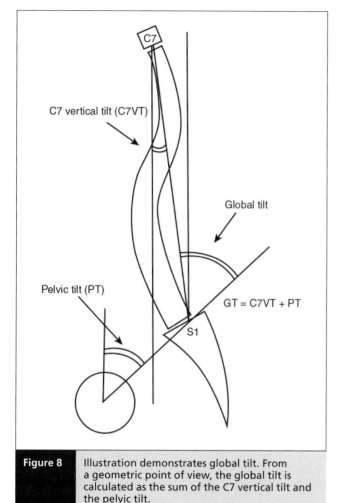

Figure 8 Illustration demonstrates global tilt. From a geometric point of view, the global tilt is calculated as the sum of the C7 vertical tilt and the pelvic tilt.

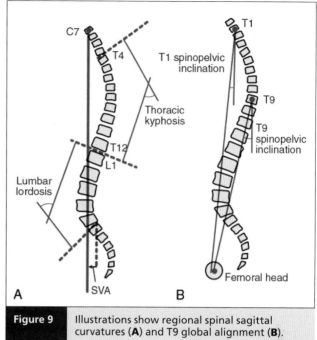

Figure 9 Illustrations show regional spinal sagittal curvatures (**A**) and T9 global alignment (**B**).

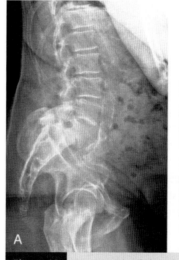
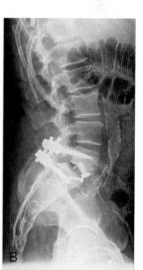

Figure 10 Preoperative (**A**) and postoperative (**B**) lateral radiographs show spondylolisthesis, a local sagittal abnormality, treated with an anterior-posterior spinal fusion.

apex. CT can be helpful for detailing the osseous anatomy and degenerative segmental bridging. The initial treatment almost always is nonsurgical and includes exercise, aerobic conditioning, and the judicious use of NSAIDs. Prolonged narcotic use or bracing is unlikely to be beneficial.[12,42]

Surgery can be considered after unsuccessful nonsurgical treatment, particularly if there is progression of the kyphosis. The surgical procedure exposes the patient to substantial blood loss, neurologic risk, fluid shifts, metabolic and systemic organ stress, and pain. As before any corrective surgery for a major sagittal plane deformity, the surgeon must ascertain the patient's general medical condition and risk factors. The patient should be evaluated for cardiac and pulmonary pathologies. Nutritional status should be assessed and improved if necessary. The importance of a comorbidity such as tobacco smoking, diabetes, or obesity should be assessed.[12,42]

Surgical procedures for a regional kyphosis primarily are posterior. An adjunctive anterior procedure can be considered for spinal release, decompression of neural elements, and resection of vertebral bodies.[12,43-45] The goal is to return the spine to normal measurements (45° to 50°). A truly rigid deformity may require anterior intervertebral releases, corpectomies, or multiple posterior osteotomies. For moderate, relatively flexible curves, osteotomy techniques such as aggressive facetectomy and posterior column removal (the Ponte procedure) increasingly are favored.[43] Very large, rigid kyphotic deformities may require aggressive techniques such as pedicle subtraction

5: Spine Deformity

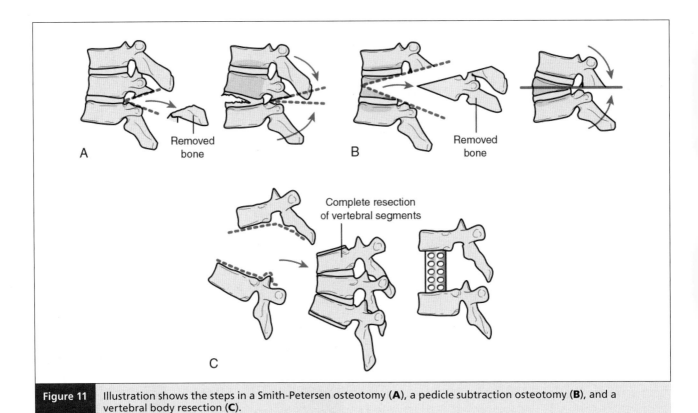

Figure 11 Illustration shows the steps in a Smith-Petersen osteotomy (**A**), a pedicle subtraction osteotomy (**B**), and a vertebral body resection (**C**).

osteotomy or vertebral resection. A posterior approach permits access for anterior and/or posterior column resection, fusions, and fixation options including the use of hooks, screws, wires, and bands. A relatively flexible kyphosis may be appropriately realigned using a combination of anesthesia, positioning, and gentle cantilever reduction with posterior instrumentation.

Overcorrection of a regional deformity such as Scheuermann kyphosis should be avoided because it can lead to the development of painful and deforming junctional kyphosis above or below the correction. In addition, the surgeon must be mindful of the patient's overall health and age.

Global Sagittal Abnormalities

In a patient with global sagittal malalignment, the head and neck lie anterior to the sacrum and pelvis. The result is pain, dysfunction, and deformity. Patients with a flexible global sagittal abnormality, such as a patient who can lie flat on the examining table, may respond to nonsurgical care. Nonsurgical modalities, such as intensive physical therapy, are less likely to be successful in patients with a rigid deformity than in those with a flexible deformity. A global spine deformity can be treated with a variety

of surgical approaches depending on the etiology and structural characteristics of the deformity; the surgeon's expertise; and the patient's expectations, health, age, bone quality, comorbidities, and surgical history. To achieve the best outcome for the patient, surgical decision making also should take into account the experience of hospital teams (including operating room, nursing, and intensive care unit staff) and available facilities. Surgical reconstruction is intended to achieve relatively pain-free positioning of the head and neck over the pelvis, limited external immobilization, and, if at all possible, maintenance of motion segments.

As the spine ages, stiffness and thoracic kyphosis increase and LL decreases. As a result, the gravity line gradually shifts forward.[8,27] The patient's deformity can be classified based on its flexibility as totally flexible and correctable, partially correctable through some mobile segments, or totally inflexible with no correctability (a fixed deformity).[46] Because the origin of a flexible deformity typically is at the disk level, reconstruction is done at the disk level in the anterior column using an anterior, lateral, or posterior approach, typically with bone graft or interbody cages. Smith-Petersen–type osteotomies (SPOs) at multiple levels are used to obtain a posteriorly based correction (**Figure 11, A**). An SPO is a wedge-shaped osteotomy of the posterior arch with ligamentum flavum excision. A formal wedge (Ponte) osteotomy also removes the facet joints. These osteotomies typically measure approximately 1 cm. Correction is obtained by closing the gap with instrumentation.[3,47] This technique relies on anterior disk flexibility and may achieve correction of up to 10° to 15° per level. The total angular correction depends on the number of levels treated. Many authors recommend secondary anterior interbody support, especially if the disks are relatively flexible.[3,12,47]

A vertebral resection is necessary to correct a fixed deformity. A pedicle subtraction osteotomy (PSO), in which a wedge of bone is removed from both the anterior and posterior columns, is used to correct a rigid global deformity, as in ankylosing spondylitis[23,47-53] (**Figure 11, B**). Stabilizing screws with connecting rods bridge the resection area to provide stability and resist inadvertent translation. The entire posterior arch and the pedicles are then removed down to the vertebral body. The vertebral body is decancellated in a wedge fashion, with the posterior wall preserved until the end of the procedure. The apex of the wedge is anterior within the vertebral body; care is taken not to resect the anterior wall itself so it will remain as a fulcrum when the wedge is closed. The size of the removed wedge to some extent depends on the necessary angular correction but typically runs from a foraminal space to the caudal space below. The ultimate maneuver involves carefully resecting the posterior wall and imploding it anteriorly into the resected area. The surgical table is extended, and sequential tightening and compression of the screw-rod construct commences. Many surgeons use a four-rod construct across the osteotomy to decrease the risk of rod failure; others prefer to use two lordotic contoured rods to control the amount of correction.

Most PSOs achieve a 30° to 45° local correction depending on the size of the wedge.[3,23,50] The greatest global correction of the C7 plumb line measurement is achieved if the osteotomy is done at a relatively caudal level (**Figure 12**). PSOs were reported to be most effective in improving PT, sacral slope, and lordosis in patients whose PI was small or moderate (less than 60°).[23]

A posterior-based vertebral body resection, which involves a resection of the posterior column and one or more vertebral bodies, is useful for treating the most severe and rigid deformities.[3,48] This procedure may be required if a rigid coronal deformity also is to be treated. An interbody cage or another form of strut graft can be used to support the defect created by the vertebral body resection and avoid buckling of the neural elements as the spinal column is shortened (**Figure 11, C**).

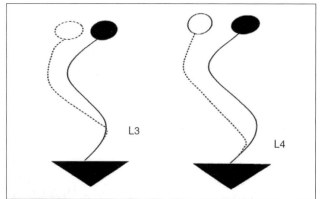

| Figure 12 | Schematic diagram showing the sagittal plumb line before (dashed lines, white circles) and after (solid lines, black circles) a posterior-based osteotomy at L3 (**A**) or L4 (**B**). (Reproduced with permission from Roussouly P, Nnadi C: Sagittal plane deformity: An overview of interpretation and management. *Eur Spine J* 2010;19[11]:1824-1836.) |

Complications

The rate of complications after surgery for correction of adult sagittal plane deformity ranges from 20% to more than 50%.[3,54-57] In 2011, the Scoliosis Research Society Morbidity and Mortality Report cited a 29.4% incidence of complications after correction of fixed thoracolumbar sagittal plane deformities.[54] The most common complications were durotomy (6%), wound infection (3.8%), new neurologic deficit (3.6%), and instrumentation failure (1.7%). The complication rate depended on the procedure and ranged from 17% after surgery without osteotomy to more than 60% after a posterior-based vertebral body resection. Bleeding in a PSO is substantially greater than in an SPO and principally is from the bony resection through the cancellous vertebral body. Leaving the osteotomy until the end of the procedure helps limit blood loss. Closure of the osteotomy itself also diminishes the active bleeding.

The risk of neurologic complications increases with the invasiveness of the corrective procedure.[46,56,58] A 7.8% rate of permanent nerve injury has been reported.[56] A 10-year study of PSOs reported an 11% rate of postoperative neurologic deficits, with permanent deficits in almost 3% of patients.[59]

Summary

The study of normal spine alignment, along with in-depth analysis of specific spinopelvic parameters, has led to an improved understanding of the importance of maintaining sagittal balance or returning the head and neck to its most economical position over the lumbosacral junction. Surgical planning should include a detailed clinical and radiographic analysis so that the procedure can be designed to restore the original delicate balance among all components of the spinal column.

Key Study Points

- PI is a measurement of the position of the sacrum within the pelvis and its relationship to the femoral heads. PI has become a vitally important measurement for treating adult spine conditions.

- PI, which does not significantly change after skeletal maturity, has a direct influence on the amount of LL necessary to maintain adequate sagittal balance.

- Sagittal plane abnormalities are categorized as local, as in spondylolisthesis; regional, as in Scheuermann kyphosis of the thoracic spine; or global, as in flatback deformity or ankylosing spondylitis.

- In a global sagittal imbalance, the degree of imbalance, the flexibility of the spine, and the biology of the bone are considered in determining whether osteotomies are needed for correction and, if so, the number and type required.

Annotated References

1. Duval-Beaupère G, Schmidt C, Cosson P: A barycentremetric study of the sagittal shape of spine and pelvis: The conditions required for an economic standing position. *Ann Biomed Eng* 1992;20(4):451-462.

2. Dubousset J: Three-dimensional analysis of the scoliotic deformity, in Weinstein SL, ed: *The Pediatric Spine: Principles and Practice* .New York, NY, Raven Press, 1994, pp 479-496.

3. Roussouly P, Nnadi C: Sagittal plane deformity: An overview of interpretation and management. *Eur Spine J* 2010;19(11):1824-1836.

4. Araújo F, Lucas R, Alegrete N, Azevedo A, Barros H: Sagittal standing posture, back pain, and quality of life among adults from the general population: A sex-specific association. *Spine (Phila Pa 1976)* 2014;39(13):E782-E794.

   The authors attempt to determine the relationship of standing sagittal posture and clinical symptoms of back pain and quality-of-life measures. In males, no consistent association was found between sagittal standing posture and quality-of-life measures. In females, a possible association was found between increased PI and sacral slope as a cause of back pain. Level of evidence: III.

5. Djurasovic M, Glassman SD: Correlation of radiographic and clinical findings in spinal deformities. *Neurosurg Clin N Am* 2007;18(2):223-227.

6. Glassman SD, Bridwell K, Dimar JR, Horton W, Berven S, Schwab F: The impact of positive sagittal balance in adult spinal deformity. *Spine (Phila Pa 1976)* 2005;30(18):2024-2029.

7. Bernhardt M, Bridwell KH: Segmental analysis of the sagittal plane alignment of the normal thoracic and lumbar spines and thoracolumbar junction. *Spine (Phila Pa 1976)* 1989;14(7):717-721.

8. Iyer S, Lenke LG, Nemani VM, et al: Variations in sagittal alignment parameters based on age: A prospective study of asymptomatic volunteers using full-body radiographs. *Spine (Phila Pa 1976)* 2016;41(23):1826-1836.

   Radiographic imaging from the occiput to the toes was performed in 115 asymptomatic volunteers. The following normative values were reported: T1-pelvis angle (r = 0.44, $P < 0.001$), knee flexion angle (r = 0.42, $P < 0.001$), global sagittal angle (r = 0.56, $P < 0.001$), and C7 SVA (r = 0.46, $P < 0.001$); all of these values increased with age. LL (r = 0.212, $P = 0.039$) decreased with age. Level of evidence: IV.

9. Roussouly P, Gollogly S, Berthonnaud E, Dimnet J: Classification of the normal variation in the sagittal alignment of the human lumbar spine and pelvis in the standing position. *Spine (Phila Pa 1976)* 2005;30(3):346-353.

10. Voutsinas SA, MacEwen GD: Sagittal profiles of the spine. *Clin Orthop Relat Res* 1986;210:235-242.

11. Vedantam R, Lenke LG, Keeney JA, Bridwell KH: Comparison of standing sagittal spinal alignment in asymptomatic adolescents and adults. *Spine (Phila Pa 1976)* 1998;23(2):211-215.

12. Macagno AE, O'Brien MF: Thoracic and thoracolumbar kyphosis in adults. *Spine (Phila Pa 1976)* 2006;31(19suppl):S161-S170.

13. Schwab F, Lafage V, Boyce R, Skalli W, Farcy JP: Gravity line analysis in adult volunteers: Age-related correlation with spinal parameters, pelvic parameters, and foot position. *Spine (Phila Pa 1976)* 2006;31(25):E959-E967.

14. Legaye J, Duval-Beaupère G, Hecquet J, Marty C: Pelvic incidence: A fundamental pelvic parameter for three-dimensional regulation of spinal sagittal curves. *Eur Spine J* 1998;7(2):99-103.

15. Boulay C, Tardieu C, Hecquet J, et al: Sagittal alignment of spine and pelvis regulated by pelvic incidence: Standard values and prediction of lordosis. *Eur Spine J* 2006;15(4):415-422.

16. Blondel B, Schwab F, Ungar B, et al: Impact of magnitude and percentage of global sagittal plane correction on

health-related quality of life at 2-years follow-up. *Neuro-surgery* 2012;71(2):341-348, discussion 348.

This multicenter study retrospectively analyzed 76 patients with adult spinal deformity (all with an SVA >80 mm) to determine the minimal clinically important difference needed to affect health-related quality of life. It was found that the likelihood of reaching a minimal clinically important difference was significantly improved for patients with a correction of greater than 120 mm but not for patients with corrections of 60 mm to 120 mm. A significantly greater likelihood of reaching minimal clinically important difference thresholds was observed for corrections greater than 66% of the patient's preoperative SVA. Level of evidence: III.

17. Mac-Thiong JM, Transfeldt EE, Mehbod AA, et al: Can C7 plumbline and gravity line predict health related quality of life in adult scoliosis? *Spine (Phila Pa 1976)* 2009;34(15):E519-E527.

18. Schwab F, Patel A, Ungar B, Farcy JP, Lafage V: Adult spinal deformity-postoperative standing imbalance: How much can you tolerate? An overview of key parameters in assessing alignment and planning corrective surgery. *Spine (Phila Pa 1976)* 2010;35(25):2224-2231.

19. Le Huec JC, Aunoble S, Philippe L, Nicolas P: Pelvic parameters: Origin and significance. *Eur Spine J* 2011;20(suppl 5):564-571.

The position of the lumbar spine is affected by the PT and sacral slope. Consequently, the pelvic parameters affect the entire underlying sagittal spinal profile. Global spinal balance involves harmonization of this lordosis (and thoracic kyphosis), taking into account these pelvic parameters.

20. Yang C, Yang M, Wei X, et al: Lumbar lordosis minus thoracic kyphosis: A novel regional predictor for sagittal balance in elderly populations. *Spine (Phila Pa 1976)* 2016;41(5):399-403.

An evaluation of standing radiographs of 129 elderly patients revealed that a value greater than 0° when thoracic kyphosis is subtracted from LL highly correlates with adequate sagittal alignment. Level of evidence: IV.

21. Lafage V, Schwab F, Vira S, Patel A, Ungar B, Farcy JP: Spino-pelvic parameters after surgery can be predicted: A preliminary formula and validation of standing alignment. *Spine (Phila Pa 1976)* 2011;36(13):1037-1045.

Full-length standing radiographs of 219 adult patients with spinal deformity were used to determine PT and global sagittal balance (measured by the SVA). Prediction models were then applied on a second group of patients to estimate postoperative radiographic parameters after PSO. This led to a predictive formula for postoperative sagittal alignment. Level of evidence: IV.

22. Legaye J, Duval-Beaupère G: Sagittal plane alignment of the spine and gravity: A radiological and clinical evaluation. *Acta Orthop Belg* 2005;71(2):213-220.

23. Cogniet A, Aunoble S, Rigal J, Demezon H, Sadikki R, Le Huec JC: Clinical and radiological outcomes of lumbar posterior subtraction osteotomies are correlated to pelvic incidence and FBI index: Prospective series of 63 cases. *Eur Spine J* 2016;25(8):2657-2667.

A prospective study of 63 patients who underwent spinal deformity correction with PSO showed the mean correction obtained after PSO was 31.7° ± 8.4°; hence, a global improvement in LL of 22° was seen. Subgroup analysis demonstrated greater improvement in PT, sacral slope, and spinal parameters of patients with a small or moderate PI. Level of evidence: III.

24. Obeid I, Boissière L, Yilgor C, et al; European Spine Study Group, ESSG: Global tilt: A single parameter incorporating spinal and pelvic sagittal parameters and least affected by patient positioning. *Eur Spine J* 2016;25(11):3644-3649.

A cohort of 22 patients with sagittal spinal malalignment was evaluated with standing lateral radiography. PT, SVA, and global tilt were measured in two positions—hands on the shoulders or attempting to lean backward. The authors concluded that global tilt appeared to be less affected by the patient's position compared with SVA or PT. Level of evidence: IV.

25. Rigoard P, Blond S, David R, Mertens P: Pathophysiological characterisation of back pain generators in failed back surgery syndrome: Part B. *Neurochirurgie* 2015;61(suppl 1):S35-S44.

Results of a search of the literature between 1930 and 2013 suggest that nociceptive fibers innervating any anatomic structure can play a role in the pathogenesis of the low back pain component of failed back surgery syndrome. The main spinal pain generators include muscle spasm, the facet joints, the disk complex, and sagittal imbalance. These pain generators should be carefully reviewed before making a diagnosis of failed back surgery syndrome.

26. Bridwell K: Spine osteotomy and resection, in DeWald RL, Arlet V, Carl AL, O'Brien MF, eds: *Spinal Deformities: The Comprehensive Text*. New York, NY, Thieme Medical Publishers, 2003, pp 551-561.

27. Hammerberg EM, Wood KB: Sagittal profile of the elderly. *J Spinal Disord Tech* 2003;16(1):44-50.

28. Liu N, Wood KB, Schwab JH, et al: Utility of flexion-extension radiographs in lumbar spondylolisthesis: A prospective study. *Spine (Phila Pa 1976)* 2015;40(16):E929-E935.

A comparison of flexion and extension mobility of a listhetic segment of the lumbar spine demonstrated more motion when using supine MRI and upright plain radiography versus upright flexion-extension lateral radiography. Level of evidence: II.

29. Glassman SD, Carreon LY, Shaffrey CI, et al: The costs and benefits of nonoperative management for adult scoliosis. *Spine (Phila Pa 1976)* 2010;35(5):578-582.

30. Bridwell KH, Glassman S, Horton W, et al: Does treatment (nonoperative and operative) improve the two-year quality

5: Spine Deformity

of life in patients with adult symptomatic lumbar scoliosis: A prospective multicenter evidence-based medicine study. *Spine (Phila Pa 1976)* 2009;34(20):2171-2178.

31. Curfs I, Grimm B, van der Linde M, Willems P, van Hemert W: Radiological prediction of posttraumatic kyphosis after thoracolumbar fracture. *Open Orthop J* 2016;10:135-142.

    A retrospective analysis of thoracolumbar fractures seen between 2004 and 2011 revealed that patients with AO-type A3 fractures (burst) appear to be at greatest risk for posttraumatic kyphosis. Localization at T12-L1 and age older than 50 years also seem to be risk factors for posttraumatic kyphosis. Level of evidence: IV.

32. Pizones J, Zúñiga L, Sánchez-Mariscal F, Alvarez P, Gómez-Rice A, Izquierdo E: MRI study of post-traumatic incompetence of posterior ligamentous complex: Importance of the supraspinous ligament. Prospective study of 74 traumatic fractures. *Eur Spine J* 2012;21(11):2222-2231.

    A prospective study of 74 acute vertebral fractures evaluated using radiography and MRI found that although the presence of interspinous ligament edema on magnetic resonance images correlated surgically with intact ligaments or laxity, interspinous ligament edema is not enough to define posterior tension band incompetence without supraspinous ligament rupture. Level of evidence: IV.

33. Schoenfeld AJ, Wood KB, Fisher CF, et al: Posttraumatic kyphosis: Current state of diagnosis and treatment. Results of a multinational survey of spine trauma surgeons. *J Spinal Disord Tech* 2010;23(7):e1-e8.

34. Malcolm BW, Bradford DS, Winter RB, Chou SN: Post-traumatic kyphosis: A review of forty-eight surgically treated patients. *J Bone Joint Surg Am* 1981;63(6):891-899.

35. Wang SJ, Han YC, Liu XM, et al: Fusion techniques for adult isthmic spondylolisthesis: A systematic review. *Arch Orthop Trauma Surg* 2014;134(6):777-784.

    This systematic review examined the best treatment for adult isthmic spondylolisthesis. Compared with other fusion techniques, transforaminal lumbar interbody fusion had fewer complications, anterior lumbar interbody fusion achieved better sagittal alignment, and circumferential fusion achieved better fusion rates. However, it is difficult to make recommendations regarding the best treatment because of methodologic variances in the evaluated studies.

36. Kwon BK, Hilibrand AS, Malloy K, et al: A critical analysis of the literature regarding surgical approach and outcome for adult low-grade isthmic spondylolisthesis. *J Spinal Disord Tech* 2005;(18suppl):S30-S40.

37. Boachie-Adjei O, Do T, Rawlins BA: Partial lumbosacral kyphosis reduction, decompression, and posterior lumbosacral transfixation in high-grade isthmic spondylolisthesis: Clinical and radiographic results in six patients. *Spine (Phila Pa 1976)* 2002;27(6):E161-E168.

38. Boos N, Marchesi D, Zuber K, Aebi M: Treatment of severe spondylolisthesis by reduction and pedicular fixation: A 4-6-year follow-up study. *Spine (Phila Pa 1976)* 1993;18(12):1655-1661.

39. Hu SS, Bradford DS, Transfeldt EE, Cohen M: Reduction of high-grade spondylolisthesis using Edwards instrumentation. *Spine (Phila Pa 1976)* 1996;21(3):367-371.

40. Bradford DS, Boachie-Adjei O: Treatment of severe spondylolisthesis by anterior and posterior reduction and stabilization: A long-term follow-up study. *J Bone Joint Surg Am* 1990;72(7):1060-1066.

41. Petraco DM, Spivak JM, Cappadona JG, Kummer FJ, Neuwirth MG: An anatomic evaluation of L5 nerve stretch in spondylolisthesis reduction. *Spine (Phila Pa 1976)* 1996;21(10):1133-1138, discussion 1139.

42. Hu SS, Berven SH: Preparing the adult deformity patient for spinal surgery. *Spine (Phila Pa 1976)* 2006;31(19suppl):S126-S131.

43. Geck MJ, Macagno A, Ponte A, Shufflebarger HL: The Ponte procedure: Posterior only treatment of Scheuermann's kyphosis using segmental posterior shortening and pedicle screw instrumentation. *J Spinal Disord Tech* 2007;20(8):586-593.

44. Lowe TG: Scheuermann's kyphosis. *Neurosurg Clin N Am* 2007;18(2):305-315.

45. Cho WJ, Kang CN, Park YS, Kim HJ, Cho JL: Surgical correction of fixed kyphosis. *Asian Spine J* 2007;1(1):12-18.

46. Bridwell KH: Decision making regarding Smith-Petersen vs. pedicle subtraction osteotomy vs. vertebral column resection for spinal deformity. *Spine (Phila Pa 1976)* 2006;31(19suppl):S171-S178.

47. Cho KJ, Bridwell KH, Lenke LG, Berra A, Baldus C: Comparison of Smith-Petersen versus pedicle subtraction osteotomy for the correction of fixed sagittal imbalance. *Spine (Phila Pa 1976)* 2005;30(18):2030-2037, discussion 2038.

48. Chen Z, Zeng Y, Li W, Guo Z, Qi Q, Sun C: Apical segmental resection osteotomy with dual axial rotation corrective technique for severe focal kyphosis of the thoracolumbar spine. *J Neurosurg Spine* 2011;14(1):106-113.

    The authors report on their experiences with 23 patients with severe apical kyphotic spinal deformities treated with apical segmental resection osteotomy with dual axial rotation correction and instrumented anterior column reconstruction and fusion. Although a high rate of success and neurologic improvement were reported, transient neurologic deficits occurred. Level of evidence: IV.

49. Berven SH, Deviren V, Smith JA, Emami A, Hu SS, Bradford DS: Management of fixed sagittal plane deformity: Results of the transpedicular wedge resection osteotomy. *Spine (Phila Pa 1976)* 2001;26(18):2036-2043.

5: Spine Deformity

50. Bridwell KH, Lewis SJ, Lenke LG, Baldus C, Blanke K: Pedicle subtraction osteotomy for the treatment of fixed sagittal imbalance. *J Bone Joint Surg Am* 2003;85(3):454-463.

51. Chen IH, Chien JT, Yu TC: Transpedicular wedge osteotomy for correction of thoracolumbar kyphosis in ankylosing spondylitis: Experience with 78 patients. *Spine (Phila Pa 1976)* 2001;26(16):E354-E360.

52. Danisa OA, Turner D, Richardson WJ: Surgical correction of lumbar kyphotic deformity: Posterior reduction "eggshell" osteotomy. *J Neurosurg* 2000;92(1suppl):50-56.

53. McMaster MJ: A technique for lumbar spinal osteotomy in ankylosing spondylitis. *J Bone Joint Surg Br* 1985;67(2):204-210.

54. Smith JS, Sansur CA, Donaldson WF III, et al: Short-term morbidity and mortality associated with correction of thoracolumbar fixed sagittal plane deformity: A report from the Scoliosis Research Society Morbidity and Mortality Committee. *Spine (Phila Pa 1976)* 2011;36(12):958-964.

    A review of the Scoliosis Research Society database from 2004 to 2007 found 170 complications in 132 patients who underwent correction for thoracolumbar fixed sagittal plane deformity. Three deaths occurred (0.5%). The most common complications were durotomy (5.9%), wound infection (3.8%), and new neurologic deficit (3.8%). Cases involving an osteotomy had a higher complication rate (34.8%) than cases not involving an osteotomy (17.0%, $P < 0.001$).

55. Kim KT, Suk KS, Cho YJ, Hong GP, Park BJ: Clinical outcome results of pedicle subtraction osteotomy in ankylosing spondylitis with kyphotic deformity. *Spine (Phila Pa 1976)* 2002;27(6):612-618.

56. Willems KF, Slot GH, Anderson PG, Pavlov PW, de Kleuver M: Spinal osteotomy in patients with ankylosing spondylitis: Complications during first postoperative year. *Spine (Phila Pa 1976)* 2005;30(1):101-107.

57. Van Royen BJ, De Gast A, Smit TH: Deformity planning for sagittal plane corrective osteotomies of the spine in ankylosing spondylitis. *Eur Spine J* 2000;9(6):492-498.

58. Bridwell KH, Lewis SJ, Edwards C, et al: Complications and outcomes of pedicle subtraction osteotomies for fixed sagittal imbalance. *Spine (Phila Pa 1976)* 2003;28(18):2093-2101.

59. Buchowski JM, Bridwell KH, Lenke LG, et al: Neurologic complications of lumbar pedicle subtraction osteotomy: A 10-year assessment. *Spine (Phila Pa 1976)* 2007;32(20):2245-2252.

5: Spine Deformity

Chapter 26

Spondylolisthesis in Children and Young Adults

Stefan Parent, MD, PhD   Hubert Labelle, MD   Jean-Marc Mac-Thiong, MD, PhD

Abstract

Spondylolisthesis in children and adults has been the topic of intense research during the past two decades in an attempt to gain a better understanding of the effects of sacropelvic morphology on pelvic balance and global sagittal balance. This new understanding of sagittal balance, both in normal and affected individuals, has led to the development of a comprehensive classification system that can help guide treatment of patients with low- and high-grade spondylolisthesis.

Keywords: adolescents; children; sagittal balance; spondylolisthesis; spondylolysis

Dr. Parent or an immediate family member has received royalties from EOS Imaging; serves as a paid consultant to AO Spine, DePuy, EOS Imaging, and Medtronic; has stock or stock options held in Spinologics; has received research or institutional support from DePuy, EOS Imaging, the Orthopaedic Research and Education Foundation, the Rick Hansen Institute, and the Setting Scoliosis Straight Foundation. Dr. Labelle or an immediate family member is a member of a speakers' bureau or has made paid presentations on behalf of DePuy; has stock or stock options held in Spinologics; and serves as a board member, owner, officer, or committee member of the Scoliosis Research Society. Dr. Mac-Thiong or an immediate family member has stock or stock options held in Spinologics; has received research or institutional support from Medtronic; and has received nonincome support (such as equipment or services), commercially derived honoraria, or other non–research-related funding (such as paid travel) from Medtronic.

Introduction

Spondylolysis is a defect in the pars articularis of a vertebra. It can occur independently or in association with spondylolisthesis and very often occurs at the L5-S1 level. Spondylolisthesis is the forward displacement of one vertebra with respect to the adjacent caudal vertebra. Spondyloptosis is defined as a 100% translation of one vertebra over the next caudal vertebra.

Epidemiology

Isthmic spondylolisthesis in children occurs principally at L5-S1 (87%), but also has been reported at L4-L5 (10%) and L3-L4 (3%).[1] A defect in the pars interarticularis has never been reported in a newborn. In a prospective study of 500 children, a prevalence of spondylolysis of 4.4% by age 6 years, 5.2% by age 12 years, 5.6% by age 14 years, and 6% in adulthood was reported.[2] In the children with bilateral spondylolysis, 68% of the children had spondylolisthesis by age 6 years and 74% had the condition by age 18 years. A 45-year follow-up study of 30 participants in whom spondylolysis had been diagnosed during childhood showed that spondylolisthesis did not develop in 8 of the study participants with unilateral defects, whereas 22 of the participants with bilateral spondylolysis had spondylolisthesis.[3] In these study participants, a slowing of slip progression occurred with each decade up to the age of 50 years.

Spondylolysis is highly prevalent in some Native American populations.[4] An increased prevalence of spondylolysis and spondylolisthesis also has been reported in athletes in certain sports such as gymnastics;[5] however, a more recent study did not observe this association between increased occurrence and participation in gymnastics.[6]

5: Spine Deformity

Etiology

The exact etiology of spondylolysis and spondylolisthesis is unknown, but it is most likely multifactorial. Various hereditary, traumatic, biomechanical, growth, and morphologic factors have been proposed to play a role.

Hereditary Predisposition

It is believed that spondylolisthesis is related to an autosomal dominant genetic predisposition with incomplete penetrance.[7,8] An increased prevalence of spondylolisthesis has been reported in members of the same family, ranging from 19% to 69% in first-degree relatives.[2,7] In addition, high-grade spondylolisthesis has been reported in identical twins.[9]

Traumatic and Biomechanical Factors

Repetitive microtrauma has been suggested as a cause for spondylolisthesis via the creation of a stress fracture of the pars interarticularis.[10] The pars interarticularis (the weakest region of the posterior neural arch) is subjected to high shear, compressive, and tensile loads during flexion and extension movements.[11] Athletes who participate in sports that involve recurrent alternating flexion-extension spinal loading have a higher risk for the development of spondylolysis and spondylolisthesis. The prevalence of spondylolisthesis is increased in this population.[5]

Under normal conditions, the facet joints at L5-S1 resist most of the shear force, whereas most of the compression force passes through the disks. The facet joints are not functional in patients with spondylolysis; thus, most of the shear stresses at L5-S1 are transferred to the disk, which predisposes the patient to disk degeneration and subsequent spondylolisthesis. In addition, forward displacement of the body of L5 distracts the pars defect because the posterior elements of L5 stay strongly attached to the posterior ligaments and erector spinae muscles. As spondylolisthesis progresses, a further decrease in disk stiffness occurs, and stresses increase across the lumbosacral junction.[12] Varying degrees of facet, laminar, and end plate dysplasia are common in spondylolisthesis and disturb the normal posterior bony hook/catch at the lumbosacral junction.[2,13,14] In some cases of spondylolisthesis, the initially present pars defect heals with elongation of the posterior elements.[11]

Morphology and Spinopelvic Balance

The alignment of the lumbar spine and, subsequently, the mechanical stresses at the lumbosacral junction are altered by the morphology of the sacrum and pelvis. Sagittal plane sacropelvic morphology and orientation are routinely measured using pelvic incidence (PI), sacral slope (SS), and pelvic tilt (PT) (**Figure 1**). The PI, as a morphologic parameter, is specific to each individual and unaffected by changes in body position. The PI represents the arithmetic sum of the PT and SS. PI is described as a line drawn from the center of the femoral heads to the midpoint of the sacral end plate and a line perpendicular to the center of the sacral end plate. SS is defined as the angle subtended by the horizontal plane and the upper sacral end plate. PT is defined as the angle created by a line from the midpoint of the sacral end plate to the center femoral heads and a vertical plumb line.

In children and adolescents without spondylolisthesis, sacropelvic morphology regulates the sacropelvic orientation, which in turn greatly affects the shape and orientation of the spine, especially lumbar lordosis.[15,16] Sacropelvic morphology is different in healthy control subjects than in patients with spondylolisthesis.[17] The PI also increases in direct linear proportion to the severity of the spondylolisthesis.[17] With the increasing severity of the spondylolisthesis, the close relationship between sacropelvic and lumbar geometry typical of normal healthy individuals is disturbed.[16]

In control subjects with abnormal sacropelvic morphology, there appears to be a predisposition to altered mechanical stresses in the lumbar spine and lumbosacral junction. These individuals also seem to be at a higher risk for the development of spondylolysis and spondylolisthesis. The shear stress on the L5-S1 disk tends to be increased by a high PI associated with a high SS. This induces increased loading on the L5 pars articularis.[18] A low PI can lead to repetitive impingement of the pars interarticularis of L5 by the posterior facets of L4 and S1 during extension movements.[18]

Lumbosacral alignment and global sagittal alignment may be altered in the presence of abnormal sacropelvic balance and progressive spondylolisthesis. In addition to the translational slip of L5 on top of S1, an angular deformity appearing as lumbosacral kyphosis can occur. Forward global spinal balance (as measured by a plumb line from C7 to the sacrum) and forward spinopelvic balance (as measured by a plumb line from C7 to the hip axis) also can be observed, particularly in patients with high-grade spondylolisthesis.[16] In response to progressively abnormal sacropelvic, lumbosacral, and global balance, the center of gravity of the torso tends to be displaced anteriorly. This anterior displacement causes forward displacement of the anterior part of L5, whereas the posterior part of L5 stays attached to the posterior soft tissues and the L5-S1 facet.

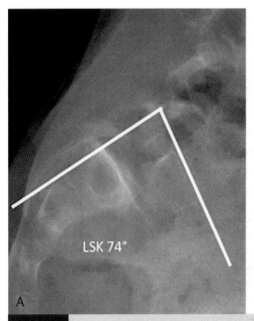
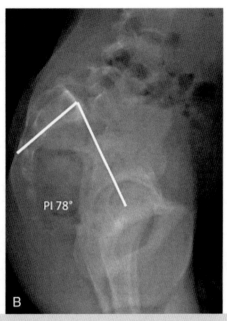
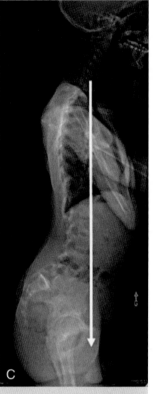

| Figure 1 | Radiographic studies from a patient with high-grade spondylolisthesis. **A,** Lateral radiograph shows characteristic local deformity associated with high-grade spondylolisthesis, including slippage, sacral doming, and lumbosacral kyphosis (LSK). **B,** Increasing pelvic tilt and pelvic incidence (PI) occur as the patient tries to compensate by retroverting the pelvis. **C,** Global sagittal balance can be evaluated with a full-length standing radiograph. Sagittal imbalance and hip flexion occur as the patient tries to compensate globally for the high degree of slip. |

Classification Systems

Meyerding Classification

The Meyerding system is the simplest classification of spondylolisthesis.[19] The classification is based on the percentage of translation. Grade I means a translation of the cranial vertebra of 0 to 25%, grade II a translation of 26% to 50%, grade III a translation of 51% to 75%, and grade IV a translation of 76% to 99%. Grade V was later added to describe ptosis of the cranial vertebra.

Wiltse Classification

The Wiltse classification divides spondylolisthesis into five major types (and several subtypes) based on radiologic findings[20] (**Figure 2**). The five types are as follows: dysplastic, isthmic, degenerative, traumatic, and pathologic. In the dysplastic type, there is a congenital defect of the lumbosacral facet joints and the translation is secondary to an abnormal neural arch. In the isthmic type, the lumbosacral facets are normal but the spondylolisthesis is caused by a defect in the pars interarticularis. The isthmic type can be further subdivided based on whether the pars

fracture is lytic, elongated, or acute. Degenerative spondylolisthesis results from chronic instability and intersegmental degenerative changes. Traumatic spondylolisthesis results from an acute fracture of posterior elements other than the pars interarticularis. The pathologic type is associated with diffuse or local disease that compromises the usual structural integrity that prevents slippage.

Although this classification system is usefulness in classifying spondylolisthesis by defect type, it is not helpful in treatment planning.

Marchetti and Bartolozzi Classification

The Marchetti and Bartolozzi classification is an etiology-based prognosis system of spondylolisthesis that divides types into two broad categories—developmental and acquired.[21] Based on the severity of bony dysplasia in the L5 and S1 vertebrae and the risk of further slippage, developmental spondylolisthesis is categorized into two major types–high dysplastic and low dysplastic. Dysplastic characteristics commonly seen in both variants include dysplastic facet joints; however, high dysplastic spondylolisthesis also is associated with

5: Spine Deformity

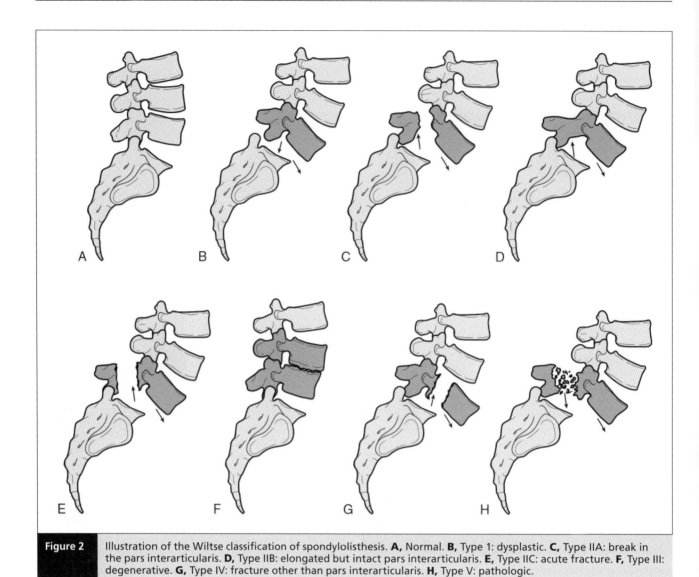

Figure 2 Illustration of the Wiltse classification of spondylolisthesis. **A,** Normal. **B,** Type 1: dysplastic. **C,** Type IIA: break in the pars interarticularis. **D,** Type IIB: elongated but intact pars interarticularis. **E,** Type IIC: acute fracture. **F,** Type III: degenerative. **G,** Type IV: fracture other than pars interarticularis. **H,** Type V: pathologic.

substantial lumbosacral kyphosis, trapezoidal L5 vertebra, hypoplastic transverse processes, and sacral doming with verticalization of the sacrum. Characteristics of low dysplastic spondylolisthesis include preservation of the shape of the L5 vertebral body and sacral dome, a relatively normal lumbosacral profile, and preservation of a flat SI upper end plate.

Acquired spondylolisthesis occurs secondary to trauma, surgery, a pathologic disease, or a degenerative process. Traumatic spondylolisthesis can result from an acute or a stress fracture. A stress fracture typically occurs in young athletes and is distinct from isthmic dysplastic spondylolisthesis.

Sagittal Spinopelvic Classification

The aforementioned classification systems are of little help in determining surgical treatment. In 2011, the Spinal Deformity Study Group (SDSG) developed a classification system that incorporated sagittal spinopelvic balance and recognized six types of spondylolisthesis[22] (**Figure 3**). This classification is based on the following four important characteristics that can be assessed on weight-bearing sagittal radiographs of the spine and pelvis: (1) low- or high-grade slip, (2) low, normal, or high PI, (3) balanced or unbalanced spinopelvic balance, and (4) low or high lumbosacral kyphosis.

To classify spondylolisthesis, the slip grade is measured on a lateral standing radiograph of the patient's spine to determine if it is low grade (Meyerding grades 0, 1, and 2 or slip <50%) or high grade (grades 3, 4, and spondyloptosis or slip ≥50%). The sagittal balance is then measured by determining the sacropelvic and spinopelvic alignment, using measurements of PI, SS, PT, and the C7 plumb line.

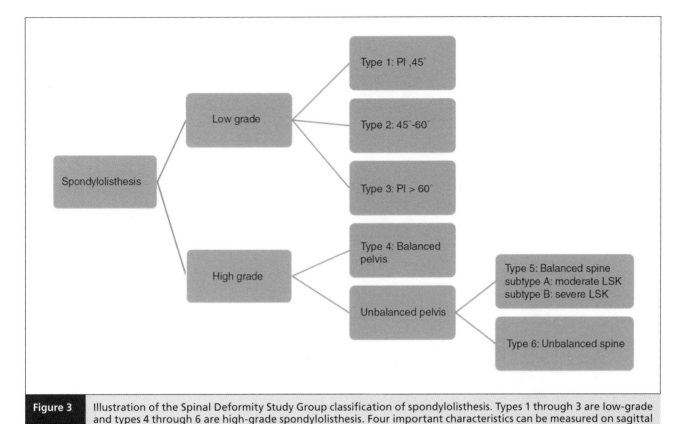

Figure 3 Illustration of the Spinal Deformity Study Group classification of spondylolisthesis. Types 1 through 3 are low-grade and types 4 through 6 are high-grade spondylolisthesis. Four important characteristics can be measured on sagittal radiographs— slip, pelvic incidence (PI), spinopelvic balance, and lumbosacral kyphosis (LSK).

There are three types of low-grade spondylolisthesis. Type 1, the nutcracker type, has a low PI (<45°) and low SS. Type 2 has a normal PI (between 45° and 60°). Type 3, the shear type, has a high PI (>60°) and a high SS.

There also are three types of high-grade spondylolisthesis. First, each patient is classified as having a balanced or an unbalanced sacropelvic relationship using PT and SS values or using a nomogram from a 2007 study that found that PT and SS values were similar in control subjects, but patients with an unbalanced pelvis had sagittal spinal alignment that differed from that of the group with a balanced plevis.[23] When the SS is greater than the PT or when the pelvis remains within normal values for asymptomatic patients, the spine is classified as balanced, whereas when the SS is less than the PT or when the SS and PT are below normal values for asymptomatic patients, the spine is classified as unbalanced (**Figure 4**). Spinopelvic balance is then determined using the C7 plumb line. If this line falls over or behind the femoral heads, the spine is balanced, whereas if the line lies in front of the femoral heads, the spine is unbalanced. The spine is typically balanced in patients with low-grade spondylolisthesis and in those with high-grade spondylolisthesis if sacropelvic balance exists. The three types of high-grade spondylolisthesis are

as follows: type 4, balanced pelvis; type 5, unbalanced pelvis with a balanced spine, and type 6, unbalanced pelvis with unbalanced spine. In addition, type 5 spondylolisthesis has the following two subtypes: type 5A, which is associated with normal or low lumbosacral kyphosis (as measured by Dubousset lumbosacral angle ≥80°) and type 5B, which is associated with high lumbosacral kyphosis (as measured by Dubousset lumbosacral angle <80°). Spinal balance should be measured principally in patients with high-grade deformities and an unbalanced pelvis (types 5 and 6).

Patients with L5-S1 spondylolisthesis are a heterogeneous group with various postural adaptations that require consideration during assessment and treatment. Abnormal spinopelvic balance changes the biomechanical stresses at the lumbosacral junction and affects the compensation mechanisms used to maintain adequate posture.

Clinical Presentation and Physical Examination

A careful history and physical examination are important for determining the clinical extent of a deformity. Even in the presence of high-grade spondylolisthesis, patients

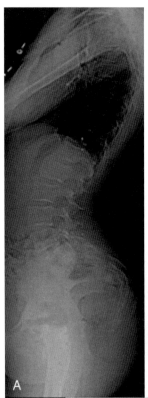
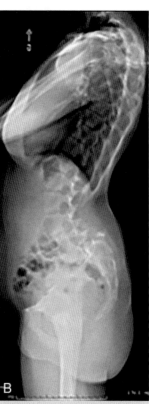

Figure 4   Weight-bearing radiographs show high-grade spondylolisthesis with a balanced pelvis (**A**) and an unbalanced pelvis (**B**).

who do not exhibit substantial symptoms can be treated nonsurgically.

Patients with low-grade spondylolisthesis usually have a normal gait and posture. As the slip progresses, increased lumbar lordosis with a prominent abdomen, heart-shaped buttocks, shortened-appearing trunk, and a rib cage approaching the iliac crests may be noticed. The classic Phalen-Dickson sign occurs when the hips and knees flex to compensate for the forward position of the trunk caused by anterior displacement of the body center of gravity.[24] A palpable step-off may exist at the lumbosacral junction. A scoliotic deformity may be observed and may be secondary to nerve root tension or compression, muscle spasm (antalgic scoliosis), asymmetric slippage in the frontal plane (olisthetic scoliosis), or concomitant idiopathic scoliosis. The extension range of motion is often painful and stiff in symptomatic patients with spondylolisthesis. In some patients, tight hamstrings may be caused by knee flexion or nerve root tension/compression, particularly at L5. The straight-leg raise test and/or the Lasègue sign are usually positive in patients with L5 or S1 nerve root tension. It is essential to perform a careful neurologic examination to find signs of nerve root compression or cauda equina syndrome.

Diagnostic Methods

Plain Radiography

The clinician should obtain lateral and PA plain standing radiographs of the lumbosacral spine when evaluating a patient for spondylolysis and spondylolisthesis. Dysplastic posterior elements or an associated scoliosis are best seen on a PA view. Preoperatively, a Ferguson AP view taken parallel to the L5-S1 disk can improve the visualization of the L5 pedicles, transverse processes, and sacrum to look for dysplastic features. Postoperatively, this view may help in the evaluation of a fusion mass. The lateral radiographic view shows the spondylolisthesis and allows identification of the pars defect and wedging of the L5 vertebral body and sacral dysplasia. Oblique views often allow better detection of unilateral lesions in patients with spondylolysis. Oblique views are ordered if suspicion of lysis cannot be excluded based on lateral radiographs.

In the presence of a spondylolisthesis, long cassette standing PA and lateral radiographs of the spine and pelvis, including the femoral heads, are recommended to evaluate coronal and sagittal trunk balance. Long cassette PA views are used to detect associated scoliosis. Coronal balance is measured by the C7 plumb line with respect to the center of the upper end plate of S1. Sacropelvic morphology and orientation and lumbar lordosis and thoracic kyphosis are assessed with a long cassette lateral view. Overall sagittal balance is assessed using the C7 plumb line with respect to the sacrum or to the hip axis.

Computed Tomography

In children with back pain and no clinical radiographic findings, CT is useful for identifying a pars interarticularis defect. Preoperatively, CT can be used to evaluate the bony architecture of the lumbosacral junction, with particular attention to the size of the transverse processes at L4 and L5 if posterior-only fusion is being considered.

Bone Scans and Single Photon Emission Computed Tomography

To distinguish an acute fracture of the pars interarticularis from a longstanding defect, a bone scan can be helpful. A bone scan can help distinguish between patients with an established defect nonunion and those in whom healing is still progressing and who may benefit from immobilization.[25] Single photon emission computed tomography (SPECT) may be more accurate and sensitive than a planar bone scan[26] because SPECT provides more contrast and sensitivity and improves anatomic localization of skeletal lesions without exposing the patient to additional radiation.

Magnetic Resonance Imaging

MRI is advantageous because the spine can be imaged in any plane without exposure to radiation, and the cauda equina and nerve roots can be assessed in patients with neurologic compromise. Particular attention is given to the evaluation of the L5 nerve roots in the L5-S1 foramen and cauda equina, especially in the presence of an elongated healed pars interarticularis. In patients with high-grade spondylolisthesis, preoperative MRI is recommended for the assessment of neuroanatomic relationships and adjacent disks.

Treatment

Nonsurgical

Asymptomatic individuals with an incidental finding of spondylolysis or low-grade low-dysplastic developmental spondylolisthesis require no treatment or activity restrictions. However, these patients are at greater risk for progression and should be seen at regular intervals (6 months) for radiographic surveillance until skeletal maturity.

In the skeletally immature patient with a slip less than 50%, nonsurgical treatment is recommended. Usually, a good or excellent outcome is achieved and the patient can return to sports participation. Nonsurgical management of acute symptoms includes primarily rest, physical therapy (lumbar and abdominal muscle training), hamstring stretching, mild analgesics, and NSAIDs. Symptomatic patients with focal increased uptake on a bone scan, SPECT, or MRI and, more specifically, patients with an acquired stress fracture, may respond to a trial of bracing and rest to unite the pars defect. Healing occurs infrequently, but is more likely to occur in acute and unilateral defects. Defects associated with spondylolisthesis and L5-S1 defects are less likely to heal. Bracing in neutral lordosis with a thoracolumbosacral orthosis worn full time for 2 to 3 months is recommended and can be tried for pain alleviation in some symptomatic patients with chronic spondylolysis. Unfortunately, no high-level evidence exists on which to base specific recommendations or protocols for nonsurgical treatment.

Surgical

Indications

The goals of surgical treatment of pediatric spondylolisthesis are pain relief, prevention of progression, and improvement in function. Surgical treatment is indicated for slips greater than 50% in growing children and greater than 75% in mature adolescents, in patients with documented slip progression of more than 30%, persistent functional impairment, pain or neurologic symptoms despite appropriate nonsurgical treatment, and progressive postural deformity or gait abnormality. Patients with slip grades of 3 or higher are usually candidates for surgery.

Because some asymptomatic patients may not seek medical treatment when surgical stabilization is needed, it is important to ensure reliable monitoring of these patients.[27] Surgery may be appropriate for an asymptomatic patient if careful monitoring is not possible.

Low-Grade Spondylolisthesis

Low-grade spondylolisthesis usually can be treated with postural reduction and in situ fusion. The need for decompression can be determined based on the patient symptoms and physical examination findings, with additional information obtained from advanced imaging studies (CT and/or MRI). Central canal stenosis and/or foraminal stenosis should be ruled out and, if present, formal or indirect decompression should be performed. In situ fusion can be achieved either through a Wiltse approach (when no formal central decompression is required) or through a central midline approach. Posterolateral fusion with autologous iliac crest bone graft remains the procedure of choice for in situ fusion. If feasible, spinal instrumentation reduces the need for prolonged immobilization; however, the space available for bone grafting is reduced.

High-Grade Spondylolisthesis

The treatment of high-grade spondylolisthesis remains somewhat controversial. Some historical cohort studies reported high complication rates with attempted reduction.[28,29] In addition, excellent clinical outcomes at long-term follow-up of in situ fusion have been recently reported.[30] With advancements in neuromonitoring, surgical instrumentation, and the understanding of normal and pathologic sagittal balance, it is increasingly likely that a subset of patients with high-grade spondylolisthesis can benefit from reduction procedures. A clear distinction must be made between a well-balanced, high-grade spondylolisthesis (type 4) and an unbalanced high-grade spondylolisthesis (types 5 or 6). The balanced type 4 spondylolisthesis can potentially be fused in situ after postural reduction on the operating table with the addition of pedicle and iliac screws. The fusion can be strengthened by a fibular strut graft and/or by intervertebral screws spanning the L5-S1 space from an S1 posteriorly based starting point.

5: Spine Deformity

In patients with a high-grade spondylolisthesis with pelvic retroversion with or without sagittal spinal imbalance (types 5 or 6), normal sagittal balance cannot be restored without correcting the lumbosacral kyphosis and decreasing the PT or retroversion. The most important technical points are that the L5 nerve root should be widely decompressed and well visualized before any attempted reduction, and every effort should be made to correct lumbosacral kyphosis to decrease tension on the nerves and facilitate reduction. A sacral dome osteotomy may be required to help with lumbosacral kyphosis reduction. Complete reduction of the slip is not mandatory. To help reduce the risk of pseudarthrosis, anterior support in the form of an interbody cage is often used with posteriorly based pedicle screws, with or without additional iliac fixation.

Spondyloptosis

Spondyloptosis (complete slippage of L5 over S1) is the most severe type of translational spine deformity, and severe neurologic symptoms usually develop. Spondyloptosis is one of the most challenging surgical problems. Because the slippage is complete, surgical reduction of L5 over S1 is usually not possible. Proposed treatments include in situ fusion versus complete L5 vertebrectomy and reduction of L4 over S1. This is a high-risk procedure with substantial complications. If sagittal balance is preserved (ie, a balanced spine with minimal sagittal imbalance), the safest treatment is likely in situ fusion with a fibular graft placed through the vertebral body of S1 into the inferior end plate of L5, with supplemental pedicle screw instrumentation to L4 and iliac screw fixation.

Complications

Surgical treatment of spondylolisthesis in children and adolescents is a relatively uncommon procedure, representing only 2.4% of spine procedures. In one large surgeon-reported morbidity database, the overall rate of complications was 10.4%, with neurologic deficit representing the most common complication (5% rate).[28] Other complications included a dural tear (1.3% rate) and wound infection (2% rate).

Summary

It is helpful for spine surgeons and others who treat children and adolescents with spondylolysis and spondylolisthesis to be aware of the latest concepts regarding the biomechanics, clinical presentations, imaging modalities, diagnostic strategies, and nonsurgical and surgical treatments of these conditions. Treatment is aimed at preventing slip progression, restoring spinopelvic balance, and minimizing complications to achieve optimal patient outcomes.

Key Study Points

- Spondylolisthesis in children and young adults can cause profound discomfort as well as neurologic symptoms if not treated properly.
- Treatment goals are to prevent further slip progression and restore spinopelvic balance while minimizing the complications associated with spondylolisthesis reduction.
- A good understanding of spinopelvic sagittal balance is essential to provide personalized surgical treatment to patients with spondylolisthesis.

Annotated References

1. Eisenstein S: Spondylolysis: A skeletal investigation of two population groups. *J Bone Joint Surg Br* 1978;60(4):488-494.

2. Fredrickson BE, Baker D, McHolick WJ, Yuan HA, Lubicky JP: The natural history of spondylolysis and spondylolisthesis. *J Bone Joint Surg Am* 1984;66(5):699-707.

3. Beutler WJ, Fredrickson BE, Murtland A, Sweeney CA, Grant WD, Baker D: The natural history of spondylolysis and spondylolisthesis: 45-year follow-up evaluation. *Spine (Phila Pa 1976)* 2003;28(10):1027-1035, discussion 1035.

4. Stewart TD: The age incidence of neural-arch defects in Alaskan natives, considered from the standpoint of etiology. *J Bone Joint Surg Am* 1953;35:937-950.

5. Letts M, Smallman T, Afanasiev R, Gouw G: Fracture of the pars interarticularis in adolescent athletes: A clinical-biomechanical analysis. *J Pediatr Orthop* 1986;6(1):40-46.

6. Toueg C-W, Mac-Thiong J-M, Grimard G, Poitras B, Parent S, Labelle H: Spondylolisthesis, sacro-pelvic morphology, and orientation in young gymnasts. *J Spinal Disord Tech* 2015;28(6):E358-E364.

   The authors present a cross-sectional evaluation of sacropelvic parameters and morphology in a cohort of 92 young gymnasts. A prevalence of spondylolisthesis of 6.5% was reported, which is similar to that of the general population. The authors concluded that the prevalence of spondylolisthesis was not higher in this population. Gymnasts with spondylolisthesis showed abnormal pelvic indices.

7. Wynne-Davies R, Scott JH: Inheritance and spondylolisthesis: A radiographic family survey. *J Bone Joint Surg Br* 1979;61(3):301-305.

8. Haukipuro K, Keränen N, Koivisto E, Lindholm R, Norio R, Punto L: Familial occurrence of lumbar spondylolysis and spondylolisthesis. *Clin Genet* 1978;13(6):471-476.

9. Moke L, Debeer P, Moens P: Spondylolisthesis in twins: Multifactorial etiology. A case report and review of the literature. *Spine (Phila Pa 1976)* 2011;36(11):E741-E746.

   The authors report on two sets of identical twins from two different families with high-dysplastic developmental spondylolisthesis.

10. Farfan HF, Osteria V, Lamy C: The mechanical etiology of spondylolysis and spondylolisthesis. *Clin Orthop Relat Res* 1976;117:40-55.

11. Hammerberg KW: New concepts on the pathogenesis and classification of spondylolisthesis. *Spine (Phila Pa 1976)* 2005;30(suppl 6):S4-S11.

12. Natarajan RN, Garretson RB III, Biyani A, Lim TH, Andersson GB, An HS: Effects of slip severity and loading directions on the stability of isthmic spondylolisthesis: A finite element model study. *Spine (Phila Pa 1976)* 2003;28(11):1103-1112.

13. Mac-Thiong J-M, Labelle H, Parent S, et al: Assessment of sacral doming in lumbosacral spondylolisthesis. *Spine (Phila Pa 1976)* 2007;32(17):1888-1895.

14. Pawar A, Labelle H, Mac-Thiong J-M: The evaluation of lumbosacral dysplasia in young patients with lumbosacral spondylolisthesis: Comparison with controls and relationship with the severity of slip. *Eur Spine J* 2012;21(11):2122-2127.

    Radiographs were evaluated for the presence of dysplasia in 120 normal control subjects, 91 patients with low-grade spondylolisthesis, and 40 patients with high-grade spondylolisthesis. The authors found that dysplastic features were more common in patients with spondylolisthesis and that their presence was more common and more severe in those with high-grade spondylolisthesis.

15. Mac-Thiong J-M, Labelle H, Berthonnaud E, Betz RR, Roussouly P: Sagittal spinopelvic balance in normal children and adolescents. *Eur Spine J* 2007;16(2):227-234.

16. Mac-Thiong J-M, Wang Z, de Guise JA, Labelle H: Postural model of sagittal spino-pelvic alignment and its relevance for lumbosacral developmental spondylolisthesis. *Spine (Phila Pa 1976)* 2008;33(21):2316-2325.

17. Labelle H, Roussouly P, Berthonnaud E, et al: Spondylolisthesis, pelvic incidence, and spinopelvic balance: A correlation study. *Spine (Phila Pa 1976)* 2004;29(18):2049-2054.

18. Roussouly P, Gollogly S, Berthonnaud E, Labelle H, Weidenbaum M: Sagittal alignment of the spine and pelvis in the presence of L5-S1 isthmic lysis and low-grade spondylolisthesis. *Spine (Phila Pa 1976)* 2006;31(21):2484-2490.

19. Meyerding HW: Spondylolisthesis. *Surg Gynecol Obstet* 1932;54:371-377.

20. Wiltse LL, Newman PH, Macnab I: Classification of spondylolisis and spondylolisthesis. *Clin Orthop Relat Res* 1976;117:23-29.

21. Marchetti PG, Bartolozzi P: Classification of spondylolisthesis as a guideline for treatment, in Bridewell KH, DeWald RL, Hammerberg KW, eds: *The Textbook of Spinal Surgery*, ed 2. Philadelphia, PA, Lippincott-Raven, 1997, pp 1211-1254.

22. Labelle H, Mac-Thiong J-M, Roussouly P: Spino-pelvic sagittal balance of spondylolisthesis: A review and classification. *Eur Spine J* 2011;20(suppl 5):641-646.

    The authors review of the role of spinopelvic sagittal balance in patients with spondylolisthesis and present a new classification for the treatment of spondylolisthesis based on spinopelvic balance, spinal balance, and grade. The classification is designed to guide surgical decision-making in providing a rationale for the need of reduction versus in situ fusion.

23. Hresko MT, Labelle H, Roussouly P, Berthonnaud E: Classification of high-grade spondylolistheses based on pelvic version and spine balance: Possible rationale for reduction. *Spine (Phila Pa 1976)* 2007;32(20):2208-2213.

24. Phalen GS, Dickson JA: Spondylolisthesis and tight hamstrings. *J Bone Joint Surg Am* 1961;43(4):505-512.

25. van den Oever M, Merrick MV, Scott JH: Bone scintigraphy in symptomatic spondylolysis. *J Bone Joint Surg Br* 1987;69(3):453-456.

26. Lusins JO, Elting JJ, Cicoria AD, Goldsmith SJ: SPECT evaluation of lumbar spondylolysis and spondylolisthesis. *Spine (Phila Pa 1976)* 1994;19(5):608-612.

27. Bourassa-Moreau É, Mac-Thiong JM, Joncas J, Parent S, Labelle H: Quality of life of patients with high-grade spondylolisthesis: Minimum 2-year follow-up after surgical and nonsurgical treatments. *Spine J* 2013;13(7):770-774.

    The authors report on 28 pediatric patients with high-grade spondylolisthesis who underwent either surgical (23 patients) or nonsurgical treatment (5 patients). Patients with lower baseline Health-Related-Quality-of-Life scores benefited most from surgery. In selected patients with good baseline Health-Related-Quality-of-Life scores and no neurologic impairment, nonsurgical care with close observation was a safe treatment option.

28. Fu K-M, Smith JS, Polly DW Jr, et al: Morbidity and mortality in the surgical treatment of six hundred five pediatric patients with isthmic or dysplastic spondylolisthesis. *Spine (Phila Pa 1976)* 2011;36(4):308-312.

5: Spine Deformity

The authors queried a large mortality and morbidity database of the Scoliosis Research Society for complications associated with the surgical treatment of isthmic spondylolisthesis. They found that this procedure is relatively rare, representing only 2.4% of cases, and has relatively high morbidity. The nature of this surgeon–self-reported database for complications may underestimate the real complication rate associated with this procedure.

29. Sansur CA, Reames DL, Smith JS, et al: Morbidity and mortality in the surgical treatment of 10,242 adults with spondylolisthesis. *J Neurosurg Spine* 2010;13(5):589-593.

30. Joelson A, Hedlund R, Frennered K: Normal health-related quality of life and ability to work twenty-nine years after in situ arthrodesis for high-grade isthmic spondylolisthesis. *J Bone Joint Surg Am* 2014;96(12):e100.

The authors present the long-term results of in situ fusion for high-grade spondylolisthesis. Clinical outcomes for 35 of 40 consecutive patients that underwent in situ fusion at the mean age of 15 years were reviewed. Results showed good outcomes in health-related quality of life, disability, pain, and agility up to 29 years after surgery. Level of evidence: IV.

Section 6

Trauma

SECTION EDITOR:

Jeffrey C. Wang, MD

Chapter 27

Initial Management of the Patient With Spine Trauma

Brian K. Kwon, MD, PhD, FRCSC   Étienne Bourassa-Moreau, MD, MSc

Abstract

The appropriate initial treatment of patients with spine trauma is critical for achieving the best clinical outcomes. Spine immobilization to protect the spinal cord from further injury is required until unstable injury is ruled out and a definitive treatment plan is determined. Resuscitation of patients having spinal cord injuries requires careful attention to the unique pathophysiologic considerations associated with neurologic impairment. Spine clearance protocols incorporate information from the patient's history, physical examination, and imaging studies. MRI has an important role in evaluating the integrity of soft-tissue structures that stabilize the spinal column and the spinal cord. Recent clinical data support the benefits of early surgical decompression after spinal cord injury. It is helpful to be familiar with the important principles of early care of spine trauma along with recent developments within this field.

Keywords: initial resuscitation; neurologic assessment; spine imaging; spine immobilization; traumatic spinal cord injury

Introduction

Early recognition of spine trauma is critical for the initiation of appropriate care that protects the spinal cord from

Dr. Kwon or an immediate family member serves as a paid consultant to Acorda Therapeutics. Neither Dr. Bourassa-Moreau nor any immediate family member has received anything of value from or has stock or stock options held in a commercial company or institution related directly or indirectly to the subject of this chapter.

further injury. Physicians caring for such patients early after their injury may be responsible for immobilizing the patient appropriately, examining and documenting the degree of neurologic impairment, obtaining the necessary imaging studies, characterizing the nature of the spine injury, and organizing specialized care if necessary. This chapter reviews the basic principles of early management of spine trauma, with an emphasis on incorporating recent knowledge in the field.

Epidemiology and Demographics

The annual incidence of spinal column trauma is estimated at 640 cases per million individuals, whereas the incidence of traumatic spinal cord injury (SCI) is much lower at approximately 54 cases per million individuals in North America. Although the incidence of traumatic SCI is relatively low in the general population, in the setting of those sustaining blunt trauma, SCI occurs in up to 10% of patients.[1] Although a reduction in complete SCIs in young adults resulting from motor vehicle crashes has occurred in the past decades, the incidence of incomplete tetraplegia in the elderly population after blunt trauma (particularly from falls) is increasing.[2]

Advanced Trauma Life Support Protocol: Special Considerations

Patients with spine injuries are trauma patients first and therefore need to be initially evaluated and resuscitated per the Advanced Trauma Life Support (ATLS) protocol. While adhering to the ATLS principles, clinicians must also maintain the assumption that an unstable traumatic SCI is present; such awareness is essential to avoid further damage to the spinal column or cord, efficiently identify such injuries, and initiate appropriate management. The ATLS protocol has unique considerations specific to the management of spine injuries.

Airway Control and Cervical Spine Protection

The possibility that a trauma patient has sustained an unstable cervical spine injury mandates cervical spine immobilization and protection during early airway management. If intubation is necessary, it should be performed with the spine maintained in neutral alignment and with as little movement as possible. The trauma team should anticipate situations in which intubation with cervical spine immobilization may be challenging and ensure that appropriate expertise for securing the airway (such as anesthesiology) is available.

Breathing

The presence of obvious quadriplegia on initial assessment, such as that often provided by the paramedic staff, is an important consideration for the ATLS assessment of breathing. With injuries at C3 or higher, patients may experience acute respiratory arrest at the injury scene, which requires urgent intubation and ventilation. Individuals with lower cervical SCI (C3 through T1) may have impaired intercostal muscle function, increasing the delay in ventilatory failure.

Circulation

Hypotension in the patient with acute trauma is assumed to have a hemorrhagic etiology until proved otherwise. If all sources of bleeding are excluded and the patient is hypotensive with bradycardia, neurogenic shock from SCI is likely. Neurogenic shock occurs typically in SCIs rostral to T4 as a result of disrupted sympathetic tone in the peripheral vasculature and heart. Irrespective of etiology, hypotension must be aggressively corrected to minimize secondary ischemic damage to the spinal cord and other sensitive organs. Once the patient is normovolemic, maintaining mean arterial pressure (MAP) at 85 to 90 mm Hg for 5 to 7 days has been recommended. Although the specific MAP goal of 85 to 90 mm Hg is not based on strong clinical evidence, recent observational studies suggest that vigilant maintenance of MAP and the avoidance of hypotension may be associated with improved neurologic recovery, especially in complete SCI.[3-5] However, maintaining such a MAP target with vasopressors is often challenging to achieve in practice, and so vigilance on behalf of the clinical team is needed.[6]

Disability and Exposure

After management of the airway, breathing, circulation and all life-threatening injuries, the patient's level of consciousness should be documented. The presence of voluntary movement in the four extremities should be established after full exposure of the patient. The patient should be log rolled to inspect and palpate the spine to provide important information about the spinal column (**Figure 1**). The presence of tenderness, swelling, or a step deformity can suggest the presence of a posterior ligamentous injury and warrants advanced imaging. The final component of the log roll is the digital rectal examination. This is arguably the most important component of the neurologic examination in a patient with an SCI. Perianal and anal sensation, anal tone, and voluntary contraction, as well as the bulbocavernosus reflex, should all be documented. An absent bulbocavernosus reflex means that spinal shock is still present, and the true extent of the neurologic impairment may not be fully appreciated. The diagnosis of a complete SCI should be made after spinal shock resolves, which is operationally defined as the return of the bulbocavernosus reflex (usually within 48 to 72 hours after injury). Characterizing the true extent of neurologic impairment in the early stages after injury is frequently complicated by concomitant injuries (including brain injury), pharmacologic sedation, or intoxication.[7]

Neurologic Assessment of the Traumatic SCI

A detailed neurologic assessment early after SCI is critical for treatment planning, prognosis, communication, and outcome measurement. The International Standards for the Neurological Classification of Spinal Cord Injury (ISNCSCI) is the globally accepted method for clinically measuring motor and sensory impairment after SCI and communicating the severity of neurologic injury. Motor function is assessed by measuring strength in five key muscle groups in the upper extremities and five key groups in the lower extremities. Sensory assessment of light touch and pinprick sensation is completed throughout 28 dermatomes. The interpretation of the completeness of injury is based on the presence of perianal and anal sensation, anal tone and voluntary contraction, and the bulbocavernosus reflex. Although the ISNCSCI is an invaluable clinical tool, the examination requires considerable time to perform carefully and comprehensively and requires patient participation in detailed motor and sensory assessments. The time required is challenging in the setting of acute trauma for surgeons whose time is limited, and patient participation is frequently impossible because of concomitant injuries, intoxication and/or sedation, or even language barriers. The limitations of ISNCSCI have motivated interest in finding objective biomarkers of SCI severity that use biochemical features within the cerebrospinal fluid and blood or imaging modalities such as MRI.[8,9]

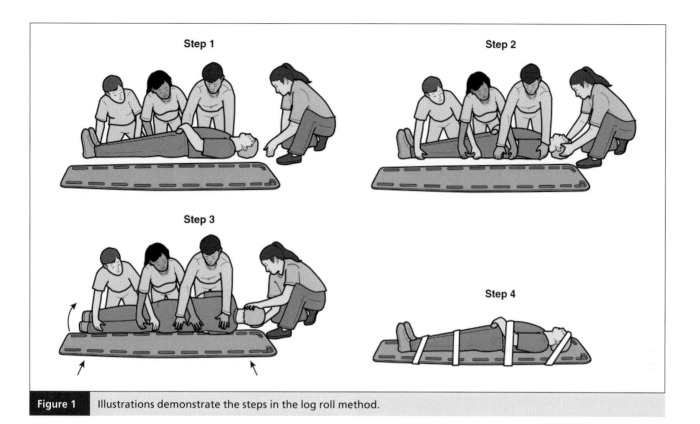

Figure 1   Illustrations demonstrate the steps in the log roll method.

Imaging Assessment for Spine Trauma

In the trauma setting, the first question is whether imaging is actually required. To guide decision making, the Canadian C-Spine (cervical spine) Rule and the National Emergency Xray Utilization Study (NEXUS) criteria are widely used. Recent literature has suggested that the Canadian C-Spine Rule has slightly better diagnostic accuracy than the NEXUS protocol.[10]

For patients who require imaging, it is challenging for the clinician to rule out unstable, clinically important injuries while responsibly using the available imaging resources. AP, lateral, and open-mouth odontoid radiographs have been traditionally used to rule out injuries from the occiput to T1. However, the poor sensitivity of conventional radiography to diagnose injuries of the cervical spine has resulted in the widespread use of CT, with excellent resolution of osseous anatomy and better visualization of both occipitocervical and cervicothoracic junctions. The superior diagnostic quality of CT must be weighed against the much higher radiation exposure than that associated with conventional radiography; however, because fractures are often undetected on radiographs, CT is gradually becoming the standard for diagnostic imaging of the cervical spine after trauma. Although the use of CT for evaluating osseous detail and spine alignment is unmatched, MRI provides an unparalleled assessment of soft tissues, including the neurologic elements. MRI can demonstrate the status of the spinal cord and the degree to which it is compromised by intervertebral disk, ligamentum flavum, or epidural hematoma. This information helps guide surgeons planning a closed reduction of a facet dislocation or selection of the approach for surgical decompression and stabilization (**Figure 2**). MRI, especially sagittal short tau inversion recovery sequences, also can help assess the integrity of ligaments when bony alignment on CT scans and the mechanism of trauma suggest disruption. Recent studies showed that the addition of MRI to CT may increase the detection of posterior ligamentous complex disruption in one-third of thoracolumbar trauma, and consequently change the classification of these injuries and potentially the decision making for treatment.[11,12] However, in the setting of cervical trauma, it is unclear if MRI combined with CT is better able to determine ligamentous stability compared with CT alone.[13]

In the setting of minor spine trauma in elderly patients, the clinician must determine whether a compression fracture is related to osteoporosis or if it is a pathologic fracture resulting from metastasis. MRI can provide critical radiologic clues that suggest a pathologic fracture, including involvement of the entire vertebral body, abnormal bone marrow signal in multiple vertebrae, convex

6: Trauma

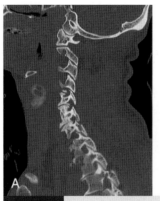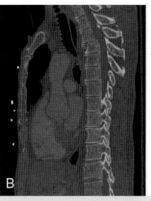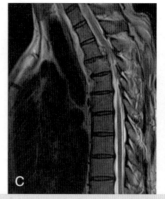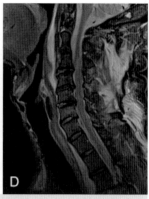

Figure 2 Images of the spine of a 53-year-old man who sustained an incomplete cervical spinal cord injury after a motor vehicle crash. **A,** Parasagittal cervical CT scan shows a C7 bilateral facet fracture. **B,** Midsagittal thoracic CT scan shows a T3-T4 flexion distraction fracture. **C,** Thoracic midsagittal T2-weighted magnetic resonance image shows T3-T4 disk material abutting against the spinal cord. **D,** Cervical midsagittal short tau inversion recovery magnetic resonance image shows multilevel cervical spinal stenosis. Selection of the appropriate levels for surgical decompression and the approach can be made only after evaluating the information provided by the MRI studies.

appearance of the posterior wall, and enhancement of surrounding soft tissue.[14]

Cervical Spine Clearance

Arguably, no other topic has raised as much concern and anxiety in the setting of spinal trauma than how to clear the cervical spine in the obtunded, unexaminable patient, and specifically, what imaging studies are required to achieve reasonable assurance for cervical collar removal from such patients. The prevailing concern has been the possibility of occult ligamentous disruption causing instability and potential spinal cord compromise despite negative findings on high-quality (<3-mm cut) CT scans. The use of MRI in this clinical setting has generated much controversy in the literature. Recent studies have provided some guidance.

A single-center prospective study of 830 patients with blunt trauma and cervical spine tenderness showed no added benefits of MRI for the detection of clinically important cervical injury compared with CT alone.[15] In a recent prospective North American multicenter study on 10,276 patients with blunt trauma and positive NEXUS criteria to warrant imaging, 198 patients had SCI substantial enough to require surgical or halo stabilization; 3 of these patients had normal CT findings despite abnormal MRI (sensitivity, 98.5%; negative predictive value, 99.97%).[16] Each of these 3 patients had focal neurologic deficits that would alert the physician to the possibility of an unstable SCI.

Although contemporary CT is a powerful tool to help rule out cervical spine injury, MRI provides more information about the status of the discoligamentous soft-tissue stabilizing structures. The challenges for using MRI as a screening tool for cervical trauma are the well-documented concerns that MRI is not only costly but also oversensitive, which can generate many false-positive findings.[17,18] Also, injuries detected using MRI alone (not with CT) may be so subtle as to not be clinically significant.[19-21] In addition, moving an obtunded, intubated, and potentially hemodynamically unstable patient from a highly supervised intensive care unit to an MRI machine puts the patient at some risk.

In the past 5 years, several studies have suggested that it is safe to rule out clinically significant traumatic instability using a normal, high-quality CT scan alone.[15,16,18] However, cervical clearance protocols vary among institutions, depending on available resources and the local tolerance to risk. A 2015 systematic review and practice management guideline from the Eastern Association for Surgery of Trauma suggested that imaging protocols should consider imaging quality, the presence of spine pathology confounders, the level of detail for neurologic examination, the process and availability for spine specialist consultation, and distinct reasons for using imaging adjuncts such as MRI.[22]

Initial Imaging for Thoracolumbar Trauma

Most of the literature regarding imaging of spine trauma is specific to the cervical region, although thoracic and thoracolumbar trauma have similar issues. Recent data suggest that when screening for patients at risk of thoracolumbar trauma, it is crucial to consider the clinical evaluation, the patient's age, and mechanism of trauma to optimize the sensitivity of detection.[23,24] Trauma patients

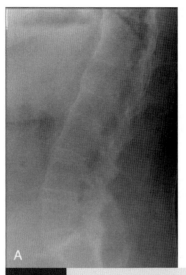 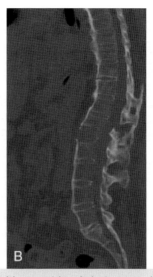 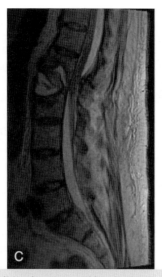 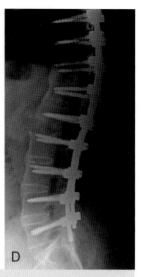

Figure 3   Images from a 49-year-old man with ankylosing spondylitis who reported low back pain after a minor fall. The patient was discharged from an outpatient clinic after radiography. **A,** Lateral radiograph of the lumbar spine shows no obvious fracture. The patient reported gradually worsening pain and saddle paresthesia over the following 2 weeks. **B,** Midsagittal lumbar CT scan shows a grossly displaced fracture through the L1-L2 ossified disk and interspinous ligaments. **C,** Midsagittal T2-weighted magnetic resonance image shows local compression of the conus medullaris. **D,** Lateral lumbar radiograph obtained following posterior decompression and long (T9-L5) instrumented fusion.

undergoing visceral CT can undergo a prompt thoracolumbar spine evaluation. Visceral CT scans are sufficient to clear the thoracolumbar spine without the use of plain radiography.[25] In addition, visceral CT can use adequate reconstruction algorithms to produce thoracolumbar spine imaging essentially equivalent to that of specific CT of the spine.[26]

Spine Ankylosis

The extensive literature regarding imaging and the assessment of stability is based on displacement and ligamentous integrity. It is important to recognize that much of this information does not apply to patients with spine ankylosis. Fractures of any degree in the ankylosed spine can be potentially highly unstable because of the long lever arms being applied to the fracture site. In cases of ankylosing spondylitis or diffuse idiopathic skeletal hyperostosis, low-velocity injury (such as a fall from a standing height) can result in fractures that may seem trivial but are potentially highly unstable.

In principle, the patient presenting with neck or back pain who is found to have spine ankylosis on imaging must be considered to have sustained an unstable spine fracture until proved otherwise. This degree of vigilance is critical in the assessment of these patients because initial imaging studies may not reveal the fracture, which, by virtue of the ankylosis, must completely disrupt both the anterior and posterior columns, as with a long bone fracture. High-quality, thin-slice CT scans with sagittal and coronal reconstructions may be necessary to identify a possible nondisplaced crack in the ankylosed spine.[27] MRI and nuclear medicine bone scanning may also help in situations in which uncertainty exists after CT scanning about the presence of a fracture in the ankylosed spine. It is important to recognize spine ankylosis and to be vigilant about ruling out an occult injury (**Figure 3**).

In patients with spine ankyloses, the entire spine must be fully imaged because concomitant spine fractures are common and the history and physical examination are often unreliable. It is important to remember that the spine should be immobilized in the patient's normal physiologic position, which may be much more kyphotic than the typical alignment. Individualized immobilization using sandbags, beanbags, towels, and straps is safer than using standard collars and braces, which may further extend and displace a fracture originally caused by hyperextension. Patients with ankylosing spondylitis should be closely monitored because of the high risk of epidural hematoma and associated delayed neurologic injury. Anesthesiology consultation is advised if any surgery is planned because of the difficulty in securing the airway.

Therapeutic Modalities in Spine Trauma

After a spine injury has been identified, the surgeon must assess the degree of instability to determine whether surgical fixation is required or external immobilization

6: Trauma

with some form of orthosis will be sufficient. Clearly, not all spine fractures require surgical intervention, and the decision making regarding surgery typically considers the need to provide stability, the need to decompress neurologic elements, and patient factors that may influence the choice of surgical or nonsurgical treatment (such as medical comorbidities and body habitus). Classification systems such as the Subaxial Cervical Spine Injury Classification were established to help guide the clinician in this decision-making process by accounting for the degree of mechanical instability and the extent of neurologic impairment.[28] The more recently established AOSpine classification systems for cervical[29] and thoracolumbar[30] injuries are based on injury morphology and are not necessarily meant to guide treatment in the way that the Subaxial Cervical Spine Injury Classification was designed, but are likely to become widely used in the future.

Bracing and External Immobilization

Bracing remains a common definitive treatment of many spine injuries deemed sufficiently stable to heal without surgical fixation. In the cervical spine, many types of commercially available braces are available. A 2016 systematic review reported on the effectiveness of cervical orthoses for immobilizing the spine.[31] Various cervical orthoses were classified as cervical devices (soft collar), cervicothoracic devices, or craniothoracic devices.[32] The results of the review suggest that a soft collar does not reliably restrict range of motion and cervicothoracic devices can limit flexion and extension by 40% to 60% of normal motion, but restrict lateral flexion and rotation less than 20%. By comparison, craniothoracic devices restrict 60% to 80% of cervical motion in all directions.[31] Because studies that evaluate the immobilization effectiveness of cervical collars typically use healthy, noninjured volunteers, extrapolating these data to individuals with unstable cervical injuries may be challenging.[33] Moreover, prolonged use of a poorly fitted spinal collar can cause local pain and pressure ulcers that can be confounded with vertebral pain.[34,35] Cervicothoracic devices should be used judiciously in craniocervical and atlantoaxial injuries because they do not provide substantial immobilization of the upper cervical spine; craniothoracic devices such as a halo vest are preferred for such upper cervical injuries. Caution should be exercised for applying halo vests in the elderly population because these devices have been associated with significant complications, including aspiration, pneumonia, cardiorespiratory events, and death.[36]

The role of bracing in thoracolumbar trauma remains controversial, particularly for thoracolumbar burst fractures and compression fractures in neurologically intact patients.[37] In the setting of stable thoracolumbar burst fractures in neurologically intact patients, two recent randomized trials have shown that bracing may not offer any clinical or radiographic advantage over mobilization without bracing.[38,39] In a compression fracture (an injury more stable than a burst fracture), bracing is not needed for stability but can be used for patient comfort. Similarly, for an osteoporotic compression fracture, an external orthosis is an acceptable treatment option, although strong clinical evidence to support its use is lacking.[40,41] For patients with a compression fracture, the ideal brace should be lightweight, comfortable, easy to apply, and well-fitting to optimize patient compliance and avoid pressure ulcer, respiratory compromise, and axial muscle weakness.

Closed Reduction of Spine Fractures and Dislocations

The goal of closed reduction is to realign a dislocated spine and potentially relieve any ongoing spinal cord compression. When and how to reduce a cervical facet dislocation continues to be discussed because of the possibility that a disk herniation could be displaced into the spinal cord.[42]

It can be argued that in a neurologically intact patient there is no immediate need to obtain a closed reduction, so waiting to perform MRI to assess the disk is warranted. The decision is more complex in neurologically impaired patients. In a patient with complete quadriplegia and ongoing cord compression, a rapid closed reduction without delay for imaging may provide substantial relief, particularly if performed very early after injury.[43] In the setting of incomplete quadriplegia with ongoing cord compression, the decision is more difficult. Immediate closed reduction of the dislocation may worsen the patient's condition because of disk herniation; however, waiting to perform MRI may potentially miss the opportunity to improve function because of prolonged compression of the spinal cord. This decision must be based on the clinician's assessment of the patient and available resources. MRI may be readily available in the emergency department at some institutions, but it also can take many hours and result in prolonged duration of cord compression. At some institutions, it may be faster to perform an anterior cervical diskectomy and open reduction than to set up the necessary equipment and assemble the required staff to conduct a closed reduction in an awake patient.

The technique for closed reduction of a cervical facet dislocation in an awake, cooperative individual involves pharmacologic sedation, muscle relaxation, close monitoring of respiratory status, traction, and repeated radiographic evaluation. Traction weights of 15 lb for the head and an additional 10 lb per level above the dislocation have been recommended, but safe reduction with weights well over 100 lb also have been described.[44] Distraction of the dislocated level by using traction is an important component, not just for clearing the tips of the dislocated facets to reduce them, but also to potentially draw disk material that has herniated up behind the supradjacent vertebral body (where it may be pushed into the spinal cord on reduction) back down into the intervertebral space. This important aspect of the reduction was revealed by an important study that reported on performing closed reductions in the MRI machine to visualize the effect on the disk when applying traction to the dislocated level.[45]

Surgical Intervention

Arguably, the most significant development in the field in the past 5 years relates to the timing of surgical decompression for cervical SCI and the need for urgent transport of such neurologically impaired individuals to centers that commonly manage such injuries.[46]

The Surgical Timing in Acute Spinal Cord Injury Study was a prospective observational study that suggested surgery performed within 24 hours after cervical SCI improved the likelihood of regaining two or more American Spinal Injury Association Impairment Scale (AIS) grades.[47] Prospectively collected registry data from Canada reported that early surgery (within 24 hours) was associated with greater motor score improvement (approximately 5 points) in patients with incomplete SCI, but did not alter motor score improvement in complete (AIS grade A) injuries.[48] Aside from neurologic recovery, early surgical decompression in SCI has been shown to decrease postoperative complications and reduce the length of hospital stay.[49] Although a prospective randomized trial is unlikely to be performed to address this question, the emerging trend is that early surgery at the very least is safe and may be associated with better neurologic and clinical outcomes.[50] Interestingly, recent studies have explored even earlier time windows of intervention and have suggested that decompression within 8 hours may be even more beneficial.[51,52]

Current and Future Neuroprotective Strategies

Methylprednisolone is the only pharmacologic agent currently used as a neuroprotective agent in acute SCI. Although the National Acute Spinal Cord Injury Study (II and III) generated clinical enthusiasm regarding the efficacy of high-dose methylprednisolone, the conduct and interpretation of those studies have been subjected to substantial scrutiny, and complications such as infection, hyperglycemia, respiratory compromise, and gastrointestinal hemorrhage have been highlighted. Guidelines published in 2013 by the American Association of Neurological Surgeons/Congress of Neurological Surgeons Joint Guidelines Committee have recommended that methylprednisolone not be administered in acute SCI, which represents a strong (and controversial) statement about what had been generally accepted as only a treatment option and not a standard of care.[53] Variations in practice patterns, perspectives on the risk and/or benefit, and fear of litigation will undoubtedly result in ongoing methylprednisolone administration in acute SCI and the controversy surrounding its use will likely continue.

In addition to methylprednisolone, many other approaches are being evaluated as neuroprotective agents for acute SCI.[53] Currently, approaches including riluzole, minocycline, systemic hypothermia, and a rho inhibitor are being actively studied in acute traumatic SCI.[54] These approaches appear to be safe, and early studies have provided some evidence that they will be neurologically efficacious. The definitive clinical trials to establish this efficacy in a prospective randomized manner are ongoing, and results will likely be available in the future.

Summary

The management of traumatic SCI begins in the field, with a high index of suspicion and safe spine immobilization. Emergency management of a patient with an unstable spinal column and SCI requires specific care related to airway control, breathing support, and hemodynamic stabilization. Appropriate imaging should be performed to rule out spine trauma, assess for spine instability, determine pattern of neurologic compression, and identify pathologic fracture. Timely initiation of spine care is critical to avoid neurologic deterioration, medical complications, or worsening of instability.

Key Study Points

- The capability of bracing to immobilize the spine varies greatly, depending on the level of injury and the design of the brace.
- A high-quality, normal CT scan is sufficient to rule out ligamentous injury in most clinical scenarios.
- MRI is an invaluable tool to assess neurologic tissue compromise, discoligamentous integrity, and to identify pathologic fracture in spine trauma.
- Management of spine trauma should be initiated in a timely fashion, especially in the setting of SCI, in which all attempts should be made to minimize surgical delays.

6: Trauma

Annotated References

1. Hasler RM, Exadaktylos AK, Bouamra O, et al: Epidemiology and predictors of spinal injury in adult major trauma patients: European cohort study. *Eur Spine J* 2011;20(12):2174-2180.

   This epidemiologic study reviewed a prospective European cohort of 250,584 major trauma patients from 1988 to 2009. The risk factors for spine injury were male sex, age younger than 45 years, Glasgow Coma Scale score less than 15, concomitant chest injury, and high-velocity mechanism.

2. Oliver M, Inaba K, Tang A, et al: The changing epidemiology of spinal trauma: A 13-year review from a Level I trauma centre. *Injury* 2012;43(8):1296-1300.

   This epidemiologic single-center retrospective study of a spine trauma population demonstrated a decrease in mortality and SCIs related to motor vehicle accidents between 1996 and 2008. In addition, multilevel SCI after blunt trauma became more common in elderly patients.

3. Catapano JS, John Hawryluk GW, Whetstone W, et al: Higher mean arterial pressure values correlate with neurologic improvement in patients with initially complete spinal cord injuries. *World Neurosurg* 2016;96:72-79.

   This retrospective study investigated the MAP values in relation to neurologic recovery in traumatic SCI. A positive correlation was found between MAP and neurological recovery for AIS grades A, B, and C, but not D. Level of evidence: III.

4. Hawryluk G, Whetstone W, Saigal R, et al: Mean arterial blood pressure correlates with neurological recovery after human spinal cord injury: Analysis of high frequency physiologic data. *J Neurotrauma* 2015;32(24):1958-1967.

   This retrospective study on the MAP value after traumatic SCI showed a correlation between higher MAP during the first 2 to 3 days after injury and early neurologic recovery. Higher proportion of MAP decreasing beyond 85 mm Hg also was correlated with poorer outcome. Level of evidence: III.

5. Casha S, Christie S: A systematic review of intensive cardiopulmonary management after spinal cord injury. *J Neurotrauma* 2011;28(8):1479-1495.

   This literature review supports cardiopulmonary management for acute SCI in specifically monitored intensive care units. Weak evidence supports the maintenance of MAP greater than 85 mm Hg for 1 week.

6. Kong CY, Hosseini AM, Belanger LM, et al: A prospective evaluation of hemodynamic management in acute spinal cord injury patients. *Spinal Cord* 2013;51(6):466-471.

   This single-center prospective study investigated the intrathecal pressure in relation with MAP for traumatic SCI. Even in the best clinical setting, the actual MAP can frequently decrease beyond the intended target.

7. Lee RS, Noonan VK, Batke J, et al: Feasibility of patient recruitment into clinical trials of experimental treatments for acute spinal cord injury. *J Clin Neurosci* 2012;19(10):1338-1343.

   The results of this study suggest that many patients with SCI are not candidates for clinical trial because a reliable classification using the International Standards for Neurological Classification of Spinal Cord Injury is not made early after their injury or because they arrived too late at the trauma center.

8. Kwon BK, Streijger F, Fallah N, et al: Cerebrospinal fluid biomarkers to stratify injury severity and predict outcome in human traumatic spinal cord injury. *J Neurotrauma* 2016 [Epub ahead of print].

   This prospective study of cerebrospinal fluid analysis in acute SCI suggest that these markers have a valuable diagnostic and prognostic value for recovery. Level of evidence: I.

9. Freund P, Weiskopf N, Ashburner J, et al: MRI investigation of the sensorimotor cortex and the corticospinal tract after acute spinal cord injury: A prospective longitudinal study. *Lancet Neurol* 2013;12(9):873-881.

   This prospective analysis of brain and spinal cord MRI obtained after SCI revealed substantial spinal cord atrophy and corticospinal tract atrophy above the injured level. Level of evidence: I.

10. Michaleff ZA, Maher CG, Verhagen AP, Rebbeck T, Lin CW: Accuracy of the Canadian C-spine rule and NEXUS to screen for clinically important cervical spine injury in patients following blunt trauma: A systematic review. *CMAJ* 2012;184(16):E867-E876.

    This systematic literature review suggested that the Canadian C-Spine Rule may have better diagnostic accuracy than the National Emergency X-Radiography Utilization Study criteria.

11. Pizones J, Izquierdo E, Alvarez P, et al: Impact of magnetic resonance imaging on decision making for thoracolumbar traumatic fracture diagnosis and treatment. *Eur Spine J* 2011;20(suppl 3):390-396.

    This prospective study found MRI results changed the classification of thoracolumbar injury in 24% of patients and changed the therapeutic management in 16% of patients. Level of evidence: I.

12. Winklhofer S, Thekkumthala-Sommer M, Schmidt D, et al: Magnetic resonance imaging frequently changes classification of acute traumatic thoracolumbar spine injuries. *Skeletal Radiol* 2013;42(6):779-786.

    This retrospective radiographic analysis study revealed that MRI changed the AO classification in 31% of patients with thoracolumbar injury by improving detection of soft-tissue injury compared with CT. Level of evidence: III.

13. Mascarenhas D, Dreizin D, Bodanapally UK, Stein DM: Parsing the utility of CT and MRI in the Subaxial Cervical

Spine Injury Classification (SLIC) System: Is CT SLIC enough? *AJR Am J Roentgenol* 2016;206(6):1292-1297.

This retrospective radiographic/clinical study suggests that MRI adds little to surgical decision making compared with CT alone. Level of evidence: III.

14. Kumar Y, Hayashi D: Role of magnetic resonance imaging in acute spinal trauma: A pictorial review. *BMC Musculoskelet Disord* 2016;17:310.

This pictorial review highlights the important role of MRI in spine trauma for assessing ligamentous injury, neurologic compression, and clarifying the etiology of a fracture.

15. Resnick S, Inaba K, Karamanos E, et al: Clinical relevance of magnetic resonance imaging in cervical spine clearance: A prospective study. *JAMA Surg* 2014;149(9):934-939.

This prospective observational study suggests that in adults eligible for evaluation of neurologic deficit or pain, CT was effective for the detection cervical spine injury requiring surgical stabilization or halo placement. MRI did not provide any clinically relevant information. Level of evidence: I.

16. Inaba K, Byerly S, Bush LD, et al; WTA C-Spine Study Group: Cervical spinal clearance: A prospective Western Trauma Association Multi-institutional Trial. *J Trauma Acute Care Surg* 2016;81(6):1122-1130.

This prospective multicenter observational study from the Western Trauma Association suggested that CT has a sensitivity of 98.5% to help rule out clinically significant cervical blunt trauma, but MRI is necessary for patients with normal CT findings but abnormal neurologic examination results. Level of evidence: II.

17. Muchow RD, Resnick DK, Abdel MP, Munoz A, Anderson PA: Magnetic resonance imaging (MRI) in the clearance of the cervical spine in blunt trauma: A meta-analysis. *J Trauma* 2008;64(1):179-189.

18. Malhotra A, Wu X, Kalra VB, et al: Utility of MRI for cervical spine clearance after blunt traumatic injury: A meta-analysis. *Eur Radiol* 2017;27(3):1148-1160.

This systematic review found that the number of patients with unstable injuries detected on MRI but missed on CT was extremely low (16 of 5,286 trauma patients). The rate of false-positive findings with MRI might outweigh the detection rate.

19. Schuster R, Waxman K, Sanchez B, et al: Magnetic resonance imaging is not needed to clear cervical spines in blunt trauma patients with normal computed tomographic results and no motor deficits. *Arch Surg* 2005;140(8):762-766.

20. Tomycz ND, Chew BG, Chang YF, et al: MRI is unnecessary to clear the cervical spine in obtunded/comatose trauma patients: The four-year experience of a level I trauma center. *J Trauma* 2008;64(5):1258-1263.

21. James IA, Moukalled A, Yu E, et al: A systematic review of the need for MRI for the clearance of cervical spine injury in obtunded blunt trauma patients after normal cervical spine CT. *J Emerg Trauma Shock* 2014;7(4):251-255.

This literature review suggested that 0.7% of obtunded patients had unstable cervical injuries detected on MRI but missed on CT scan. There is a role for cervical spine MRI in obtunded patients with no possible neurologic examination, but when gross motor function is intact, CT alone may be sufficient.

22. Patel MB, Humble SS, Cullinane DC, et al: Cervical spine collar clearance in the obtunded adult blunt trauma patient: A systematic review and practice management guideline from the Eastern Association for the Surgery of Trauma. *J Trauma Acute Care Surg* 2015;78(2):430-441.

This systematic literature review suggests that a cervical collar can be removed after a high-quality CT scan shows negative results in obtunded adults with blunt trauma.

23. Inaba K, Nosanov L, Menaker J, et al; AAST TL-Spine Multicenter Study Group: Prospective derivation of a clinical decision rule for thoracolumbar spine evaluation after blunt trauma: An American Association for the Surgery of Trauma Multi-Institutional Trials Group Study. *J Trauma Acute Care Surg* 2015;78(3):459-465, discussion 465-467.

When screening for trauma patients at risk of thoracolumbar spine injury, clinical examination combined with age older than 60 years and a high-risk mechanism resulted in a sensitivity of 98.9% for clinically significant thoracolumbar injury and 100% for thoracolumbar injury requiring surgery. Level of evidence: III.

24. Cason B, Rostas J, Simmons J, Frotan MA, Brevard SB, Gonzalez RP: Thoracolumbar spine clearance: Clinical examination for patients with distracting injuries. *J Trauma Acute Care Surg* 2016;80(1):125-130.

This retrospective cohort study investigated the performance of clinical examination to clear thoracolumbar trauma in patients with distractive injuries. The sensitivity of clinical evaluation clearance was 75% for all thoracolumbar injury and 89% for significant injury requiring surgery or bracing. Level of evidence: IV.

25. Inaba K, Munera F, McKenney M, et al: Visceral torso computed tomography for clearance of the thoracolumbar spine in trauma: A review of the literature. *J Trauma* 2006;60(4):915-920.

26. Kim S, Yoon CS, Ryu JA, et al: A comparison of the diagnostic performances of visceral organ-targeted versus spine-targeted protocols for the evaluation of spinal fractures using sixteen-channel multidetector row computed tomography: Is additional spine-targeted computed tomography necessary to evaluate thoracolumbar spinal fractures in blunt trauma victims? *J Trauma* 2010;69(2):437-446.

27. Harrop JS, Sharan A, Anderson G, et al: Failure of standard imaging to detect a cervical fracture in a patient

6: Trauma

with ankylosing spondylitis. *Spine (Phila Pa 1976)* 2005;30(14):E417-E419.

28. Vaccaro AR, Hulbert RJ, Patel AA, et al; Spine Trauma Study Group: The subaxial cervical spine injury classification system: A novel approach to recognize the importance of morphology, neurology, and integrity of the disco-ligamentous complex. *Spine (Phila Pa 1976)* 2007;32(21):2365-2374.

29. Vaccaro AR, Koerner JD, Radcliff KE, et al: AOSpine subaxial cervical spine injury classification system. *Eur Spine J* 2016;25(7):2173-2184.

30. Vaccaro AR, Oner C, Kepler CK, et al; AOSpine Spinal Cord Injury & Trauma Knowledge Forum: AOSpine thoracolumbar spine injury classification system: Fracture description, neurological status, and key modifiers. *Spine (Phila Pa 1976)* 2013;38(23):2028-2037.

This article describes a morphologic classification system, the AOSpine subaxial cervical spine injury system, which demonstrated substantial interobserver and intraobserver reliability.

31. Holla M, Huisman JM, Verdonschot N, Goosen J, Hosman AJ, Hannink G: The ability of external immobilizers to restrict movement of the cervical spine: A systematic review. *Eur Spine J* 2016;25(7):2023-2036.

This systematic literature review found that cervicothoracic external immobilization devices restricted some flexion and extension but does not immobilize lateral flexion and rotation as well as craniothoracic devices.

32. Holla M, Huisman JM, Hosman AJ: A validated classification for external immobilization of the cervical spine. *Evid Based Spine Care J* 2013;4(2):72-77.

This study presents a classification for external cervical immobilization that appeared clinically useful and had almost perfect intrarater and interrater agreement.

33. Horodyski M, DiPaola CP, Conrad BP, Rechtine GR II: Cervical collars are insufficient for immobilizing an unstable cervical spine injury. *J Emerg Med* 2011;41(5):513-519.

This cadaver study shows that cervical collar use did not effectively reduce cervical motion when an unstable spine injury is present.

34. Ham W, Schoonhoven L, Schuurmans MJ, Leenen LP: Pressure ulcers from spinal immobilization in trauma patients: A systematic review. *J Trauma Acute Care Surg* 2014;76(4):1131-1141.

This systematic literature review suggests an increased risk of pressure ulcer development with external immobilization devices.

35. Ham WH, Schoonhoven L, Schuurmans MJ, Leenen LP: Pressure ulcers, indentation marks and pain from cervical spine immobilization with extrication collars and headblocks: An observational study. *Injury* 2016;47(9):1924-1931.

This prospective observational study on trauma patients in the emergency department found substantial grade 1 and 2 pressure ulcers as well as shoulder and chest pain associated with the use of extrication collars and headblocks. Level of evidence: II.

36. Majercik S, Tashjian RZ, Biffl WL, Harrington DT, Cioffi WG: Halo vest immobilization in the elderly: A death sentence? *J Trauma* 2005;59(2):350-356, discussion 356-358.

37. Chang V, Holly LT: Bracing for thoracolumbar fractures. *Neurosurg Focus* 2014;37(1):E3.

This review highlights the ideal characteristics of bracing for thoracolumbar injuries.

38. Bailey CS, Urquhart JC, Dvorak MF, et al: Orthosis versus no orthosis for the treatment of thoracolumbar burst fractures without neurologic injury: A multi-center prospective randomized equivalence trial. *Spine J* 2014;14(11):2557-2564.

This randomized clinical trial compared brace use with no brace for nonsurgical management of thoracolumbar burst fracture type AO-A3. Brace use did not improve Roland Morris Disability Questionnaire score at 3 months. Level of evidence: I.

39. Shamji MF, Roffey DM, Young DK, Reindl R, Wai EK: A pilot evaluation of the role of bracing in stable thoracolumbar burst fractures without neurological deficit. *J Spinal Disord Tech* 2014;27(7):370-375.

This small multicenter randomized controlled trial for type AO-A3 thoracolumbar injury compared nonsurgical treatment with and without bracing and found similar radiographic and clinical outcomes but longer hospital lengths of stay with bracing. Level of evidence: I.

40. Esses SI, McGuire R, Jenkins J, et al: American Academy of Orthopaedic Surgeons clinical practice guideline on: The treatment of osteoporotic spinal compression fractures. *J Bone Joint Surg Am* 2011;93(20):1934-1936.

This article reviews the American Academy of Orthopaedic Surgeons clinical practice guideline on the treatment of osteoporotic spinal compression fractures.

41. Longo UG, Loppini M, Denaro L, Maffulli N, Denaro V: Conservative management of patients with an osteoporotic vertebral fracture: A review of the literature. *J Bone Joint Surg Br* 2012;94(2):152-157.

This review suggests no evidence exists for or against the use of external orthoses for treatment of vertebral compression fracture.

42. Eismont FJ, Arena MJ, Green BA: Extrusion of an intervertebral disc associated with traumatic subluxation or dislocation of cervical facets. Case report. *J Bone Joint Surg Am* 1991;73(10):1555-1560.

43. Newton D, England M, Doll H, Gardner BP: The case for early treatment of dislocations of the cervical spine with

cord involvement sustained playing rugby. *J Bone Joint Surg Br* 2011;93(12):1646-1652.

This retrospective cohort study of 57 cervical facet dislocations sustained by rugby players suggests reduction within 4 hours after injury can dramatically improve neurologic recovery in complete SCI. Level of evidence: IV.

44. Cotler JM, Herbison GJ, Nasuti JF, Ditunno JF Jr, An H, Wolff BE: Closed reduction of traumatic cervical spine dislocation using traction weights up to 140 pounds. *Spine (Phila Pa 1976)* 1993;18(3):386-390.

45. Darsaut TE, Ashforth R, Bhargava R, et al: A pilot study of magnetic resonance imaging-guided closed reduction of cervical spine fractures. *Spine (Phila Pa 1976)* 2006;31(18):2085-2090.

46. Parent S, Barchi S, LeBreton M, Casha S, Fehlings MG: The impact of specialized centers of care for spinal cord injury on length of stay, complications, and mortality: A systematic review of the literature. *J Neurotrauma* 2011;28(8):1363-1370.

This literature review suggests that patients with traumatic SCI should be transferred to specialized centers early after trauma to decrease length of stay, mortality, and severity of complications.

47. Fehlings MG, Vaccaro A, Wilson JR, et al: Early versus delayed decompression for traumatic cervical spinal cord injury: Results of the Surgical Timing in Acute Spinal Cord Injury Study (STASCIS). *PLoS One* 2012;7(2):e32037.

This multicenter prospective cohort of 313 cervical trauma SCIs suggests surgical decompression within 24 hours can be performed safely and is associated with improvement of at least two AIS grades at 6-month follow-up. Level of evidence: II.

48. Dvorak MF, Noonan VK, Fallah N, et al; RHSCIR Network: The influence of time from injury to surgery on motor recovery and length of hospital stay in acute traumatic spinal cord injury: An observational Canadian cohort study. *J Neurotrauma* 2015;32(9):645-654.

This prospective Canadian cohort of traumatic SCI reported that surgery less than 24 hours after injury improved motor recovery in incomplete traumatic SCI but not in complete traumatic SCI, and reduces length of stay. Level of evidence: II.

49. Bourassa-Moreau E, Mac-Thiong JM, Feldman DE, Thompson C, Parent S: Non-neurological outcomes after complete traumatic spinal cord injury: The impact of surgical timing. *J Neurotrauma* 2013;30(18):1596-1601.

This retrospective cohort study of complete American Spinal Injury Association grade A SCI showed reduced acute hospitalization complication rates and costs with surgery performed earlier than 24 hours after injury. Level of evidence: III.

50. Battistuzzo CR, Armstrong A, Clark J, et al: Early decompression following cervical spinal cord injury: Examining the process of care from accident scene to surgery. *J Neurotrauma* 2016;33(12):1161-1169.

This retrospective study on cervical SCI shows that delays in surgical decompression decreased significantly between 2010 and 2013. An association was found between shorter surgical timing and significant neurological recovery. Level of evidence: III.

51. Jug M, Kejžar N, Vesel M, et al: Neurological recovery after traumatic cervical spinal cord injury is superior if surgical decompression and instrumented fusion are performed within 8 hours versus 8 to 24 hours after injury: A single center experience. *J Neurotrauma* 2015;32(18):1385-1392.

This prospective cohort study on cervical traumatic SCI showed that surgical delay less than 8 hours after trauma resulted in greater improvement than when surgery was performed between 8 and 24 hours. Level of evidence: II.

52. Grassner L, Wutte C, Klein B, et al: Early decompression (<8 h) after traumatic cervical spinal cord injury improves functional outcome as assessed by spinal cord independence measure after one year. *J Neurotrauma* 2016;33(18):1658-1666.

This retrospective study showed that surgery performed for traumatic cervical SCI within 8 hours of trauma had better SCI independence measure scores and greater improvement in American Spinal Injury Association grades. Level of evidence: III.

53. Hurlbert RJ, Hadley MN, Walters BC, et al: Pharmacological therapy for acute spinal cord injury. *Neurosurgery* 2013;72(suppl 2):93-105.

This literature review on high-dose methylprednisolone and ganglioside reported no evidence supports their use in patients with traumatic SCI.

54. Ahuja CS, Fehlings M: Concise review: Bridging the gap. Novel neuroregenerative and neuroprotective strategies in spinal cord injury. *Stem Cells Transl Med* 2016;5(7):914-924.

This article reviews the important neuroprotective interventions currently applied in clinical practice, those under clinical investigation, and potential future neuroregenerative therapies.

6: Trauma

Chapter 28

Occipitocervical and Subaxial Cervical Trauma

Paul A. Anderson, MD   Raymond J. Hah, MD

Abstract

Cervical spine trauma can be a devastating injury that is often associated with delays in diagnosis and subsequent neurologic deficits. The number of injuries in the upper cervical spine is increasing, mostly occurring in the geriatric population. Many new classification systems provide more exact differentiation of stability and may help guide treatment. For atlas and axis fractures, several techniques of osteosynthesis have been proposed rather that atlantoaxial fusion. In the subaxial spine, hyperextension injuries with spinal cord injuries and fractures through an ankylosed spine are increasing in frequency, and evidence suggests early surgery provides optimum outcomes. Other common injuries are lateral mass and facet fractures, with newer evidence suggesting that surgical treatment is better than nonsurgical treatment.

Keywords: atlas fractures; axis fractures; craniocervical dissociation; lower cervical spine injuries; occipital condyle fractures; upper cervical spine trauma

Dr. Anderson or an immediate family member has received royalties from Pioneer and Stryker; serves as a paid consultant to Globus Medical; serves as an unpaid consultant to and has stock or stock options held in Expanding Orthopedics, SI Bone, Spartec, and Titan Surgical; and serves as a board member, owner, officer, or committee member of the American Academy of Orthopaedics Surgeons, the American Orthopaedic Association, the ASTM, the Lumbar Spine Research Society, the North American Spine Society, the Spine Arthroplasty Society, Spine Section of the American Association of Neurological Surgeons, and Congress of Neurological Surgeons. Dr. Hah or an immediate family member serves as a paid consultant to Flospine.

Introduction

Cervical spine trauma results in complex, heterogeneous injury patterns that can devastate a patient's quality of life and hasten death. Early identification and classification of injury patterns is essential and possible by using critical physical examination and modern imaging. The use of protocols to identify substantial injury can result in fewer delays and missed diagnoses. Most injuries have multiple treatment options, and treatment should be individualized.

Epidemiology

Cervical spine injuries occur in 3% to 5% of all blunt trauma patients; fewer than 25% of these patients sustain spinal cord injuries.[1] A bimodal distribution exists, with an increased incidence in younger patients (age range, 16 to 25 years) and in patients older than 65 years. Although the geriatric population is increasing in number, the rate of spine fractures in these patients appears to be increasing at a greater rate.[2] Older patients may sustain cervical spine trauma with lower-energy mechanisms, but the mortality rate is still as high as 25%.[3]

Cervical spine trauma is often grouped into upper and subaxial injuries. Upper cervical injuries occur between the occiput and C2; subaxial injuries are found between C3 and T1. In all cervical injuries, 65% of fractures and 75% of dislocations occur in the subaxial cervical spine.[4]

Fatal vehicular trauma is often associated with upper cervical injury. In a report of 69 individuals with cranial cervical disassociation in a single county in Washington state over a 5-year period, two-thirds of the individuals died at the scene and one-third survived to reach the hospital.[5] A review of cervical spine injuries reported that atlanto-occipital dislocation occurred in 0.6% of blunt trauma patients, was the strongest predictor of mortality, and was missed in 25% of patients, all of whom died.[6]

6: Trauma

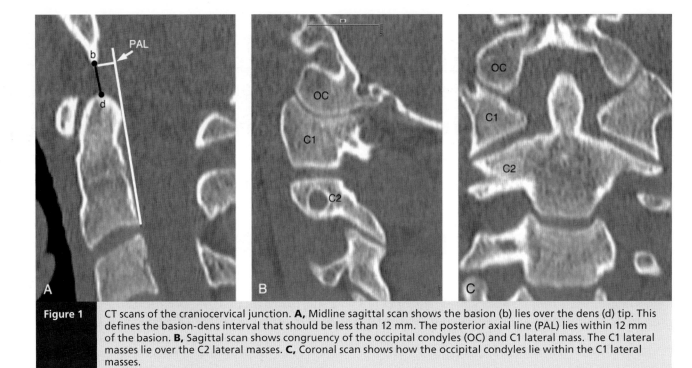

| Figure 1 | CT scans of the craniocervical junction. **A,** Midline sagittal scan shows the basion (b) lies over the dens (d) tip. This defines the basion-dens interval that should be less than 12 mm. The posterior axial line (PAL) lies within 12 mm of the basion. **B,** Sagittal scan shows congruency of the occipital condyles (OC) and C1 lateral mass. The C1 lateral masses lie over the C2 lateral masses. **C,** Coronal scan shows how the occipital condyles lie within the C1 lateral masses. |

Diagnosis

Protocols for the initial evaluation of cervical spine injuries have been described previously.[7,8] Patients should be evaluated quickly and the cervical spine appropriately immobilized. In those with suspected or known injury, evaluation includes a thorough history, physical examination, and appropriate imaging, which may include radiography, CT, and/or MRI. CT has largely replaced plain radiography in the evaluation of most trauma patients because of its increased availability, speed, and accuracy.

Conventional radiographs are quickly and easily obtained. Lateral radiographs have 85% sensitivity, increasing to 92% with the addition of AP and open-mouth views.[9] In low-risk patients with adequate imaging (visualization from C1-T1), radiographs may be sufficient for clearance. Flexion-extension views may be additionally helpful in diagnosing cervical instability in the subacute setting, but are not cost effective or easily obtained in the acute setting. In addition, they may be associated with the risk of spinal cord injury.[7] In high-risk patients or when radiography is inadequate, CT is recommended because it has a diagnostic sensitivity higher than 99% and provides excellent osseous anatomic detail.[9] MRI allows additional visualization of soft-tissue structures. The main indication for MRI is the presence of neurologic deficit because it allows accurate diagnosis of the cause and location of neurologic compression, including osseous fragments, disk herniation, epidural hematoma, and spontaneously reduced instability. One meta-analysis reported that MRI also is sensitive for ligamentous injury on short tau inversion recovery or fat-suppressed T2-weighted images and is most sensitive within 72 hours after injury.[10] When there is high clinical suspicion of cervical spine instability or when a patient is unevaluable, MRI is the preferred imaging modality. MRI allowed identification of 20.9% of patients with cervical injuries not diagnosed by using radiography and/or CT.[10]

Anatomy

Craniocervical Junction

The craniocervical junction includes the occipitoatlantal and atlantoaxial articulations. The occipital condyles project downward, creating a "cup" that lies within the concavity (saucer) created by the atlantal lateral masses (**Figure 1**). Thus, spinal column stability exists if gravity and the alar ligaments, which project laterally and slightly cranially from the dens to the anterior-medial edge of the foramen magnum, and the tectorial membrane ligaments hold the occipital condyles downward. The tectorial membrane, which is the thickened continuation of the posterior longitudinal ligament spanning between the dens and the foramen magnum, is the other essential restraining ligament.

The atlas is a ring-like structure with large lateral masses connected by a short anterior arch and a longer posterior arch. The posterior arch is notched on its superior surface by the vertebral artery, which can be considered a weak location where fractures can occur. The inferior surface of the atlantal lateral masses is semiconvex and located directly above a similar facet articulation of the axis. These articulations have no bony stability to allow gliding and rotation needed for atlantoaxial rotation. The axis has a large body and large spinous processes. Most conspicuous is the dens or odontoid process, which projects in a cranial direction behind the atlantal anterior arch. Forward translation is prevented by the transverse ligament and secondarily by the alar ligaments. Biomechanically, the atlas acts as a bushing while the stabilizing ligaments extend from the axis to the occiput.

The other important craniocervical ligament is the cruciate ligament. This structure thickens horizontally, creating the transverse ligament that spans behind the dens and attaches to tubercles on the atlas. The transverse ligament prevents anterior atlantoaxial subluxation by maintaining the dens in apposition to the atlantal anterior arch. The anterior atlantal ligament extends from the posterior aspect of the atlantal anterior arch to the ventral aspect of the dens.[11] The authors of a 2012 study reported that the cruciate ligament was present in 81.3% of anatomic specimens and measured 4 × 4 × 4 mm. It was thought to tighten before the alar ligaments during atlantoaxial rotation. It also prevented posterior displacement of the dens.

Subaxial Anatomy

The subaxial cervical vertebrae have similar morphology, although they become larger caudally. Short, obliquely oriented pedicles connect the vertebral body to the lateral masses. The lateral masses are rhomboid shaped when viewed laterally and square shaped when viewed dorsally. The upward and downward projections of the lateral masses are the superior and inferior facets, respectively. Posteriorly, the lateral masses are connected by thin lamina that thickens in the midline. The spinous processes extend posteriorly from the lamina. The spinous processes are bifid from C3 to C5, and in most instances, C6.

Three articulations are present between each vertebra. The disk consists of the nucleus and anulus fibrosus. The anulus fibrosus has a strong collagenous structure and is important for stability. Two-paired synovial facet joints are oriented upward and help prevent anterior translation. The anterior and posterior longitudinal ligaments are broad and these ligaments are located on the anterior and posterior vertebral bodies, respectively. Posteriorly, the ligamentum flava spans between the lamina. The nuchal ligaments are the ligamentum nuchae, which strongly attach to the external occipital protuberance, C2, C7, and T1, and the supraspinatus and interspinous ligaments. The intervertebral joints are reinforced with facet capsules.

Occipital Condyle Fractures

Occipital condyle fractures occur in 1% to 3% of patients with blunt craniocervical trauma; in patients with an initial Glasgow Coma Scale score of 3 to 6, the incidence is reported as high as 4.4%.[12,13] The diagnosis is usually made using head or cervical spine CT scans. MRI studies are rarely required, although they will show intramedullary hemorrhage, epidermal hematoma, or disrupted ligaments and joint capsules. Impaired consciousness limits physical examination, but abnormalities in cranial nerve function suggest occipital condyle fractures.

The occipital condyles are perforated by the hypoglossal nerve (cranial nerve XII); just lateral to this is the jugular foramen containing cranial nerves IX, X, and XI. Injury to these nerves in combination is called Collet-Sicard syndrome.[14] One study reported that cranial nerve injuries occur in 40% of patients with occipital condyle fracture.[15] Cranial nerve deficits frequently occur or are recognized in a delayed fashion; the delay is associated with misdiagnosis or lack of proper treatment.[16] Because of associated head trauma, mortality occurs in up to 20% of patients.[17]

Fracture/Injury Classification

Occipital condyle fractures are classified based on morphology[18] (**Figure 2**). Type I fractures are comminuted without displacement. Type II fractures are associated skull base injuries that may or may not be displaced. Type III fractures are avulsion fractures from the alar ligaments. Occipital condyles may be bilateral, which suggests craniocervical dissociation (CCD). The critical determination of stability is based on displacement between the occipital condyles and C1 lateral masses. Type I and nondisplaced type II and III fractures are stable injuries; any associated displacement indicates an unstable injury.

Treatment

Stable injuries are managed with a cervical collar.[19] Unstable and displaced injuries should be treated as described for CCD, usually with occipital cervical fusion. Treatment with a halo vest may be considered for patients with less severe injuries. A study of 31 patients with occipital condyle fracture with a 27-month follow-up found low levels of disabilities, but 21% of patients had moderate or severe disability.[17] The disability was not thought to be directly caused by the occipital condyle fracture; rather, it resulted from the overall pattern of injury. Another study reported

6: Trauma

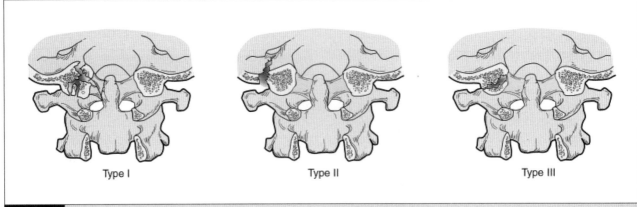

Figure 2 Illustrations demonstrate occipital condyle fracture classification. See text for details.

similar results in 28 patients with nondisplaced fractures treated nonsurgically.[19]

Craniocervical Dissociation

CCDs are injuries between the occiput atlas and axis, including atlanto-occipital dislocations and atlantoaxial diastasis. As with other areas of the spine, injuries represent a continuum of stability. CCD results from disruption of the ligaments spanning the craniocervical junction. This injury continues to be difficult to diagnose, and failure to make a diagnosis results in neurologic injury or death.[20]

Associated neurologic deficits are common, including traumatic brain injury in more than 50% of injuries and cranial nerve deficits in 48% of injuries.[6] The most frequent cranial nerve deficits are VI, X, and XII. Carotid and vertebral artery injuries are seen in 10% to 50% of CCDs; stroke occurs in 20% of patients with vascular injuries.[21,22] Screening with CT angiography is recommended for all patients with CCD.

Diagnosis

Most patients who have sustained blunt trauma undergo CT that includes the craniocervical junction. The anatomy of the craniocervical junction is complex, and the essential stabilizing structures are ligaments that are poorly visualized on CT and even on MRI. Various radiographic parameters aid in the diagnosis of CCD. The most sensitive is the occipital condyle–C1 interval (CCI),[23] which defines the apposition of the occipital condyle convexity to the concavity in the atlantal lateral mass. This articulation should always be congruent and symmetric. A threshold level of greater than 1.5 mm in adults indicates instability.[24] In addition to diastasis between the occipital condyles and atlantal lateral masses, abnormal displacement may occur between the atlas and axis. MRI findings aid in the diagnosis of ligamentous disruption.[25] Important findings include diastasis of either the occipital-C1 or atlantoaxial joints and disruption of the cruciate ligament.[26] Injury of these articulations may occur together.

Classification

Injuries are traditionally classified by direction, which is not clinically helpful because the direction of displacement simply reflects the head position relative to the thoracic spine.[25] A more functional classification based on CT and MRI findings has been proposed.[27] Type 1 injuries are stable and have suspected ligamentous injury on MRI studies, but normal alignment on CT scans and traction radiographs. Type 2 injuries also have normal CT findings, but have displacement greater than 2 mm on a traction test. Type 3 injuries are unstable and are displaced on CT, MRI, or static imaging. A new classification of CCD separates injuries that occur only at the atlanto-occipital joint, those only at the atlantoaxial joint, and those that occur at both locations.[26]

Initial Treatment

CCD requires immediate treatment to avoid displacement and neurologic deterioration (**Figure 3**). Patients are immobilized with a collar, and transportation within the hospital should be limited. Traction is contraindicated because of potential neurologic deterioration. In displaced craniocervical injuries, reduction and stabilization may be achieved with a halo vest.[24] Immobilization and use of an external orthosis while awaiting early surgery is not associated with risk of neurologic injury.[25] An upright position of 30° to 40° allows gravity to aid reduction when vertical diastasis is present. For displaced injuries, urgent surgery should be considered.

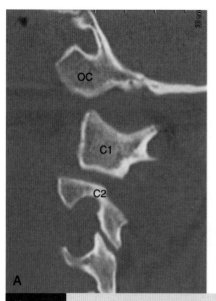 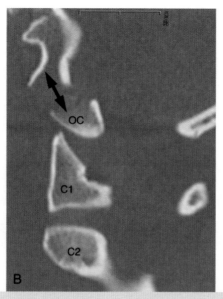 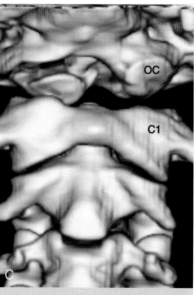

Figure 3 Images from a 24-year-old man who sustained injuries to cranial nerves VI and XII and incomplete spinal cord injury after a motorcycle crash. Sagittal CT scans show dislocation of left occipitoatlantal joints (**A**) and a displaced type II occipital condyle (OC) with dislocation on the right side (**B**). **C,** Frontal view of three-dimensional CT reconstruction shows anterior atlanto-occipital dislocation.

Definitive Treatment

For displaced injuries, occipitocervical fusion is recommended. A systematic review found that neurologic worsening developed in only 1 patient of 29 treated with early surgery; of 12 patients treated nonsurgically, treatment was successful in 5 and neurologic injury or inability to achieve stability occurred in 7 patients.[24] A knowledge gap exists in recommending the best treatment of patients with less severe injuries such as minimally displaced subluxations (Bellabarba type 2 injuries) because nonsurgical treatment outcomes are unknown.

In a report of 31 patients with craniocervical dislocation, 23 survived with treatment by occipitocervical fusion;[6] improved neurologic function was seen in 5 patients, 9 had no change, and 9 remained neurologically intact. Patient-reported outcomes showed persistent functional disabilities in survivors, but low levels of chronic pain. One-half of patients returned to work and one-half were disabled.

Atlas Fractures

Atlas fractures are common injuries, occurring in 10% of all cervical spine fractures.[28] As with other cervical injuries, the frequency is increasing, especially in the elderly population. Atlas fractures occur in combination with axis fractures in approximately 20% of patients.[5]

Classification

No new morphologic description has been proposed, and atlas fractures are evaluated by location (**Figure 4**). Type I injuries are stable anterior and posterior arch fractures. Type II injuries are combined anterior and posterior arch fractures (such as Jefferson fractures). Type IIA fractures have intact transverse ligaments, and type IIB have disrupted transverse ligaments. Type III fractures are lateral mass fractures that may have associated transverse ligament injury. One study noted that type III lateral mass split fractures with rupture of the transverse atlantal ligament (TAL) are at risk for progressive displacement.[29] The status of the TAL is an important measure of atlas fracture stability; these ligaments are considered to be disrupted when the lateral spread of the lateral masses exceeds 6.9 mm. The TAL injury can be an avulsion (type I) or midsubstance (type II).[30]

Treatment

Nonsurgical treatment is appropriate for stable and minimally displaced fractures with or without TAL injury. However, review of long-term outcomes showed poorer quality of life after an atlas fracture, which was independent of the treatment given.[31] In most instances, a collar can be used. Radiographs should be scrutinized for displacement of the lateral masses, which is seen best on the open-mouth view.

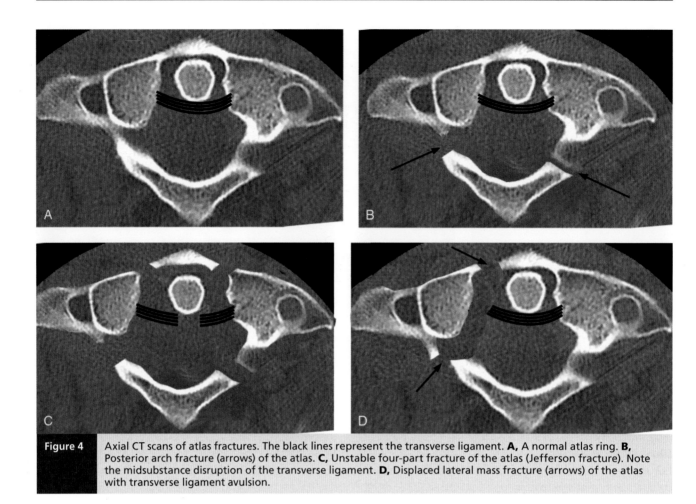

Figure 4 Axial CT scans of atlas fractures. The black lines represent the transverse ligament. **A,** A normal atlas ring. **B,** Posterior arch fracture (arrows) of the atlas. **C,** Unstable four-part fracture of the atlas (Jefferson fracture). Note the midsubstance disruption of the transverse ligament. **D,** Displaced lateral mass fracture (arrows) of the atlas with transverse ligament avulsion.

Outward displacement of the lateral masses results in loss of craniocervical and atlantoaxial motion and, rarely, cranial migration of the dens into the foramen magnum. The possibility of lateral mass screw fixation to maintain alignment is appealing because it results in osteosynthesis without fusion. Several techniques are possible, including posterior, transoral, transnasal, and transcervical.

One study reviewed 22 patients treated with posterior fixation at 2-year follow-up.[32] Fracture healing in all patients and satisfactory pain outcomes were reported, with mean visual analog scale scores decreased from 7.2 to 1.9. No loss of reduction or hardware failure was noted. In unstable burst-type fractures, the transverse ligament is disrupted and may not adequately heal despite direct fixation of the atlas ring, resulting in delayed C1-C2 instability. A review of 11 patients with atlas fractures with TAL injuries treated by posterior fixation reported no delayed instability;[30] in a systematic review, no such cases were reported in the literature.[33]

Atlantoaxial Instability

Atlantoaxial instability occurs when there is displacement of the C1-C2 articulations in any direction. Most commonly, this occurs following fractures, including odontoid, atlas, and occipital condyle fractures, as well as injuries to the transverse ligament. These injuries result in an increase in the atlanto-dens interval and have a poor prognosis for healing. Isolated transverse ligament injuries are best treated surgically with atlantoaxial fusion. However, atlantoaxial instability is often associated with CCD; if CCD is present, occipitocervical fusion is recommended.

Rotatory subluxation of C1-2 is a rare traumatic event, except in children, and is usually associated with TAL injury (**Figure 5**). In children, a trial of nonsurgical treatment by reduction and immobilization is recommended. In adults, atlantoaxial fusion should be performed for injury to the TAL.

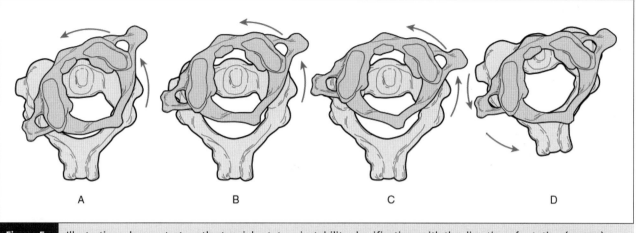

Figure 5 Illustrations demonstrates atlantoaxial rotatory instability classification, with the direction of rotation (arrows). Illustrations demonstrates atlantoaxial rotatory instability classification, with the direction of rotation (arrows). **A,** Type I: normal physiologic rotation of C1-C2. The atlas rotates around the dens and the transverse ligament is intact. **B,** Type II: rotatory fixation associated with a deficiency of the transverse ligament and 3- to 5-mm anterior displacement of the atlas. **C,** Type III: greater than 5-mm anterior displacement of the atlas on the axis. This type of instability is associated with both transverse ligament and alar ligament insufficiency. **D,** Type IV: posterior displacement of the atlas on the axis resulting from a deficient dens.

Axis Fractures

Axis fractures occur in 10% to 20% of all cervical fractures. Three injury types are considered: traumatic spondylolisthesis of the axis, odontoid fractures, and C2 body fractures. In addition, axis fractures occur frequently in combination with atlas and other cervical spine injuries.

Traumatic Spondylolisthesis of the Axis

Traumatic spondylolisthesis of the axis is a common fracture and has many variants. Initially described as a pars interarticularis fracture secondary to judicial hangings, traumatic spondylolisthesis occurs more frequently from hyperextension mechanisms. This injury is a traumatic separation of the anterior elements from the posterior elements. Classically, fractures occur in the pars interarticularis, but many variations are present. Other fracture locations include the pedicles, posterior vertebral bodies, and laminae. Fracture involving the posterior wall is termed the atypical hangman's fracture; rarely, an associated C2-C3 facet dislocation occurs. Anterior displacement at C2-C3 may occur when the anulus fibrosus is injured. These fractures may be associated with additional C2 body and type III odontoid fractures. The fractures may not be symmetric between the sides, implying an oblique vector mechanism.

Classification

Fractures are usually classified by the Levine system (**Figure 6**). Type I is a nondisplaced posterior element fracture. Type IIA has no displacement but significant angulation, and type IIB has more than 3 mm of anterior displacement. Type III is associated with C2-C3 facet dislocations. The atypical hangman's fracture is a fracture that involves the posterior vertebral body and is present in almost two-thirds of cases.[34]

Treatment

Type I fractures are stable and healing occurs in 10 to 12 weeks with nonsurgical treatment using a collar or orthosis. There is no consensus on the best treatment of type II fractures.[35] If nonsurgical treatment is attempted and displacement or angulation occurs, surgery can be considered. Rarely, displaced hangman's fractures can result in nonunion or malunion with nonsurgical treatment.

Recently, small case series have focused on various surgical techniques: anterior C2-C3 fusion with plate, osteosynthesis fixation with a C2 pedicle screw, C2-C3 fixation using pedicle screws, and posterior C1-C3 fusion.[36] Other series have proposed combining anterior fusion of C2-C3 with posterior fixation when adequate reduction cannot be achieved.[37] Anterior C2-C3 fusion has proved reliable for this injury and does not increase risk of vertebral artery injury.[36] Osteosynthesis using a posterior screw has the advantage of sparing motion, although the C2-C3 discoligamentous injury often results in anterior fusion. In one report of 23 patients treated with primary fixation, all experienced healing.[38] Translation and angulation were reduced, and patients had minimal disability on the Neck Disability Index. Pedicle screw fixation

6: Trauma

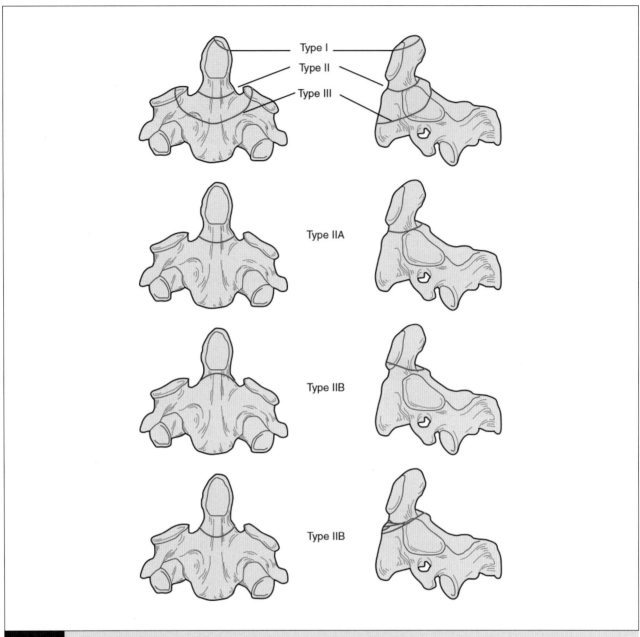

Type I
Type II
Type III

Type IIA

Type IIB

Type IIB

Figure 6   Illustrations demonstrate the classification of traumatic spondylolisthesis of the axis. See text for details.

across the fracture combined with C3 pedicle or lateral mass screws has been shown to be safe and effective.[39]

Type III fractures include dislocations of the C2-C3 facet articulations. This narrows the spinal canal, and spinal cord injury may occur. The treatment requires open reduction; the facet dislocations cannot be reduced with closed traction because of the pars interarticularis fractures. After open reduction, a C2-C3 posterior fusion with screw fixation is performed. Treatment of the traumatic spondylolisthesis component of this injury can be nonsurgical or by using pedicular fixation.

Odontoid Fractures
Classification
The classic Anderson and Alonzo system provides excellent prognostication and defines treatment pathways.[40] Type I fractures are avulsions of the dens tip from the alar ligaments, which are rare and may be associated with CCD. Type II injuries are fractures through the dens waist and have a relatively poor prognosis. On the open-mouth or coronal CT view, the fracture is superior to the atlantoaxial articulations. Type III injuries are transverse fractures into the body and enter the atlantoaxial articulations.

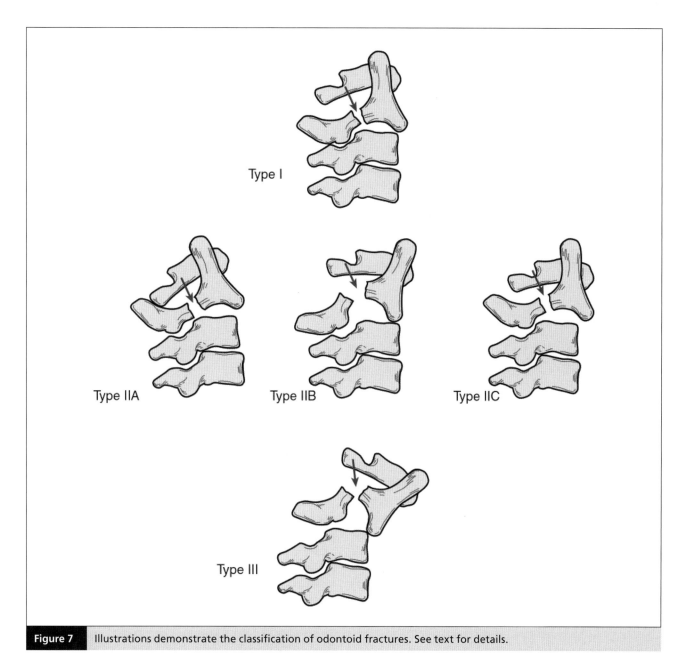

Figure 7 Illustrations demonstrate the classification of odontoid fractures. See text for details.

Fractures treated nonsurgically have a relatively good prognosis. A modification was proposed to help determine the treatment of type II fractures[41] (**Figure 7**). Type IIA injuries are transverse fractures. Type IIB injuries have an oblique fracture line from anterior-cranial to posterior-caudal that favors odontoid screw fixation. Type IIC injuries are comminuted or have an unfavorable obliquity for odontoid screw fixation. Odontoid fractures in geriatric patients are associated with erosive atlantoaxial arthrosis, which weakens the dens, and thus are considered insufficiency fractures.[42] Many of these injuries are stable because all soft tissues remain intact.

Treatment

All treatment decisions are based on low-quality evidence because a Cochrane systematic review could not identify any studies with criteria of high-enough quality on which to base treatment decisions for any fracture type.[43] Type I fractures should be investigated for any signs of CCD; fractures without CCD are stable and can be treated in collar. Type I injuries associated with CCD with minimal displacement may be treated nonsurgically, and displaced fractures are treated with occipitocervical fusion.

Type II odontoid fractures can be unstable and have high rates of nonunion (range, 25% to 50%) when treated nonsurgically.[35] Risk factors for nonunion are initial

6: Trauma

displacement of 5 mm or greater, angulation of 11° or greater, fracture comminution, instability despite immobilization, and a patient of advanced age.[35]

No consensus exists regarding optimal treatment.[35] Options include collar or halo vest immobilization, posterior fusion, and anterior screw fixation. The special cases of geriatric fractures are discussed later in this chapter. Evidence-based guidelines recommend external immobilization unless initial displacement is greater than 5 mm, angulation is greater than 11°, or when reduction cannot be maintained.[35] For displaced fractures or for those patients who cannot tolerate external immobilization, surgery should be considered.

A retrospective review reported the results of nonsurgical treatment of 66 patients with type II odontoid fractures.[44] Two-thirds were treated with halo vest immobilization; the rest were treated with a collar or custom brace. At 64-month follow-up, 92% had bony healing, 4% had fibrous pseudarthrosis, and 4% had unstable pseudarthrosis. Patients had mild to moderate symptoms of pain, functional disability, and psychologic disturbance based on health-related quality of life.

The odontoid screw provides the advantage of stability to allow healing without loss of atlantoaxial motion. A systematic review of odontoid screw fixation reported a 10% nonunion rate, a 10% rate of revision surgery, and a 10% incidence of persistent dysphagia.[45] Risk of poor outcomes was higher in geriatric patients. The use of one versus two screws remains controversial. One biomechanical study found no difference when comparing fixation with one versus two screws;[46] another study reported higher fusion rates in a clinical series using two screws.[47]

Posterior atlantoaxial fusion is an alternative procedure that provides stronger fixation than odontoid screws, but patients will lose 50% of head rotation. Several techniques can be used and must be tailored to the patient's anatomy and body habitus. The Magerl C1-C2 transarticular fixation and C1 lateral mass screws with C2 pedicle screws are the most common methods.[18] Prior to surgery, the vascular anatomy needs to be studied to plan screw trajectories to decrease the risk of injury to the vertebral artery. For cases in which bony anomalies exist, CT angiography should be performed because vascular anomalies also are frequently identified.[48] Using translaminar C2 screws is an alternative fixation method to lower the risk of vertebral artery injury, although these interfere with decortication for onlay bone grafting. Fusion rates are higher with the posterior technique compared with the anterior odontoid screws, but comparisons of clinical outcomes are lacking.[49]

Nonsurgical treatment of type III fractures (whether by using a collar or a halo vest) results in healing in approximately 85% of patients.[35] Therefore, the initial treatment is a trial of external immobilization and surgery is reserved for those whose alignment cannot be maintained or when initial displacement is greater than 5 mm.

Combined Atlas and Axis Injuries

Combined atlas and axis injuries are common, occurring in 25% of injuries in the upper cervical spine and 3% to 4% of all cervical injuries.[50] Management options include halo vest immobilization, cervical orthosis, and posterior fusion. The latter is reserved for those patients who cannot be managed nonsurgically or who have substantial displacement of the axis. The indications for surgery are similar to those for type II odontoid fractures. The surgical procedure needs to be individualized depending on fracture morphology and can include Magerl transarticular screws, the Harms technique, or occipitocervical fusion.

Fractures in Geriatric Patients

Odontoid fractures in elderly patients are reaching epidemic proportions and are recognized as resulting in high rates of morbidity, mortality, and poor quality of life.[2] A review of three centers found a 30-day mortality rate of 14.7% and a long-term mortality rate of 47.7% at a mean follow-up of 2.5 years.[51] Risk factors were older age, male sex, and increased patient comorbidities. Nonsurgical care was associated with higher mortality than surgical treatment. Increasingly, odontoid fractures are being recognized as insufficiency fractures, with erosive disease contributing to fracture in more than 50% of patients.[42]

No consensus exists on the optimal treatment of geriatric odontoid fractures. One study reported that nonsurgical care was associated with nonunion in 20% of patients compared with only 5% in surgically treated patients.[52] Despite attempted nonsurgical treatment, 25% of patients required surgery. Treatment failure, either death or worsening of disability, occurred in more than 50% of patients and in both treatment groups. Poorer health-related outcomes were associated with treatment failure. One study reported that patients in whom nonunion developed after nonsurgical treatment had similar outcomes to those who experienced union.[53] However, most patients required surgical treatment. Late neurologic deficits were not observed. A 2013 study found that surgically treated patients had improved health-related outcomes and lower mortality than nonsurgically treated patients.[54] Systematic reviews and meta-analyses comparing surgical and nonsurgical care published conflicting evidence of whether surgery offers advantages.[35,55,56] Currently, surgery for geriatric odontoid fractures should be considered for those patients with active lifestyles, without substantial comorbidities, and without impaired cognitive function.

Axis Body Fractures

Fractures of the axis body are a heterogeneous group of injuries that are usually stable and have a good prognosis. A systematic review classified these injuries by orientation of the fracture planes.[57] Vertically oriented fractures are type I when in the sagittal plane and type II when in the coronal plane. Type III injuries are transversely oriented. A rostral type III injury is equivalent to the type III odontoid fracture; a more caudal fracture may be associated with C2-C3 subluxation. Nonsurgical treatment was successful in most type I and type II injuries. Approximately 25% of type III injuries were treated surgically, and the most common indication was initial fracture displacement.

Lower Cervical Spine Injuries

Classification

Many classification systems for lower cervical spine injuries have been described based on presumed mechanism and morphologic characteristics. Recent advances focus on quantification of stability, modern imaging, and better predictive models to aid decision making for treatment.

Allen and Ferguson Classification

The Allen and Ferguson system is a mechanistic classification with the major patterns of compressive flexion, vertical compression, distractive flexion, compressive extension, distractive extension, and lateral flexion. Subcategories are based on the degree of anatomic disruption.[58] Interobserver reliability is only moderate when the major classifications are used.[59]

Cervical Spine Injury Severity Score

The Cervical Spine Injury Severity Score is based on a scoring system for the four columns of the cervical spine: anterior, posterior, and two lateral columns. Disruption of each column is graded on a scale of 0 to 5 and the sum of scores ranges from 0 to 20, with a sum greater than 7 generally requiring surgical treatment.[60] Intraobserver and interobserver reliability is high; however, the score does not provide a system to classify injuries.[59,61]

Subaxial Cervical Spine Injury Classification

The Subaxial Cervical Spine Injury Classification (SLIC) system is based on the injury morphology, the neurologic status of the patient, and the integrity of the discoligamentous complex.[62] Points are given for each category;

a higher point total represents a more severe injury and need for surgery. Moderate interobserver reliability has been demonstrated.

AOSpine Subaxial Cervical Spine Injury Classification

A recent update to the AOSpine Subaxial Cervical Spine Injury Classification system is based on injury morphology, facet injury, neurologic status, and case-specific modifiers.[63] Injuries are divided into type A, compression; type B, distraction; and type C, translation rotation. Intraobserver and interobserver reliability were shown to be substantial.[64,65] Additional studies are required to evaluate the clinical utility of the AOSpine Subaxial Cervical Spine Injury Classification.

Cervical Spine Instability

The classic definition of spinal instability is "the loss of the ability of the spine under physiologic loads to maintain its pattern of displacement so that there is no initial or additional neurological deficit, no major deformity, and no incapacitating pain."[66] This is a binary definition, but the clinical presentation of instability may be more nuanced. Checklists have been proposed, incorporating the variables of anterior or posterior column injury, translation, excessive angulation, distraction, and neurologic injury, but these have not shown substantial clinical use or validity.[66] The SLIC and Cervical Spine Injury Severity Score offer quantification of instability over a continuous range and may be used to aid in decision making.[67]

Treatment

The goals of surgery are to decompress neural elements when needed, reduce and maintain spinal alignment, and stabilize the spine until bony healing is achieved. Long-term goals are to maximize neurologic recovery while providing lasting stability to the injured segment. In addition to avoidance of further complications, the number of treated levels should be minimized, as should postoperative immobilization. Although algorithms may assist in the decision-making process, optimal treatment depends not only on neurologic status, the severity of injury, and the injury type, but also on concomitant injuries, comorbidities, and other patient-specific factors.[68]

General Principles of Nonsurgical Care

Nonsurgical care is warranted for patients who have stable fractures. Prolonged traction should be avoided. The use of the halo vest is limited because of poor patient acceptance and its limited effectiveness in the lower cervical spine. Most patients with stable injuries are treated with a hard collar or cervicothoracic orthosis; it is recommended that these devices be applied by a certified orthotist. Padding

6: Trauma

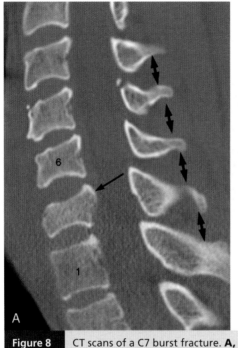
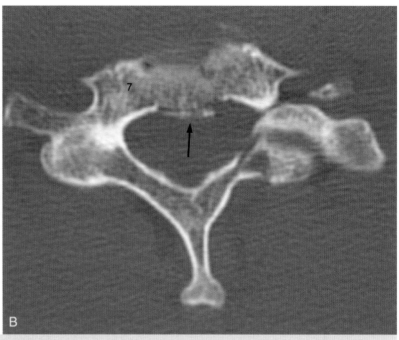

Figure 8	CT scans of a C7 burst fracture. **A,** Sagittal scan shows a C7 burst fracture (arrow) in a 22-year-old patient. The double arrows show that there is symmetric spread between the spinous processes indicating the absence of posterior ligamentous injury. **B,** Axial scan shows a lateral mass fracture (arrow) of C7 is present.

should wick away fluids and be able to be changed regularly. In cognitively impaired patients, the risk of decubitus ulceration is present; therefore, skin checks should be performed frequently. After orthosis application, the patient can be mobilized and an upright radiograph obtained, which is essential to confirm the efficacy of nonsurgical management. Displacement, angulation, development of increased pain, or any neurologic change indicates treatment failure and may require surgical treatment, which occurs in approximately 5% to 10% of patients. Education of the patient and family is essential to ensure proper brace management. Geriatric patients may have dysphagia when in an orthosis with aspiration risk, and a swallow consultation should be obtained before feeding. Because activities of daily living may be compromised, an occupational therapy consultation is recommended.

Management of Specific Types of Injuries
Type A Injuries
The treatments described in this section are based on the AOSpine Subaxial Cervical Spine Injury classification scheme. Type A0 injuries have no bony injury such as a central cord syndrome or have isolated process fractures. Isolated lamina fractures are uncommon and have fracture lines medial to the facet but lateral to the spinous process.[69] In the absence of neurologic or ligamentous injury, the injuries can be treated with a rigid orthosis

alone. Ventral displacement into the spinal canal with associated neurologic deficit has been described. In these cases, posterior decompression and stabilization is recommended. Spinous process fractures may be avulsion injuries of the lower cervical or upper thoracic levels from the pull of the supraspinous ligament[58] or a result of impaction occurring during hyperextension. Management is immobilization with a cervical orthosis. However, there may be associated posterior ligamentous disruption; therefore, vigilance is required to ensure maintenance of alignment with orthotic treatment.

Transverse process fractures are defined as a fracture of any portion of the transverse process and can extend into the foramen transversarium.[69] These injuries do not require immobilization and are associated with satisfactory outcomes.[70] Propagation into the foramen transversarium above C7 increases concern for vertebral artery injury.

Type A1 injuries are compression fractures involving a single end plate; type A2 fractures involve both end plates. Type A3 are burst fractures involving a single end plate with retropulsion of the posterior wall into the spinal canal (**Figure 8**). Type A4 are burst fractures involving two end plates. Type A fractures associated with flexion-distraction injuries are classified as type B injuries.

Type A1 and A2 fractures are uncommon in the cervical spine and usually are secondary to low-energy trauma

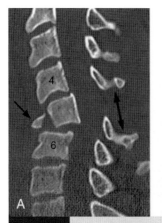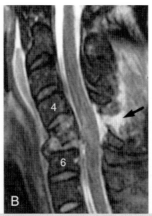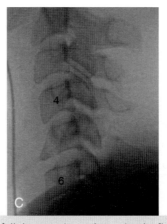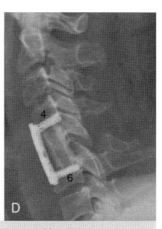

Figure 9   Images obtained from a 45-year-old woman who fell down stairs and sustained a flexion-axial loading injury to C5. **A,** Sagittal CT scan shows a teardrop fragment from the anteroinferior corner of the vertebral body (arrow), which has rotated into the spinal canal. The double arrow shows the spread in the spinous process. The patient presented with progressive neurologic deterioration. **B,** Sagittal T2-weighted fat-suppressed MRI shows complete posterior ligamentous disruption (arrow). The spinal cord is compressed and edema is seen within the ventral aspect of the spinal cord. **C,** Lateral fluoroscopic view obtained after C5 corpectomy and plate reconstruction. Cranial-tong traction (60 lb) shows excellent reduction of fracture. **D,** Lateral radiograph shows excellent realignment following anterior corpectomy with strut grafting and application of an anterior plate.

in the presence of osteoporosis. Isolated type A1 and A2 injuries are treated with cervical immobilization.

Type A3 and A4 burst fractures without posterior osteoligamentous involvement occur as a result of axial loading and are associated with the risk of neurologic injury. No new information is available on the best treatment of these injuries. In the absence of substantial retropulsion or neurologic injury, they may be managed in a rigid orthosis with close radiographic follow-up. If neurologic injury is present, surgical treatment with anterior corpectomy, strut grafting, and plating should be performed.[71] Nonsurgical treatment of type A4 injuries with more comminution of the body is theoretically more likely to fail.

Type B Injuries
Type B1 injuries are distraction injuries through the posterior bony structures. Type B2 injuries have posterior ligamentous disruption, resulting in kyphosis. The anulus fibrosus of the disk and posterior longitudinal ligament may be involved. Type B3 injuries are anterior tension band injuries usually resulting from hyperextension forces. All three injury types may have associated anterior body injuries, but the predominant nature of the injury distraction is either posterior or anterior. A type A3 burst fracture often has a posterior ligamentous injury and thus is classified as type B2 (the more severe component of the injury).

For type B1 bony injuries that theoretically have a high likelihood of healing, nonsurgical treatment may be attempted. If displacement occurs, either anterior or posterior fixation would be recommended.

Type B2 injuries are more common, with poor potential for healing. MRI with fat suppression is useful to determine the extent of ligamentous injury. Isolated posterior ligamentous injuries may have attempted closed treatment with an orthosis. Type B2 injuries are often associated with complex injuries such as flexion teardrop fractures (also called flexion axial loading injuries) and burst fractures.

The flexion teardrop fracture is a vertebral body fracture with a triangular or quadrangular anteroinferior vertebral body fragment with associated anterior cranial-caudal vertebral body height loss[69] (**Figure 9**). The fracture results from axial loading in combination with a flexion moment and common mechanisms include motor vehicle crash, diving into shallow water, and football spear tackling injuries. Instability varies widely and correlates with the degree of propagation through middle and posterior columns.

Stable injuries may present as isolated superior end plate fractures and can be treated with a hard cervical orthosis and close follow-up. Superior end plate fractures with neurologic injury may represent spontaneous relocation of a more unstable injury and mandate advanced imaging to evaluate for disk herniation or discoligamentous complex injury. Teardrop fractures with neurologic injury, vertebral displacement, or disruption of the discoligamentous complex are unstable and require surgical treatment. If displacement and spinal cord injury exist, awake closed reduction should be attempted using traction with Gardner-Wells tongs under radiographic guidance. If complete reduction is obtained and no persistent

6: Trauma

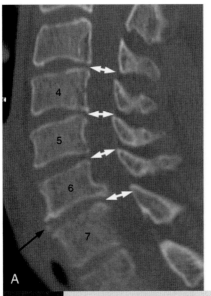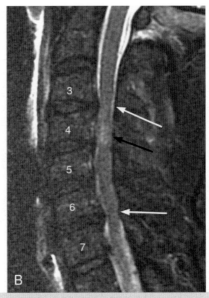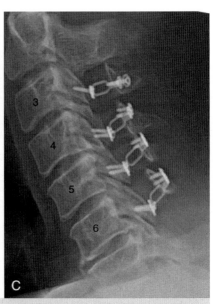

Figure 10 Images from a 57-year-old man who fell, hitting his face and hyperextending his neck. The patient had incomplete quadriplegia with no hand movement and grade 2 to 3 motor strength in the lower extremities. **A,** Sagittal CT scan shows spinal canal stenosis (white arrows) and possible fracture at C6-7 disk space (black arrow). **B,** MRI was performed because of an unexplained neurologic deficit. Spinal cord compression from stenosis is present from C3-4 to C6-7 (white arrows) as seen on sagittal T2-weighted MRI. Substantial spinal cord edema is noted at C4-5 (black arrow). **C,** The patient underwent plate laminoplasty and reconstruction. Postoperatively, the patient had an excellent neurologic recovery and regained all strength in his legs and upper extremities.

cord compression exists, posterior-only lateral mass screw-and-rod fixation may be sufficient.[72] If retrolisthesis persists after closed reduction, anterior corpectomy with strut graft and plating should be performed for adequate decompression and anterior column support. Effective treatment by using corpectomy and anterior plate fixation was reported in 21 patients.[73] Posterior fixation may be necessary based on the degree of posterior disruption. The burst fracture with posterior ligamentous disruption is treated similarly to the flexion teardrop fracture.

Type B3 injuries are disk distraction injuries and have an increasing incidence, especially in older patients who sustain falls that create extension forces to the cervical spine. In the mobile spine, hyperextension may result in failure of the anterior longitudinal ligament and disk tension. Subtle findings may include anterior soft-tissue swelling or anteroinferior avulsion fractures, whereas more severe injuries may reveal segmental hyperlordosis. However, the presentation of extension injuries varies and depends on the initial stiffness of the spine.

Hyperextension injuries in elderly patients with spondylotic and stenotic spines may result in spinal cord injury without overt structural instability (**Figure 10**). This often manifests as a central cord syndrome with disproportionate involvement of the upper extremities compared with the lower extremities. No consensus exists for the timing of intervention in patients with central cord syndrome.

Some authors advocate for initial nonsurgical management with subsequent decompression performed for inadequate recovery; others advocate for aggressive surgical decompression to potentially hasten recovery, shorten the length of hospitalization, and reduce associated morbidity.[74,75] Two recent systematic reviews reported that decompression performed within 24 hours of injury was safe and effective, but no recommendations could be made because of the lack of high-quality evidence.[75,76]

The ideal surgical technique for the treatment of central cord syndrome depends on cervical alignment and the number of stenotic segments. Single-level distraction-extension injuries such as type B3 injuries are treated with anterior diskectomy and fusion using a plate. Multilevel pathology in patients with lordotic or neutral alignment of the disks can generally be treated with laminoplasty or laminectomy and fusion (**Figure 10**). With focal kyphosis or stenosis, anterior decompression and fusion is recommended, although combined anterior and posterior approaches may be required to achieve adequate decompression and stability.

In patients with spinal ankylosis, the initial diagnosis is paramount because the diagnosis of patients is often delayed, causing neurologic deterioration, which results in death.[77,78] CT should be performed in patients with ankylosing spondylitis or those with diffuse idiopathic skeletal hyperostosis with spinal pain after trauma. MRI

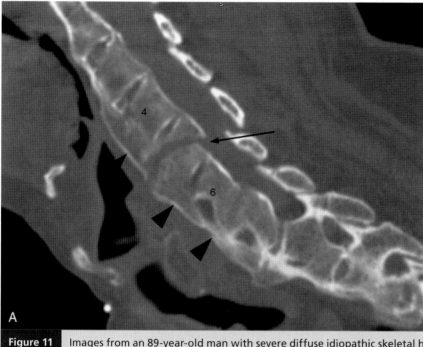
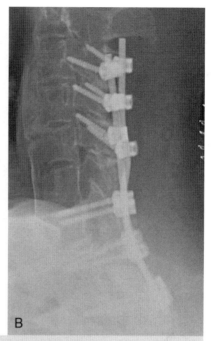

Figure 11 Images from an 89-year-old man with severe diffuse idiopathic skeletal hyperostosis who sustained a hyperextension injury. **A,** Sagittal CT scan shows large osteophytes, which are seen throughout the cervical spine (arrowheads). Note the posterior displaced fracture through C5 with complete spinal cord injury (arrow). **B,** Lateral radiograph obtained after placement of C3-T2 posterior instrumentation.

may be required if CT is inconclusive. Surgical treatment of subaxial cervical fractures in patients with ankylosing spondylitis is recommended unless medically contraindicated.[78,79] Nonsurgical treatment has a high incidence of displacement, kyphosis, and/or neurologic deterioration.[78] Long-segment posterior fixation is generally recommended to resist failure from long lever arm, but circumferential treatment may be required[80] (**Figure 11**).

Type C Injuries

Type C injuries are unstable and have displacement along any vertebral axis. These injuries are associated with many type A and B injuries but are classified as type C because of the displacement of one vertebra relative to another. Most type C injuries have facet fracture and dislocations.

Facet Injuries

Facet injuries are common and often result in vertebral subluxation, narrowing of the spinal canal, and spinal cord or nerve root injury. Whether facet fractures are unilateral or bilateral has a substantial influence on prognosis and treatment decisions. Type F1 facet injuries are nondisplaced facet fractures involving less than 40% of the facet or are less than 1 cm in height from the fracture to the tip of the facet and have low potential for subluxation. Type F2 facet injuries are fractures that involve more than

40% of the facet or are less than 1 cm in height from the fracture to the tip of the facet and have increased potential for displacement. Type F3 facet fractures also are known as fracture separation of the lateral mass. In this injury pattern, the lateral mass becomes free floating as a result of an ipsilateral pedicle and a laminar fracture. The mass can rotate forward, allowing subluxation of both cranial and caudal facet joints. Type F4 facet injuries are facet subluxations and dislocations with or without fracture. These can be combined with other vertebral body fractures or can be posterior subluxation from hyperextension vectors.

The treatment of type F1 and F2 lesions remains controversial. Surgical and nonsurgical treatment was compared in 40 patients with nondisplaced unilateral facet fractures.[81] Nonsurgical treatment was unsuccessful in 9 of 15 patients as a result of progressive subluxation; all but 1 patient treated surgically had successful healing. Unilateral facet injuries frequently result in rotational instability. These injuries are associated with discoligamentous injury.[81,82] Another study reported that 3 of 15 patients treated nonsurgically healed, and 20 of 24 surgically treated patients had good outcomes.[82] Attempts at nonsurgical management had no adverse effect on final pain scores.

Type F3 fracture-separation of the lateral masses may destabilize at the cranial or caudal level or both (**Figure 12**). A 2016 study reviewed 60 cases of cervical

6: Trauma

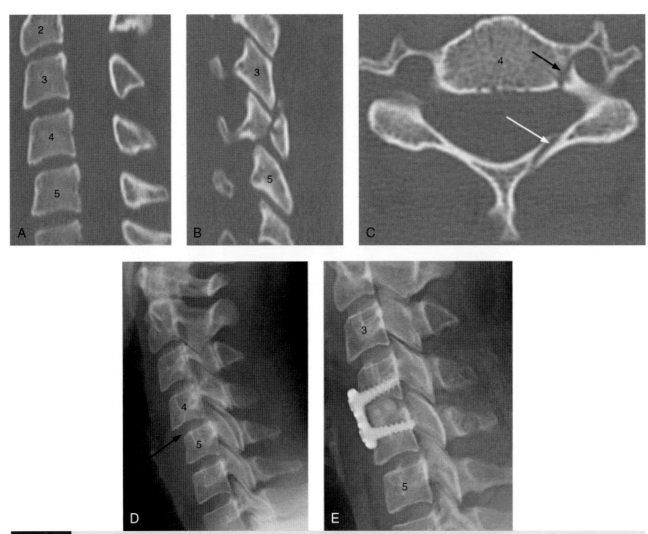

Figure 12 Images of a fracture-separation from a neurologically intact 25-year-old man. **A,** Sagittal CT shows no fracture or displacement. **B,** Sagittal CT obtained in the plane of the facets demonstrates a superior facet fracture exceeding 40% of the facet. **C,** Axial CT scan shows fracture-separation of the lateral mass of C4. The separation is created by pedicle fracture (black arrow) and fracture lamina (white arrow). **D,** Lateral weight-bearing radiograph demonstrates subluxation. The patient was treated with anterior diskectomy and plate fusion. **E,** Postoperative lateral radiograph shows excellent alignment.

fracture separations.[83] Associated injuries to the intervertebral disk and posterior ligamentous complex were present in more than 50% of cases. Disk injuries occurred much more frequently at the caudal level. Given the location of the vertebral artery within the lateral mass, vertebral artery injuries were noted in 22% of cases, although no patient experienced a stroke. Subluxation developed in all eight nonsurgically treated patients and six went on to surgery. Of the six patients initially treated with single-level fusion, subluxation developed in five at the cranial level. All two-level fusions treated with anterior or posterior approaches went on to heal, and none developed further subluxation. Fracture-separations were considered best treated with two-level fusions.

The treatment of type F4 facet injuries depends on the severity of the injury, the presence of neurologic injury, the location of neural compression, and whether the comminution is anterior or posterior. Unilateral facet dislocations without fracture that have been reduced with traction may be treated nonsurgically, although outcomes appear to be better with surgical treatment.[8,72,82,84] A systematic review of displaced unilateral and bilateral facet fractures found that surgical radiographic outcomes were superior, with 91% successful outcomes compared with 43% for nonsurgical care.[85] The data did not support superiority of an anterior or a posterior approach. This is consistent with previous randomized trials that showed similar results between anterior and posterior approaches.[72,84]

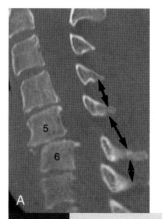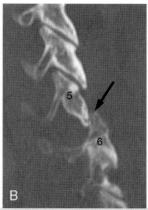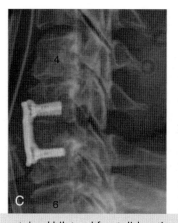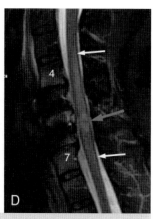

Figure 13 Images obtained from a 54-year-old woman who sustained bilateral facet dislocation at C5-6 and complete respiratory-dependent quadriplegia after vehicular trauma. **A,** Sagittal CT scan shows 30% subluxation, kyphosis, and widening of interspinous ligaments (arrows). The patient underwent immediate surgery for reduction and anterior cervical diskectomy and fusion at C5-C6. **B,** Sagittal scan of lateral masses shows facet dislocation at C5-C6 (arrow). **C,** Postoperative lateral radiograph demonstrates anterior fusion. **D,** Postoperative sagittal MRI demonstrates higher level of neurologic injury. Note extensive edema from C3-4 to C7 (white arrows). At the zone of injury, there appears to be hemorrhage and large area of edema (gray arrow).

The initial management of facet subluxation or dislocation is controversial.[86] Disk herniation can occur in 56% of unilateral and 82.5% of bilateral dislocations, and it has the potential to cause neurologic deterioration after reduction.[86] In patients who are neurologically intact or incomplete, two strategies have been used. The first is to obtain an MRI study before any reduction attempt. If a disk herniation is present, open reduction with anterior diskectomy, interbody fusion, and instrumentation is recommended. The other strategy is closed reduction with cranial tong traction, which can be used with an alert, cooperative patient. A postreduction MRI should be performed before surgical intervention to assess for residual stenosis. In patients with complete spinal cord injury and facet dislocation, realigning the spine with early closed reduction is recommended before obtaining MRI. Because no consensus exists, both patient and institutional factors must be considered when choosing the best treatment. Adequate staffing and equipment, ease of obtaining MRI, and operating room availability are all important factors to consider; expedient treatment of the patient is paramount.

Closed traction with Gardner-Wells tongs should be performed in a setting with appropriate monitoring. Initially, 10- to 15-lb weights should be used, with additional weight added under guidance of serial examinations and lateral imaging. Up to 140 lb of weight in larger patients at lower cervical levels has been used safely. Flexion or rotation maneuvers may be necessary in some patients to disengage the facets. Adequate visualization of the involved level is essential, and other levels also should be carefully examined for distraction of previously undetected injuries. After reduction is obtained, the traction weights usually can be decreased; however, larger weights may be necessary to maintain reduction in high-grade injuries or with facet fracture-dislocations. Neurologic deterioration during reduction requires slow removal of weight, emergent MRI to evaluate for etiology, and surgical decompression and stabilization.

Bilateral facet dislocations almost always require surgical treatment (**Figure 13**). Because either anterior or posterior fixation can yield successful results for the treatment of flexion-distraction injuries, the choice of approach is usually determined by the location of compression pathology and osseous comminution. A circumferential procedure may be required in severely comminuted injuries or with extreme ligamentous disruption.

Vertebral Artery Injury

Vertebral artery injuries are present in up to 11% of cervical spine injuries, and 75% of blunt vertebral artery injuries are associated with cervical spine fractures.[87] Common injury patterns that require screening with CT angiography or magnetic resonance angiography are complete cord injuries, CCD, atlantoaxial fractures, any fracture through the foramen transversarium, and facet fractures or subluxations. Symptomatic vertebral artery injuries are managed with anticoagulation and vascular or neurosurgery consultation. Endovascular procedures may be useful. The treatment of asymptomatic lesions is controversial but antiplatelet therapy is recommended.

Summary

Cervical spine injuries are common, occurring in 3% to 5% of all trauma patients. Patients must be rapidly evaluated and treated, with attention given to the prevention of further injury. A thorough history and physical examination along with appropriate imaging is mandatory. Injury classification systems with emphasis on fracture stability are evolving and are used to guide treatment and offer a common language to study these injuries. Ideal treatment maintains the structural and neurologic stability of the patient, while preserving motion segments and allowing for rapid mobilization. Surgical treatment may involve anterior, posterior, or circumferential treatment and depends on injury type, location of neurologic compression, and extent of comminution or ligamentous disruption.

Key Study Points

- Cervical spine injuries are common in patients sustaining blunt trauma, occurring in 3% to 5% of these patients.
- Identification of cervical spine injury and correct classification are essential to provide optimum management.
- Treatment is largely based on the presence of neurologic deficits and fracture stability.
- The goals of treatment are to protect the neural elements from further injury, stabilize fractures and dislocations, and provide long-term spinal stability.
- New surgical treatments that minimize fusion and soft-tissue trauma are available, but further research is needed.

Annotated References

1. Oliver M, Inaba K, Tang A, et al: The changing epidemiology of spinal trauma: A 13-year review from a Level I trauma centre. *Injury* 2012;43(8):1296-1300.

    The authors report on a retrospective review performed over a 13-year period at a level 1 trauma center. An increased frequency of spine injury occurred over the period, but the incidence of spinal cord injury and mortality decreased. Mortality decreased because injuries caused by motor vehicle crashes declined and injuries caused by falls increased.

2. Zusman NL, Ching AC, Hart RA, Yoo JU: Incidence of second cervical vertebral fractures far surpassed the rate predicted by the changing age distribution and growth among elderly persons in the United States (2005-2008). *Spine (Phila Pa 1976)* 2013;38(9):752-756.

    Using the Medicare database from 2006 to 2009, the authors of this study found that C2 fractures increased by 22% in the geriatric population, which was 2.5 times faster than population growth of that group. The greatest increase occurred in octogenarians.

3. Damadi AA, Saxe AW, Fath JJ, Apelgren KN: Cervical spine fractures in patients 65 years or older: A 3-year experience at a level I trauma center. *J Trauma* 2008;64(3):745-748.

4. Goldberg W, Mueller C, Panacek E, Tigges S, Hoffman JR, Mower WR; NEXUS Group: Distribution and patterns of blunt traumatic cervical spine injury. *Ann Emerg Med* 2001;38(1):17-21.

5. Cooper Z, Gross JA, Lacey JM, Traven N, Mirza SK, Arbabi S: Identifying survivors with traumatic craniocervical dissociation: A retrospective study. *J Surg Res* 2010;160(1):3-8.

6. Mendenhall SK, Sivaganesan A, Mistry A, Sivasubramaniam P, McGirt MJ, Devin CJ: Traumatic atlantooccipital dislocation: Comprehensive assessment of mortality, neurologic improvement, and patient-reported outcomes at a level 1 trauma center over 15 years. *Spine J* 2015;15(11):2385-2395.

    The authors of this study performed a retrospective study of 31 patients with atlanto-occipital injury. Eight patients died within 90 days, all of whom had received a delayed diagnosis. Higher Injury Severity Score and higher American Spinal Injury Association impairment scores were associated with a missed diagnosis. Follow-up disability and pain were moderate in survivors. Level of evidence: III.

7. Anderson PA, Gugala Z, Lindsey RW, Schoenfeld AJ, Harris MB: Clearing the cervical spine in the blunt trauma patient. *J Am Acad Orthop Surg* 2010;18(3):149-159.

8. Theodore N, Hadley MN, Aarabi B, et al: Prehospital cervical spinal immobilization after trauma. *Neurosurgery* 2013;72(suppl 2):22-34.

    This is an updated evidence-based guideline for the prehospital immobilization of patients with spinal cord injury. Based on moderate evidence, the authors recommend that all trauma patients with suspected spinal cord injury be immobilized using a hard collar and placed on a backboard. Patients who are awake, not intoxicated, without neck pain or tenderness, a normal neurologic examination, and no distracting injuries do not require immobilization. Level of evidence: IV.

9. Munera F, Rivas LA, Nunez DB Jr, Quencer RM: Imaging evaluation of adult spinal injuries: Emphasis on multidetector CT in cervical spine trauma. *Radiology* 2012;263(3):645-660.

    This review discusses the role of multidetector CT in identifying patients with blunt spinal injuries. CT has a sensitivity and specificity greater than 99%, which far exceeds plain radiography. X-ray reduction sequences to limit irradiation also are reviewed.

10. Muchow RD, Resnick DK, Abdel MP, Munoz A, Anderson PA: Magnetic resonance imaging (MRI) in the clearance of the cervical spine in blunt trauma: A meta-analysis. *J Trauma* 2008;64(1):179-189.

11. Tubbs RS, Mortazavi MM, Louis RG, et al: The anterior atlantodental ligament: Its anatomy and potential functional significance. *World Neurosurg* 2012;77(5-6):775-777.

    The anterior atlantodental ligament spanning between the dens and posterior aspect of the anterior atlas arch was identified in 13 of 16 cadaver specimens. It appears to resist posterior displacement of the dens and, with the alar ligaments, resist atlantoaxial rotation.

12. Dhall SS, Hadley MN, Aarabi B, et al: Nutritional support after spinal cord injury. *Neurosurgery* 2013;72(suppl 2):255-259.

    Guidelines regarding nutritional support after spinal cord injury were created after an evidence-based review. Based on level III evidence, the study authors recommend that nutritional support begin soon after injury, although its effect on neurologic recovery and risk of complications is unknown. Level of evidence: V.

13. Theodore N, Aarabi B, Dhall SS, et al: Occipital condyle fractures. *Neurosurgery* 2013;72(suppl 2):106-113.

    This updated evidence-based guideline on the diagnosis and management of occipital condyle fractures provides a level II recommendation (moderate evidence) that CT be used to establish the diagnosis and a level III (low evidence) recommendation for MRI to assess craniocervical ligaments. Only a weak level III recommendation was made for treatment of patients with stable injuries with an orthosis and those with displaced or unstable injuries with a halo vest or occipitocervical fusion.

14. Domenicucci M, Mancarella C, Dugoni ED, Ciappetta P, Paolo M: Post-traumatic Collet-Sicard syndrome: Personal observation and review of the pertinent literature with clinical, radiologic and anatomic considerations. *Eur Spine J* 2015;24(4):663-670.

    The authors present a case report and review of the literature of 14 patients who sustained occipital condyle and atlas fractures combined with injuries to the lower four cranial nerves. Three patients with neurologic injuries did not improve, whereas 11 had modest to complete recovery. Patients with neurologic injuries associated with atlas fractures did better than those with occipital condyle fractures. Level of evidence: IV.

15. Utheim NC, Josefsen R, Nakstad PH, Solgaard T, Roise O: Occipital condyle fracture and lower cranial nerve palsy after blunt head trauma: A literature review and case report. *J Trauma Manag Outcomes* 2015;9:2.

    The authors of this study review a case of occipital condyle fractures following the development of delayed palsies of cranial nerves IX through XII. The literature was reviewed and pertinent anatomy was discussed to explain cranial deficits and possible mechanisms for delayed presentations.

16. Rué M, Jecko V, Dautheribes M, Vignes JR: Delayed hypoglossal nerve palsy following unnoticed occipital condyle fracture. *Neurochirurgie* 2013;59(6):221-223.

    A case report of a missed diagnosis of an occipital condyle fracture with a hypoglossal nerve injury occurring 15 days later is presented. The authors emphasize the importance of cranial nerve examination of all trauma patients. Level of evidence: IV.

17. Mueller FJ, Fuechtmeier B, Kinner B, et al: Occipital condyle fractures: Prospective follow-up of 31 cases within 5 years at a level 1 trauma centre. *Eur Spine J* 2012;21(2):289-294.

    Of 31 patients with occipital condyle fracture, 22 survivors were evaluated at 1-year follow-up. One patient with atlanto-occipital instability underwent fusion and all others were treated nonsurgically. Moderate neck disability and poor health-related quality of life was observed, but this was considered to be a result of associated injuries. Level of evidence: IV.

18. Bransford RJ, Alton TB, Patel AR, Bellabarba C: Upper cervical spine trauma. *J Am Acad Orthop Surg* 2014;22(11):718-729.

    The authors provide a narrative review of upper cervical trauma. Level of evidence. V.

19. Maddox JJ, Rodriguez-Feo JA III, Maddox GE, Gullung G, McGwin G, Theiss SM: Nonoperative treatment of occipital condyle fractures: An outcomes review of 32 fractures. *Spine (Phila Pa 1976)* 2012;37(16):E964-E968.

    The authors of this study performed a retrospective study of 28 patients with occipital condyle fractures. Neck disability was mild and pain was usually described as a headache. In the absence of ligamentous injury, occipital condyle fractures can be managed nonsurgically. Level of evidence: IV.

20. Reis A, Bransford R, Penoyar T, Chapman JR, Bellabarba C: Diagnosis and treatment of craniocervical dissociation in 48 consecutive survivors. *Evid Based Spine Care J* 2010;1(2):69-70.

21. Mueller FJ, Kinner B, Rosskopf M, Neumann C, Nerlich M, Fuechtmeier B: Incidence and outcome of atlanto-occipital dissociation at a level 1 trauma centre: A prospective study of five cases within 5 years. *Eur Spine J* 2013;22(1):65-71.

    The authors reviewed five cases of atlanto-occipital dislocation (which occurs in 0.2% of all trauma cases) occurring over a 5-year period. Three patients died, one was quadriplegic, and one could ambulate and care for himself but had posttraumatic stress disorder. These poor outcomes emphasize the severity and critical location of this type of injury. Level of evidence: IV.

22. Vilela MD, Kim LJ, Bellabarba C, Bransford RJ: Blunt cerebrovascular injuries in association with craniocervical distraction injuries: A retrospective review of consecutive cases. *Spine J* 2015;15(3):499-505.

6: Trauma

Of 29 patients with unstable CCD who were evaluated for blunt cerebrovascular injury, 30 injuries were identified in 15 patients, and strokes were present in 20% of cases. Screening was recommended in all patients with CCD. Level of evidence: III.

23. Martinez-del-Campo E, Kalb S, Soriano-Baron H, et al: Computed tomography parameters for atlantooccipital dislocation in adult patients: The occipital condyle-C1 interval. *J Neurosurg Spine* 2016;24(4):535-545.

    In 81 patients, 22 of whom had atlanto-occipital dislocation and 59 who did not, an evaluation of the diagnostic effect of the occipital condyle–C1 interval, condylar sum, the Wholey and Harris intervals, Powers and Sun ratios, Wackenheim line, and Lee X-lines was performed using thin-slice CT. The threshold of 1.5 mm for the occipital condyle–C1 interval and 3 mm for the condylar sum had the highest sensitivity and specificity. Level of evidence: II.

24. Theodore N, Aarabi B, Dhall SS, et al: The diagnosis and management of traumatic atlanto-occipital dislocation injuries. *Neurosurgery* 2013;72(suppl 2):114-126.

    This updated evidence-based guideline for the diagnosis and management of atlanto-occipital dislocation injuries concluded that CT is the best diagnostic modality and the condyle–C1 interval was the most sensitive radiologic parameter. Based on weak evidence, posterior occipital fusion with instrumentation is recommended. The use of traction is not recommended because it is associated with a risk of neurologic deterioration. Level of evidence: IV.

25. Roy AK, Miller BA, Holland CM, Fountain AJ Jr, Pradilla G, Ahmad FU: Magnetic resonance imaging of traumatic injury to the craniovertebral junction: A case-based review. *Neurosurg Focus* 2015;38(4):E3.

    The study authors reviewed MRI and CT results from eight patients with traumatic injury to the craniocervical junction and performed a literature review. They found that specific anatomic measurements from CT were not reliable, and MRI should be performed when the diagnosis is considered. Level of evidence: III.

26. Radcliff K, Kepler C, Reitman C, Harrop J, Vaccaro A: CT and MRI-based diagnosis of craniocervical dislocations: The role of the occipitoatlantal ligament. *Clin Orthop Relat Res* 2012;470(6):1602-1613.

    In a review of 18 cases of craniocervical dislocation, the authors found that diastasis between the occipital condyles did not occur in isolation, whereas isolated diastasis between the atlantoaxial joints occurred in 5 patients; 6 patients had both occipitoatlantal and atlantoaxial joint displacement. MRI was useful in identifying associated soft-tissue ligamentous injury. Level of evidence: III.

27. Bellabarba C, Mirza SK, West GA, et al: Diagnosis and treatment of craniocervical dislocation in a series of 17 consecutive survivors during an 8-year period. *J Neurosurg Spine* 2006;4(6):429-440.

28. Matthiessen C, Robinson Y: Epidemiology of atlas fractures: A national registry-based cohort study of 1,537 cases. *Spine J* 2015;15(11):2332-2337.

    Using the Swedish National Patient Registry, the annual incidence and mortality of atlas fractures from 1997 to 2011 was determined. The overall incidence doubled; the incidence in 2011 was 17 per 1 million. Atlas fractures were more common in older patients, accounted for 10.6% of all cervical fractures, and were associated with axis fractures in 195 cases.

29. Bransford R, Falicov A, Nguyen Q, Chapman J: Unilateral C-1 lateral mass sagittal split fracture: An unstable Jefferson fracture variant. *J Neurosurg Spine* 2009;10(5):466-473.

30. Shatsky J, Bellabarba C, Nguyen Q, Bransford RJ: A retrospective review of fixation of C1 ring fractures: Does the transverse atlantal ligament (TAL) really matter? *Spine J* 2016;16(3):372-379.

    Twelve patients with atlas fractures and TAL disruptions were treated with posterior osteosynthesis. At follow-up, no patient had late atlantoaxial instability. Pain was minimal at final follow-up. Level of evidence: IV.

31. Dvorak MF, Johnson MG, Boyd M, Johnson G, Kwon BK, Fisher CG: Long-term health-related quality of life outcomes following Jefferson-type burst fractures of the atlas. *J Neurosurg Spine* 2005;2(4):411-417.

32. He B, Yan L, Zhao Q, Chang Z, Hao D: Self-designed posterior atlas polyaxial lateral mass screw-plate fixation for unstable atlas fracture. *Spine J* 2014;14(12):2892-2896.

    The study authors present a retrospective review of 22 cases of posterior fixation with a polyaxial screw-plate construct for unstable atlas fractures. At 12 months, all fractures had healed based on CT. The technique proved effective and safe. Level of evidence: IV.

33. Bednar DA, Almansoori KA: Solitary C1 posterior fixation for unstable isolated atlas fractures: Case report and systematic review of the literature. *Global Spine J* 2016;6(4):375-382.

    The authors performed a retrospective literature review identifying posterior fixation of atlas fractures. Results were satisfactory, with high a healing rate, and the procedure was safe. The authors concluded that despite good results, further research is needed in patients treated in such a manner who also have a transverse ligament injury. Level of evidence: IV.

34. Al-Mahfoudh R, Beagrie C, Woolley E, et al: Management of typical and atypical hangman's fractures. *Global Spine J* 2016;6(3):248-256.

    In this retrospective review of 41 patients with hangman's fractures, 3 patients were treated surgically and the rest were treated with an orthosis or a halo vest. All experienced healing. Nonsurgical treatment was concluded as appropriate for most patients. Level of evidence: IV.

35. Ryken TC, Hadley MN, Aarabi B, et al: Management of isolated fractures of the axis in adults. *Neurosurgery* 2013;72(suppl 2):132-150.

This updated evidence-based guideline for the management of combined atlas and axis fractures concluded, based on weak evidence, that treatment in most patients is determined by specifics of the axis fracture. In most cases nonsurgical treatment is the optimal treatment. Displaced axis fractures greater than 5 mm and those with excessive angulation (>11°) should be considered for surgery. Level of evidence: IV.

36. Schleicher P, Scholz M, Pingel A, Kandziora F: Traumatic spondylolisthesis of the axis vertebra in adults. *Global Spine J* 2015;5(4):346-358.

The authors performed a systematic review of management of traumatic spondylolisthesis of the axis. They could not identify high-quality evidence on which to base treatment decisions because most decisions are based on expert opinion and theoretic considerations.

37. Xie N, Khoo LT, Yuan W, et al: Combined anterior C2-C3 fusion and C2 pedicle screw fixation for the treatment of unstable hangman's fracture: A contrast to anterior approach only. *Spine (Phila Pa 1976)* 2010;35(6):613-619.

38. Shin JJ, Kim SH, Cho YE, Cheshier SH, Park J: Primary surgical management by reduction and fixation of unstable hangman's fractures with discoligamentous instability or combined fractures: Clinical article. *J Neurosurg Spine* 2013;19(5):569-575.

The authors of this study report that posterior reduction and screw fixation can be used to attempt to achieve stability in patients with a hangman's fracture and discoligamentous instability or in those with combined fractures. Level of evidence: IV.

39. Ma W, Xu R, Liu J, et al: Posterior short-segment fixation and fusion in unstable Hangman's fractures. *Spine (Phila Pa 1976)* 2011;36(7):529-533.

The authors retrospectively reviewed 35 patients with unstable hangman's fractures treated by posterior C2-C3 fixation. Healing occurred in all patients, but CT demonstrated screw malposition towards the vertebral artery and towards the spinal canal at C3 in 12 patients. Level of evidence: IV.

40. Anderson LD, D'Alonzo RT: Fractures of the odontoid process of the axis. *J Bone Joint Surg Am* 1974;56(8):1663-1674.

41. Grauer JN, Shafi B, Hilibrand AS, et al: Proposal of a modified, treatment-oriented classification of odontoid fractures. *Spine J* 2005;5(2):123-129.

42. Shinseki MS, Zusman NL, Hiratzka J, Marshall LM, Yoo JU: Association between advanced degenerative changes of the atlanto-dens joint and presence of dens fracture. *J Bone Joint Surg Am* 2014;96(9):712-717.

The authors compared CT scans of the cervical spine in 56 patients older than 55 years with a dens fracture with CT scans from a large group without a dens fracture. Erosive degenerative changes, including intraosseous cysts, were seen in 64% of the group with a dens fracture compared with only 16% of group without a dens fracture. The authors concluded that the erosive changes and cyst formation were associated with dens fracture. Level of evidence: II.

43. Shears E, Armitstead CP: Surgical versus conservative management for odontoid fractures. *Cochrane Database Syst Rev* 2008;4:CD005078.

44. Butler JS, Dolan RT, Burbridge M, et al: The long-term functional outcome of type II odontoid fractures managed non-operatively. *Eur Spine J* 2010;19(10):1635-1642.

45. Tian NF, Hu XQ, Wu LJ, et al: Pooled analysis of nonunion, re-operation, infection, and approach related complications after anterior odontoid screw fixation. *PLoS One* 2014;9(7):e103065.

A retrospective review of 14 cases of posterior fixation of hangman's fractures assisted by an intraoperative three-dimensional fluoroscopy-based navigation showed that all patients healed and no complications occurred. Screw malposition occurred in five patients but resulted in no clinical consequences.

46. Feng G, Wendlandt R, Spuck S, Schulz AP: One-screw fixation provides similar stability to that of two-screw fixation for type II dens fractures. *Clin Orthop Relat Res* 2012;470(7):2021-2028.

The authors conducted a biomechanical experiment comparing a single screw with two screws for simulated odontoid fracture fixation. They found a similar stabilizing effect from both techniques, although neither restored normal resistance to shear or torsion.

47. Dailey AT, Hart D, Finn MA, Schmidt MH, Apfelbaum RI: Anterior fixation of odontoid fractures in an elderly population. *J Neurosurg Spine* 2010;12(1):1-8.

48. Yamazaki M, Okawa A, Furuya T, et al: Anomalous vertebral arteries in the extra- and intraosseous regions of the craniovertebral junction visualized by 3-dimensional computed tomographic angiography: Analysis of 100 consecutive surgical cases and review of the literature. *Spine (Phila Pa 1976)* 2012;37(22):E1389-E1397.

Of 100 consecutive patients treated with craniocervical instrumentation and evaluated for bony and vascular anomalies, 10 had vascular anomalies. Thirty-one cases had a high-riding vertebral artery in C2 that was at risk surgically, although no vascular injuries occurred. Increased vascular anomalies were associated with bony anomalies. Level of evidence: III.

49. Shen Y, Miao J, Li C, et al: A meta-analysis of the fusion rate from surgical treatment for odontoid factures: Anterior odontoid screw versus posterior C1-C2 arthrodesis. *Eur Spine J* 2015;24(8):1649-1657.

This meta-analysis found a higher fusion rate with a posterior approach using an odontoid screw in older patients, but not in younger patients. However, substantial heterogeneity was present, limiting the strength of conclusions. Functional outcome and pain were not evaluated.

50. Ryken TC, Hadley MN, Aarabi B, et al: Management of acute combination fractures of the atlas and axis in adults. *Neurosurgery* 2013;72(suppl 2):151-158.

   The management of acute combination fractures of the atlas and axis through 2010 was summarized. Combination injuries are relatively frequent and have an increased incidence of neurologic deficit compared with isolated injury. Axis fracture subtype usually determines the management strategy. Level III evidence supports that most injuries are treated with external immobilization. C1 with type II odontoid combination fractures with an atlantodental ratio of 5 mm or greater and C1 with hangman's combination fractures with C2-C3 angulation of 11° or greater should be considered for surgical treatment.

51. Chapman J, Smith JS, Kopjar B, et al: The AOSpine North America Geriatric Odontoid Fracture Mortality Study: A retrospective review of mortality outcomes for operative versus nonoperative treatment of 322 patients with long-term follow-up. *Spine (Phila Pa 1976)* 2013;38(13):1098-1104.

   This retrospective review of 322 patients age 65 years or older with type II odontoid fractures demonstrated that surgically treated patients had a 30-day survival advantage and trend toward improved long-term survival compared with nonsurgically treated patients. Surgically treated patients had longer hospital and intensive care unit stays and were more likely to receive a feeding tube. Level of evidence: IV.

52. Fehlings MG, Arun R, Vaccaro AR, Arnold PM, Chapman JR, Kopjar B: Predictors of treatment outcomes in geriatric patients with odontoid fractures: AOSpine North America multi-centre prospective GOF study. *Spine (Phila Pa 1976)* 2013;38(11):881-886.

   This multicenter prospective cohort study examined 159 elderly patients with type II odontoid fractures for predictors of treatment failure. Older age, initial nonsurgical treatment, and male sex were associated with failure of treatment, as defined by death, decline in neck disability by 9.5 points, or major treatment-related complication. One-year mortality was 18.2%. Level of evidence: I.

53. Smith HE, Kerr SM, Fehlings MG, et al: Trends in epidemiology and management of type II odontoid fractures: 20-year experience at a model system spine injury tertiary referral center. *J Spinal Disord Tech* 2010;23(8):501-505.

54. Vaccaro AR, Kepler CK, Kopjar B, et al: Functional and quality-of-life outcomes in geriatric patients with type-II dens fracture. *J Bone Joint Surg Am* 2013;95(8):729-735.

   Validated clinical measures were used to assess outcomes and complications in 159 patients with type II dens fracture who were treated surgically (101 patients) and nonsurgically (58 patients). The patients who received surgical treatment had significantly better outcomes than the nonsurgical group. Although the rate of complications was similar in both groups, patients who received surgical treatment had a significantly lower nonunion rate.

55. Schroeder GD, Kepler CK, Kurd MF, et al: A systematic review of the treatment of geriatric type II odontoid fractures. *Neurosurgery* 2015;77(suppl 4):S6-S14.

   This systematic review of type II odontoid fractures in patients older than 60 years resulted in 21 articles with 1,233 patients. Short-term and long-term mortality were lower in patients who underwent surgical treatment versus nonsurgical treatment, and no differences were reported in the rates of complications between the two groups. Choice of surgical approach (anterior or posterior) and type of external orthosis (hard collar or halo vest) did not affect rates of complications or mortality.

56. Yang Z, Yuan ZZ, Ma JX, Ma XL: Conservative versus surgical treatment for type II odontoid fractures in the elderly: Grading the evidence through a meta-analysis. *Orthop Traumatol Surg Res* 2015;101(7):839-844.

   This meta-analysis reviewed 12 studies with 730 elderly patients with type II odontoid fractures (441 treated nonsurgically and 289 treated surgically). No difference was found between the surgical and nonsurgical groups regarding mortality, but nonsurgical treatment had a higher rate of nonunion.

57. Kepler CK, Vaccaro AR, Fleischman AN, et al: Treatment of axis body fractures: A systematic review. *Clin Spine Surg* 2016 [Epub ahead of print].

   In this study, 920 patients with C2 body fractures from 52 studies were systematically reviewed. Most fractures were treated nonsurgically, but a trend toward increasing surgical intervention was noted. The overall union rate was 91%. The risk of nonunion included higher degrees of subluxation, displacement, comminution, concomitant injury, delay in treatment, and older age.

58. Allen BL Jr, Ferguson RL, Lehmann TR, O'Brien RP: A mechanistic classification of closed, indirect fractures and dislocations of the lower cervical spine. *Spine (Phila Pa 1976)* 1982;7(1):1-27.

59. Stone AT, Bransford RJ, Lee MJ, et al: Reliability of classification systems for subaxial cervical injuries. *Evid Based Spine Care J* 2010;1(3):19-26.

60. Anderson PA, Moore TA, Davis KW, et al; Spinal Trauma Study Group: Cervical spine injury severity score: Assessment of reliability. *J Bone Joint Surg Am* 2007;89(5):1057-1065.

61. Zehnder SW, Lenarz CJ, Place HM: Teachability and reliability of a new classification system for lower cervical spinal injuries. *Spine (Phila Pa 1976)* 2009;34(19):2039-2043.

62. Vaccaro AR, Hulbert RJ, Patel AA, et al; Spine Trauma Study Group: The subaxial cervical spine injury classification system: A novel approach to recognize the importance of morphology, neurology, and integrity of the disco-ligamentous complex. *Spine (Phila Pa 1976)* 2007;32(21):2365-2374.

63. Vaccaro AR, Koerner JD, Radcliff KE, et al: AOSpine subaxial cervical spine injury classification system. *Eur Spine J* 2016;25(7):2173-2184.

A subaxial cervical spine injury classification was developed by experts using a consensus process. The classification is based on three injury morphologies: A, compression; B, tension band; and C, translation with additional descriptors for facet injury, patient factors, and neurologic status. Intraobserver and interobserver reliability were substantial across all subtypes.

64. Silva OT, Sabba MF, Lira HI, et al: Evaluation of the reliability and validity of the newer AOSpine subaxial cervical injury classification (C-3 to C-7). *J Neurosurg Spine* 2016;25(3):303-308.

Fifty-one patients were reviewed by five surgeons in a study to evaluate the reliability and validity of the AOSpine Subaxial Cervical Injury classification. General reliability was acceptable for the major group classifications, but limitations for subgroups were identified. Only mild (type A0) and severe (type C) had a high rate of interobserver agreement and type B injuries were rarely diagnosed. Level of evidence: II.

65. Urrutia J, Zamora T, Campos M, et al: A comparative agreement evaluation of two subaxial cervical spine injury classification systems: The AOSpine and the Allen and Ferguson schemes. *Eur Spine J* 2016;25(7):2185-2192.

Imaging of 65 patients with subaxial cervical spine injuries were reviewed by six evaluators to compare agreement evaluation of the AOSpine and Allen and Ferguson classification systems. For interobserver agreement, the main AO injury types had substantial agreement, AO subtypes showed moderate agreement, and the Allen and Ferguson classification had significantly lower agreement. Intraobserver reliability was substantial for all classification schemes. No differences were found between level of training or by specific injury type. Level of evidence: II.

66. White AA III, Panjabi MM: Update on the evaluation of instability of the lower cervical spine. *Instr Course Lect* 1987;36:513-520.

67. Dvorak MF, Fisher CG, Fehlings MG, et al: The surgical approach to subaxial cervical spine injuries: An evidence-based algorithm based on the SLIC classification system. *Spine (Phila Pa 1976)* 2007;32(23):2620-2629.

68. Gelb DE, Aarabi B, Dhall SS, et al: Treatment of subaxial cervical spinal injuries. *Neurosurgery* 2013;72(suppl 2):187-194.

This summary of level III evidence and treatment recommendations for subaxial cervical spinal injuries reported that the broad spectrum of injuries requires tailored treatment, but the goals remain decompression of the spinal cord and stable immobilization to allow for early mobilization and rehabilitation. Both anterior and posterior approaches are acceptable in patients not requiring specific ventral or dorsal decompression. Patients with ankylosed spines should undergo advanced imaging routinely, even after minor trauma. Surgical treatment should be either long-segment posterior fixation or combined anterior and posterior fixation to avoid failure.

69. Bono CM, Schoenfeld A, Gupta G, et al: Reliability and reproducibility of subaxial cervical injury description system: A standardized nomenclature schema. *Spine (Phila Pa 1976)* 2011;36(17):E1140-E1144.

Eleven injury types and definitions were established and refined for subaxial cervical spine injuries. Eighteen cases were reviewed and moderate interrater and substantial intrarater agreement were demonstrated; however, only four injury subtypes demonstrated greater than 50% interrater agreement (burst, lateral mass, flexion teardrop, and anterior distraction injuries). Level of evidence: III.

70. Schotanus M, van Middendorp JJ, Hosman AJ: Isolated transverse process fractures of the subaxial cervical spine: A clinically insignificant injury or not? A prospective, longitudinal analysis in a consecutive high-energy blunt trauma population. *Spine (Phila Pa 1976)* 2010;35(19):E965-E970.

71. Koivikko MP, Myllynen P, Karjalainen M, Vornanen M, Santavirta S: Conservative and operative treatment in cervical burst fractures. *Arch Orthop Trauma Surg* 2000;120(7-8):448-451.

72. Brodke DS, Anderson PA, Newell DW, Grady MS, Chapman JR: Comparison of anterior and posterior approaches in cervical spinal cord injuries. *J Spinal Disord Tech* 2003;16(3):229-235.

73. Kim HJ, Lee KY, Kim WC: Treatment outcome of cervical tear drop fracture. *Asian Spine J* 2009;3(2):73-79.

74. Brodell DW, Jain A, Elfar JC, Mesfin A: National trends in the management of central cord syndrome: An analysis of 16,134 patients. *Spine J* 2015;15(3):435-442.

In a cohort of 16,134 patients with central cord syndrome from the nationwide inpatient sample, 39.7% underwent surgical treatment, most commonly anterior cervical decompression and fusion, then posterior cervical decompression and fusion, and posterior cervical decompression. Surgical management increased over the study period. Inpatient mortality was 2.6%. Risk factors for mortality included increased age, medical comorbidities, rural hospitals, and low income.

75. Aarabi B, Hadley MN, Dhall SS, et al: Management of acute traumatic central cord syndrome (ATCCS). *Neurosurgery* 2013;72(suppl 2):195-204.

This summary of level III evidence through 2011 on the treatment of acute traumatic central cord syndrome supports aggressive medical management, including intensive care unit care and mean arterial pressure goals of 85 to 90 mm Hg after the initial injury. Level III evidence supports that surgery is safe and effective. Early reduction of fracture-dislocation and surgical decompression of ongoing spinal cord compression is recommended.

76. Anderson KK, Tetreault L, Shamji MF, et al: Optimal timing of surgical decompression for acute traumatic central

6: Trauma

cord syndrome: A systematic review of the literature. *Neurosurgery* 2015;77(suppl 4):S15-S32.

This systematic review was performed to determine if timing of surgery for traumatic central cord syndrome is important for neurologic outcome, length of hospital stay, and complications. Earlier surgery (either less than 24 hours or less than 2 weeks) seemed to improve recovery compared with later surgery and was not associated with increased length of hospital stay or mortality; however, levels of evidence for these recommendations were low.

77. Schiefer TK, Milligan BD, Bracken CD, et al: In-hospital neurologic deterioration following fractures of the ankylosed spine: A single-institution experience. *World Neurosurg* 2015;83(5):775-783.

Patients with vertebral fractures in the setting of diffuse idiopathic skeletal hyperostosis or ankylosing spondylitis were retrospectively reviewed. Neurologic deterioration after initial presentation occurred in 8.6% of patients. Postoperative neurologic deterioration occurred in 7.6% of surgically managed patients; 1-year mortality was 23%. Older age and higher presenting neurologic function predicted 1-year functional outcome.

78. Caron T, Bransford R, Nguyen Q, Agel J, Chapman J, Bellabarba C: Spine fractures in patients with ankylosing spinal disorders. *Spine (Phila Pa 1976)* 2010;35(11):E458-E464.

79. Robinson Y, Willander J, Olerud C: Surgical stabilization improves survival of spinal fractures related to ankylosing spondylitis. *Spine (Phila Pa 1976)* 2015;40(21):1697-1702.

A review of the Swedish mortality registry identified 919 patients with ankylosing spondylitis, with 1,131 spinal fractures. Surgical treatment was associated with improved survival. Spinal cord injury was the highest predictor of mortality. Level of evidence: III.

80. Robinson Y, Robinson AL, Olerud C: Complications and survival after long posterior instrumentation of cervical and cervicothoracic fractures related to ankylosing spondylitis or diffuse idiopathic skeletal hyperostosis. *Spine (Phila Pa 1976)* 2015;40(4):E227-E233.

Forty-one patients with cervical and cervicothoracic fractures were followed prospectively after posterior instrumentation. Complication rates were high and included five with surgical site infection, three with pneumonia, two who required tracheostomy, and one cerebrospinal fluid leak. No cases of implant failure or nonunion were reported. Survival was affected by age, sex, smoking, and presence of spinal cord injury. Level of evidence: III.

81. Aarabi B, Mirvis S, Shanmuganathan K, et al: Comparative effectiveness of surgical versus nonoperative management of unilateral, nondisplaced, subaxial cervical spine facet fractures without evidence of spinal cord injury: Clinical article. *J Neurosurg Spine* 2014;20(3):270-277.

Outcomes of 25 patients with unilateral, nondisplaced, subaxial facet fractures, 10 of whom were surgically treated and 15 of whom were nonsurgically treated, were analyzed. Fractures occurred most commonly at C7.

Nonsurgical treatment and younger patient age predicted treatment failure irrespective of fracture plane, instability, and SLIC scores. Level of evidence: IV.

82. Lee SH, Sung JK: Unilateral lateral mass-facet fractures with rotational instability: New classification and a review of 39 cases treated conservatively and with single segment anterior fusion. *J Trauma* 2009;66(3):758-767.

83. Manoso MW, Moore TA, Agel J, Bellabarba C, Bransford RJ: Floating lateral mass fractures of the cervical spine. *Spine (Phila Pa 1976)* 2016;41(18):1421-1427.

A retrospective study of 60 patients who sustained fracture separation of the lateral mass was performed. Subluxation developed in all the patients who were treated nonsurgically, and 75% of those patients ultimately required surgery. Single-level anterior cervical fusion was associated with the development of subluxation at the adjacent level, whereas two-level fusions had the best clinical and radiographic results. Level of evidence: IV.

84. Kwon BK, Fisher CG, Boyd MC, et al: A prospective randomized controlled trial of anterior compared with posterior stabilization for unilateral facet injuries of the cervical spine. *J Neurosurg Spine* 2007;7(1):1-12.

85. Kepler CK, Vaccaro AR, Chen E, et al: Treatment of isolated cervical facet fractures: A systematic review. *J Neurosurg Spine* 2015;1-8.

A systematic review of facet fractures found that surgical treatment was associated with improved clinical and radiographic outcomes. Anterior fusion achieved better results than posterior fusion; however, many of the studies reporting on posterior fusion used outmoded wire fixation. Level of evidence: IV.

86. Ryken TC, Hurlbert RJ, Hadley MN, et al: The acute cardiopulmonary management of patients with cervical spinal cord injuries. *Neurosurgery* 2013;72(suppl 2):84-92.

This updated, evidence-based guideline for acute cardiopulmonary management in patients with spinal cord injury concluded (based on weak evidence) that patients should be monitored in an intensive care unit and have immediate restoration of systolic blood pressure to at least 90 mm Hg. The study authors recommended that the mean arterial blood pressure be maintained between 85 and 90 mm Hg for 7 days. Level of evidence: IV.

87. Harrigan MR, Hadley MN, Dhall SS, et al: Management of vertebral artery injuries following non-penetrating cervical trauma. *Neurosurgery* 2013;72(suppl 2):234-243.

The authors present an updated, evidence-based guideline for managing vertebral artery injury associated with nonpenetrating cervical trauma. Based on strong evidence, patients who meet the modified Denver Criteria should undergo CT angiography. If not available, or when interventional care is considered, conventional angiography can be considered. Treatment by antiplatelet or anticoagulation should be individualized. The role of endovascular treatment has yet to be defined in this population. Level of evidence: IV.

Chapter 29

Thoracolumbar and Lumbosacral Trauma

John G. DeVine, MD   Uzondu F. Agochukwu, MD   Keith L. Jackson II, MD

Abstract

The evaluation and treatment of thoracolumbar and lumbosacral fractures have evolved over the past decade. Imaging standards in most trauma centers include the use of CT facilitated with MRI when necessary. Classification systems have been developed that afford both a common language for morphologic descriptions and treatment guidelines for management. Treatment guidelines are based on severity scores that take into account injury morphology and neurologic status. Most thoracolumbar and lumbosacral injuries can be managed nonsurgically; however, when surgical treatment is indicated, goals should include neurologic decompression when required, reduction, and spinal and/or pelvic stabilization. The timing of surgery is dependent on several variables, including patient comorbidities and polytrauma, but should be approached with urgency in the setting of an incomplete spinal cord injury.

Keywords: lumbopelvic disassociation; lumbosacral trauma; sacral fracture; thoracolumbar trauma

Dr. DeVine or an immediate family member is a member of a speakers' bureau or has made paid presentations on behalf of Globus Medical and Ulrich Medical USA; serves as a paid consultant to FacetLink, Spinal Elements, and Ulrich Medical USA; and served as a board member, owner, officer, or committee member of AOSpine North America Education Committee, 2012-2014. Neither of the following authors nor any immediate family member has received anything of value from or has stock or stock options held in a commercial company or institution related directly or indirectly to the subject of this chapter: Dr. Agochukwu and Dr. Jackson.

Introduction

Thoracolumbar and lumbosacral fractures range from insufficiency and fragility fractures, which are associated with metabolic bone disorders, to high-energy fractures and dislocations, which are associated with neurologic injury. This chapter primarily focuses on high-energy injuries. These fractures are grouped anatomically as pure thoracic (T1-T9), thoracolumbar (T10-L2), low lumbar (L3-L5), and sacral (S1-S5) injuries. Thoracolumbar fractures are the most common and are morphologically classified as compression, distraction, or translational-rotational. Sacral fractures can be associated with injury to the pelvic ring or lumbosacral junction. Most sacral fractures are intrinsic to the sacrum and are stable; however, vertical fractures parallel to the long axis of the sacrum can result in an unstable pelvic ring. Complex multiplanar sacral fractures may be associated with spinopelvic dissociation.

It is important to be familiar with several key concepts in the initial management of a patient with spinal trauma. The patient is turned once using a formal log rolling technique to allow inspection and palpation of the posterior integument and spine. Sentinel examination findings include swelling, ballottable subcutaneous fluid, overt soft-tissue disruption, crepitus, and bony malalignment. A formal neurologic examination that includes a rectal examination for voluntary tone and bulbocavernosus reflex should be performed. Specific assessments of motor, reflex, and sensory components of the lumbosacral and sacral plexus should be recorded. Screening for overt or occult blood in the urethral meatus, rectum, or vaginal vault can be done during the initial neurologic examination. Some findings of the initial evaluation are particularly valuable and prognostic. In a patient with a neurologic deficit, the absence of the bulbocavernosus reflex indicates spinal shock; therefore, a spinal cord syndrome cannot be classified. The bulbocavernosus reflex generally returns within 72 hours, but it may not return in patients who sustain an injury to the conus. In a patient with a neurologic deficit, intact pinprick sensation in the lower sacral dermatome distribution portends a favorable prognosis for recovery of bladder function. Sacral sparing on the return of the bulbocavernosus reflex is the most important predictor of a favorable neurologic outcome. Priapism signifies a complete spinal cord injury because it indicates loss of sympathetic tone to the genitalia in the presence of intact and unregulated parasympathetic input.

Thoracolumbar Trauma

Classification

Thoracolumbar Injury Classification and Severity Scale

Over time, the classification of thoracolumbar injuries has evolved.[1] Recent systems, including the Thoracolumbar Injury Classification and Severity (TLICS) Scale and the AOSpine Thoracolumbar Spine Injury Classification System, provide the most comprehensive classifications to date. These classification systems allow a common language and provide treatment recommendations.

The scoring system of the TLICS Scale attempts to predict the natural history and clinical outcome of various spinal injury patterns. The variables critical to decision making are injury morphology, the integrity of the posterior ligamentous complex (PLC), and the neurologic status of the patient[2] (**Figure 1**). The three main injury categories are assigned a numerical value. The higher the number, the more likely it is that the injury affects mechanical or neurologic stability. In the presence of more than one injury (noncontiguous or contiguous), the most severely involved level is scored.

Thoracolumbar injuries are first grouped into the following categories based on morphology: compression, translation/rotation, or distraction. These groups are given a score of 1 to 4 points. The integrity of the PLC is then assessed with the assignment of another score (0 to 3 points). A final score (0 to 3 points) is assigned based on the patient's neurologic findings. When the comprehensive severity score is 3 points or less, nonsurgical treatment is suggested. Surgical treatment is considered for patients with a score of 5 or more points. Injuries with a score of 4 points may be treated surgically or nonsurgically.[3]

The TLICS Scale also provides suggestions on the appropriate surgical approach, which is largely based on the integrity of the PLC and the neurologic status of the patient. The general guidelines are as follows: (1) an incomplete neurologic injury requires an anterior procedure if neural compression from anterior anatomic structures is present after attempts at reduction, (2) PLC disruption requires a posterior procedure to restore the tension band, and (3) a combined anterior and posterior approach is recommended for a combination of incomplete neurologic injury and PLC disruption.

It is important to note that the TLICS Scale does not take into account systemic factors (eg, rheumatoid arthritis, ankylosing spondylitis, or osteoporosis) or local factors (eg, extreme kyphosis or collapse, inability to allow bracing, adjacent rib fractures, or open fractures). The decision to treat a fracture anteriorly or posteriorly should be based largely on the experience of the treating surgeon.

Posterior Ligamentous Complex

The importance of the PLC in overall spinal column stability has been well described in the literature. The PLC, which is composed of the facet joint capsules, interspinous ligament, supraspinous ligament, and ligamentum flavum, protects the spine from excessive translation, rotation, flexion, and distraction. If the PLC is disrupted, the use of supplementary posterior instrumentation after anterolateral decompression and instrumentation for thoracolumbar burst fractures should be considered.[4]

Although accurate assessment of the PLC is important in decision making, the best method of injury identification remains unclear. Palpation on physical examination is unreliable. Plain radiography and CT can identify PLC injuries by the anatomic manifestation of instability, including facet joint diastasis, sagittal translation, increased interspinous distance, horizontal translation, and rotation of the vertebrae.[5] MRI allows the visualization of the components of the PLC; however, unless clear disruption of the ligaments is visualized, a change in PLC signal intensity alone is graded as indeterminate.

AOSpine Thoracolumbar Spine Injury Classification System

Critics of the TLICS Scale question the feasibility and reproducibility of evaluating the integrity of the PLC using MRI.[6] In addition, the TLICS Scale does not offer a definitive treatment recommendation for a neurologically intact patient with a thoracolumbar burst fracture and an indeterminate PLC disruption (assigned 4 points on the TLICS Scale).[7] Introduced in 2013, the AOSpine Thoracolumbar Spine Injury Classification System sought to address these concerns through the evaluation of the morphologic classification of a fracture, the neurologic status of the patient, and clinical modifiers.[6]

Thoracolumbar injury morphology is classified based on the mode of failure of the spinal column. Type A injuries are compression injuries; type B injuries are characterized by failure of the posterior or anterior tension band, without evidence of either gross translation or the potential for gross translation; and type C injuries result from the failure of all stabilizing elements,

Injury morphology		Qualifier	Points
Compression	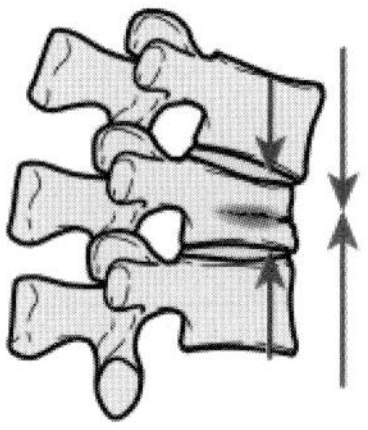	–	1
		Burst	+1
Rotation-translation	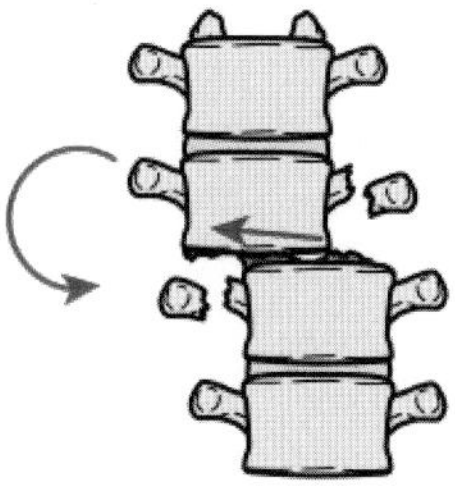	–	3
Distraction	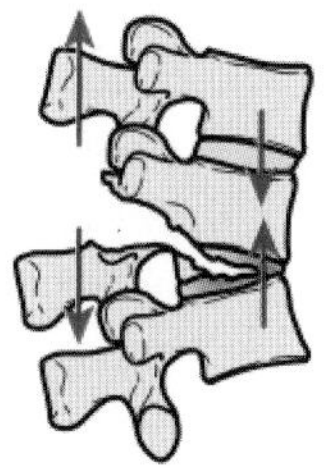	–	4
Neurologic status			
Intact		–	0
Nerve root		–	2
Spinal cord/conus medullaris		Incomplete	3
		Complete	2
Cauda equina		–	3
Posterior ligaments			
Intact		–	0
Suspected/indeterminate		–	1
Disrupted		–	2

Figure 1   Listing of the Thoracolumbar Injury Classification and Severity Scale with schematic drawings showing compression, rotation-translation, and distraction injury morphology; the arrows indicate the direction of force. The overall score consists of the total of the injury morphology, neurologic status, and posterior ligamentous complex status subscores.

which leads to dislocation or displacement in any plane or complete disruption of a soft-tissue hinge (even in the absence of translation). These injuries are further subdivided based on severity. Neurologic status is graded with a six-part system (N0 through N5), with NX used to designate patients who cannot be examined because of either head injury or another condition that does not allow a complete neurologic examination. In some cases, modifiers (M1 and M2) can be used to further describe the injury. M1 is used to designate fractures with an indeterminate injury to the tension band, and M2 is used to designate a patient-specific comorbidity, which may serve as an indication for or against surgery. Although a spinal injury score is not established in the AOSpine classification, a linked surgical algorithm provides treatment recommendations. The AOSpine

6: Trauma

Thoracolumbar Spine Injury Classification System has been validated and has good intraobserver and interobserver reliability.[8]

Neurologic Injury

The incidence of neurologic deficit associated with thoracolumbar fractures varies based on the injury pattern. Individuals involved in motor vehicle crashes are at higher risk of neurologic injury if they are very young or very old, are underweight or overweight, were not restrained by a seat belt, and were involved in a crash with a great change in impact velocity.[9] Patients with an incomplete spinal cord injury have a better prognosis for neurologic recovery than those with a complete injury. The timing of surgery remains controversial.[10] A systematic review of the literature, including studies of thoracic and lumbar fractures, demonstrated that early fixation leads to a lower complication rate and shorter length of intensive care and hospital stays, but does not necessarily improve the neurologic outcome.[11] Surgical intervention should be performed as soon as the patient is medically stable.

Compression Fractures

Most compression fractures are stable, and fractures without neurologic or posterior ligamentous injury can be managed nonsurgically. Injuries cranial to T11 do not require bracing because of support provided by the rib cage. Although evidence is mixed, most thoracolumbar compression fractures are managed with a brace for 6 to 12 weeks.

Despite the relatively subtle findings associated with compression fractures, the patient should be thoroughly examined for other contiguous and noncontiguous spinal and nonspinal injuries. In the absence of high-energy trauma, other causes of fracture, including osteoporosis, primary or metastatic cancer, and other endocrine abnormalities, should be considered.

Burst Fractures

Burst fractures are characterized by disruption of the posterior wall of the vertebral body, which differentiates them from compression fractures. The etiology is typically related to a powerful axial load. Lamina fractures also may occur (notably vertical laminar fractures in the lower lumbar spine) and do not necessarily render the spine unstable. Burst fractures with less than 20% height loss or 20° local kyphosis are typically considered stable. In neurologically intact patients, the assessment of stability of more severe injuries is informed by the status of the PLC. Although MRI may be the optimal imaging modality, evidence also supports the use of CT.[8]

Nonsurgical Treatment

Most neurologically intact patients with thoracolumbar burst fractures without PLC disruption can be managed nonsurgically. In a prospective study in which patients with thoracolumbar burst fractures without neurologic injury were randomized to surgical or nonsurgical treatment, analysis at 4 years after injury revealed few differences between the groups. However, long-term follow-up (16 to 22 years) found that patients who were managed nonsurgically reported less pain and better function compared with those who were treated surgically.[11] Several similar studies, however, do not differentiate between burst fractures with and without injury to the PLC. Patients with burst fractures and PLC injury are at risk for progressive kyphosis, which can result in pain, functional impairment, and neurologic injury.

In most studies comparing nonsurgical and surgical treatment, an orthosis is used as the basis of nonsurgical care. However, brace treatment has not been proved an effective technique. A review of randomized controlled trials comparing clinical and radiologic outcomes of patients with thoracolumbar burst fractures treated with or without an orthosis reported no significant differences between the groups regarding loss of kyphotic angle, failure of nonsurgical management requiring subsequent surgery, and levels of disability and pain.[12] Although data suggest no difference in outcomes, a brace is prescribed for most patients for comfort.

Surgical Treatment

The surgical approach for treating thoracolumbar burst fractures varies depending on surgeon training and region. The goals of surgery should be at the forefront of decision making. For unstable fractures with neurologic injury, the procedure best suited to allow adequate decompression of the neural elements and stabilization should be selected. The surgeon's familiarity with a procedure and patient factors such as comorbidities and polytrauma also should be considered.

Posterior Approach

In general, the advantages of the posterior approach include surgeon familiarity, lower risk to vascular and visceral anatomy, and ease of reexploration. Indirect reduction often can be achieved with ligamentotaxis. If ligamentotaxis does not provide acceptable reduction, direct decompression may be achieved through a posterior transpedicular approach. Although laminectomy is a useful adjunct to direct decompression or to address traumatic dural tears at the level of the fracture, its use in isolation is an inadequate means for decompressing the neural elements.

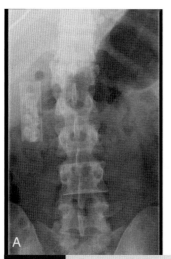 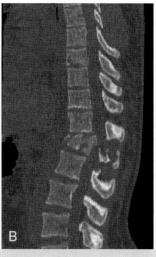 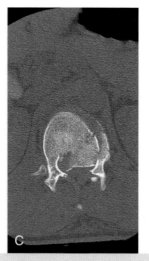 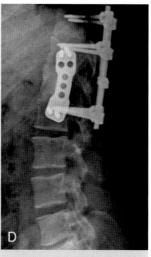

Figure 2 Imaging studies from a 26-year-old man with a thoracolumbar burst fracture with an incomplete spinal cord injury sustained in a high-speed motor vehicle crash. **A,** AP radiograph shows the L1 fracture with loss of height and interpedicular widening. **B,** Midsagittal CT scan shows the displaced L1 fracture fragment in the spinal canal and an associated contiguous fracture of the T12 superior end plate. **C,** Axial CT scan of L1 shows 75% canal intrusion of the fracture fragment. **D,** Lateral radiograph after posterior pedicle fixation at T11-L2 and anterior corpectomy with reconstruction using structural allograft.

Traditionally recommended constructs include pedicle screw stabilization two to three levels cephalad and caudal to the level of injury. Although biomechanical studies have demonstrated that shorter segment instrumentation is less rigid than the intact spine, the number of instrumented levels for optimal fixation remains controversial. Clinically, a load-sharing classification score of more than 6 points was found to predict construct failure in short-segment posterior instrumentation. In patients with greater comminution and fragment displacement and, therefore, lower load-sharing capability, supplemental anterior reconstruction or long-segment posterior instrumentation was recommended. Recently, however, short-segment posterior fixation with intermediate screws placed at the level of the fractured vertebrae were found to adequately maintain reduction in burst fractures with a load-sharing classification score of 7 or more points.[13] None of the patients in the study had postoperative implant failure at final follow-up. In the current era of evolving fracture fixation concepts and implant design advancements, the relevance of load-sharing classification scores in the management of unstable burst fractures is debatable.

Anterior Approach
In theory, anterior surgery should offer superior neural element decompression in burst fractures, particularly at the level of the conus medullaris. However, the benefits of anterior decompression over transpedicular or indirect decompression by ligamentotaxis have not been established. An anterior-only approach is particularly concerning in patients with PLC injury because the absence of a posterior tension band may result in a higher failure rate. In these patients, supplemental posterior fixation is recommended. Few randomized controlled trials have been performed to assess the optimal approach in thoracolumbar fracture management. A systematic review of the literature comparing anterior to posterior approaches in patients with thoracolumbar fractures reported no significant differences between groups regarding the Cobb angle, Frankel classification, American Spinal Injury Association (ASIA) and Japanese Orthopaedic Association motor scores, complications, and number of patients returning to work.[14] In the subgroup of patients with a burst fracture, surgical times were substantially shorter and perioperative blood loss was less in the group treated with the posterior approach. Because no consensus exists in the literature, the surgical approach should take into account the goals of surgery, including neural decompression and restoration of spine stability, as well as surgeon familiarity with the approach and patient comorbidities. In some instances, a combined approach may be optimal (**Figure 2**).

Distraction Injuries
Distraction injuries are characterized by separation of bony or ligamentous structures, which results in destruction of the functional spinal unit. These injuries are considered unstable in multiple classification systems, and surgical stabilization is indicated. In the past, extension

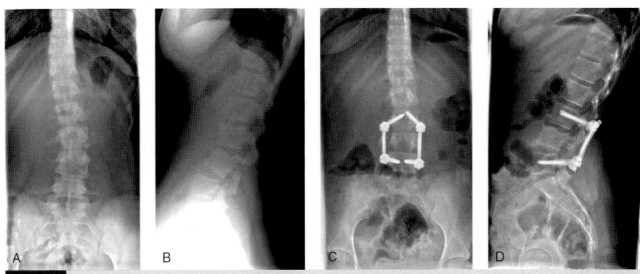

Figure 3 Radiographs from a 17-year-old girl with a distraction injury with an intact anterior column with dense nerve root injury to L4 and L5 bilaterally. **A,** AP radiograph shows an interpedicular fracture in the horizontal plane and an increase in the interspinous distance between L3 and L4. **B,** Lateral radiograph of the distraction injury via the L4 pedicle and exiting the superior end plate. AP **(C)** and lateral **(D)** radiographs show reduction of the fracture with short-segment posterior fixation.

brace management has been considered for injuries involving the vertebral bone only (bony Chance fracture). In the absence of a neurologic injury or PLC involvement, a TLICS Scale score of 4 points would be given. Acceptable outcomes have been reported in noncomparative studies for this unique subset of patients. However, comparative studies assessing nonsurgical and surgical management have reported worsened kyphosis, pain, and functional outcomes at 1-year follow-up in the nonsurgical cohort.[15]

Posterior segmental fixation with pedicle screw and rod constructs is the most established surgical treatment, especially when there is evidence of PLC involvement or neurologic injury (TLICS Scale score >4 points). The number of segments treated varies depending on the morphology of the distraction. Short-segment stabilization has been reported as a modality of treatment, most notably in the setting of an undamaged anterior vertebral body with an intact anterior longitudinal ligament and anulus fibrosis (**Figure 3**). In distraction injuries that compromise the anterior column, long-segment instrumentation spanning two to three levels caudal and cephalad is recommended.

The use of percutaneous fixation in the setting of flexion-distraction injuries of the thoracolumbar spine has been compared with open treatment.[16] There were no statistically significant differences in the ASIA score or the degrees of kyphotic angulation between the minimally invasive and open surgery groups. There was a trend toward shorter surgical time and less blood loss in patients undergoing minimally invasive fixation. However, it

should be noted that percutaneous approaches do not allow posterolateral bone grafting. The ramifications of instrumentation without arthrodesis are not clear in this setting.

Translational Injuries

An injury with translation only and no interspinous widening is considered a translation-only injury. In the presence of substantial ligamentous damage or neurologic injury, a translational injury is considered unstable and requires surgical intervention. Rotatory injuries are relatively rare, although they are very unstable. Rotational instability can be best seen as a horizontal rotation of the spinous processes and pedicles on an AP radiograph or an axial CT scan. An isolated bilateral facet fracture or dislocation with translation commonly results in a complete spinal cord injury caused by the pincer effect of the displaced yet intact neural arches. This injury typically involves disruption of the PLC and corresponds to a TLICS Scale score of 5 points or more. Reduction and instrumented fusion two to three levels caudal and cephalad from a posterior approach is the recommended treatment (**Figure 4**).

Lumbosacral Trauma

Classification of Lower Lumbar Spine Injuries

Lower lumbar fractures have been classified using the same systems as the more cephalad thoracolumbar injuries mentioned previously in this chapter. However, with an

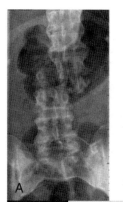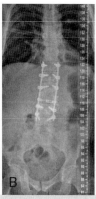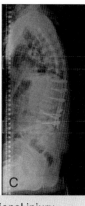

Figure 4 Radiographs showing a translational injury through the L1-L2 functional spinal unit and shortening of the spinal column associated with cauda equina syndrome. **A,** AP radiograph shows the translational injury at L1-L2. AP (**B**) and lateral (**C**) radiographs show reduction and long-segment posterior fixation.

average 49.2° lordosis from L4-S1, injuries in this region can have a substantial effect on sagittal balance.[17] Because current classification schemes do not consider sagittal balance, their use in the lower lumbar spine may be limited.[18,19] To date, a comprehensive classification for injuries of the lower lumbar spine has not been presented.

Classification of Sacral Injuries

The AO/Orthopaedic Trauma Association classification categorizes sacral fractures in the context of overall pelvic stability as 61-A3, 61-B1 to 61-B3, and 61-C1 to 61-C3 (**Figure 5**). A 61-A3 fracture does not compromise the integrity of the posterior pelvic ring. A 61-B injury represents an incomplete disruption of the osseoligamentous integrity of the posterior pelvic ring, with an intact pelvic floor and, therefore, no vertical displacement. A 61-C injury is a so-called vertical shear injury and involves complete loss of osseoligamentous stability of the posterior arch and disruption of the pelvic floor.

The Denis classification specifically focuses on sacral fractures (**Figure 6**). This widely used system correlates anatomic factors with neurologic injury risk on a progressive severity scale. The Denis system differentiates alar fracture (zone 1); transforaminal fracture (zone 2); and central fracture, which includes any fracture extending into the spinal canal (zone 3).[20] Lumbosacral stability is not taken into account, however.

Classification of Lumbopelvic Dissociation

Spinopelvic dissociation is characterized by a bilateral vertical fracture, which often is connected by a somewhat transverse fracture line or a series of comminuted fracture lines. In descriptive terms, the result is a U-type fracture or, if the vertical fracture lines extend and exit caudal to the sacroiliac joint, an H-type (bilateral pelvic instability) or Y-type (unilateral pelvic instability) fracture or a similar permutation. Unfortunately, these classifications do not take into account the mechanism of injury or the type, magnitude, or directions of fracture displacement. The Roy-Camille subclassification of Denis zone 3 injuries and sacral fracture-dislocations associated with spinopelvic dissociation describes three types of transversely oriented sacral fractures that are classified according to injury severity and the presumed likelihood of neurologic injury.[21] The model of a single transverse fracture line connecting two longitudinally oriented fractures is overly simple; the fracture pattern usually is more complex, and comminution is more extensive.

Major limitations of each of these historic classification systems are their descriptive nature, lack of validity, and failure to account for important treatment considerations. In an attempt to address these shortcomings, the Lumbosacral Injury Classification System (LSICS) was introduced.[22] Similar to the TLICS Scale system, the LSICS accounts for injury morphology, neurologic status, and integrity of the PLC to derive a composite score. (**Tables 1, 2,** and **3.**) This composite score then can be used to help determine treatment. The cumulative score from each category represents the total LSICS score. Surgical intervention should be considered in patients with an LSICS score of 5 points or higher in patients without other contraindications to surgery.

Neurologic Injury

Formal testing of neurologic function should be performed using ASIA principles. The examination should include assessment of the motor, reflex, and sensory components of the lumbosacral and sacral plexuses. A rectal examination also helps quantify voluntary sphincter contraction as well as light touch and pinprick sensation to the lower sacral dermatomes. Bowel, bladder, or sexual dysfunction generally involves bilateral injury to the S2-S4 roots. In unilateral Denis zone 1 and 2 fractures, the neurologic deficits generally are limited to the lower extremities. Six percent of zone 1 injuries are associated with sensorimotor deficits and primarily involve the L5 nerve root distribution, which is located in a vulnerable position along the sacral ala. Lower extremity neurologic deficits occur in 28% of zone 2 injuries and may affect multiple nerve roots, depending on the involved foramina. The likelihood of neurologic deficits in a zone 3 injury is 57%, and 75% of these deficits involve a loss of bowel, bladder, or sexual function (probably resulting from bilateral root injury).[20] In fractures with a transverse component, the most common neurologic

6: Trauma

Groups:
Type A fracture: pelvis, ring, stable (61-A)

1. Fracture of innominate bone, avulsion (61-A1)

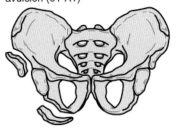

2. Fracture of innominate bone, direct blow (61-A2)

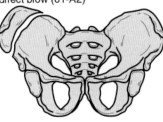

3. Transverse fracture of sacrum and coccyx (61-A3)

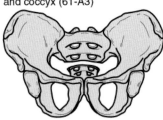

Type B fracture: pelvis, ring, partially stable (61-B)

1. Unilateral, partial disruption of posterior arch, external rotation ("open-book" injury) (61-B1)

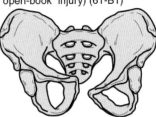

2. Unilateral, partial disruption of posterior arch, internal rotation (lateral compression injury) (61-B2)

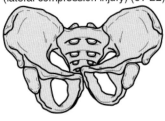

3. Bilateral, partial lesion of posterior arch (61-B3)

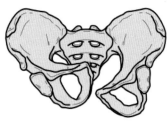

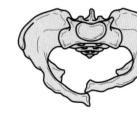

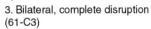

Type C fracture: pelvis, ring, complete disruption of posterior arch unstable (61-C)

1. Unilateral, complete disruption of posterior arch (61-C1)

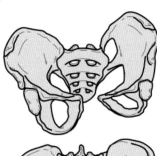

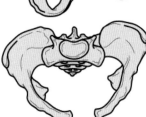

2. Bilateral, ipsilateral complete, contralateral incomplete (61-C2)

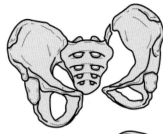

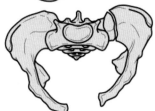

3. Bilateral, complete disruption (61-C3)

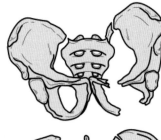

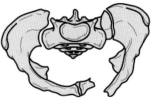

Figure 5   Illustration of the AO/Orthopaedic Trauma Association classification of pelvic fractures. (Reproduced from Wright RD: Pelvic, acetabular, and sacral fractures, in Boyer MI, ed: *AAOS Comprehensive Orthopaedic Board Review*, ed 2. Rosemont, IL, American Academy of Orthopaedic Surgeons, 2014, pp 363-386.)

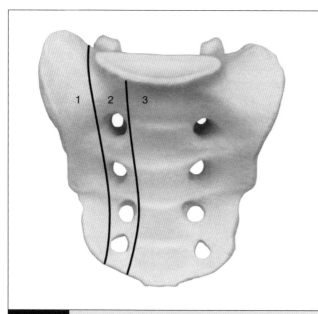

Figure 6 Illustration of the Denis classification of sacral fractures, in which zone 1 is alar, zone 2 is transforaminal, and zone 3 extends into the spinal canal. (Reproduced from Bellabarba C, Schildhauer TA, Chapman JR: Fractures of the sacrum, in Rao RD, Smuck M, eds: *Orthopaedic Knowledge Update Spine 4*. Rosemont, IL, American Academy of Orthopaedic Surgeons, 2012, pp 251-262.)

Table 1

Lumbosacral Injury Classification System: Injury Morphology

Type	Points
Flexion compression	
≤20° kyphosis	1
>20° kyphosis	2
Axial compression (comminution of upper sacrum)	
Without sacral canal or neuroforaminal encroachment	2
With sacral canal or neuroforaminal encroachment	3
Translation/rotation	3
Anterior or posterior translation of upper sacrum	
Lumbosacral facet injury or dislocation	
Vertical translation or instability	
Blast/shear (severe comminution or segmental bone loss)	4

Reproduced with permission from Lehman RA, Kang DG, Bellabarba C: A new classification for complex lumbosacral injuries. *Spine* 2012;12(7):612-628.

Table 2

Lumbosacral Injury Classification System: Integrity of the Posterior Ligamentous Complex

Posterior Ligamentous Complex Status	Points
Intact	0
Indeterminate	1
Disrupted	2

Reproduced with permission from Lehman RA, Kang DG, Bellabarba C: A new classification for complex lumbosacral injuries. *Spine* 2012;12(7):612-628.

Table 3

Lumbosacral Injury Classification System: Neurologic Status

Severity	Points
Intact	0
Paresthesia only	1
Lower extremity motor deficit	2
Bowel/bladder dysfunction	3
Progressive neurologic deficit	4

Reproduced with permission from Lehman RA, Kang DG, Bellabarba C: A new classification for complex lumbosacral injuries. *Spine* 2012;12(7):612-628.

injury is cauda equina syndrome.[23] The lack of motor or sensory deficits in the lower extremities associated with these injuries heightens the importance of examining the rectal tone and the perianal sensation at the time of the initial examination. Approximately 80% of patients with neurologic deficits have improvement after a sacral fracture-dislocation, regardless of treatment.[24,25] Specific mechanisms of nerve root injuries range from compression or traction to transection or avulsion. The specific type of injury to the nerve root likely has a major role in determining a patient's overall neurologic improvement.

Imaging

The initial evaluation of a patient with a lumbosacral injury may include AP and lateral pelvic radiographs. Findings consistent with H-type or U-type fractures on the AP view include vertical fracture lines or a sacral inclination so great that it gives the appearance of an inlet view of the S1 vertebral body (a so-called paradoxic inlet). A lateral view of the sacrum may help identify a transverse sacral fracture or fracture-dislocation not visible on plain pelvic radiographs. In many medical centers, pelvic CT has become the primary radiographic screening tool for patients with a suspected sacral fracture and is

6: Trauma

typically necessary to fully define the fracture pattern. Axial images often are sufficient for identifying a simple fracture pattern such as a vertical Denis zone 1 or 2 injury, although CT reconstruction of inlet and outlet pelvic views may be useful. The acquisition of 2-mm or thinner slices allows high-quality sagittal and coronal reformation, which provides comprehensive visualization of the sacral anatomy and identification of lumbosacral pathology. MRI is helpful in determining the etiology of a neurologic deficit and in assessing the integrity of the PLC. Specific findings that may indicate PLC disruption on MRI include disruption or attenuation of the supraspinous or infraspinous ligaments, ligamentum flavum disruption, facet capsular disruption, or widening of the facet joint.

Nonsurgical Treatment

Nonsurgical treatment is generally recommended for neurologically intact patients with a sacral fracture that does not compromise pelvic or spinopelvic stability, such as a transverse fracture below the sacroiliac joints. Nonsurgical treatment also is appropriate for an incomplete, unilateral sacral fracture (Denis zone 1 or 2) involving either the ventral or dorsal cortex, but not both. Nonsurgical management consists of a short period of bed rest followed by early mobilization and protected weight bearing on the injured side, with or without the use of an orthotic device.[25-27] Unfortunately, little consensus exists on the tolerable extent of fracture displacement or the definition of sacral instability. An analysis of long-term functional outcomes after surgical or nonsurgical treatment of sacral fractures reported a high rate of fair or poor results.[28] These outcomes were unrelated to the magnitude of residual displacement and believed to result from pain or a radicular lesion. Severe comminution, relative osteopenia of the sacral ala, the anatomic complexity of the sacrum, and the absence of instrumentation well suited to this region are among the specific challenges associated with achieving stable fixation of the sacrum in a zone 3 sacral U-type fracture variant. In the past, such factors may have contributed to a reluctance to treat the fracture surgically; however, surgical intervention is recommended for these injuries because nonsurgical treatment requires 8 to 12 weeks of bed rest and distal femoral skeletal traction and has a high risk of complications, including skin breakdown at the apex of the sacral kyphosis.[29]

Surgical Treatment

The decision for surgical treatment is based on a combination of fracture characteristics and the patient's neurologic status, concomitant injuries, and comorbidities. The LSICS offers an algorithm to guide treatment of these injuries[22] (**Figure 7**). Although controversy exists regarding specific surgical parameters, fracture reduction with or without direct neural decompression and stabilization is typically the treatment of choice for a patient with a displaced sacral fracture with soft-tissue compromise or neurologic deficits. In these patients, early fracture reduction with fixation can facilitate neural decompression and mobilization and can prevent progressive lumbosacral deformity[30,31] (**Figure 8**).

Open Fracture and Substantial Soft-Tissue Injury

An open fracture or substantial soft-tissue injury requires special consideration. Initial management should consist of early wound irrigation and débridement of all nonviable tissue, with meticulous dead-space closure and drainage. Gynecologic or urologic consultation is advised in patients with genitourinary involvement. Bowel perforation often requires early colonic diversion to prevent further contamination. In these cases, the patient should receive 24 to 48 hours of broad-spectrum empirical antibiotic coverage. Flap coverage may be required if there is substantial soft-tissue loss.[22] Depending on the fracture type, initial stabilization may include anterior pelvic ring external fixation and placement of a percutaneous iliosacral screw in the posterior pelvis.[32,33] Definitive sacral fracture stabilization can be performed when the soft tissues are viable and progressively healing. Stabilization of the fracture is of the utmost importance in the treatment of soft-tissue injury. The degree of mechanical stability was identified as the only variable factor statistically associated with infection in open pelvic fractures; a mechanically unstable pelvis, as determined by physical examination, was associated with a tenfold increase in the risk of infection.[34]

Timing of Surgery

To date, there have been no large, well-designed studies demonstrating better neurologic outcomes with early decompression; however, many investigators suggest decompressive surgery within 2 weeks of injury in patients with a neurologic deficit and ongoing compressive pathology.[22,23] Neurologic decompression can be accomplished either indirectly with fracture reduction, before hematoma consolidation, or with direct decompression through sacral laminectomy and ventral foraminotomy. A multilevel sacral laminectomy is necessary for a complex sacral fracture involving extensive areas of the sacral spinal canal. The quality of reduction, particularly the elimination of residual postoperative translation and kyphosis, appears to correlate with outcomes based on the postoperative Pelvic Outcomes Scale.

Traumatic dural tears are relatively common. Suture repair is undertaken if possible. Otherwise, the patching

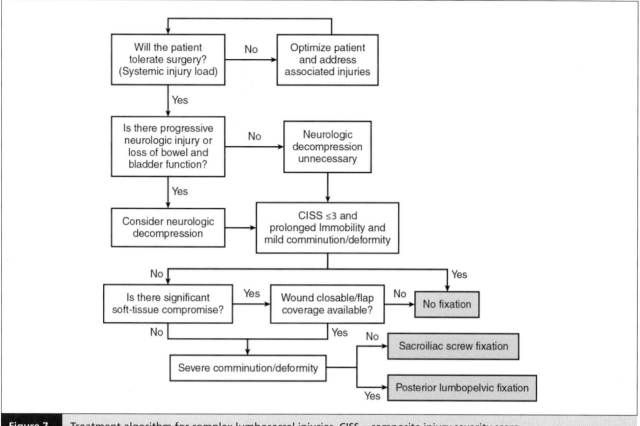

Figure 7 Treatment algorithm for complex lumbosacral injuries. CISS = composite injury severity score.

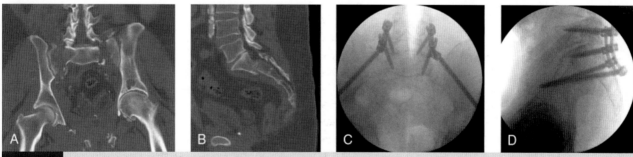

Figure 8 CT images from a patient with a sacral H-type fracture and a Lumbosacral Injury Classification System score of 8 (injury morphology, 4 points; integrity of the posterior ligamentous complex, 1 point; neurologic status, 3 points). **A**, Coronal CT scan shows a bilateral vertical sacral fracture and displacement (61-C3). **B**, Sagittal CT scan shows the horizontal sacral fracture with minimal kyphosis and anterior displacement. AP (**C**) and lateral (**D**) CT images after open reduction, decompression, and lumbopelvic fixation.

technique should involve the use of a dural allograft, collagen matrix, or biologic sealant.

Complications in Thoracolumbar and Lumbosacral Trauma

Wound-related complications are relatively common after the surgical treatment of thoracolumbar and sacral fractures. Wound drainage resulting from seroma and pseudomeningocele formation requires

surgical reexploration. If infection occurs, treatment also includes intravenous antibiotics for at least 6 weeks and nutritional support.

Decubitus ulcers may develop over prominent bone or hardware. In the patient with a spinal cord injury, insensate areas are at increased risk for the development of ulcers.

Implant failure can occur before or after fracture healing. Rod or screw breakage may not be associated with symptoms; however, in the early postoperative period,

6: Trauma

such failure may be associated with loss of reduction or progressive kyphosis.

Summary

The evaluation and treatment of thoracolumbar and lumbosacral fractures have evolved considerably as imaging standards have improved and new fracture stabilization concepts and techniques have been developed. Recent classification systems have afforded both a common language for descriptive purposes and treatment guidelines for management. Surgical treatment, when indicated, should be focused on neurologic decompression when required and on reduction and stabilization based on the principles outlined in this chapter. Surgical timing is dependent on several variables, including patient comorbidities and the presence of polytrauma, but should be approached with urgency in the setting of an incomplete spinal cord injury.

Key Study Points

- Classification systems have evolved for both thoracolumbar and lumbosacral injuries that offer treatment guidelines based on severity scores that take into account injury morphology and neurologic status.
- The goals of surgical treatment of both thoracolumbar and lumbosacral fractures are neural decompression, fracture reduction, and spinal and/or pelvic stabilization.
- Surgical timing is dependent on several variables in the polytrauma patient with thoracolumbar or lumbosacral injuries, but should be approached with urgency in the setting of an incomplete spinal cord injury.

Annotated References

1. Azam MQ, Sadat-Ali M: The concept of evolution of thoracolumbar fracture classifications helps in surgical decisions. *Asian Spine J* 2015;9(6):984-994.

   The authors provide a concise review of thoracolumbar classification systems from 1929 to the present.

2. Vaccaro AR, Lehman RA Jr, Hurlbert RJ, et al: A new classification of thoracolumbar injuries: The importance of injury morphology, the integrity of the posterior ligamentous complex, and neurologic status. *Spine (Phila Pa 1976)* 2005;30(20):2325-2333.

3. Pneumaticos SG, Karampinas PK, Triantafilopoulos G, Koufos S, Polyzois V, Vlamis J: Evaluation of TLICS for thoracolumbar fractures. *Eur Spine J* 2016;25(4):1123-1127.

   This study demonstrated that nonsurgical treatment of patients with a TLICS Scale score of 4 points is safe and equally as effective as nonsurgical treatment for patients with scores of 3 points or less.

4. Chen J, Jia YS, Sun Q, et al: Multivariate analysis of risk factors for predicting supplementary posterior instrumentation after anterolateral decompression and instrumentation in treating thoracolumbar burst fractures. *J Orthop Surg Res* 2015;10:17.

   In this retrospective review of 238 patients who underwent anterolateral surgery for a thoracolumbar burst fracture, 27 patients (11.3%) required supplemental posterior fixation. Older age and disruption of the PLC were independent risk factors predicting the need for supplementary posterior fixation.

5. Barcelos AC, Joaquim AF, Botelho RV: Reliability of the evaluation of posterior ligamentous complex injury in thoracolumbar spine trauma with the use of computed tomography scan. *Eur Spine J* 2016;25(4):1135-1143.

   In this study, the use of CT as the only diagnostic tool in patients with thoracolumbar spine trauma resulted in the identification of PLC injury in most patients and demonstrated satisfactory reliability.

6. Vaccaro AR, Oner C, Kepler CK, et al; AOSpine Spinal Cord Injury & Trauma Knowledge Forum: AOSpine thoracolumbar spine injury classification system: Fracture description, neurological status, and key modifiers. *Spine (Phila Pa 1976)* 2013;38(23):2028-2037.

   The authors introduce an internationally devised comprehensive yet simple classification of thoracolumbar spine injuries. The classification has acceptable intraobserver and interobserver reliability for use in both clinical practice and research. Level of evidence: IV.

7. Schroeder GD, Vaccaro AR, Kepler CK, et al: Establishing the injury severity of thoracolumbar trauma: Confirmation of the hierarchical structure of the AOSpine Thoracolumbar Spine Injury Classification System. *Spine (Phila Pa 1976)* 2015;40(8):E498-E503.

   The authors report on a survey of spine surgeons from regions around the world to grade the severity of each variable of the AOSpine Thoracolumbar Spine Injury Classification System. No regional or experiential difference in perceived severity of thoracolumbar trauma was found, and the classification was confirmed as a logical approach to assessing these injuries.

8. Rajasekaran S, Vaccaro AR, Kanna RM, et al: The value of CT and MRI in the classification and surgical decision-making among spine surgeons in thoracolumbar spinal injuries. *Eur Spine J* 2016.

   This study demonstrated that radiographs alone were insufficient for accurate classification of thoracolumbar spinal injuries, except for C-type injuries. CT was mandatory for accurately classifying these injuries. MRI did confer a modest gain in sensitivity in B2-type injuries. The authors concluded that the need for MRI for classifying or assessing instability is not supported.

9. Mukherjee S, Beck C, Yoganandan N, RaoRD: Incidence and mechanism of neurologic deficit after thoracolumbar fractures sustained in motor vehicle collisions. *J Neurosurg Spine* 2016;24(2):323-331.

    This study determined the incidence of and assessed the risk factors associated with neurologic injury to motor vehicle occupants who sustain fractures of the thoracolumbar spine. Crash data elements from the Crash Injury Research and Engineering Network were used.

10. Xing D, Chen Y, Ma JX, et al: A methodological systematic review of early versus late stabilization of thoracolumbar spine fractures. *Eur Spine J* 2013;22(10):2157-2166.

    This review concluded that a definite recommendation could not be made for or against early stabilization in thoracolumbar fractures secondary to the heterogeneity of the included studies and low-level evidence. However, the study authors agreed that early stabilization may reduce hospital length of stay, intensive care length of stay, ventilator days, morbidity, and hospital expenses, particularly for patients with thoracic injuries.

11. Wood KB, Buttermann GR, Phukan R, et al: Operative compared with nonoperative treatment of a thoracolumbar burst fracture without neurological deficit: A prospective randomized study with follow-up at sixteen to twenty-two years. *J Bone Joint Surg Am* 2015;97(1):3-9.

    The authors report on long-term follow-up of a previously published study in which analysis at 4 years after treatment of a thoracolumbar burst fracture without neurologic deficit found few differences between surgical and nonsurgical management. However, at a 16- to 22-year follow-up, the nonsurgical group reported less pain and better function compared with the surgically treated cohort.

12. Alcalá-Cerra G, Paternina-Caicedo AJ, Díaz-Becerra C, Moscote-Salazar LR, Fernandes-Joaquim A: Orthosis for thoracolumbar burst fractures without neurologic deficit: A systematic review of prospective randomized controlled trials. *J Craniovertebr Junction Spine* 2014;5(1):25-32.

    The evidence from two randomized controlled trials revealed no significant differences in loss of kyphotic angle, pain, or length of the hospital stay between patients with a thoracolumbar burst fracture without neurologic deficit who were treated with or without an orthosis. Higher Medical Outcomes Study 36-Item Short Form scores in the physical and mental domains were found in the group treated without an orthosis.

13. Kanna RM, Shetty AP, Rajasekaran S: Posterior fixation including the fractured vertebra for severe unstable thoracolumbar fractures. *Spine J* 2015;15(2):256-264.

    The authors present a review of 32 patients with an unstable burst fracture and load-sharing classification scores of 7 or higher for whom anterior reconstruction historically would have been recommended, who were treated with short-segment posterior fixation, including the fractured vertebrae. Reduction was achieved and maintained, which avoided the need for anterior reconstruction.

14. Zhu Q, Shi F, Cai W, Bai J, Fan J, Yang H: Comparison of anterior versus posterior approach in the treatment of thoracolumbar fractures: A systematic review. *Int Surg* 2015;100(6):1124-1133.

    The authors discuss their systematic review of 3 randomized controlled trials and 11 clinically controlled trials comparing the anterior versus the posterior approach for treating thoracolumbar fractures. No significant differences between the groups were found in the Cobb angle, the Frankel classification, ASIA and Japanese Orthopaedic Association motor scores, complications, and the number of patients who were able to return to work

15. Lopez AJ, Scheer JK, Smith ZA, Dahdaleh NS: Management of flexion distraction injuries to the thoracolumbar spine. *J Clin Neurosci* 2015;22(12):1853-1856.

    A review of the literature regarding the management of flexion-distraction injuries is presented. The available evidence, which was low-level evidence, strongly supports management with long-segment posterior fixation with or without fusion using open or percutaneous surgery.

16. Grossbach AJ, Dahdaleh NS, Abel TJ, Woods GD, Dlouhy BJ, Hitchon PW: Flexion-distraction injuries of the thoracolumbar spine: Open fusion versus percutaneous pedicle screw fixation. *Neurosurg Focus* 2013;35(2):E2.

    A nonrandomized comparison of flexion-distraction injuries treated with posterior stabilization is presented. Open arthrodesis was performed in 27 patients, whereas 11 patients were treated with percutaneous stabilization without arthrodesis. No difference was found in ASIA score or the degree of kyphotic angulation; a trend toward shorter surgical time for the percutaneous group was noted.

17. Abdel MP, Bodemer WS, Anderson PA: Supine thoracolumbar sagittal spine alignment: Comparing computerized tomography and plain radiographs. *Spine (Phila Pa 1976)* 2012;37(4):340-345.

    This study compared plain radiography versus CT with regard to thoracolumbar sagittal spine alignment in supine patients. Results provided supine references for sagittal spine alignment using the Cobb method. A high degree of reliability for both radiography and CT was reported.

18. Schroeder GD, Kepler CK, Koerner JD, et al: Can a thoracolumbar injury severity score be uniformly applied from T1 to L5 or are modifications necessary? *Global Spine J* 2015;5(4):339-345.

    After a review of the literature, the authors concluded that the new AOSpine Thoracolumbar Spine Injury Classification System does not necessarily apply to injuries at the cervicothoracic and lumbosacral junctions because of the unique morphologic properties at those locations.

19. Moore TA, Bransford RJ, France JC, et al: Low lumbar fractures: Does thoracolumbar injury

6: Trauma

classification and severity score work? *Spine (Phila Pa 1976)* 2014;39(17):E1021-E1025.

Low lumbar fractures were classified using the TLICS Scale system. Fair reliability was found among reviewers, which revealed the presence of factors that were not inclusive to the TLICS Scale for these injuries. Maintenance of lordosis and global sagittal alignment are important factors in treating these injuries, but they were not considered in the TLICS Scale system.

20. Denis F, Davis S, Comfort T: Sacral fractures: An important problem. Retrospective analysis of 236 cases. *Clin Orthop Relat Res* 1988;227(227):67-81.

21. Roy-Camille R, Saillant G, Gagna G, Mazel C: Transverse fracture of the upper sacrum: Suicidal jumper's fracture. *Spine (Phila Pa 1976)* 1985;10(9):838-845.

22. Lehman RA Jr, Kang DG, Bellabarba C: A new classification for complex lumbosacral injuries. *Spine J* 2012;12(7):612-628.

    The LSICS is based on morphology, posterior ligamentous integrity, and neurologic status. An algorithm is presented to define optimal treatment.

23. Yi C, Hak DJ: Traumatic spinopelvic dissociation or U-shaped sacral fracture: A review of the literature. *Injury* 2012;43(4):402-408.

    The authors report on a literature review of spinopelvic dissociation or U-shaped sacral fractures, which are rare high-energy injury patterns characterized by a transverse sacral fracture in conjunction with bilateral vertical sacral fracture-dislocations. These injuries are associated with a high incidence of neurologic complications. This review describes the incidence, clinical evaluation, treatment, and outcomes of this injury pattern, with an emphasis on lumbopelvic fixation to restore stability.

24. Kim MY, Reidy DP, Nolan PC, Finkelstein JA: Transverse sacral fractures: Case series and literature review. *Can J Surg* 2001;44(5):359-363.

    A review of the incidence, evaluation, and treatment methods for transverse sacral fractures is presented. The relatively new techniques of lumbopelvic fixation and triangular osteosynthesis to restore stability to the lumbosacral junction are highlighted.

25. Phelan ST, Jones DA, Bishay M: Conservative management of transverse fractures of the sacrum with neurological features: A report of four cases. *J Bone Joint Surg Br* 1991;73(6):969-971.

26. Strange-Vognsen HH, Lebech A: An unusual type of fracture in the upper sacrum. *J Orthop Trauma* 1991;5(2):200-203.

27. Sabiston CP, Wing PC: Sacral fractures: Classification and neurologic implications. *J Trauma* 1986;26(12):1113-1115.

28. Dujardin FH, Hossenbaccus M, Duparc F, Biga N, Thomine JM: Long-term functional prognosis of posterior injuries in high-energy pelvic disruption. *J Orthop Trauma* 1998;12(3):145-150, discussion 150-151.

29. Chapman JR, Schildauer TA, Bellabarba C, Nork SE, Mirza SK: Treatment of sacral fractures with neurologic injuries. *Top Spinal Cord Inj Rehabil* 2002;8:59-78.

30. Fardon DF: Displaced fracture of the lumbosacral spine with delayed cauda equina deficit: Report of a case and review of literature. *Clin Orthop Relat Res* 1976;120:155-158.

31. Carl A, Delman A, Engler G: Displaced transverse sacral fractures: A case report, review of the literature, and the CT scan as an aid in management. *Clin Orthop Relat Res* 1985;194:195-198.

32. Bellabarba C, Stewart JD, Ricci WM, DiPasquale TG, Bolhofner BR: Midline sagittal sacral fractures in anterior-posterior compression pelvic ring injuries. *J Orthop Trauma* 2003;17(1):32-37.

33. Nork SE, Jones CB, Harding SP, Mirza SK, Routt ML Jr: Percutaneous stabilization of U-shaped sacral fractures using iliosacral screws: Technique and early results. *J Orthop Trauma* 2001;15(4):238-246.

34. Woods RK, O'Keefe G, Rhee P, Routt ML Jr, Maier RV: Open pelvic fracture and fecal diversion. *Arch Surg* 1998;133(3):281-286.

Chapter 30

Whiplash and Whiplash-Associated Disorders

Jerome Schofferman, MD

Abstract

Whiplash is the term used to describe neck pain after a motor vehicle collision, and whiplash-associated disorders refer to the myriad of other symptoms that might develop. Chronic pain develops in as many as 50% of patients who sustain acute whiplash injury, and significant chronic pain and disability develop in as many as 4% to 16% of these patients. It has been suggested that the type of early care does not affect outcomes. For chronic pain, exercise and body mechanics training are the most commonly prescribed remedies, but improvements are often small. The cervical facet joints are the structural cause most readily identified in patients with refractory pain. When such pain is present, treatment with radiofrequency neurotomy can be beneficial. Medications may be indicated for patients with refractory pain, although data are lacking. Surgery is reserved for those rare patients with severe refractory pain who do not improve with other treatments, are psychologically healthy, and have an identifiable structural injury such as an injured disk that can potentially be improved with surgery.

Keywords: motor vehicle collision; neck pain; whiplash-associated disorders; whiplash injury

Introduction

Whiplash and whiplash-associated injury are the terms used to describe a neck injury resulting from an acceleration and/or deceleration injury caused by a motor vehicle collision (MVC) or other forms of indirect

Dr. Schofferman or an immediate family member serves as a board member, owner, officer, or committee member of the North American Spine Society.

trauma.[1] Whiplash-associated disorders is the general term used to describe other symptoms in patients with whiplash.

Symptoms of Whiplash Injury

Neck Pain

Neck pain is the predominant symptom of whiplash injury and is seen in 84% to 95% of patients who are symptomatic after an MVC.[2,3] In one-third of patients, neck pain occurs immediately following the MVC. In 90% of patients, pain begins within the first 24 hours, but occasionally the onset of symptoms is delayed. Neck pain can be unilateral or bilateral. It is commonly referred to the trapezius, interscapular area, arms (diffusely or focally), and posterior occipital region. Pain can be constant or intermittent, and the severity varies. It has been unequivocally established that neck pain can be a result of a facet joint injury, and it is inferred from the best available evidence that chronic neck pain also can be caused by a disk injury, a nerve root injury attributable to sudden narrowing of the neural canal during the collision, and perhaps ligament and muscle damage.[4,5]

Headache

Headache resulting from neck injury (cervicogenic headache) occurs in 72% to 81% of patients with whiplash injury and might be considered the most cephalad presentation of axial neck pain.[2,3] Pain is usually suboccipital and may radiate to one or both temporal regions, the frontal regions, and crown of the head. It can be unilateral or bilateral and vary in severity and frequency, even in the same individual. Cervicogenic headache is often confused with migraine or tension-type headaches. It is often precipitated or worsened by prolonged static neck position or repeated end-range flexion, extension, or axial rotation.

6: Trauma

Symptoms and Causes of Acute and Chronic Whiplash-Associated Disorders

Most patients with whiplash injury have multiple areas of pain. In the past, the experience of widespread pain and perhaps unexpected symptoms had been considered to have a predominantly psychological cause, or what had been called somatization illness. Currently, these symptoms can be explained by the combination of a broader view of whiplash-associated disorders and central sensitization with hyperalgesia and allodynia.

Low Back Pain

Low back pain is seen in more than 50% of patients with acute whiplash injury. In 30% to 42% of these patients, low back pain is still present 6 months later.[2,6] The primary structures associated with chronic low back pain resulting from MVC are lumbar disks, facet joints, and sacroiliac joints.[7]

Midback or Thoracic Pain

Midback or thoracic pain occurs after MVC in approximately 55% of patients with whiplash injury, and 23% still have midback pain 1 year later.[3] Thoracic pain can result from disk injury or herniation, and presumably from thoracic facet joints and less often, costovertebral joints.[8]

Shoulder Pain

Shoulder pain can be referred from the neck, can be a result of an impingement syndrome,[9] and perhaps more often can be referred pain from deeper cervical spine structures to muscles in the shoulder area.

Soft-Tissue Injury

Soft-tissue injury is a nonspecific term that has little clinical value and has been used to minimize the cause of a patient's complaints of pain in the medicolegal context. Soft tissues are muscles and ligaments. Certainly, pain can be felt after acute whiplash injury that emanates from these soft tissues.[4] However, these injuries are expected to heal in 6 to 8 weeks. When pain persists, it is most likely a result of other structural problems. Chronic muscular pain might be better attributed to either excess strain when muscles overwork to compensate for injuries to deeper structures or to poor posture as the body attempts to minimize stress and pain.

Dizziness

Dizziness and unsteadiness, sometimes accompanied by visual disturbances, are described by 40% to 75% of patients with chronic whiplash.[10] The dizziness is not vertiginous; instead, it is a feeling of general lightheadedness or unsteadiness. The symptoms are seen more often in patients with moderate to severe neck pain.

Fibromyalgia

Fibromyalgia is a condition in which widespread pain is felt in muscles, tendons, joints, and bones that occurs on both sides of the body above and below the waist and lasts longer than 3 months. True fibromyalgia is rare following an MVC.

Facial Pain

Facial pain, which often manifests as dysesthesia or paresthesia, is theorized to be a result of alterations in the trigeminal nerve complex, and it appears more commonly in patients with upper cervical spine injuries.[11]

Psychological Symptoms

Psychological symptoms are common. No characteristic psychological profile exists for whiplash. Approximately 13% of patients with acute whiplash demonstrate moderate to severe stress response.[12] Posttraumatic stress disorder develops in approximately 17% of patients.[13] One study reported the development of depressive symptoms in 42% of individuals without preexisting psychological illness within 6 weeks of injury and in another 18% of individuals later than 6 weeks after injury.[14] Persistent or recurrent depressive symptoms were seen in 38%.

If a psychological disorder occurs secondary to pain and impairment, then the psychological disorder would be expected to improve if pain is effectively treated. In patients with abnormal psychological test results, the results often normalize after a successful cervical radiofrequency neurotomy (RFN) but regress when pain recurs. If a repeated RFN is successful, psychological test results return to normal again.[15,16]

Structural Causes of Whiplash Injury

The only structure that can be identified or excluded with assurance is the facet joint.[4] The attribution of chronic pain to other causes is inferred from autopsy studies, retrospective case series, biomechanical work, and cadaver studies. These tissue causes may involve disks (particularly anterior anulus tears), anterior longitudinal ligament, dorsal root ganglia, vascular systems, and muscles.[4,5,17] The history, examination, and imaging studies are of little value in the elucidation of the specific structural cause of axial neck pain.

Facet Joints

Compelling biomechanical, autopsy, and clinical research evidence exists that cervical facet joints can be a source of pain. Multiple types of lesions that occur within the facet joint can cause acute or chronic pain[18] (**Figure 1**). These include rupture or tear of the facet joint capsule and contusion of the intra-articular meniscus.

Facet joints are the source of pain in 25% to 54% of patients with neck pain after whiplash.[19,20] In cervicogenic headache, the prevalence of C2-C3 facet joint pain was 53%.[21]

Cervical facet pain can be unilateral or bilateral and is usually located just off the midline. Pain is often precipitated or worsened by movement and referred to the trapezius interscapular areas. Upper facet joint pain can cause headache. No specific findings exist for facet joint pain on history, physical examination, or radiologic studies. Facet joint pain can only be diagnosed by using medial branch blocks.[4]

Disks

Anatomic, biomechanical, and autopsy studies show that disks can be injured along with the anterior longitudinal ligament during the abnormal hyperextension phase of whiplash.[4,5,17] Potential disk injuries include anulus fibrosus tears and end plate avulsions[18] (**Figure 1**). Disk pain can be localized to the level of the injured disk and often is referred to the areas of the trapezius and interscapular region. The mapping pattern of referral from disks overlaps the referral patterns of the facet joints. One recent study suggested that open disk stimulation via tapping the spinous processes can identify a painful disk. Subsequent arthrodesis of the presumed painful disk relieved the neck pain, which, if generalizable, implies the disk can be a source of pain.[22]

Atlanto-occipital and Atlantoaxial Joints

The atlanto-occipital and atlantoaxial joints have been shown to be a cause of headache by the provocation of concordant head pain during injection of the joint with local anesthetic, which is followed by relief of the presenting pain immediately afterward.[23] The pain is suboccipital and can be unilateral or bilateral; it is typically an aching pain and can be quite severe. Pain from these joints (or upper cervical facet joints) is frequently mistaken for occipital neuralgia because of the pain distribution, but neuralgic pain is electric or shock-like in nature rather than aching.

Shoulder Joint, Shoulder Muscles, and Peripheral Nerve Injury or Entrapment

Peripheral nerve injuries and entrapments occur in almost 10% of patients with whiplash. Median nerve injury is most likely a result of blunt nerve trauma from the steering wheel or dashboard. Impingement has been noted in some patients.[9]

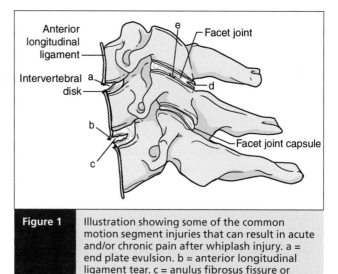

Figure 1 Illustration showing some of the common motion segment injuries that can result in acute and/or chronic pain after whiplash injury. a = end plate evulsion. b = anterior longitudinal ligament tear. c = anulus fibrosus fissure or tear. d = facet joint capsule tear. e = facet joint meniscus damage.

Muscle Pain

Muscle pain occurs in the acute phase. If chronic pain is attributed to muscles, it most likely is referred pain or pain attributable to muscle strain that occurs from compensating for injured deep structures. However, fatty infiltration of muscles does occur, especially in patients with more severe pain and disability. The clinical importance is not clear.

Other Potential Causes/Mediators of Whiplash Injury and Whiplash-Associated Disorders

Psychological Factors

A substantial number of patients with whiplash have psychological distress compared with individuals who are uninjured in crashes and control subjects.[24] Psychological problems, including anxiety disorder, depression, and posttraumatic stress disorder (PTSD) after an MVC, are more likely to develop in individuals who sustain whiplash in comparison with individuals who are not injured. Individuals with preexisting mental health problems are more susceptible to the development of chronic whiplash symptoms than those who do not have a history of mental health problems.

Other important issues are fear avoidance (fear of movement), catastrophizing (exaggerated negative beliefs or interpretations of current or anticipated pain), and dysfunctional coping style.[25] Interwoven with these issues are the patient's expectations for recovery, anger, blame, and, in the opinion of some investigators, the role of litigation. Fear avoidance is the avoidance of activity because of fear of increasing pain, worsening an injury,

6: Trauma

or causing reinjury.[25] The fear might be conscious or unconscious. The fear avoidance can result in disuse and worsening disability and can progress to mood disorder. Catastrophizing can play a role in both acute and chronic whiplash. Coping style is the way an individual copes with his or her injury symptoms cognitively, behaviorally, and emotionally. Patients with active coping styles tend to do better than those with passive coping styles. PTSD is a pathologic anxiety state resulting from a direct or indirect traumatic event, has specific clusters of diagnostic criteria, and causes substantial distress or impairment of function. PTSD occurs in up to 23% of patients after an MVC.

Central Hyperexcitability (Sensitization)

Central nervous system sensitization with hyperexcitability and hyperalgesia sometimes develops in patients with chronic whiplash. This partly explains the widespread pain and pain response to usually innocuous (endogenous and exogenous) stimuli. The cycle of abnormal events begins with tissue injury that causes the release of multiple mediators that results in the sensitization process and changes in the peripheral and central nervous system that result in abnormal pain processing.[26]

Cognitive Impairment

Many patients with whiplash-associated disorders report difficulties with memory, concentration, and simple calculations, often associated with emotional lability and excessive irritability. Such findings are consistent with minimal traumatic brain injury (coup-contrecoup injury) but also with chronic pain, medications, and PTSD. Psychological evaluation is indicated in the presence of these findings.

Litigation

The role of litigation and compensation is often misunderstood both in the medicolegal context and in the evaluation, treatment, and expectation of outcome. The hypothesis that individuals with whiplash injury are "cured by verdict" has been clearly disproven.[27] No good evidence exists that the potential for litigation results in worse health.[28] Most studies do not address reverse causation, such as whether severe or ongoing symptoms influence the decision to pursue compensation or vice versa.

Mechanism of Whiplash Injury

After a rear-end collision, the torso is forced upward and forward while the head initially remains stationary, which results in relative anterior translation of the torso with respect to the head as well as an abnormal upward force.

To compensate for this differential motion between the torso and head, the uppermost spinal segments flex while the distal segments move into extension distally, creating an S-shaped curve (**Figure 2**). Most injuries occur during this phase because of the abnormal and nonphysiologic shear and compression forces.[29]

Most of this biomechanical information has been obtained from simulated rear-impact studies; however, whiplash injury can occur from front-end impact as well.[30-32] Approximately 50% of injuries occur in rear-impact collisions, 27% in front-end impact, and 16% in side impact.[31] Front or side impact can result in the same symptoms as rear impact collisions.[31] Based on bioengineering studies, the disks and anterior longitudinal ligament are susceptible to injury in a frontal impact crash.[30]

Natural History of Whiplash Injury

Most individuals involved in an MVC do not sustain injury. The natural history of those who sustain injury is discouraging.[33-35] Of those who are injured, the consensus is that 50% do not recover fully.[34,35] Of those who recover, most do better within the first 3 to 6 months; only a small percentage of patients fully recover after 6 months.[33,34] Those who do not recover are left with mild to moderate pain, but 4% to 16% have moderate to severe pain, with the potential for substantial disability.[33,35]

Prognostic Factors

Risks for Initial Injury

Conflicting evidence exists regarding crash risk factors for initial injury. In typical lower-speed crashes, it is unlikely that a change in velocity less than 9 km/hr will result in substantial injury, although the relationship between the change in velocity and injury threshold has not been established.[29] However, short-term cervical, lumbar, and thoracic symptoms can occur at a change in velocity as low as 6.3 km/hr.[36,37] Other factors for injury for which the evidence is somewhat conflicting include being the driver or front seat passenger, neck pain prior to the collision, female sex, older age, head rotated at impact, head restraint that is too low, and awareness of impending collision.

Risks for Chronic Pain and Disability

Inconsistency exists regarding most risk factors for a poor prognosis; however, virtually all investigators agree that a high level of initial pain is associated consistently with a poor prognosis. Hypothetically, this could mean that more initial pain implies greater injury that might

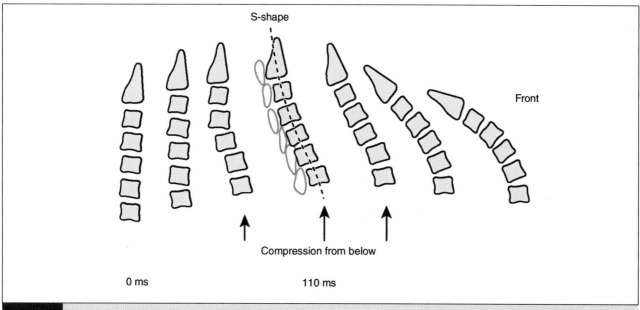

S-shape

Front

Compression from below

0 ms   110 ms

| **Figure 2** | Illustration of abnormal movement of the cervical spine after a rear-end motor vehicle collision (impact from the left in this figure). After collision, the thorax moves anteriorly and upward, compressing the cervical spine from below and causing abnormal deformation and an S-shaped curvature. |

be more likely to result in chronicity, recognizing that, most often, the structural etiology cannot be definitively identified. Consistent with the greater injury hypothesis, a 2016 study reported that approximately 45% of the patients with initial mild pain and disability recovered fully, the 39% who had early moderate pain and disability improved but eventually had mild levels of pain and disability, and 16% of the patients with initial severe pain and disability eventually had chronic moderate to severe levels of pain and disability.[35] In addition to the initial degree of pain, consensus is good that a high level of early neck-related disability and early widespread pain also predict a poor prognosis.[34,36]

The psychological factors often but not consistently linked to a poor prognosis include poor mental health prior to the MVC and postcollision PTSD, catastrophizing, passive coping, low expectations of recovery, expectations of long recovery time, and high levels of anxiety.[25,36,38]

No good relationship has been shown between vehicle damage and occupant injury.[39]

Treatment: Acute Neck Pain

The goals of early treatment of whiplash injury are to reduce pain, maintain function, and decrease the likelihood of progression to chronic pain and disability. No treatment protocol meets these goals. Perhaps most discouraging is that individualized treatment that allowed

pharmacologic intervention, multimodal physical therapy, and psychotherapy according to each patient's individual needs achieved no better outcomes than those achieved with typical care.[39,40] Furthermore, it appears that the more aggressive the early treatment, the worse the prognosis.[41]

The Ontario Protocol for Traffic Injury Management (OPTIMa) Collaboration recommends that major structural or medical illness be ruled out first.[42] Clinicians should educate patients on the typically benign causes of the neck pain and that it is best to continue normal activities.[43] The authors of the OPTIMa Collaboration study believed it is reasonable to prescribe structured education, but only in combination with supervised strength training, or range-of-motion exercises with mobilization or manipulation, and perhaps muscle relaxants.[42] Immobilization in a cervical orthosis delays recovery.

Medications are often prescribed for acute whiplash injury. High-dose methylprednisolone administered within 8 hours of injury has been shown to reduce the level of pain, total number of sick days taken, and sick leave profile, but its use seems to be rare.[44] NSAIDs might be more effective than placebo, but many patients have adverse side effects. The choice of medication is empiric and based on the level of pain and amount of impairment.

As a practical matter, it is important that the clinician takes some action. Given the lack of high-level evidence, it is reasonable that the patient be reassured that the pain is not dangerous and activity will not worsen the problem.

6: Trauma

The patient should be informed that substantial improvement is likely and the best outcome is seen in those who maintain a high level of function despite the pain. In the absence of neurologic abnormalities, imaging studies are not indicated or necessary. The choice of which drug to use depends on the individual patient's risk factors, prior medication use, and the severity of the pain. For mild to moderate pain, an NSAID seems appropriate for patients at low risk of complications, perhaps combined with a short course of a skeletal muscle relaxant. To maintain function in patients with severe pain, short-acting opioids can be used for 7 to 10 days, with no refills until the patient is seen again by his or her physician. Some physicians believe that the first refill is the one that must be most carefully considered. Another option, with no data for oral use, is to add an oral corticosteroid such as prednisone or an equivalent for 7 to 10 days, starting with approximately 60 mg, with the dose tapering off after approximately 3 days.

It is important to schedule a follow-up visit, at which time physical therapy can be considered, if only to try to avoid catastrophizing and fear avoidance and to reevaluate the patient's medications. The patient should be reevaluated regularly. If no meaningful improvement occurs by 3 to 4 months, more aggressive evaluation and treatment are indicated. MRI and radiography can be performed, and the patient should be referred for physical therapy with neck-specific exercises.

Treatment: Chronic Neck Pain

Exercise Therapy

Exercise therapy remains the first choice of treatment for chronic whiplash injury, at least theoretically, because of the known changes often seen with respect to neck muscle function and fatty infiltration of muscles.[45] However, the evidence of efficacy for neck-specific exercises is not consistent. Clearly, despite a good rehabilitation program, a substantial number of patients will continue to have pain and disability that might require interventional or pharmacologic treatments.

A supervised exercise program that emphasizes strength and endurance training appears to be helpful in patients with chronic neck pain after whiplash injury.[45,46] A 2016 study reported that neck-specific exercises with and without a behavioral approach by a physical therapist have resulted in some reduced disability and pain compared with instructions to exercise.[47] However, only 61% of the patients achieved a 50% reduction in pain. Patients with greater initial pain and disability tended to have more functional improvement. Benefits are no longer apparent at 2 years, so patients need to be instructed that they must continue to exercise. Other advantages of exercise can include reduced fear avoidance, improved coping abilities, and decreased catastrophizing. Other patients have found intensive exercise no better than advice.[48]

Spinal manipulative therapy combined with exercise is beneficial for chronic mechanical neck pain when combined with neck-specific exercises in some patients.[49] Manual therapy plus neck-specific exercises are better than usual care by general practitioners for patients with mechanical neck pain.[49]

Interventional Treatments

RFN is the interventional treatment with the best evidence of efficacy for neck pain resulting from whiplash. RFN is applicable only to those patients with proven facet joint pain. When relief is achieved after a diagnostic medial branch block, long-term relief can be obtained in more than 70% of patients after RFN. Improvement is maintained for approximately 10 months.[4,50] When benefits dissipate, repeat RFN is usually successful.[9]

In addition to pain relief, advantages include alleviation of disability and improvement of cervical range of motion, psychological distress, and pain catastrophizing, all of which returned to baseline when the benefits of the RFN diminished at approximately 10 months.[50] RFN produced no improvement in PTSD symptoms.[16]

No evidence exists that cervical epidural corticosteroid injections help relieve axial neck pain. Intra-articular injections of corticosteroids are not effective for the long-term treatment of cervical facet joint pain but can provide short-term relief. Evidence is mixed for the efficacy of botulinum toxin injections.

Medication management has not been studied at all for chronic whiplash pain, and no good evidence exists to make recommendations, which, as a result, are empiric. Treatment recommendations are usually extrapolated from studies of the use of medications in patients with lumbar spine pain. Long-term NSAID use is probably not a good choice when weighing the small benefits versus the high risks, especially in older patients and in those with medical illnesses. Acetaminophen should be used in doses at 2 g per day or less because of the risk of hepatic dysfunction.

If rehabilitation or therapeutic injections are not successful, or response to other medications and psychological treatment is poor, opioid analgesics may be used in carefully selected patients. Such treatment should be guided by an experienced specialist in pain medicine who will evaluate the patient thoroughly and guide treatment carefully.

The use of anticonvulsants and antidepressants has not been studied in whiplash injury, but these drugs have been useful in patients with neuropathic pain. Some patients with whiplash display evidence of central sensitization, which could be considered a type of neuropathic pain.[26]

Surgery

Surgery is rarely indicated in the treatment of patients with chronic whiplash and dominant axial neck pain but can be considered after unsuccessful high-quality rehabilitation, interventions, and pharmacologic care in a patient in a healthy psychologic state. A recent study suggested that arthrodesis had better results than those of a good multimodal rehabilitation program.[22]

Summary

Whiplash and whiplash-associated disorders must be taken seriously. Only 50% of patients with whiplash injury recover completely, and a meaningful percentage of patients have significant long-term pain and disability. Because the medical evidence for many treatment options is lacking or of low quality, clinicians must rely on best available evidence. Although it does not appear that any type of early care for acute neck pain is superior to others or improves the natural history, many treatments can provide short-term relief. For chronic neck pain, exercise and body mechanics training are usually recommended, but improvements are usually small and supporting data are mixed. The facet joints are commonly injured and might be amenable to treatment with RFN.

Key Study Points

- The natural history of patients with neck pain, headache, or other symptom after whiplash injury is not benign.
- Perhaps the most important aspects of early care for patients with acute whiplash injury are education and encouragement to remain active.
- Chronic neck pain after whiplash injury might respond to exercise, but improvements are small or moderate and data are mixed.
- Because facet joints are a common source of pain and often can be treated with RFN, patients who are not improving might be offered medial branch blocks followed by RFN if medial branch blocks are helpful.

Annotated References

1. Spitzer WO, Skovron ML, Salmi LR, et al: Scientific monograph of the Quebec Task Force on Whiplash-Associated Disorders: Redefining "whiplash" and its management. *Spine (Phila Pa 1976)* 1995;20(8suppl):1S-73S.

2. Hincapié CA, Cassidy JD, Côté P, Carroll LJ, Guzmán J: Whiplash injury is more than neck pain: A population-based study of pain localization after traffic injury. *J Occup Environ Med* 2010;52(4):434-440.

3. Johansson MS, Boyle E, Hartvigsen J, Jensen Stochkendahl M, Carroll L, Cassidy JD: A population-based, incidence cohort study of mid-back pain after traffic collisions: Factors associated with global recovery. *Eur J Pain* 2015;19(10):1486-1495.

   This study included longitudinal data obtained from all traffic injuries occurring in Saskatchewan, Canada, during a 2-year period. A high prevalence of midback pain was found. The median time to recovery was 101 days; 23% of patients had not recovered at 1 year. Level of evidence: I.

4. Curatolo M, Bogduk N, Ivancic PC, McLean SA, Siegmund GP, Winkelstein BA: The role of tissue damage in whiplash-associated disorders: Discussion paper 1. *Spine (Phila Pa 1976)* 2011;36(25suppl):S309-S315.

   This article is a narrative review of the proven causes of tissue damage after whiplash injury. The anatomic, autopsy, and biomechanical hypotheses for other potential pain generators are discussed. Level of evidence: V.

5. Elliott J: The evidence for pathoanatomical lesions, in Sterling M, Kenardy J, eds: *Whiplash: Evidence Base for Clinical Practice.* Sydney, Australia, Elsevier, 2011, pp 29-39.

   This review of the pathomechanics of whiplash injury is followed by a discussion of the anatomic, biomechanical, theoretic, and autopsy findings.

6. Cassidy JD, Carroll L, Côté P, Berglund A, Nygren A: Low back pain after traffic collisions: A population-based cohort study. *Spine (Phila Pa 1976)* 2003;28(10):1002-1009.

7. De Palma M, Ketchum J, Saullo T, Schofferman J: Structural etiology of chronic low back pain due to motor vehicle collision. *Pain Med* 2011;12(11):1622-1627.

   This study reviewed patients with low back pain after whiplash injury using medial branch blocks, sacroiliac joint blocks, and diskography to determine the anatomic causes of low back pain. The causes were similar to those of patients with low back pain who were not in an MVC. Level of evidence: IV.

8. Dreyfuss P, Tibiletti C, Dreyer SJ: Thoracic zygapophyseal joint pain patterns: A study in normal volunteers. *Spine (Phila Pa 1976)* 1994;19(7):807-811.

6: Trauma

9. Abbassian A, Giddins GE: Subacromial impingement in patients with whiplash injury to the cervical spine. *J Orthop Surg Res* 2008;3:25.

10. Treleaven J: Dizziness, visual and sensorimotor control disturbances following whiplash injury, in Sterling M, Kenardy J, eds: *Whiplash: Evidence Base for Clinical Practice*. Sydney, Australia, Elsevier, 2011, pp 69-84.

   This chapter is an authoritative detailed discussion of the types of dizziness seen after whiplash injury. The causes are explored, including damage to the peripheral vestibular system, the possible role of stress, and the effects within the central nervous system.

11. Haldeman S, Dagenais S: Cervicogenic headaches: A critical review. *Spine J* 2001;1(1):31-46.

12. Kongsted A, Bendix T, Qerama E, et al: Acute stress response and recovery after whiplash injuries: A one-year prospective study. *Eur J Pain* 2008;12(4):455-463.

13. Buitenhuis J, de Jong P, Jaspers J, Kenardy J: Psychological aspects of whiplash associated disorders, in Sterling M, Kenardy J, eds: *Whiplash: Evidence Base for Clinical Practice*. Sydney, Australia, Elsevier, 2011, pp 85-92.

   This chapter provides a discussion of which types of psychological distress are associated with chronic whiplash symptoms. The acute stress disorder that can result in PTSD is discussed. Important modifiers such as anger, forms of coping, catastrophizing, fear avoidance, and expectations are detailed.

14. Carroll LJ, Cassidy JD, Côté P: Frequency, timing, and course of depressive symptomatology after whiplash. *Spine (Phila Pa 1976)* 2006;31(16):E551-E556.

15. Wallis BJ, Lord SM, Bogduk N: Resolution of psychological distress of whiplash patients following treatment by radiofrequency neurotomy: A randomised, double-blind, placebo-controlled trial. *Pain* 1997;73(1):15-22.

16. Smith AD, Jull G, Schneider GM, Frizzell B, Hooper RA, Sterling M: Modulation of cervical facet joint nociception and pain attenuates physical and psychological features of chronic whiplash: A prospective study. *PM R* 2015;7(9):913-921.

   Patients were assessed for disability and psychological issues before and after successful RFN. When pain improved, the disability, psychological distress, and catastrophizing all improved, but returned after the benefits of RFN diminished. Level of evidence: IV.

17. Siegmund GP, Winkelstein BA, Ivancic PC, Svensson MY, Vasavada A: The anatomy and biomechanics of acute and chronic whiplash injury. *Traffic Inj Prev* 2009;10(2):101-112.

18. Barnsley L, Lord S, Bogduk N: Whiplash injury. *Pain* 1994;58(3):283-307.

19. Barnsley L, Lord SM, Wallis BJ, Bogduk N: The prevalence of chronic cervical zygapophysial joint pain after whiplash. *Spine (Phila Pa 1976)* 1995;20(1):20-25, discussion 26.

20. Persson M, Sörensen J, Gerdle B: Chronic whiplash associated disorders (WAD): Responses to nerve blocks of cervical zygapophyseal joints. *Pain Med* 2016;17(12):2162-2175.

   In this study, 47 patients with chronic whiplash pain underwent medial branch block, starting with the most likely level (based on localization of pain and pain maps) and moving proximally and distally until pain improved by 50% or all joints were anesthetized. A positive response was noted in 29% of the patients. Level of evidence: IV.

21. Govind J, King W, Bailey B, Bogduk N: Radiofrequency neurotomy for the treatment of third occipital headache. *J Neurol Neurosurg Psychiatry* 2003;74(1):88-93.

22. Nyström B, Svensson E, Larsson S, Schillberg B, Mörk A, Taube A: A small group whiplash-associated-disorders (WAD) patients with central neck pain and movement induced stabbing pain, the painful segment determined by mechanical provocation: Fusion surgery was superior to multimodal rehabilitation in a randomized trial. *Scand J Pain* 2016;12:33-42.

   Patients with refractory neck pain were selected for randomization to multimodal rehabilitation versus fusion. The surgical level was selected by open spinous tapping. The surgery group did better in both intention and as-treated analyses. Level of evidence: II.

23. Dreyfuss P, Michaelsen M, Fletcher D: Atlanto-occipital and lateral atlanto-axial joint pain patterns. *Spine (Phila Pa 1976)* 1994;19(10):1125-1131.

24. Craig A, Tran Y, Guest R, et al: Psychological impact of injuries sustained in motor vehicle crashes: Systematic review and meta-analysis. *BMJ Open* 2016;6(9):e011993.

   Psychological distress is common after whiplash neck injury and whiplash-associated disorders. Most studies show the distress is still present after 3 years. Preventive strategies are needed for successful treatment. Level of evidence: II.

25. Buitenhuis J, de Jong PJ: Fear avoidance and illness beliefs in post-traumatic neck pain. *Spine (Phila Pa 1976)* 2011;36(25suppl):S238-S243.

   In this brief review of the fear-avoidance cycle, pain resulted in catastrophizing, which led to incorrect and dysfunctional beliefs followed by negative expectations regarding timing and degree of recovery, followed by fear avoidance. Providers might be able to interrupt this cycle by asking about patient's beliefs and offering good explanations.

26. Van Oosterwijck J, Nijs J, Meeus M, Paul L: Evidence for central sensitization in chronic whiplash: A systematic literature review. *Eur J Pain* 2013;17(3):299-312.

Central nervous system mechanisms, referred to as central sensitization, are involved in sustaining some pain in certain patients with whiplash. These central nervous system mechanisms partly explain the widespread pain as well as pain in the absence of known stimuli. Underlying mechanisms are not yet clear. Level of evidence: II.

27. Spearing NM, Gyrd-Hansen D, Pobereskin LH, Rowell DS, Connelly LB: Are people who claim compensation "cured by a verdict"? A longitudinal study of health outcomes after whiplash. *J Law Med* 2012;20(1):82-92.

    The possibility for compensation can cause patients to overstate their problems. An examination of claim settlement versus continuation of symptoms showed that removing the financial incentive to overreport has no effect on pain. Claimants do not appear to be "cured by verdict." Level of evidence: III.

28. Spearing NM, Connelly LB: Whiplash and the compensation hypothesis. *Spine (Phila Pa 1976)* 2011;36(25suppl):S303-S308.

    This systematic review examined studies using health outcomes, not proxy, and reported strong evidence of no association between litigation and poor outcomes after whiplash.

29. Stemper B, Yoganandan N, Pintar F, Maiman D: Mechanism of injury, in Sterling M, Kenardy J, eds: *Whiplash: Evidence Base for Clinical Practice*. Sydney, Australia, Elsevier, 2011, pp 16-28.

    This chapter provides an excellent review of the mechanisms of injury to the cervical spine after rear-end MVCs.

30. Ito S, Ivancic PC, Pearson AM, et al: Cervical intervertebral disc injury during simulated frontal impact. *Eur Spine J* 2005;14(4):356-365.

31. Siknov V, Tortolani P: Whiplash-associated disorders, in Rao RD, Smuck M, eds: *Orthopaedic Knowledge Update: Spine 4*. Rosemont, IL, American Academy of Orthopaedic Surgeons, 2011, pp 273-279.

    This chapter highlights important studies published from 2005 through 2010 concerning whiplash-associated injuries.

32. Panjabi MM, Ito S, Pearson AM, Ivancic PC: Injury mechanisms of the cervical intervertebral disc during simulated whiplash. *Spine (Phila Pa 1976)* 2004;29(11):1217-1225.

33. Radanov BP, Sturzenegger M, Di Stefano G: Long-term outcome after whiplash injury: A 2-year follow-up considering features of injury mechanism and somatic, radiologic, and psychosocial findings. *Medicine (Baltimore)* 1995;74(5):281-297.

34. Carroll LJ, Holm LW, Hogg-Johnson S, et al: Course and prognostic factors for neck pain in whiplash-associated disorders (WAD): Results of the Bone and Joint Decade 2000-2010 Task Force on Neck Pain and Its Associated Disorders. *J Manipulative Physiol Ther* 2009;32(2suppl):S97-S107.

35. Ritchie C, Sterling M: Recovery pathways and prognosis after whiplash injury. *J Orthop Sports Phys Ther* 2016;46(10):851-861.

    This study was one of the first to correlate initial symptoms after injury with outcomes. Three general pathways are suggested: mild pain, good recovery; moderate pain and disability, fair recovery; and severe pain and disability, poor recovery. Level of evidence: I.

36. Williamson E, Williams MA, Gates S, Lamb SE: Risk factors for chronic disability in a cohort of patients with acute whiplash associated disorders seeking physiotherapy treatment for persisting symptoms. *Physiotherapy* 2015;101(1):34-43.

    Of 430 patients with acute whiplash, chronic disability developed in 136 (32%). Factors suggesting disability outcome were high baseline disability, longer predicted patient recovery time, psychological distress, passive coping, and greater number of symptoms. Level of evidence: I.

37. Bartsch AJ, Gilbertson LG, Prakash V, Morr DR, Wiechel JF: Minor crashes and 'whiplash' in the United States. *Ann Adv Automot Med* 2008;52:117-128.

38. Guest R, Tran Y, Gopinath B, Cameron ID, Craig A: Psychological distress following a motor vehicle crash: A systematic review of preventative interventions. *Injury* 2016;47(11):2415-2423.

    This systematic review of treatments to prevent psychological distress after whiplash injury reported that preventive interventions were not effective. Treatment results for depression were mixed; cognitive-behavioral therapy showed the best results. Level of evidence: II.

39. Croft AC, Freeman MD: Correlating crash severity with injury risk, injury severity, and long-term symptoms in low velocity motor vehicle collisions. *Med Sci Monit* 2005;11(10):RA316-RA321.

40. Jull G, Kenardy J, Hendrikz J, Cohen M, Sterling M: Management of acute whiplash: A randomized controlled trial of multidisciplinary stratified treatments. *Pain* 2013;154(9):1798-1806.

    This randomized study of acute whiplash compared individualized multidisciplinary care with usual care. At 6 and 12 months, no difference was noted in pain or disability. In both groups, more initial disability acutely predicted more disability at 6 and 12 months. Level of evidence: I.

41. Skillgate E, Côté P, Cassidy JD, Boyle E, Carroll L, Holm LW: Effect of early intensive care on recovery from whiplash-associated disorders: Results of a population-based cohort study. *Arch Phys Med Rehabil* 2016;97(5):739-746.

    The number of visits by 5,204 patients to healthcare providers was tracked for 42 days after collision. In those with higher utilization of health care, recovery was slower. This study suggests that "less is more," and patients should be offered only essential early care. Level of evidence: I.

42. Côté P, Wong JJ, Sutton D, et al: Management of neck pain and associated disorders: A clinical practice

guideline from the Ontario Protocol for Traffic Injury Management (OPTIMa) Collaboration. *Eur Spine J* 2016;25(7):2000-2022.

This study reported on guidelines for neck pain and associated disorders that were developed based on literature review.

43. Pape E, Hagen KB, Brox JI, Natvig B, Schirmer H: Early multidisciplinary evaluation and advice was ineffective for whiplash-associated disorders. *Eur J Pain* 2009;13(10):1068-1075.

44. Pettersson K, Toolanen G: High-dose methylprednisolone prevents extensive sick leave after whiplash injury: A prospective, randomized, double-blind study. *Spine (Phila Pa 1976)* 1998;23(9):984-989.

45. Peolsson A, Landén Ludvigsson M, Tigerfors AM, Peterson G: Effects of neck-specific exercises compared to waiting list for individuals with chronic whiplash-associated disorders: A prospective, randomized controlled study. *Arch Phys Med Rehabil* 2016;97(2):189-195.

   In this comparison of patients randomized to neck-specific exercises or a waiting list, between-group analysis showed the neck-specific exercise group had substantially less disability but not less pain. In an intragroup analysis, the neck-specific exercise group improved in all measures, and the waitlist group worsened in most measures. Level of evidence: II.

46. Standaert CJ, Kumbhare DA: Second-order peer reviews of clinically relevant articles for the physiatrist: What works for chronic whiplash-associated disorders. Neck-specific exercises with or without behavioral modification? *Am J Phys Med Rehabil* 2016;95(4):e53-e56.

   This study rereviewed a 2016 study by Ludvigsson and associates and noted improvement, but gains were small. Other studies on exercise after whiplash also were examined.

47. Ludvigsson ML, Peterson G, Dedering Å, Peolsson A: One- and two-year follow-up of a randomized trial of neck-specific exercise with or without a behavioural approach compared with prescription of physical activity in chronic whiplash disorder. *J Rehabil Med* 2016;48(1):56-64.

   In this study, 216 patients performed neck-specific exercises with or without behavioral intervention versus a physical activity prescription. At 1-year follow-up, both neck-specific exercise groups did better with less disability and less pain, but no difference was noted between them. At 2-year follow-up, both neck-specific exercise groups had less disability, but improvements in pain were not significant. Level of evidence: I.

48. Michaleff ZA, Maher CG, Lin CW, et al: Comprehensive physiotherapy exercise programme or advice for chronic whiplash (PROMISE): A pragmatic randomised controlled trial. *Lancet* 2014;384(9938):133-141.

   This study of comprehensive exercise versus advice showed no difference between groups at each data point up to 12 months. PTSD did not change the effects of treatment. Level of evidence: I.

49. Sutton DA, Côté P, Wong JJ, et al: Is multimodal care effective for the management of patients with whiplash-associated disorders or neck pain and associated disorders? A systematic review by the Ontario Protocol for Traffic Injury Management (OPTIMa) Collaboration. *Spine J* 2016;16(12):1541-1565.

   The authors of this systematic review reported that multimodal care may be beneficial for patients with early or recalcitrant symptoms after whiplash-associated disorders or associated disorders with neck pain. Any one type of multimodal care was not found to be superior to others.

50. Husted DS, Orton D, Schofferman J, Kine G: Effectiveness of repeated radiofrequency neurotomy for cervical facet joint pain. *J Spinal Disord Tech* 2008;21(6):406-408.

Chapter 31

Principles of Spinal Cord Injury Rehabilitation

Michelle Gittler, MD

Abstract

The paralysis that accompanies spinal cord injury is only one aspect of postinjury consequences and care. Acute management includes the airway and respiration, cardiovascular resuscitation, spinal shock, and bowel and bladder function. After medical, surgical, and vertebral stability are achieved, the patient is typically transferred from the surgical intensive care unit; rehabilitation then begins, with a focus on maximizing functional independence with therapy and education. Issues to be addressed include impaired mobility and self-care; respiratory dysfunction; autonomic dysreflexia; venous thromboembolism; risk of pressure ulcers; pain; neurogenic bowel and bladder conditions; sexual dysfunction; and other secondary conditions, which may include spasticity, heterotopic ossification, syrinx, nerve entrapment/compression, osteoporosis, abnormalities of carbohydrate and lipid metabolism, and a myriad of (preventable) causes of early death.

Keywords: complete and incomplete spinal cord injuries; neurogenic bladder; neurogenic bowel; neuropathic pain; paraplegia; tetraplegia

Introduction

Although there have been no incidence studies of spinal cord injury (SCI) in the United States since the 1990s, it is estimated that there are approximately 12,000 new cases annually.[1] Over the years, the average age at the time of injury has increased from 29 years during the 1970s to 42 years during the period from 2010 to 2015.

Dr. Gittler or an immediate family member serves as a board member, owner, officer, or committee member of the American Academy of Physical Medicine and Rehabilitation.

Overall, the mean age is 34 years, with the most frequent age at SCI being 19 years. SCI occurs most often in males (80%), with a disproportionate share of these injuries (23%) occurring in black Americans, who represent only 12% of the general population. Motor vehicle crashes are the leading cause of injury, followed by falls, violently acquired injuries (primarily gunshot wounds), and sports injuries (with diving remaining the most common sport associated with spinal injury). The most frequent neurologic category is incomplete tetraplegia (45%), followed by incomplete paraplegia (21%). The least frequent neurologic presentation is complete tetraplegia. Although the life expectancy for individuals with SCI is still less than the life expectancy for those without SCI, individuals surviving at least 1 year after injury may live an additional 50 years, which necessitates ongoing management by a physician skilled in SCI medicine.[1]

Traumatic Injury

Outcomes for patients with SCI are tracked by the National Spinal Cord Injury Statistical Center, which manages the world's largest SCI database and is the hub of the SCI model care system. However, because only approximately 13% of patients with SCI receive care in a model system, much of what is known about outcomes is extrapolated from a small population of patients.[1]

Traumatic SCI, as differentiated from medical SCI such as spinal cord compression secondary to metastatic disease, hematoma, and infection, is initiated by a sudden blow or rupture to the spine or spinal cord that may or may not fracture and dislocate vertebrae. Damage begins at the moment of primary injury when the cord itself is damaged, either directly or as a result of bone fragments or disk material. SCI also can occur without structural damage to the cord, such as secondary injury from the blast effect. Within minutes, subsequent swelling within the spinal canal increases pressure on the cord and may cut blood flow to spinal cord tissue. As a result of SCI and spinal shock, the body loses its ability to regulate blood

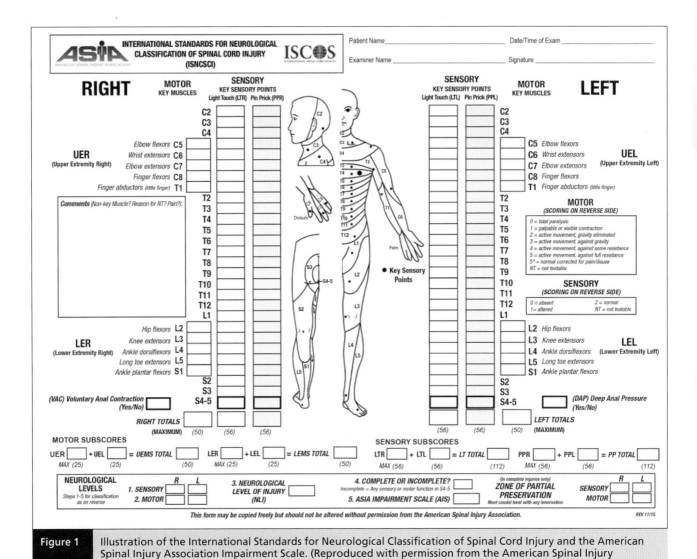

Figure 1 Illustration of the International Standards for Neurological Classification of Spinal Cord Injury and the American Spinal Injury Association Impairment Scale. (Reproduced with permission from the American Spinal Injury Association: *International Standards for Neurological Classification of Spinal Cord Injury*. Available at: http://asia-spinalinjury.org/wp-content/uploads/2016/02/International_Stds_Diagram_Worksheet.pdf. Accessed March 9, 2017.)

pressure, which may cause profound hypotension. Some controversy exists about the extent and even definition of spinal shock. During spinal shock, the entire spinal cord below the level of injury becomes temporarily disabled, with loss of all reflexes in addition to paralysis and loss of sensation. The cascade of biochemical and cellular events kills neurons, destroys myelin, and triggers an inflammatory immune response, which is the beginning of the secondary injury process. This process can result in an increased area of cord destruction.

Classification

Injuries are classified as complete or incomplete based on the International Standards for Neurological Classification of Spinal Cord Injury, which measures the extent of

neurologic injury after SCI. The American Spinal Injury Association (ASIA) Impairment Scale helps to further classify an injury (**Figure 1**).

An incomplete injury means that the ability of the spinal cord to convey messages to or from the brain is not completely lost. In a complete injury, there is no communication from the brain and spinal cord to parts of the body below the level of the injury. Based on the ASIA Impairment Scale definition, some motor or sensory function must be present in the sacral segments (S4-S5) for an injury to be described as incomplete.

Terminology

Precision is important in communication and documentation of SCI. The term tetraplegia is preferred over

Muscle Function Grading

0 = total paralysis

1 = palpable or visible contraction

2 = active movement, full range of motion (ROM) with gravity eliminated

3 = active movement, full ROM against gravity

4 = active movement, full ROM against gravity and moderate resistance in a muscle specific position

5 = (normal) active movement, full ROM against gravity and full resistance in a functional muscle position expected from an otherwise unimpaired person

5* = (normal) active movement, full ROM against gravity and sufficient resistance to be considered normal if identified inhibiting factors (i.e. pain, disuse) were not present

NT = not testable (i.e. due to immobilization, severe pain such that the patient cannot be graded, amputation of limb, or contracture of > 50% of the normal ROM)

Sensory Grading

0 = Absent

1 = Altered, either decreased/impaired sensation or hypersensitivity

2 = Normal

NT = Not testable

When to Test Non-Key Muscles:

In a patient with an apparent AIS B classification, non-key muscle functions more than 3 levels below the motor level on each side should be tested to most accurately classify the injury (differentiate between AIS B and C).

Movement	Root level
Shoulder: Flexion, extension, abduction, adduction, internal and external rotation **Elbow:** Supination	C5
Elbow: Pronation **Wrist:** Flexion	C6
Finger: Flexion at proximal joint, extension **Thumb:** Flexion, extension and abduction in plane of thumb	C7
Finger: Flexion at MCP joint **Thumb:** Opposition, adduction and abduction perpendicular to palm	C8
Finger: Abduction of the index finger	T1
Hip: Adduction	L2
Hip: External rotation	L3
Hip: Extension, abduction, internal rotation **Knee:** Flexion **Ankle:** Inversion and eversion **Toe:** MP and IP extension	L4
Hallux and Toe: DIP and PIP flexion and abduction	L5
Hallux: Adduction	S1

ASIA Impairment Scale (AIS)

A = Complete. No sensory or motor function is preserved in the sacral segments S4-5.

B = Sensory Incomplete. Sensory but not motor function is preserved below the neurological level and includes the sacral segments S4-5 (light touch or pin prick at S4-5 or deep anal pressure) AND no motor function is preserved more than three levels below the motor level on either side of the body.

C = Motor Incomplete. Motor function is preserved at the most caudal sacral segments for voluntary anal contraction (VAC) OR the patient meets the criteria for sensory incomplete status (sensory function preserved at the most caudal sacral segments (S4-S5) by LT, PP or DAP), and has some sparing of motor function more than three levels below the ipsilateral motor level on either side of the body.
(This includes key or non-key muscle functions to determine motor incomplete status.) For AIS C – less than half of key muscle functions below the single NLI have a muscle grade ≥ 3.

D = Motor Incomplete. Motor incomplete status as defined above, with at least half (half or more) of key muscle functions below the single NLI having a muscle grade ≥ 3.

E = Normal. If sensation and motor function as tested with the ISNCSCI are graded as normal in all segments, and the patient had prior deficits, then the AIS grade is E. Someone without an initial SCI does not receive an AIS grade.

Using ND: To document the sensory, motor and NLI levels, the ASIA Impairment Scale grade, and/or the zone of partial preservation (ZPP) when they are unable to be determined based on the examination results.

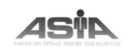

INTERNATIONAL STANDARDS FOR NEUROLOGICAL CLASSIFICATION OF SPINAL CORD INJURY

Steps in Classification

The following order is recommended for determining the classification of individuals with SCI.

1. Determine sensory levels for right and left sides.
The sensory level is the most caudal, intact dermatome for both pin prick and light touch sensation.

2. Determine motor levels for right and left sides.
Defined by the lowest key muscle function that has a grade of at least 3 (on supine testing), providing the key muscle functions represented by segments above that level are judged to be intact (graded as a 5).
Note: in regions where there is no myotome to test, the motor level is presumed to be the same as the sensory level, if testable motor function above that level is also normal.

3. Determine the neurological level of injury (NLI)
This refers to the most caudal segment of the cord with intact sensation and antigravity (3 or more) muscle function strength, provided that there is normal (intact) sensory and motor function rostrally respectively.
The NLI is the most cephalad of the sensory and motor levels determined in steps 1 and 2.

4. Determine whether the injury is Complete or Incomplete.
(i.e. absence or presence of sacral sparing)
*If voluntary anal contraction = **No** AND all S4-5 sensory scores = **0** AND deep anal pressure = **No**, then injury is **Complete.***
*Otherwise, injury is **Incomplete.***

5. Determine ASIA Impairment Scale (AIS) Grade:

Is injury **Complete?** If YES, AIS=A and can record ZPP (lowest dermatome or myotome on each side with some preservation)

NO ↓

Is injury Motor **Complete?** If YES, AIS=B
(No=voluntary anal contraction OR motor function more than three levels below the motor level on a given side, if the patient has sensory incomplete classification)

NO ↓

Are <u>at least</u> half (half or more) of the key muscles below the neurological level of injury graded 3 or better?

NO → AIS=C   YES → AIS=D

If sensation and motor function is normal in all segments, AIS=E
Note: AIS E is used in follow-up testing when an individual with a documented SCI has recovered normal function. If at initial testing no deficits are found, the individual is neurologically intact; the ASIA Impairment Scale does not apply.

Figure 1	(*Continued*) Illustration of the International Standards for Neurological Classification of Spinal Cord Injury and the American Spinal Injury Association Impairment Scale. (Reproduced with permission from the American Spinal Injury Association: *International Standards for Neurological Classification of Spinal Cord Injury*. Available at: http://asia-spinalinjury.org/wp-content/uploads/2016/02/International_Stds_Diagram_Worksheet.pdf. Accessed March 9, 2017.)

quadriplegia. Tetraplegia refers to impairment or loss of motor and/or sensory function in the cervical segments of the spinal cord. Paraplegia refers to impairment or loss of motor and/or sensory function in the thoracic, lumbar, or sacral segments of the spinal cord. The term paraplegia also is used in referring to cauda equina and conus medullaris injuries. The terms tetraparesis and paraparesis should not be used because they are imprecise.

Examination Findings and Rehabilitation Goals

The initial ASIA examination should be completed as soon as possible after injury. Because the patient must be alert enough to participate in the examination, the time frame for administering the examination depends on the patient's medical condition. An accurate clinical examination will result in an appropriate diagnosis, can predict recovery, can frame rehabilitation and health care planning, and is essential for research. The examination should be performed within 72 hours of injury unless factors, including sedation for ventilation, intoxication, severe pain, psychiatric disorder, or head injury, preclude an examination. The International Standards Training e-Learning Program (InSTeP) is designed to teach clinicians how to perform an accurate neurologic examination of a patient with an SCI.[2] Completion of this program has resulted in excellent interrater examination reliability.

The level of an injury and the completeness or incompleteness of an injury guide the rehabilitation goals and expected functional outcome. The Consortium for Spinal

6: Trauma

Cord Medicine, funded by the Paralyzed Veterans of America, has created a series of evidence-based clinical practice guidelines (and companion consumer guides) that have been graded for scientific strength and methodology.[3] For example, one guideline predicts what equipment will be needed, how much assistance is needed, and the expected functional outcome based on each neurologic level of injury.[4]

Strategies and Treatment

Current research through the National Institute of Neurological Disorders and Stroke, a part of the National Institutes of Health, is being done to understand and treat SCIs. Research is focused on the following four key principles: neurologic protection, regeneration, cell replacement, and retraining central nervous system circuits and plasticity.[5]

Strategies involving neurologic protection are aimed at preventing cell death and limiting inflammation. Although steroids have frequently been used to suppress activities of immune cells, steroid therapy has not been approved by the FDA for treatment of acute SCI. The Congress of Neurological Surgeons and the American Association of Neurological Surgeons cite level I evidence that the administration of methylprednisolone for acute SCI is not recommended because there is no class I or II evidence of benefit; however, class I, II, and III evidence exists that high-dose steroids are associated with harmful side effects.[6] This recommendation is a change from the prior 2002 recommendation that considered methylprednisolone as a treatment option.

In animal models of SCI, antibiotics, which can cross the blood-brain barrier, have been shown to improve motor function, decrease lesion size, and reduce cell death.[5]

The safety and effectiveness of different durations of hypothermia after SCI currently are being explored. In animal models and limited human studies, hypothermia has been shown to reduce damage to susceptible neurons in the primary injury site, reduce damage to microvasculature, and improve functional outcome.[5]

The buildup of sodium and glutamate after an SCI can lead to cell damage. Riluzole, which slows the progression of amyotrophic lateral sclerosis, has been shown in animal models to reduce cell death after SCI. An experimental drug, HP 184, blocks the entry of sodium into cells (which can impair nerve function) and may enhance cell signaling and axon survival. Drugs that can reduce glutamate binding after SCI are being evaluated because excess glutamate leads to cell death and blocks the transmission of signals across nerve synapses.[5]

Neurons have limited capacity to regenerate. Several approaches exist for repairing damaged axons through remyelination and new growth, including anti-inflammatory drugs, which inhibit amino acid toxicity and cell death that occurs after initial injury. Rolipram encourages axonal regeneration in animal models of SCI. Nogo-A is a monoclonal antibody that blocks proteins that inhibit the sprouting and regeneration of axons after spinal injury. Anti–myelin-associated glycoprotein (anti-MAG) is an antibody designed to counteract protein-sugar molecules on myelin-forming debris at the site of injury.[5]

To enable axons to advance between the tangles of inhibitory proteins and other branching molecules at the site of glial scar after SCI, a bacterial enzyme (chondroitinase ABC) is being evaluated together with cell transplants to increase functional recovery.[5]

Controversy exists concerning the benefit versus the harm of cell replacement and cell transplants, including stem cells and glial cells. Human oligodendrocyte progenitor cells have been shown to reduce secondary damage after SCI and promote functional recovery and remyelination.[5] Optimal cell delivery windows and risks of transplantation, including the formation of tumors, are being evaluated. Preclinical trials are evaluating Schwann cells taken from the individual's own body for transplantation at the site of SCI.

Nasal olfactory cells have been shown to promote axonal regeneration and remyelination at the injury site. Early trials in human patients are being conducted outside of the United States.[5]

The theory of an existing central pattern generator refers to neural networks that exist in the spinal cord that are capable of producing rhythmic movements—such as locomotion—even when there is a lack of brain and sensory input. Rats with transected spinal cords retain the ability to walk with intense step and gait training on a treadmill. This approach has shown some promise in patients with incomplete SCIs who have participated in trials using various gait training interventions such as robotic devices, body-weight–supported treadmill training, and intensive overground training.[7] The central pattern generator is theorized to exist in the T10-L2 spinal cord segment.

Neuromodulation therapy for spinal cord recovery also has been recently explored. This therapy involving a spinal cord stimulator has been used in four patients with chronic, incomplete injuries of at least 2 years' duration.[8] Some recovery of intentional movement was reported in the four patients. Other animal models have used a combination of spinal cord stimulation and neurotransmitters such as serotonin.[9]

Acute and Long-term Aspects of Care

Certain aspects of rehabilitative care should begin at the time of injury. These include preventive measures such as skin care, venous thromboembolism (VTE) prophylaxis, neurogenic bowel and bladder management, and respiratory care; all interventions should occur as soon as possible during resuscitation and stabilization.

Interdisciplinary Inpatient Rehabilitation

Comprehensive rehabilitation services should include a highly specialized interdisciplinary approach that addresses medical, physiologic, functional, psychological, and social issues. Members of the team should strive to prevent the medical complications that affect activities of daily living and functional mobility. Psychosocial effects of SCI such as issues of adjustment should be addressed. The team should formulate comprehensive discharge plans and arrange for the patient to receive lifelong follow-up to promote optimal health.[10] To optimize functional gains, the rehabilitation team will ask about the need for spinal orthoses, as these adversely affect the ability of the patient during transfers and bathing. In addition, weight-bearing restrictions and precautions may require that the individual delay comprehensive interdisciplinary rehabilitation.

Venous Thromboembolism

VTE prevention is ubiquitous in acute hospital care; however, controversy exists regarding early post–spine surgery VTE prophylaxis. This controversy is largely the result of concern about perispinal bleeding related to anticoagulant prophylaxis. Patients with traumatic SCI have the highest risk for the development of VTE within the first 2 weeks after an injury. The reported incidence of deep vein thrombosis (DVT) varies widely depending on the screening tool, with rates ranging from 9% to 100%.[11] There appears to be a DVT prophylaxis benefit to early anticoagulation in patients with acute SCI. Level II medical evidence supports beginning mechanical and chemical prophylaxis on admission after SCI and withholding chemical prophylaxis 1 day before and 1 day after surgical intervention.[12] In addition, based on level II evidence, low-dose heparin therapy alone is not recommended as a prophylactic treatment strategy and early administration of DVT prophylaxis within 72 hours is recommended. Vena cava filters are placed when there is contraindication to anticoagulation, major bleeding complications, and recurrent embolism while the patient is receiving adequate therapy. Although filters are effective in reducing the incidence of pulmonary embolism, they increase the subsequent incidence of DVT and have not been shown to increase overall survival.[13]

In 1995, pulmonary embolism was the third leading cause of death for all patients with SCI in the first year after injury, accounting for 14.9% of deaths in this group.[14] However, in the 2014 report from the National Spinal Cord Injury Statistical Center, rates of mortality attributed to pulmonary embolism had diminished to 3.3%, making pulmonary embolism the sixth leading cause of death in the first year after SCI. In addition to low-molecular-weight heparin, a clinical practice guideline suggests that direct oral anticoagulants may be considered as thromboprophylaxis during the rehabilitation phase after SCI.[14]

Respiratory Dysfunction

Pneumonia (and septicemia) have the greatest effect on reduced life expectancy for patients with SCI. Diseases of the respiratory system are the leading cause of death in patients with cervical SCI. The neurologic level of injury has a substantial effect on the function of the respiratory system. Paralysis of abdominal muscles results in an ineffective cough and impaired clearance of airway secretions. During acute injury, the forced vital capacity of patients with tetraplegia is markedly reduced, with a predicted forced vital capacity of 30%, which improves substantially by 5 weeks and continues to improve until 5 months after injury.[15] The use of an assistive cough device can help with clearance. Discussions of electric phrenic pacing and noninvasive ventilation have been documented in the literature.[15]

Neurogenic Bladder

The urologic management of patients with SCI has changed substantially over the past decades. Mortality from renal failure was 80% after World War II, but it is currently not among the leading causes of death in patients with SCI.[16] The primary goal of urologic management is to maintain renal function, which includes a low intravesical pressure.[17] After SCI, the bladder is initially areflexic and the patient is best managed with an indwelling catheter until medically and/or surgically stable. Detrusor sphincter dyssynergia develops in patients with true SCI (above the conus and below the pons). This condition may result in increased bladder pressure and incomplete bladder emptying, which can lead to vesicoureteral reflux, hydronephrosis, and subsequent renal failure. The optimal treatment plan maintains a low resting bladder pressure. Intermittent catheterization is the preferred bladder management technique after an acute injury. Bladder volumes should be kept lower than 400 mL. To maintain bladder pressures, patients may require pharmacologic management, including anticholinergic agents to relax the detrusor, alpha-blockers to

6: Trauma

lower outlet resistance, and intravesical botulinum toxin injection to relax the smooth muscle.[17]

Chronic indwelling catheters can be used when a patient cannot or will not perform intermittent catheterization; however, these catheters are associated with bladder stones, bacterial colonization, and urethral trauma such as urethral erosion, strictures, and a higher incidence of bladder cancer. Although patients are at a high risk for urinary tract infection, they more commonly have bacterial colonization. In addition to pyuria, a urinary tract infection also includes fever and constitutional symptoms. In addition, epididymitis and orchitis occur frequently in male patients with chronic indwelling catheters. Other options may include a suprapubic catheter or a continent stoma that can be catheterized.

Although electrical stimulation of the sacral roots is an effective alternative for micturition on demand, there is a risk of abolishing reflex erection and ejaculation.

Gastrointestinal System

After SCI, although the autonomic and intrinsic nervous systems of the gut preserve some intestinal coordination, colonic dysfunction can be life limiting. Fecal incontinence can occur in as many as 75% of patients.[18] Neurogenic bowel dysfunction can affect personal relationships, family life, and available free time. Scheduled bowel care after the period of spinal shock should include determination of premorbid patterns of bowel function. Previous elimination habits should be identified (morning, post meal, evening). Scheduling a bowel program for after a meal takes advantage of the gastrocolic reflex. A bowel program should be designed within the first few weeks after SCI, and may be modified throughout the patient's lifetime. Information on the neurogenic bowel is available from the Consortium for Spinal Cord Medicine.[18] The rehabilitation team will determine whether the patient has reflexic or areflexic bowel, which in turn will help direct the patient and family in establishing a bowel program.

Sexual Dysfunction

The most common self-reported problem in patients with chronic SCI is sexual dysfunction.[19] In general, men with incomplete injuries and upper motor neuron injuries have a better prognosis for achieving functional erection than men with complete injuries and lower motor neuron injuries based on self-reports; however, self-reports do not always accurately reflect the true nature of a patient's sexual status. In men with complete SCIs, reflexogenic erections tend to occur. These erections are mediated by a reflex arc exclusively in the sacral spinal cord. Tactile input passes through the pudendal nerve that accompanies the motor fibers; the efferent limb consists of preganglionic axons that travel via the pelvic nerve to the pelvic plexus to the penis, which can then result in an erection. Men with incomplete injuries may have psychogenic erections. These erections are "mentally induced" directions, which are initiated by various afferent stimuli generated or received by the brain. The brain receives afferent sensory inputs, and descending pathways from the brain control outflow from the thoracolumbar sympathetic and sacral parasympathetic plexuses to the penis. Erectile physiology in men with SCI and in healthy men is the same. Although the dominant autonomic input for tumescence is parasympathetic, whereas the input for flaccidity is sympathetic, other complicating factors are involved. Synergistic autonomic pathways compensate for each other between various neurotransmitters, including noradrenaline, acetylcholine, and nitric oxide. Pharmacotherapy uses modulators of smooth muscle by increasing erectogenic modulators and/or inhibiting erectolytic agents. Options to enhance erection include oral agents, intracavernosal injection, intraurethral suppository, constriction bands, and vacuum devices. Penile prostheses, which are used in patients with neuropathy or genitourinary reconstruction, are not used as frequently in men with SCI because of the higher infection and erosion rates in this population. Fertility in men is negatively affected after SCI, including abnormal sperm motility and morphology.

Fertility in women is generally not affected after SCI, although there is an initial acute delay in the return of ovulation cycles. Ultimately, however, there is no effect on female fertility from the injury, although this conclusion is not supported by studies comparing fertility of women with SCI with an uninjured cohort.[20] Sexual dysfunction also exists in women with SCI, although this sequela has been less studied than in men.

Spasticity

Spasticity is a velocity-dependent increase in muscle tone. Spasticity is not always a negative condition because it can be beneficial in enabling patients to bear weight during transfers and improve bed mobility. However, many uncontrolled movements can result in complications such as contractures, fracture, chronic hip dislocation, and pressure sores. In addition to range of motion, other physical modalities (eg, cold and bracing) can modify spasticity. However, pharmacologic treatment is often required to manage spasticity, including gamma-aminobutyric acid modulators and drugs that affect ion flux such as dantrolene sodium, monoamine agents, and cannabinoids. Local pharmacologic therapies may include botulinum toxin injection, which uses presynaptic inhibition of acetylcholine release to achieve effective chemical denervation of muscle fibers and prevent contraction and intrathecal infusion. Cannabis also has been studied as a treatment of spasticity.[21]

Pain Management

Perhaps the most difficult aspect of treating patients with SCI is managing pain in presumed denervated areas. Up to 75% of patients with SCI report chronic pain;[22] neuropathic pain may account for almost 50% of this pain. Neuropathic pain is cited as one of the most distressing conditions leading to poor quality of life. Neuropathic pain at or below the level of injury is often refractory to current pharmacologic and physical management.[23] In addition to neuropathic pain, patients with SCI have musculoskeletal pain that is primarily secondary to overuse of the upper extremities (shoulder); pain secondary to compressive neuropathies, including ulnar or median neuropathy; and visceral pain.

Treatment of neuropathic pain includes oral pharmacologic agents such as tricyclic antidepressants, anticonvulsants, nonsteroidal drugs, and opioid therapy. However, controversy exists regarding the effectiveness of opioid therapy in relieving neuropathic pain and its side effect of constipation, which can negatively affect a patient's bowel program and his or her quality of life. Cannabis also has been studied to address neuropathic pain.

Autonomic Dysfunction

Autonomic dysfunction is often dependent on the level of SCI. The autonomic nervous system includes sympathetic, parasympathetic, and enteric components. In upper cervical SCI, the sympathetic nervous system is decentralized and the spinal cord is no longer under the control of supraspinal structures. The cardiovascular results can be life-threatening bradycardia, hypotension, orthostasis, and autonomic dysreflexia. After upper cervical SCI, systemic arterial pressure drops secondary to a drop in cardiac output and a drop in total peripheral resistance. Interestingly, over time, patients are able to maintain blood pressure in a sitting position.

Autonomic dysreflexia (also known as autonomic hyperreflexia) manifests as hypertension, sweating above the level of injury, pounding headache, and initial bradycardia. This condition is associated with injury at or above the T6 level. Autonomic dysreflexia only occurs after spinal shock has resolved. The Consortium for Spinal Cord Medicine has published guidelines for managing this condition.[24] In general, symptoms of autonomic dysreflexia are caused by problems with urinary drainage. Untreated autonomic dysreflexia can result in death.

Osteoporosis

After SCI, regional osteoporosis syndrome may develop, with loss of 20% to 50% of bone mass in the lower extremities within the first few months. Typically, bone resorption begins at approximately week 4 after injury. Peak mobilization of calcium occurs approximately in the 16th week after injury, but it can continue for up to 2 years before a new level of bone density is established. Osteoporosis is most common in the distal femur and proximal tibia. Clinically important hypercalcemia secondary to osteoporosis can develop in some patients. There is an increased risk of fractures from disuse osteoporosis after SCI. Interestingly, SCI is not associated with osteoporosis in the spine. Femoral fractures may occur with minor trauma associated with transfers or range of motion therapy. Although orthopaedic consultation is essential, femoral fractures can be managed nonsurgically in many patients. Although some angulation may be acceptable, it is imperative that a patient can sit comfortably and avoid the development of pressure sores. Casting should be avoided because of the risk of skin breakdown, which is not recognized by the patient because of the lack of sensation.

Pressure Injury

It is estimated that up to 80% of patients with SCI will have a pressure wound at some time during their lifetime.[25] Factors that contribute to pressure wounds include (excessive) pressure, shearing, friction, and maceration. Other factors may include poor nutrition, spasticity, contractures, heterotopic ossification, and substance abuse. Pressure injuries occur over bony prominences, including the sacrum, ischium, greater trochanter, and heel. The term pressure injury has replaced the term pressure ulcer in the National Pressure Ulcer Advisory Panel Pressure Injury Staging System.[26,27] The change in terminology in the updated system more accurately describes pressure injuries to both intact and ulcerated skin (**Table 1**). In the previous staging system, stage I and deep tissue injury were used to describe injured intact skin, whereas the other stages were described as open ulcers. Confusion was created by this terminology because the definitions for each of the stages referred to the injuries as pressure ulcers. In addition to the change in terminology in the updated system, Roman numerals replaced Arabic numbers in the names of the stages. The term suspected has been removed from the deep tissue injury diagnostic label. The primary treatment of pressure ulcers is to eliminate pressure.[28]

If there is a clinical suspicion of wound infection, caution must be exercised before initiating antibiotic therapy based on wound cultures because the cultures may reflect

Table 1

Pressure Injury Staging System

Stage	Description
1: pressure injury	Nonblanchable erythema of intact skin
2: pressure injury	Partial-thickness skin loss with exposed dermis
3: pressure injury	Full-thickness skin loss
4: pressure injury	Full-thickness skin and tissue loss; if slough or eschar obscures the extent of tissue loss, this is an unstageable pressure injury
Unstageable pressure injury	Obscured full-thickness skin and tissue loss
Deep tissue pressure injury	Persistent nonblanchable deep red, maroon, or purple discoloration

colonization and cannot be considered to be the etiology of osteomyelitis.

Heterotopic Ossification

Heterotopic ossification is lamellar bone formation that occurs around a joint, often resulting in substantial loss of range of motion and sometimes resulting in incomplete ankylosis. It typically presents below the neurologic level of injury and is marked by erythema, swelling, pain, decreased range of motion, and a low-grade fever. The differential diagnosis includes DVT, cellulitis, and joint sepsis. The most common sites for heterotopic ossification in patients with SCI are the hips and knees. A triple-phase bone scan is the best method for early detection and confirmation. In a patient with heterotopic ossification, treatment with etidronate can be used if joint ankylosis has not occurred. Diphosphonate therapy prevents progression of heterotopic ossification but does not prevent the disorder. Surgery may be appropriate if heterotopic ossification is refractory to nonsurgical management. The goal of surgery is not to eradicate the ectopic bone but to allow functional range of motion. Surgery should be planned when heterotopic bone is in a quiescent state; it may take up to 18 months for the lesion to reach this active stage. Many times, the risk of heterotopic ossification resection must be weighed against the complications of pressure sores that form as a result of hip ankylosis and subsequent poor seating position. A discussion with a physiatrist for perspective on risks and benefits is critical.

Orthostatic Hypotension

Orthostatic hypotension is defined as a decrease in systolic blood pressure of 20 mm Hg or more or a reduction in diastolic blood pressure of 10 mm Hg or more with a change in body position from supine to an upright posture. Immediately after SCI, orthostatic hypotension is more common in patients with tetraplegia (prevalence as high as 82%) than in those with paraplegia (50%).[29] Orthostatic hypotension is evident in the acute period after injury and persists in a substantial number of patients for many years. Standard mobilization during therapy is reported to induce blood pressure decreases that are consistent with orthostatic hypotension in 74% of patients with SCI. Symptoms, which include dizziness, blurred vision, and syncope, occur in 59% of patients with SCI. Possible mechanisms underlying orthostatic hypotension include changes in sympathetic activity, altered baroreflex function, the lack of skeletal muscle pumping activity, cardiovascular deconditioning, and altered salt and water balance. The descending spinal cardiovascular pathways can be disrupted by SCI; this results in sympathetic hypoactivity and unopposed prevalence of intact vagal parasympathetic control.

External counterpressure applied using devices such as abdominal binders or pressure stockings may decrease capacitance within the lower extremity and abdominal vasculature beds, which are major areas of blood pooling. Functional electrical stimulation may be effective during an orthostatic challenge by redistributing blood volume from the regions of the body that are below the level of the SCI. Midodrine is the only pharmacologic intervention that has evidence for use in SCI.[30]

Upper Limb Function

The identification of appropriate candidates is the most important step in the process of restoring upper extremity function in patients with tetraplegia. A good candidate for surgical restoration of function is a patient with an ASIA motor level of at least C5 (elbow flexor [biceps and brachioradialis] strength >4/5).[31] Other criteria include neurologic stability; plateau of functional gains; good motivation, with appropriate goals for improved function; good general health; upper extremity joints with good range of motion, well-controlled spasticity, and opportunity for use of the upper extremity. To assist in surgical planning, a more comprehensive classification system of cervical SCI was developed. The International Classification for Surgery of the Hand in Tetraplegia was specifically developed to identify candidates for upper extremity restoration. In addition to moving voluntary muscles, other options for increasing function include activating paralyzed muscles with electrical stimulation.

Unfortunately, secondary complications, including urinary complications, pressure injuries, respiratory complications, contractures, bowel complications, pain, and fractures, can delay or even prevent efforts for restoring upper extremity function.

Patients with SCI who use a wheelchair or other assistive device are at risk for overuse injuries caused by cumulative trauma. Guidelines for managing acute and subacute upper limb injuries and pain; treatment of chronic musculoskeletal pain to maintain function; ergonomic recommendations; specific issues related to the shoulder, elbow, and wrist; lifetime costs; and life expectancy are available.[32]

Wheelchairs, Durable Medical Equipment, and Adaptive Equipment

To maintain independence and health, a wheelchair with the appropriate components is important to patients with SCI. Seating and mobility technologies help to maximize a patient's functional independence, through mobility, communication, and self-care. When selecting a wheelchair, the patient's needs and the wheelchair components, including cushions, molded supports, and arm and leg rests, should be considered. In addition, locations of use such as the home, work, and community environments also should be considered. A wheelchair should provide skeletal support, maintain skin integrity, and enhance function.

The choice of durable medical equipment also affects function. Assistive technologies enable a patient with tetraplegia to control an array of devices such as a computer and keyboard, television, digital video recorder, phone, lights, and doors. Durable medical equipment also includes bathroom equipment, specialty beds and mattresses, accessible vehicles, driving controls, standing frames, respiratory equipment, sexual function aids, and transfer devices.[33] Problems commonly occur in securing insurance coverage for equipment that is deemed necessary by the healthcare team and the patient.

Summary

Rehabilitation after SCI includes therapy for mobility and self-care; ongoing patient education; and assessment and advocacy to maximize functional independence, identify and address secondary conditions, and prevent secondary complications. Ideally, initial rehabilitation will occur at a center that is familiar with SCI and will include consultation with a physiatrist who has experience in acute and ongoing conditions that affect these patients.

Key Study Points

- The most straightforward aspect of SCI tends to be spine stabilization.
- As spinal stability is achieved or it is determined that surgical stabilization is not needed, the secondary conditions and complications of SCI should be addressed. These include early VTE prophylaxis, skin protection, and bladder and bowel management.
- Discussion with the treating therapists and physiatrist about orthostatic hypotension, pain management, and respiratory issues will facilitate meaningful participation in therapy and transition the patient from acute hospital care to the arena of rehabilitation.

Annotated References

1. National Spinal Cord Injury Statistical Center: *Spinal Cord Injury (SCI) Facts and Figures at a Glance.* 2016. Available at: https://www.nscisc.uab.edu/Public/Facts%20 2016.pdf. Accessed January 30, 2017

   Updated annually, this website provides statistics regarding causes of SCI, common agents of injury, and neurologic level and completeness or incompleteness of injuries. It also includes estimated lifespans, causes of death, and social factors such as marital status and employment.

2. American Spinal Injury Association: *ASIA Learning Center.* Available at: http://asia-spinalinjury.org/learning/. Accessed January 30, 2017.

   This website is an online learning resource for individuals and healthcare professions to enhance knowledge about SCI and the use of the impairment scale to accurately assess SCIs.

3. Paralyzed Veterans of America. *Clinical Practice Guidelines (CPGs).* Available at: http://www.pva.org/site/c. ajIRK9NJLcJ2E/b.8907633/k.4A9/PDFs_Clinical_ Practice_Guidelines_CPGs.htm. Accessed January 30, 2017.

4. Consortium for Spinal Cord Medicine: *Outcomes Following Traumatic Spinal Cord Injury: Clinical Practice Guidelines for Health-Care Professionals.* 1999. Available at: http://www.pva.org/atf/cf/%7BCA2A0FFB-6859- 4BC1-BC96-6B57F57F0391%7D/CPG_outcomes%20 following%20traumatic%20SCI.pdf. Accessed January 30, 2017.

5. National Institute of Neurological Disorders and Stroke: *Spinal Cord Injury: Hope Through Research.* 2016. Available at: https://www.ninds.nih.gov/Disorders/ Patient-Caregiver-Education/Hope-Through-Research/

6: Trauma

Spinal-Cord-Injury-Hope-Through-Research. Accessed January 30, 2017.

An update is presented on all active SCI research that is being funded by the National Institute of Neurologic Disorders and Stroke.

6. Resnick DK: Updated guidelines for the management of acute cervical spine and spinal cord injury. *Neurosurgery* 2013;72(suppl 2):1.

    These updated guidelines describe the state of the literature on patient's with cervical spine injuries and SCIs. The authors acknowledge that recommendations cannot exceed the strength of the literature. Multiple topics are reviewed, including prehospital cervical spine mobilization, transportation, clinical assessments, radiographic assessments, initial closed reduction, acute cardiopulmonary management, and pharmacologic therapy. Several articles looking at management of various fracture levels are included.

7. Rossignol S, Martinez M, Escalona M, et al: The "beneficial" effects of locomotor training after various types of spinal lesions in cats and rats. *Prog Brain Res* 2015;218:173-198.

    Evidence on the recovery of hind limb locomotion in cats with SCI is reviewed along with the role of the central pattern generator and the beneficial effects of locomotor training. Various lesions and improvements in deficits through locomotor training are described. The authors found that neuroplastic changes occur after a second SCI in a more rapid fashion if there has been locomotor training after a first injury.

8. Angeli CA, Edgerton VR, Gerasimenko YP, Harkema SJ: Altering spinal cord excitability enables voluntary movements after chronic complete paralysis in humans. *Brain* 2014;137(5):1394-1409.

    This is a follow-up study performed after a report of one patient with sensory incomplete SCI who regained voluntary movement after 7 months of epidural stimulation and body-weight–supported standing. This study reports on three more patients treated with implantation of epidural stimulators who regained volitional control of paralyzed muscles. A home-based stimulation protocol was developed to allow the patients to use the stimulator for approximately 1 hour while practicing intentional movements. Although the patients had some volitional movement, none of them were functional ambulators. There was no evidence of improvement in functional mobility.

9. Courtine G, Gerasimenko Y, van den Brand R, et al: Transformation of nonfunctional spinal circuits into functional states after the loss of brain input. *Nat Neurosci* 2009;12(10):1333-1342.

10. Emerich L, Parsons KC, Stein A: Competent care for persons with spinal cord injury and dysfunction in acute inpatient rehabilitation. *Top Spinal Cord Inj Rehabil* 2012;18(2):149-166.

    The authors outline resources necessary for healthcare providers to provide competent care for patients in the first stage of acute inpatient rehabilitation for SCI. The outline is not meant to present a guideline or standard of care, but rather is a description of the services necessary to provide rehabilitative care for a patient with an acute SCI.

11. Christie S, Thibault-Halman G, Casha S: Acute pharmacological DVT prophylaxis after spinal cord injury. *J Neurotrauma* 2011;28(8):1509-1514.

    Based on a literature review, the authors attempt to determine the ideal time for initiation of DVT prophylaxis with low-molecular-weight heparin in patients with SCI and specifically in patients undergoing surgery for SCI. Strong recommendation with weak data indicated that DVT prophylaxis should be initiated within 72 hours of SCI, and low-molecular-weight heparin should be withheld the morning of surgery and resumed within 24 hours after surgery.

12. American Association of Neurological Surgeons; Congress of Neurological Surgeons: Deep venous thrombosis and thromboembolism in patients with cervical spinal cord injuries, in *Guidelines for the Management of Acute Cervical Spine and Spinal Cord Injuries.* March 2013. US Department of Health and Human Services; Agency for Healthcare Research and Quality; National Guideline Clearing House. Available at: https://www.guideline.gov/summaries/summary/44342. Accessed January 30, 2017.

    This article specifically looked at VTE in patients with cervical spine injuries. Based on level I evidence, VTE prophylaxis is recommended for patients with severe motor deficits. The use of low-molecular-weight heparin or low-dose heparin combined with pneumatic compression stockings or electrical stimulation is recommended. Level II evidence concludes that oral anticoagulants alone are not recommended as prophylactic treatment. Early administration of prophylaxis within 72 hours of injury is recommended.

13. Tapson VF: Acute pulmonary embolism. *N Engl J Med* 2008;358(10):1037-1052.

14. Consortium for Spinal Cord Medicine: *Prevention of Venous Thromboembolism in Individuals With Spinal Cord Injury: Clinical Practice Guideline for Health Care Providers,* ed 3. 2016. Available at: http://www.pva.org/atf/cf/%7BCA2A0FFB-6859-4BC1-BC96-6B57F57F0391%7D/CPG_thrombo_fnl.pdf. Accessed January 30, 2017.

    The Consortium of Spinal Cord Medicine outlines the history of VTE, including pulmonary embolism as cause of death in patients with acute SCI. A subsequent drop in VTE as a cause of death in this patient population was found when adequate prophylaxis was administered. The duration of prophylaxis for VTE and the use of inferior vena cava filters are discussed based on the level of injury and comorbidities.

15. Sasson CH, Baydur A: Respiratory dysfunction in spinal cord disorders, in Lin VW, ed: *Spinal Cord Medicine: Principles and Practice.* New York, NY, Springer, 2003, pp 155-168.

16. DeVivo MJ, Krause JS, Lammertse DP: Recent trends in mortality and causes of death among persons with spinal cord injury. *Arch Phys Med Rehabil* 1999;80(11):1411-1419.

17. Consortium for Spinal Cord Medicine: *Bladder Management for Adults With Spinal Cord Injury: Clinical Practice Guideline for Health-Care Providers.* 2006. Available at: http://www.pva.org/atf/cf/%7BCA2A0FFB-6859-4BC1-BC96-6B57F57F0391%7D/CPGBladder Manageme_1AC7B4.pdf. Accessed January 30, 2017.

18. Consortium for Spinal Cord Medicine: *Neurogenic Bowel: Management in Adults With Spinal Cord Injury.* 1999. Available at: http://www.pva.org/atf/cf/%7BCA2A0FFB-6859-4BC1-BC96-6B57F57F0391%7D/cpg_neurogenic%20bowel.pdf. Accessed March 8, 2017.

19. New PW: Secondary conditions in a community sample of people with spinal cord damage. *J Spinal Cord Med* 2016;39(6):665-670.

    Based on a survey completed by individuals who had traumatic and nontraumatic spinal cord dysfunction, it was concluded that secondary conditions after SCI/dysfunction did not appear to be influenced by the etiology of the injury.

20. DeForge D, Blackmer J, Garritty C, et al: Fertility following spinal cord injury: A systematic review. *Spinal Cord* 2005;43(12):693-703.

21. Chohan H, Greenfield AL, Yadav V, Graves J: Use of cannabinoids for spasticity and pain management in MS. *Curr Treat Options Neurol* 2016;18(1):1.

    Multiple sclerosis is acknowledged to be a spinal cord–related problem. The use of cannabinoids for secondary problems such as spasticity and pain in those with multiple sclerosis will be useful for practitioners of SCI medicine. The safety and long-term effects of cannabinoids have not been evaluated.

22. Ataoğlu E, Tiftik T, Kara M, Tunç H, Ersöz M, Akkuş S: Effects of chronic pain on quality of life and depression in patients with spinal cord injury. *Spinal Cord* 2013;51(1):23-26.

    Chronic pain was present in more than 75% of this cohort of patients with SCI. Quality of life was negatively associated with chronic pain. It was recommended that chronic pain should always be treated and should be treated in a multidisciplinary setting that includes pharmacologic, physical, and psychological therapies.

23. Burke D, Fullen BM, Stokes D, Lennon O: Neuropathic pain prevalence following spinal cord injury: A systematic review and meta-analysis. *Eur J Pain* 2017;21(1):29-44.

    This review of the literature evaluated chronic pain after SCI. An analysis was completed to estimate the prevalence of neuropathic pain and chronic pain. The overall prevalence of neuropathic pain was found to be 53%. The establishment of definitions, classification systems, and assessment tools was recommended.

24. Consortium for Spinal Cord Medicine: *Acute Management of Autonomic Dysreflexia: Individuals With Spinal Cord Injury Presenting to Health-Care Facilities. Clinical Practice Guideline for Health-Care Providers.* 2001. Available at: http://www.pva.org/atf/cf/%7BCA2A0FFB-6859-4BC1-BC96-6B57F57F0391%7D/cpg_autonomic%20 dysreflexia.pdf. Accessed January 30, 2017.

25. Lindsey L, Klebine P, Oberheu AM: *Prevention of Pressure Sores Through Skin Care: Spinal Cord Injury Infosheet #13.* Birmingham, AL, Rehabilitation Research and Training Center on Secondary Conditions of SCI and Model SCI Care Center, Office of Research Service, December 2000.

26. National Pressure Ulcer Advisory Panel: *National Pressure Ulcer Advisory Panel (NPUAP) announces a change in terminology from pressure ulcer to pressure injury and updates the stages of pressure injury.* April 13, 2016. Available at: https://www.npuap.org/national-pressure-ulcer-advisory-panel-npuap-announces-a-change-in-terminology-from-pressure-ulcer-to-pressure-injury-and-updates-the-stages-of-pressure-injury. Accessed January 30, 2017.

    The National Pressure Ulcer Advisory Panel is seeking to change the terminology from *pressure ulcer* to *pressure injury*. The staging of pressure injuries was updated.

27. National Pressure Ulcer Advisory Panel: *Governmental Agencies and Professional Organizations Support NPUAP's Pressure Injury Staging System.* August 30, 2016. Available at: http://www.npuap.org/governmental-agencies-and-professional-organizations-support-npuaps-pressure-injury-staging-system/. Accessed January 30, 2017.

    This news article explained that pressure injury staging was updated to provide healthcare providers and professionals with a "clarifying staging system to better address the different types of skin wounds commonly seen by medical professionals." The 2016 Pressure Injury Staging System is anticipated to lead to more accurate and earlier diagnosis of pressure injuries, allow for more appropriate patient care, and decrease patient suffering.

28. Consortium for Spinal Cord Medicine: *Pressure Ulcer Prevention and Treatment Following Injury: A Clinical Practice Guideline for Health-Care Providers,* ed 2. 2014. Available at: http://www.pva.org/atf/cf/%7B-CA2A0FFB-6859-4BC1-BC96-6B57F57F0391%7D/CPG_Pressure%20Ulcer.pdf. Accessed January 30, 2017.

    This clinical practice guideline makes recommendations about the prevention, assessment, and treatment of pressure ulcers in SCI.

29. Krassioukov A, Eng JJ, Warburton DE, Teasell R; Spinal Cord Injury Rehabilitation Evidence Research Team: A systematic review of the management of orthostatic hypotension after spinal cord injury. *Arch Phys Med Rehabil* 2009;90(5):876-885.

6: Trauma

30. Claydon VE, Steeves JD, Krassioukov A: Orthostatic hypotension following spinal cord injury: Understanding clinical pathophysiology. *Spinal Cord* 2006;44(6):341-351.

31. Bryden AM, Peljovich AE, Hoyen HA, Nemunaitis G, Kilgore KL, Keith MW: Surgical restoration of arm and hand function in people with tetraplegia. *Top Spinal Cord Inj Rehabil* 2012;18(1):43-49.

   The process of restoring upper extremity function in patients with SCI is outlined, with a focus on identifying appropriate candidates. Spasticity and other secondary complications, which can be barriers to restoring function, also are discussed. The authors recommend that evidence in the area of reconstructive procedures for patients with tetraplegia needs to be strengthened.

32. Consortium for Spinal Cord Medicine: *Preservation of Upper Limb Function Following Spinal Cord Injury: A Clinical Practice Guideline for Health-Care Professionals.* 2005. Available at: http://www.pva.org/atf/cf/%7 BCA2A0FFB-6859-4BC1-BC96-6B57F57F0391%7D/ cpg_upperlimb.pdf. Accessed January 30, 2017.

33. American Spinal Injury Association: *Guidelines for Use of Durable Medical Equipment for Persons With Spinal Cord Injury and Dysfunction.* Available at: http://asia-spinalinjury.org/wp-content/extras/dme.php. Accessed January 30, 2017.

6: Trauma

Neoplastic and Inflammatory Conditions

SECTION EDITOR:

Mitchel B. Harris, MD

Chapter 32

Metastatic Disease to the Spine

Marco Ferrone, MD, FRCSC

Abstract

When reviewing metastatic disease to the spine, a framework provides the background for understanding metastatic disease and outlines evaluation and treatment options that can be applied using a multidisciplinary approach.

Keywords: radiation therapy; spinal cord compression; spinal metastasis

Introduction

Because metastatic disease to the spine is a complex condition in a patient who is often fragile, an interdisciplinary approach to evaluation and management is required. All interventions need to be considered in the larger context of the patient and the disease process, because interventions for metastatic disease to the spine are generally palliative in nature. Palliative care is centered on preventing and relieving suffering. These goals must be communicated realistically to the patient and his or her family, with special consideration of the patient's expectations and wishes. The range of treatment options is best considered by a team that includes a spine surgeon, a radiation oncologist, a medical oncologist, an interventional radiologist, and a palliative care pain specialist. The factors to be weighed include the tumor type, disease burden, number and location of involved spine levels, neurologic status, ambulatory status, and overall health of the patient. The recovery period from a planned intervention should not be longer than the patient's expected lifespan. The goals are to keep the patient as comfortable, stable, and mobile as possible.

Neither Dr. Ferrone nor any immediate family member has received anything of value from or has stock or stock options held in a commercial company or institution related directly or indirectly to the subject of this chapter.

Prevalence

Cancer is a pervasive and growing problem worldwide, and it is estimated to affect one in three women and one in two men in their lifetimes according to the American Cancer Society.[1] Symptomatic metastatic spinal cord compression occurs in approximately 10% of patients with metastatic cancer.[2] The posterior two-thirds of the vertebral body are most often involved, with epidural extension of tumor. Lesions may be lytic, blastic, or mixed. The thoracic spine is most commonly involved, followed by the lumbar and cervical spines, in a ratio of approximately 4:2:1, respectively. Multicentric spinal disease is seen in as many as 40% of patients.[3]

Clinical Evaluation

A thorough evaluation is always prudent, regardless of a patient's condition at the time of the initial evaluation. Some specific evaluation points should be kept in mind when evaluating a patient with suspected metastatic disease to the spine.

History and Physical Examination

It is paramount to establish a clear diagnosis of metastatic disease; the patient's history should be used for this purpose, if possible. A history of treated cancer in a patient with a new solitary lesion requires a workup to differentiate a new cancer from metastatic disease. Establishing the type of primary cancer and its radiosensitivity will shape decision making. The history can provide important information about the types of treatments the patient has undergone that could affect surgery, including prior radiation therapy, myelosuppressive chemotherapy, or therapy with a vascular endothelial growth factor inhibitor that can influence wound healing. Determining the stage and extent of the disease will help in framing the prognosis. For example, the prognosis will likely differ in a treatment-naive patient from that of a patient who has undergone many unsuccessful rounds of chemotherapy. In addition, it is necessary to clearly establish the type of pain that the patient is experiencing. Differentiating functional or mechanical pain, night pain, and radicular pain is crucial because this information will influence the treatment modalities offered. Functional or mechanical pain suggests an element of instability, whereas night pain is often caused by periosteal stretching, and radicular pain can result from compression of the neural foramina.

The physical examination is critical and should be performed serially in patients with metastatic spinal cord compression because the disease can progress and cause dramatic changes in neurologic status. The examination should focus on the subtle and early signs of myelopathy. In addition, the pain generator should be identified, and it should be determined if there is correlation between the physical examination and radiographic findings.

Laboratory Studies

Basic laboratory tests include a complete blood cell count; erythrocyte sedimentation rate; liver function test; albumin level; serum and urine immunoelectrophoresis; and calcium, phosphorus, alkaline phosphatase, blood urea nitrogen, creatinine, and glucose measurements. The C-reactive protein level and tumor marker assays, including the alpha-fetoprotein, carcinoembryonic antigen, and prostate-specific antigen panel, can be added. Serum calcium is of particular importance because hypercalcemia can occur in as many as 30% of patients with bone metastases, and correction of this condition presents an opportunity to prevent a cardiac event.[4] These laboratory tests are not diagnostic by themselves, but findings can direct the differential diagnosis and are important in understanding the host environment.

Imaging

CT of the chest, abdomen, and pelvis with contrast is necessary for staging and/or finding the primary source of the metastasis.[5] A bone scan is useful for identifying other sites of bony disease, particularly if biopsy of a spine lesion is being considered. The bone scan may identify lesions in an extremity, where biopsy could be safer than in the spine. When serum or urine immunoelectrophoresis is positive, a skeletal survey is useful for assessing the extent of bony involvement from multiple myeloma. Bone scan results often are normal in patients with multiple myeloma.[6] Orthogonal standing (or sitting) plain radiographs are beneficial even if axial images are available, because instability may be more apparent than on radiographs taken with the patient supine. MRI, with and without gadolinium contrast, will better delineate soft-tissue components, evaluate epidural encroachment, and identify the tissue with the greatest diagnostic potential for biopsy. Myelography can be considered for patients who are unable to undergo MRI. Dedicated CT of the spine with coronal and sagittal reformatting often provides more information about bony architecture and potential instability than does MRI. Dual-energy x-ray absorptiometry does not have a specific role in the evaluation of the spine in the setting of metastatic disease. Although this modality remains valuable in the evaluation of global bone and in the pathologic conditions of osteopenia and osteoporosis, its role in fracture prediction for focal metastatic lesions has not been established.

Biopsy

In the setting of a neurologically stable patient with an unknown primary lesion and a single site of disease, a biopsy should be strongly considered. For example, a primary tumor such as a chordoma would be treated differently than a metastatic lesion for which a palliative procedure may be more appropriate. Stable patients with primary spine cancer often are transferred to specialized centers for treatment. Even if primary spine cancer is not part of the differential diagnosis, a biopsy may be performed in a neurologically and structurally stable patient to determine if the cancer can be best treated with radiation therapy alone (such as lymphoma or myeloma); this determination can prevent unnecessary surgery. The biopsy can be performed by an interventional radiologist, but is often best performed after discussion with and under the direction of the treating surgeon. This method ensures that the biopsy tract can be incorporated into the final resection if en bloc resection is necessary.

Considerations in Surgical Decision Making

Neurologic Symptoms

Neurologic deficits or impending neurologic collapse is often considered an indication for surgery. The degree of neurologic compromise is evaluated based on the physical examination and MRI findings. The Spine Oncology Study Group has proposed a six-point grading system to evaluate metastatic spinal cord compression.[7] Grade 0 is the presence of disease in the vertebral body only; grade 1a is epidural disease without deformity of the thecal sac; grade 1b is deformity of the thecal sac without cord abutment; grade 1c is disease that causes thecal sac deformity and cord abutment without cord compression; grade 2 is cord compression with visible cerebrospinal fluid; and grade 3 is cord compression without visible cerebrospinal fluid around the cord.

Studies have reported preservation or improvement in neurologic function after surgical intervention, including low rates of neurologic decline.[8-10] Evidence suggests that the longer the period of time that a neurologic deficit is present, the worse the prognosis for improvement.[10] A review of the literature showed that neurologic deficits are more often improved with surgery and radiation than with radiation only.[11] In nonambulatory patients, 64% of those treated with surgery and radiation regained the ability to ambulate, whereas only 29% of those treated with radiation alone regained the ability to ambulate.

Spinal Stability

It must be determined if a lesion has caused spinal instability. A recent classification system developed by the Spine Oncology Study Group is helpful in making this determination.[12] The spine instability neoplastic score is based on the following six lesion characteristics: (1) location, (2) pain relief with recumbency, (3) the type of bony lesion (lytic or blastic), (4) spinal alignment based on radiographic findings, (5) the extent of vertebral body collapse, and (6) involvement of the posterolateral spinal elements (**Table 1**). A score of 0 to 6 points indicates a stable spine, a score of 7 to 12 points indicates a potentially unstable spine, and a score of 13 to 18 points indicates an unstable spine. A score of 0 to 6 points indicates a stable spine, a score of 7 to 12 points indicates a potentially unstable spine, and a score of 13 to 18 points indicates an unstable spine. This system was reported to have excellent interobserver and intraobserver reliability, 95.7% sensitivity, and 79.5% specificity for predicting spinal stability.[13]

Expected Longevity

One of the main factors to consider when deciding whether a surgical intervention is appropriate is the likelihood that the patient will outlive the procedure's typical recovery period. This factor is easy to articulate, but difficult to predict. Several scoring systems have been devised to help with the decision for surgical intervention. A recent retrospective study compared seven prognostic scoring systems (Bauer, modified Bauer, Tokuhashi, Tokuhashi revised, Tomita, van der Linden, and Sioutos systems) by analyzing records from 254 patients with proven spine metastases from a variety of histologies (not including multiple myeloma).[14] Sixty-two of the patients had been treated surgically, and 192 patients had been treated nonsurgically. Each scoring system has been designed to guide treatment by predicting patient survival. The weighed factors included functional scores (Karnofsky Performance Status Scale and/or Eastern Cooperative Oncology Group Performance Status); number and sites of metastases, including the viscera; the primary site of the cancer; and the presence of neurologic signs or symptoms. Only the Bauer and modified Bauer systems achieved significance in all prediction groups; the other systems failed to significantly differentiate a good prognosis from a moderate prognosis.

Table 1	
Spine Instability Neoplastic Score	
Criterion	**Points**
Location	
Junctional (occiput-C2, C7-T2, T11-L1, L5-S1)	3
Mobile spine (C3-C6, L2-L4)	2
Semirigid spine (T3-T10)	1
Rigid spine (S2-S5)	0
Pain	
Yes	3
Occasional, but not mechanical	1
No	0
Bone lesion	
Lytic	2
Mixed (lytic and blastic)	1
Blastic	0
Radiographic spine alignment	
Subluxation or translation	4
De novo deformity (kyphosis or scoliosis)	2
Normal alignment	0
Vertebral body collapse	
More than 50%	3
Less than 50%	2
No collapse, with more than 50% of body involved	1
None	0

Reproduced with permission from Fourney DR, Franqou EM, Ryken TC, et al: Spinal instability neoplastic score: An analysis of reliability and validity from the spine oncology study group. *J Clin Oncol* 2011;29(22):3072-3077.

The simplicity of the modified Bauer score adds to its utility. The modified Bauer score omits pathologic fracture, but otherwise is identical to the original Bauer score. Four factors (absence of visceral metastasis, presence of a solitary skeletal metastasis, a primary cancer that is not lung cancer, a primary cancer that is breast or kidney cancer) are scored by assigning one point for a positive answer. Life expectancy is predicted as follows: a score of 0 or 1, 4.8 months; a score of 2, 18.2 months; and a score of 3 or 4, 28.4 months.[14]

Recent improvements in accuracy have been made with the development of the New England Spinal Metastasis Score (NESMS).[15-17] The NESMS uses the modified Bauer system and adds the parameters of serum albumin and ambulatory status (**Table 2**). The NESMS is useful in predicting 30- and 90-day mortality.

7: Neoplastic and Inflammatory Conditions

Table 2

New England Spinal Metastasis Score (NESMS) With Inclusion of Points From the Modified Bauer Score

Modified Bauer Score	Points
One point each if:	
Primary tumor is not lung	1
Primary tumor is breast or kidney	1
Solitary skeletal metastasis	1
No visceral metastasis	1
NESMS Parameters	
Modified Bauer Score is 3 or 4	2
Modified Bauer Score is 0, 1, or 2	0
Serum albumin (≥3.5 g/dL)	1
Serum albumin (<3.5 g/dL)	0
Ambulatory status intact	1
Ambulatory status impaired or nonambulatory	0

[a]Note: maximum points = 3

[a]Because NESMS of 3 and 4 have identical performance, the score is capped at 3.

Surgical Options

When surgery is deemed appropriate, the specific procedure is dictated by the indication and the pathology. For example, spinal cord compression is generally addressed with a decompressive procedure, whereas instability often requires instrumentation. The type of reconstruction has not been shown to have meaningful importance. For example, a study comparing polymethyl methacrylate to an expandable cage for anterior vertebral column reconstruction after extracavitary tumor resection found no difference in survival, estimated blood loss, pain scores, or performance status. Although the group treated with expandable cages exhibited a trend toward better kyphosis reduction, this measure did not reach statistical significance.[18] A single posterior approach may be favored because it has been shown to have fewer complications than anterior and combined approaches.[19] The pathology often dictates the requirements and the extent of a surgical procedure, and all procedures must be tailored to the needs of the individual patient.

Complications

Complications affect the cost-effectiveness of interventions for spinal metastases. The Charlson index has been used to predict complications after surgical intervention for spinal metastases.[20,21] The Charlson index assigns values to known medical comorbidities. In a 2011 study,

the authors reviewed 200 cases of spinal metastasis surgically treated at one hospital between 1999 and 2009.[20] A complication rate of 34% was reported, and the Charlson index was found to be the most robust predictor of postoperative complications in the first 30 days after surgery. The NESMS score, when applied to the National Surgical Quality Improvement Program database, also effectively predicted major systemic complications, with a 26% complication rate for an NESMS score of 0, 10% for a score of 1, 9% for a score of 2, and 8% for a score of 3.[16]

Radiation Therapy

Conventional Radiation

Conventional external beam radiation therapy remains the first-line treatment of metastatic spinal cord compression. Radiation therapy can be initiated quickly, without the complex plans required for stereotactic techniques. When discussing radiation, the term fraction generally refers to the equal portion of the total radiation dose given per day. In a comparison of a short or a long course of radiation therapy using 8 Gy in a single dose, 20 Gy in 5 fractions, 30 Gy in 10 fractions, 37.5 Gy in 15 fractions, or 40 Gy in 20 fractions, preservation of ambulatory ability and improvement in neurologic function were equivalent.[22] However, the durability of the treatments differed. Starting at 4 to 6 months after radiation therapy, the patients receiving 8 Gy in a single dose and 20 Gy in 5 fractions had significantly more recurrences with true metastatic spinal cord compression compared with those treated with longer radiation therapy regimens. Therefore, a short course of radiation therapy is usually reserved for patients with life expectancies of less than 4 to 6 months. The three-dose intense regimens (30 Gy, 37.5 Gy, and 40 Gy) have shown equivalent outcomes, supporting 30 Gy in 10 fractions as the widely accepted standard treatment of metastatic spinal cord compression.

Stereotactic Radiation Therapy

Stereotactic radiation therapy allows for the delivery of higher doses of radiation while sparing radiosensitive structures such as the spinal cord. Conventional radiation therapy is substantially less expensive than stereotactic therapy, with conventional therapy costing 29% to 71% less than stereotactic treatment.[23] Stereotactic radiation therapy has been advocated in the setting of re-treatment after prior conventional radiation therapy. This therapy also has been popularized in the setting of "separation surgery," in which less aggressive surgery to decompress the spinal cord and stabilize the spine is followed by postoperative cytotoxic doses of radiation delivered to any remaining tumor by stereotactic means, while sparing the spinal cord from radiation. A 2013 study described retrospective results of separation surgery followed by stereotactic radiation therapy delivered in one of the following three patterns: high-dose single fraction therapy, high-dose hypofractionated therapy, or low-dose hypofractionated therapy. Good local control rates were reported, with a total cumulative 1-year local progression incidence of 16.4%. When the subgroups were analyzed, the cumulative incidence of local progression at 1 year was 4.1% in the high-dose hypofractionated group, 9.0% in the high-dose single fraction group, and 22.6% in the low-dose hypofractionated group.[24] Separation surgery is becoming more popular as a durable treatment with less aggressive surgical intervention.[25]

Cost-Effectiveness of Treatment

Limited data exist on the cost-effectiveness and value of interventions for spinal metastases. A Dutch study estimated the cost associated with spinal metastases to be approximately 65% for inpatient care, 33% for outpatient services, and 3% for hospice care.[26] Admissions for spinal cord compression have been estimated to cost slightly less than $60,000, based on an analysis of Medicare claims.[27] More and costlier interventions will provide increased value only if a survival benefit can be demonstrated. More study is needed in this area.

Palliative Treatment and Quality of Life

Several authors have reported good quality of life after surgical intervention for spinal metastasis.[28-30] In a large prospective series, the authors found preoperative Karnofsky, Frankel, and EuroQol Five Dimension (EQ-5D) scores to be the best predictors of postoperative quality of life.[28] The Spine Oncology Study Group Outcomes Questionnaire and the EQ-5D have found support as good outcomes measures, with the Spine Oncology Study Group Outcomes Questionnaire currently preferred.[29,30]

Summary

General principles and available literature should be considered when treating patients with metastatic disease to the spine. There is a trend toward less invasive surgery as radiation therapy continues to evolve. Accurately predicting which patients will live long enough to benefit from surgery will establish the best outcomes for patients with spinal metastases.

Key Study Points

- Radiation therapy and stereotactic radiation therapy are likely to play a larger role in treating patients with metastatic spinal disease.
- Surgery and radiation are more effective than radiation alone in reversing neurologic deficits.
- The NESMS is a useful tool in predicting 30- and 90-day mortality after surgery for spinal metastases.

Annotated References

1. Lifetime risk of developing or dying from cancer. American Cancer Society website. Available at: https://www.cancer.org/cancer/cancer-basics/lifetime-probability-of-developing-or-dying-from-cancer.html. Accessed May 23, 2017.

   Data from 2010 through 2012 were used in preparing tables showing the lifetime risks of developing and dying from certain cancers for men and women in the United States.

2. Barron KD, Hirano A, Araki S, Terry RD: Experiences with metastatic neoplasms involving the spinal cord. *Neurology* 1959;9(2):91-106.

3. Pigott KH, Baddeley H, Maher EJ: Pattern of disease in spinal cord compression on MRI scan and implications for treatment. *Clin Oncol (R Coll Radiol)* 1994;6(1):7-10.

4. Stewart AF: Clinical practice: Hypercalcemia associated with cancer. *N Engl J Med* 2005;352(4):373-379.

5. Peabody TD, Gibbs CP Jr, Simon MA: Evaluation and staging of musculoskeletal neoplasms. *J Bone Joint Surg Am* 1998;80(8):1204-1218.

6. Ludwig H, Kumpan W, Sinzinger H: Radiography and bone scintigraphy in multiple myeloma: A comparative analysis. *Br J Radiol* 1982;55(651):173-181.

7. Bilsky MH, Laufer I, Fourney DR, et al: Reliability analysis of the epidural spinal cord compression scale. *J Neurosurg Spine* 2010;13(3):324-328.

8. Patchell RA, Tibbs PA, Regine WF, et al: Direct decompressive surgical resection in the treatment of spinal cord compression caused by metastatic cancer: A randomised trial. *Lancet* 2005;366(9486):643-648.

9. Chaichana KL, Woodworth GF, Sciubba DM, et al: Predictors of ambulatory function after decompressive surgery for metastatic epidural spinal cord compression. *Neurosurgery* 2008;62(3):683-692, discussion 683-692.

10. Bakar D, Tanenbaum JE, Phan K, et al: Decompression surgery for spinal metastases: A systematic review. *Neurosurg Focus* 2016;41(2):E2.

    The authors present a literature review that included 36 studies involving the use of decompression surgery for metastases of the spine. They found that the Karnofsky score and the ability to ambulate before surgery were the strongest predictors of the ability to achieve postoperative ambulation.

11. Kim JM, Losina E, Bono CM, et al: Clinical outcome of metastatic spinal cord compression treated with surgical excision ± radiation versus radiation therapy alone: A systematic review of literature. *Spine (Phila Pa 1976)* 2012;37(1):78-84.

    A review of the literature from 1970 to 2007 on metastatic spinal cord compression found that 64% of patients who had surgery regained the ability to ambulate, whereas 29% of those treated with radiation only regained the ability to ambulate if they were nonambulatory at the time of treatment. The surgical complication rate was 29%.

12. Fisher CG, DiPaola CP, Ryken TC, et al: A novel classification system for spinal instability in neoplastic disease: An evidence-based approach and expert consensus from the Spine Oncology Study Group. *Spine (Phila Pa 1976)* 2010;35(22):E1221-E1229.

13. Fourney DR, Frangou EM, Ryken TC, et al: Spinal instability neoplastic score: An analysis of reliability and validity from the spine oncology study group. *J Clin Oncol* 2011;29(22):3072-3077.

    This study validated the Spinal Instability Neoplastic Score for the determination of spinal stability in the setting of metastatic disease. The scoring system takes into account radiologic and neurologic factors as well as physical symptoms and alignment. Based on clinical and radiographic data, patients were classified into the following groups: stable spine, unstable spine, and potentially unstable spine.

14. Wibmer C, Leithner A, Hofmann G, et al: Survival analysis of 254 patients after manifestation of spinal metastases: Evaluation of seven preoperative scoring systems. *Spine (Phila Pa 1976)* 2011;36(23):1977-1986.

    The authors present the results of their retrospective review of patients with spinal metastases that used seven accepted scoring schemes to assess patient longevity. The modified Bauer score was found to be the most accurate.

15. Goodwin CR, Schoenfeld AJ, Abu-Bonsrah NA, et al: Reliability of a spinal metastasis prognostic score to model 1-year survival. *Spine J* 2016;16(9):1102-1108.

    This study validated the reliability of NESMS and reported that it accurately predicts postoperative survival. The study was conducted at an outside institution from where the NESMS was developed.

16. Schoenfeld AJ, Le HV, Marjoua Y, et al: Assessing the utility of a clinical prediction score regarding 30-day morbidity and mortality following metastatic spinal surgery: The New England Spinal Metastasis Score (NESMS). *Spine J* 2016;16(4):482-490.

    The NESMS was applied to the National Surgical Quality Improvement Program database. The authors report that it accurately predicted 30-day mortality and short-term major morbidity after surgery for spinal metastatic disease.

17. Schoenfeld AJ, Leonard DA, Saadat E, Bono CM, Harris MB, Ferrone ML: Predictors of 30- and 90-day survival following surgical intervention for spinal metastases: A prognostic study conducted at four academic centers. *Spine (Phila Pa 1976)* 2016;41(8):E503-E509.

    The NESMS was applied to data from four major institutions and achieved accurate prediction of both 30- and 90-day mortality. Level of evidence: III.

18. Eleraky M, Papanastassiou I, Tran ND, Dakwar E, Vrionis FD: Comparison of polymethylmethacrylate versus expandable cage in anterior vertebral column reconstruction after posterior extracavitary corpectomy in lumbar and thoraco-lumbar metastatic spine tumors. *Eur Spine J* 2011;20(8):1363-1370.

    The use of polymethyl methacrylate or an expandable cage for anterior vertebral column reconstruction after extracavitary tumor resection was compared. The authors reported no difference in survival, estimated blood loss, pain scores, function outcomes, or performance status between the groups treated with either technique.

19. Campbell PG, Malone J, Yadla S, et al: Early complications related to approach in thoracic and lumbar spine surgery: A single center prospective study. *World Neurosurg* 2010;73(4):395-401.

20. Arrigo RT, Kalanithi P, Cheng I, et al: Charlson score is a robust predictor of 30-day complications following spinal metastasis surgery. *Spine (Phila Pa 1976)* 2011;36(19):E1274-E1280.

    The Charlson score was retrospectively applied to 200 patient records to determine whether it could predict 30-day complications. Patients with a score of 2 or higher were five times more likely to have a complication compared with patients with a lower score.

21. Charlson ME, Pompei P, Ales KL, MacKenzie CR: A new method of classifying prognostic comorbidity in longitudinal studies: Development and validation. *J Chronic Dis* 1987;40(5):373-383.

22. Rades D, Stalpers LJ, Veninga T, et al: Evaluation of five radiation schedules and prognostic factors for metastatic spinal cord compression. *J Clin Oncol* 2005;23(15):3366-3375.

23. Haley ML, Gerszten PC, Heron DE, Chang YF, Atteberry DS, Burton SA: Efficacy and cost-effectiveness analysis of external beam and stereotactic body radiation therapy in the treatment of spine metastases: A matched-pair analysis. *J Neurosurg Spine* 2011;14(4):537-542.

Forty-four patients were matched for age, type of primary tumor, year of treatment, and location of metastasis to compare conventional and sterotactic radiation therapy. The outcomes were pain relief, cost-effectiveness, toxicities, and the need for further intervention. Although pain relief was equivalent, sterotactic radiation had less toxicity and less need for further treatment than conventional radiation. The cost of conventional radiation therapy was 29% to 71% less than that of sterotactic radiation therapy.

24. Laufer I, Iorgulescu JB, Chapman T, et al: Local disease control for spinal metastases following "separation surgery" and adjuvant hypofractionated or high-dose single-fraction stereotactic radiosurgery: Outcome analysis in 186 patients. *J Neurosurg Spine* 2013;18(3):207-214.

   The authors present a retrospective review of 186 patients treated with surgery followed by one of three radiation treatment plans: high-dose single fraction, high-dose hypofractionated, or low-dose hypofractionated sterotactic radiosurgery. High-dose hypofractionated sterotactic therapy had the best local control rate.

25. Gerszten PC, Mendel E, Yamada Y: Radiotherapy and radiosurgery for metastatic spine disease: What are the options, indications, and outcomes? *Spine (Phila Pa 1976)* 2009;34(22suppl):S78-S92.

26. Tipsmark LS, Bünger CE, Wang M, Morgen SS, Dahl B, Søgaard R: Healthcare costs attributable to the treatment of patients with spinal metastases: A cohort study with up to 8 years follow-up. *BMC Cancer* 2015;15:354.

   A Danish clinical database review of patients undergoing treatment of spinal metastases between January 2005 and June 2012 is presented. Cost was found to be proportional to the invasiveness of the intervention, and 65% of the costs were for the inpatient index procedure.

27. Barlev A, Song X, Ivanov B, Setty V, Chung K: Payer costs for inpatient treatment of pathologic fracture, surgery to bone, and spinal cord compression among patients with multiple myeloma or bone metastasis secondary to prostate or breast cancer. *J Manag Care Pharm* 2010;16(9):693-702.

28. Choi D, Fox Z, Albert T, et al: Prediction of quality of life and survival after surgery for symptomatic spinal metastases: A multicenter cohort study to determine suitability for surgical treatment. *Neurosurgery* 2015;77(5):698-708, discussion 708.

   A prospective cohort of 922 patients with spinal metastases who were treated surgically were analyzed with preoperative and postoperative assessments using the EQ-5D; visual analog scores for pain; and the Karnofsky physical function, complications, and survival score. The preoperative Karnofsky score best predicted postoperative quality of life and survival. The Karnofsky score, tumor type, spinal metastases, and visceral metastases were the four most important factors to consider in patient treatment.

29. Street J, Lenehan B, Berven S, Fisher C: Introducing a new health-related quality of life outcome tool for metastatic disease of the spine: Content validation using the International Classification of Functioning, Disability, and Health; on behalf of the Spine Oncology Study Group. *Spine (Phila Pa 1976)* 2010;35(14):1377-1386.

30. Janssen SJ, Teunis T, van Dijk E, et al: Validation of the Spine Oncology Study Group-Outcomes Questionnaire to assess quality of life in patients with metastatic spine disease. *Spine J* 2015;Aug 5 [Epub ahead of print].

   This study compared the Spine Oncology Study Group Outcomes Questionnaire and the EQ-5D in assessing quality of life in patients with spinal metastases. The authors found that the Spine Oncology Study Group Outcomes Questionnaire had higher internal consistency and good coverage because it had no floor or ceiling effect, whereas the EQ-5D had a 10% ceiling effect.

7: Neoplastic and Inflammatory Conditions

Chapter 33

Primary Tumors of the Spine

Joseph H. Schwab, MD, MS

Abstract

Primary tumors of the spine are rare and historically have been associated with poor outcomes. However, surgical techniques and spinal reconstruction have improved substantially, making sound oncologic procedures possible, but with high morbidity. Radiation oncology techniques have also improved, and the delivery of high doses of radiation to the tumor while sparing the spinal cord is now possible. Higher doses of radiation have been shown to be effective as a surgical adjuvant. Systemic treatments are largely lacking, but at least one breakthrough has occurred in the form of anti-receptor activator of nuclear factor kappa-B ligand therapy for giant cell tumors. Targeted therapies have substantial promise for patients with cancer, and they likely will become a more important component of the treatments available.

Keywords: en bloc resection; radiation therapy; spinal neoplasia; spine tumor; targeted therapy

Introduction

There are fewer than 4,000 new cases of primary bone tumors each year in the United States, and most occur in the extremities rather than the spine.[1] Improvements in surgical techniques and instrumentation have led to the establishment of specialized centers with substantial experience in en bloc resection for select cases. However, en bloc resections are associated with high morbidity, and effective adjuvant therapies are needed to decrease the surgical burden required by these cases. Systemic targeted interventions and radiation therapy have the potential to improve outcomes with less aggressive surgical treatment. However, the long-term effectiveness and safety profiles of these adjuvant treatments are not yet known.

Staging of Musculoskeletal Neoplasms of the Vertebrae

Vertebral neoplasm staging collates relevant clinical data to predict the risk of local and distant recurrence, inform optimal surgical approach, and guide the use of adjuvant therapy.[2] Newer, adjuvant modalities such as targeted therapies and high-precision radiation therapy have prompted surgeons to reconsider incorporating these adjuvants into the management of many primary spine tumors. Given these advances in adjuvant therapy, knowledge of the oncologic staging systems commonly used in the spine is helpful.

The behavior of tumors was stratified into six groups that formed the basis of the benign and malignant Enneking staging systems.[2] Benign lesions are subclassified into three groups: the first two are considered localized lesions, and the last group includes invasive lesions. The localized tumors are further classified as latent (stage 1) or active (stage 2) forms, which are confined to bone and are not associated with a soft-tissue mass; the aggressive (stage 3) form can have a soft-tissue component. The soft-tissue component associated with aggressive lesions can cause problems with local excision, particularly if the extraosseous component is near an important neurovascular structure. Therefore, Enneking stage 3 lesions are potentially good candidates for the appropriate adjuvant therapy.

Malignant neoplasms also are grouped into three categories, according to the risk of local and distant spread. A malignant neoplasm that is localized but associated with a relatively lower risk of regional or distant spread is considered a low-grade malignant tumor (stage I). A malignant neoplasm that is locally aggressive and associated with a high risk of regional or distant spread is a high-grade malignant tumor (stage II). The final Enneking stage includes tumors that have already metastasized (stage III). This system has proved to be practical and is commonly used to describe malignant tumors of bone.

However, one of the goals of the Enneking staging system was to inform the surgical approach. Over time, the surgical treatment of malignant primary spine neoplasms

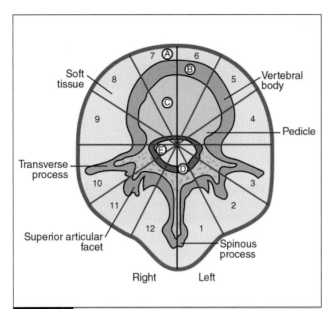

Figure 1 Illustration depicts the Weinstein-Boriani-Biagini (WBB) classification scheme that divides an axial vertebral view into 12 triangular sections to demonstrate tumor involvement. In addition, the WBB allows classification of tumor depth, including epidural soft-tissue extension. The layers of involvement are indicated by the following alphabetic designations: A = extraosseous soft tissues, B = intraosseous (superficial), C = intraosseous (deep), D = extraosseous (extradural), and E = extraosseous (intradural).

has evolved. The newer Weinstein-Boriani-Biagini (WBB) classification system was designed for spine oncologists and reflects the challenges posed by malignant spinal neoplasms[3] (**Figure 1**). The WBB uses an axial image of the tumor and divides the spine into 12 circumferential sections. Each section is further divided into image zones (A through F) based on the anatomic level of invasion. Both the Enneking and WBB systems have demonstrated only fair to moderate interobserver reliability.[4] However, the WBB provides useful information regarding surgical planning and can help inform the use of adjuvant therapy. If the tumor extends into zone D (extradural component), intraoperative radiation can be considered because the dura margin will be close or positive tumor margin.

Primary Tumors of the Spine

Giant Cell Tumor

Treatment for giant cell tumors of the spine has benefited the most from advances in both surgical techniques and targeted therapies. The advances in surgical techniques include the development of en bloc spondylectomy, which has been reported on since the late 1960s. A large 2012 series on vertebral giant cell tumors managed with en bloc spondylectomy reported effective treatment of Enneking stage 2 tumors with intralesional curettage.[5] Stage 3 tumors had high rates of local recurrence when curettage was performed, and it was concluded that en bloc resection should be considered. The potential benefits of en bloc spondylectomy regarding recurrence risk must be balanced with its increased morbidity.[6,7] This balance is particularly difficult when treating a benign but locally aggressive tumor. In some treatment centers, Enneking stage 3 giant cell tumors in the axial skeleton are considered unresectable. Specifically, the high morbidity of resection is not considered acceptable for the treatment of a benign tumor.[8] Initially, radiation therapy was used as an alternative to surgery. Late development of secondary sarcoma in the radiation field has reduced the use of this modality.[9]

As the understanding of bone physiology has improved, pharmaceutical research has developed targeted therapies for improved bone health. At one time, giant cell tumors were called osteoclastomas because it was thought that the oncologic cell was the osteoclast. Preosteoclasts express the receptor activator of nuclear factor κB (RANK) surface receptor. Inhibiting the activation of RANK by its ligand (RANKL) was meant to stop the activation of the osteoclasts. The use of a monoclonal antibody targeting RANKL (such as with denosumab) has proved effective in treating giant cell tumors. Although the antibody affects the giant cells, these cells are not the actual oncologic cells in giant cell tumors. The stromal cells remain after treatment with a RANKL inhibitor[8,10] (**Figure 2**). Therefore, after use of the RANKL inhibitor is discontinued, the tumor returns.[11,12] One of the most important effects of RANKL inhibition is the effect on soft-tissue extension. The soft-tissue mass often decreases, and in some instances, the tumor retreats to the bone of origin, which effectively changes an Enneking stage 3 tumor to a stage 2 tumor[13] (**Figure 2**). In addition to the decreased tumor volume, tumors treated with RANKL inhibition are more fibrous and less vascular.[14,15] Although RANKL inhibition seems to be an effective adjuvant therapy, which can help facilitate surgical management, the long-term effects of targeting this pathway are unknown.

Radiation in Vertebral Tumors

The most common primary malignant tumors of the vertebrae are chordoma and chondrosarcoma. Both of these tumors are resistant to nonconformal photon-based radiation therapy.[16] This method of radiation therapy is unable to selectively target the tumor. Because of the inability to shield the spinal cord, radiation oncologists have been limited to doses less than 60 Gy; however,

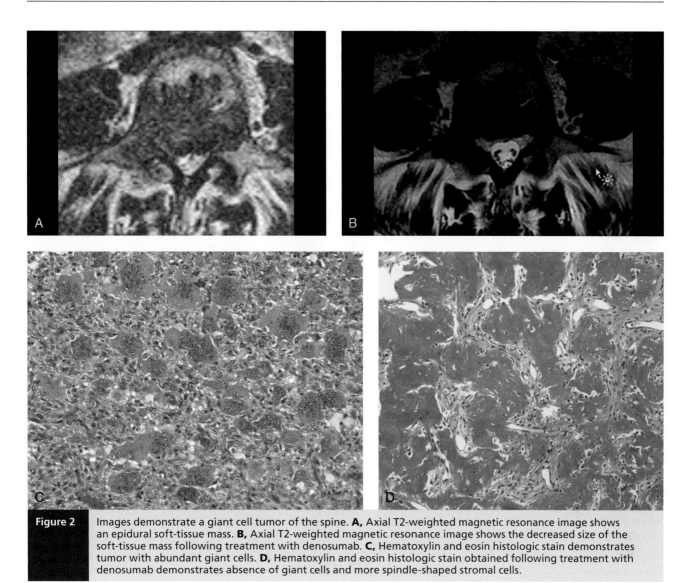

Figure 2 Images demonstrate a giant cell tumor of the spine. **A,** Axial T2-weighted magnetic resonance image shows an epidural soft-tissue mass. **B,** Axial T2-weighted magnetic resonance image shows the decreased size of the soft-tissue mass following treatment with denosumab. **C,** Hematoxylin and eosin histologic stain demonstrates tumor with abundant giant cells. **D,** Hematoxylin and eosin histologic stain obtained following treatment with denosumab demonstrates absence of giant cells and more spindle-shaped stromal cells.

newer cord-sparing methods of radiation administration allow higher doses.

Three forms of radiation are now being used to treat primary malignant spine tumors, alone or in combination with surgery: highly conformal photon radiation, proton radiation, and carbon ion radiation. Highly conformal photon radiation uses the capability to modulate the size and intensity of the photon beams in combination with radiation filters and real-time imaging. Proton and carbon ion therapy use the inherent qualities of these particles to spare noncancerous structures. Proton and carbon ion radiation both have a Bragg peak that allows the highest dose of radiation to be delivered to the target with essentially no exit dose that affects nearby healthy tissue. Radiation doses of 70 Gy or greater seem to have an effect on tumors such as chordoma and chondrosarcoma, which do not appear to respond to smaller doses.

Epidural Radiation Therapy

Staging systems are also meant to inform surgical choice. Primary tumors involving zone D (epidural soft-tissue extension) can be quite challenging. When the tumor simply effaces the dura, a marginal resection is possible. However, some tumors invade or at least adhere to the dura, which makes obtaining a negative margin challenging. In some cases, the dura can be removed with the tumor or after the main section of the tumor has been removed. Alternatively, radiation can be used to sterilize the dura instead of performing dural resection. Form-fitting plaques have been developed that can be applied directly to the dura after resection. The plaques are filled with β-emitting isotopes that deliver high doses of radiation for short distances (3 mm).[17,18] The WBB staging system could help plan for using an intraoperative plaque as an adjuvant when a close margin is anticipated.

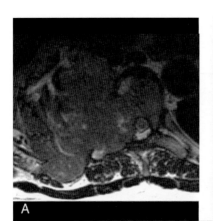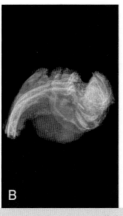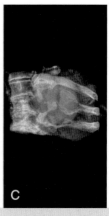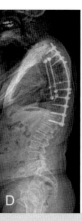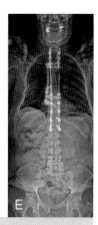

Figure 3 Images of a tumor that has invaded the chest wall, lungs, and the vertebral bodies and has compromised the spinal canal. **A,** Preoperative axial T2-weighted magnetic resonance image of the tumor. **B** and **C,** Radiographs of the specimen with surgical staples outlining the resected lung specimen. Lateral (**D**) and AP (**E**) weight-bearing radiographs obtained postoperatively show reconstruction using vascularized fibula graft.

Carbon Ion Radiation for Chordoma

Carbon ion radiation has been used to treat chordoma in the axial skeleton. One report outlined the oncologic outcomes of 188 patients with sacral chordomas treated with radiation (range, 64 to 74 Gy) with a median follow-up of 62 months.[19] The 5-year local control rate was 77% and the 10-year local control rate was 52% with carbon ions alone. This can be compared with a large, primarily surgical series in which the 5-year local control rate was 59% and the 10-year local control rate was 46%.[20] However, in the surgical series, the local control rate was 100% when a negative margin was obtained. Some data may extrapolate to the mobile spine, where the presence of the spinal cord limits both radiation delivery and surgery. Therefore, inferior local control rates would be expected in the mobile spine. A retrospective study reported the oncologic outcomes of 47 patients with sarcomas in the spine (9 of which were chordomas) treated with carbon ion therapy.[21] No recurrence was reported in eight chordoma cases at final follow-up. The report does not clearly state which patients underwent surgery or which types of surgery were performed. A case report of two patients treated with carbon ion therapy followed by en bloc spondylectomy revealed viable tumor cells in both resected specimens.[22] Definitive conclusions are difficult to determine regarding the use of carbon ion therapy for chordoma with the data available; however, the data suggest that it is more effective than conventional nonconformal radiation therapy.

Proton Radiation for Chordoma

A recent update of a phase II study provides the best data to support high-dose proton radiation therapy for chordomas and other sarcomas of the spine.[23] At 8-year follow-up, local control rates of 74% were achieved for the entire cohort of 29 chordomas, 14 chondrosarcomas, and 7 other types of sarcoma. Primary nonrecurrent tumors had local control rates of 85%. Another series of 66 chordomas of the mobile spine treated with surgery and high-dose proton radiation demonstrated that en bloc resection was superior to intralesional resection regarding local control (72% versus 54%), with a trend toward improved local control with negative margins. No local recurrence was reported in the 28 patients with primary tumors who underwent preoperative radiation and en bloc resection.[24] The largest study that evaluated definitive high-dose proton radiation without surgery included 24 patients with mobile spine and sacral chordomas that were treated with a mean radiation dose of 77.4 Gy.[25] After a median follow-up of 56 months, the local recurrence-free survival rate was 79.8%; larger tumor volume was correlated with worse survival.

Adjunctive radiation therapies result in improved local control rates. However, this benefit is balanced by the morbidity associated with the combination of radiation and surgery. In addition to the increased risk of infection, fracture rates greater than 76% have been reported after high sacrectomy.[26] In contrast, patients in the radiation-only group had a fracture rate of 22% (4 of 18 patients). Definitive radiation should be considered for patients in the higher sacrectomy group, given the higher risk of fracture and the known detrimental effect on physical function and increased pain after higher sacrectomy.[27] However, radiation alone works less well against large tumors such as those requiring high sacrectomy.[25] Radiation seems more effective for smaller tumors typically seen in the distal sacrum. However, recently reported quality-of-life and pain scores demonstrated that patients who have undergone distal sacrectomy have functional scores and pain levels comparable to those of the general population.[27]

En Bloc Resection

The techniques used for en bloc resection of mobile spine tumors have evolved, but these procedures remain technically demanding and major complications should be expected. En bloc resection should be reserved for aggressive tumors for which the systemic and local adjuvants are ineffective. En bloc resection is rarely indicated for many indolent benign tumors such as monostotic fibrous dysplasia;[28] however, en bloc resection has been shown to be an important component of local control in malignant tumors such as chondrosarcoma.[29] En bloc resection has a high rate of major complications for even the most experienced surgeons, including a mortality rate of 5%.[6,7]

Case Example

A collaborative effort among multiple surgical and non-surgical specialties is needed to perform an oncologically appropriate procedure to treat primary malignant tumor of the spine. If an oncologically sound procedure is not possible, options other than en bloc resection should be considered, given the inherent high complication rates. In this case, an active man underwent thoracic spine MRI secondary to persistent pain. T2-weighted axial views demonstrated a mass involving the vertebral body as well as the chest wall and epidural space (**Figure 3, A**). The tumor principally involved one vertebra, but both adjacent vertebrae were involved to a lesser degree. The mass also displaced the lung. A biopsy was obtained and the results were interpreted as a solitary fibrous tumor.

Preoperative proton-based radiation[24] was followed by staged en bloc resection. The posterior approach was performed first, and threadwire saws were passed at the cephalad and caudal junctions of the tumor and normal bone. The saws were placed dorsal to the great vessels. One arm of the saw was passed ventral to the spinal cord and secured to a posterior rod for use during the second stage. The patient was transferred to the intensive care unit for monitoring and resuscitation. The second surgical stage included a partial pneumonectomy and tumor removal performed by the thoracic surgery team (**Figure 3, B and C**). Radiation oncologists used a dural plaque loaded with P32 to sterilize any microscopic tumor remaining on the dura. The spine was reconstructed using a vascularized fibula graft. Additional spinal instrumentation was placed (**Figure 3, D and E**). The tumor margins were negative but would be considered marginal at the dura based on the Enneking classification.

Summary

The surgical management of primary vertebral tumors and the discipline of radiation oncology both continue to improve. Advancements in the field of radiation oncology will likely play a greater role in the management of these tumors. Systemic adjuvant therapies and the monoclonal antibody that is specific for RANKL also will play larger roles in the treatment of primary tumors of the spine.

Key Study Points

- The management of primary tumors of the spine is evolving because of improvements in adjuvant therapies.
- The collaboration of spine surgeons with colleagues in medical oncology and radiation oncology is imperative to provide the most appropriate care.
- Surgery remains an important component of care, but the type of surgery needed (ie, en bloc resection versus piecemeal resection versus stabilization) is dictated by the biology of the tumor and the availability and effectiveness of adjuvant therapy.

Annotated References

1. Siegel RL, Miller KD, Jemal A: Cancer Statistics, 2017. *CA Cancer J Clin* 2017;67(1):7-30.

   An update on the prevalence of cancer in the United States is provided.

2. William Enneking: Staging of Musculoskeletal Neoplasms, in Sundaresan N, Schmidek H, Schiller A, Rosenthal D, eds: *Tumors of the Spine Diagnosis and Clinical Management.* Philadelphia, PA, WB Saunders, 1990, p 22.

3. Boriani S, Weinstein JN, Biagini R: Primary bone tumors of the spine: Terminology and surgical staging. *Spine (Phila Pa 1976)* 1997;22(9):1036-1044.

4. Chan P, Boriani S, Fourney DR, et al: An assessment of the reliability of the Enneking and Weinstein-Boriani-Biagini classifications for staging of primary spinal tumors by the Spine Oncology Study Group. *Spine (Phila Pa 1976)* 2009;34(4):384-391.

5. Boriani S, Bandiera S, Casadei R, et al: Giant cell tumor of the mobile spine: A review of 49 cases. *Spine (Phila Pa 1976)* 2012;37(1):E37-E45.

   This retrospective study reviews the management of giant cell tumors in the mobile spine. The relative frequency of local recurrence based on the initial Enneking

7: Neoplastic and Inflammatory Conditions

classification of the tumor as well as the initial surgical treatment are discussed.

6. Amendola L, Cappuccio M, De Iure F, Bandiera S, Gasbarrini A, Boriani S: En bloc resections for primary spinal tumors in 20 years of experience: Effectiveness and safety. *Spine J* 2014;14(11):2608-2617.

   This prospective cohort study from a high-volume center reports oncologic outcomes after en bloc resection of primary tumors of the spine as well as the complications of these procedures.

7. Boriani S, Gasbarrini A, Bandiera S, Ghermandi R, Lador R: Predictors for surgical complications of en bloc resections in the spine: Review of 220 cases treated by the same team. *Eur Spine J* 2016;25(12):3932-3941.

   A detailed look at complications after en bloc spondylectomy is presented. The authors report on 226 resections in 216 patients.

8. Thomas D, Henshaw R, Skubitz K, et al: Denosumab in patients with giant-cell tumour of bone: An open-label, phase 2 study. *Lancet Oncol* 2010;11(3):275-280.

9. Rock MG, Sim FH, Unni KK, et al: Secondary malignant giant-cell tumor of bone: Clinicopathological assessment of nineteen patients. *J Bone Joint Surg Am* 1986;68(7):1073-1079.

10. Chawla S, Henshaw R, Seeger L, et al: Safety and efficacy of denosumab for adults and skeletally mature adolescents with giant cell tumour of bone: Interim analysis of an open-label, parallel-group, phase 2 study. *Lancet Oncol* 2013;14(9):901-908.

    This phase 2 study demonstrated the effect of denosumab on giant cell tumors. It provides the framework for additional studies and is helpful for understanding the effects of this new targeted therapy on giant cell tumors.

11. Lau CP, Huang L, Wong KC, Kumta SM: Comparison of the anti-tumor effects of denosumab and zoledronic acid on the neoplastic stromal cells of giant cell tumor of bone. *Connect Tissue Res* 2013;54(6):439-449.

    This study compares the effects of monoclonal antibodies and a diphosphonate (zoledronic acid) against RANKL. The mechanisms and clinical effects of these agents are discussed.

12. Mak IW, Evaniew N, Popovic S, Tozer R, Ghert M: A translational study of the neoplastic cells of giant cell tumor of bone following neoadjuvant denosumab. *J Bone Joint Surg Am* 2014;96(15):e127.

    This study explains the mechanism and effect of denosumab on giant cell tumors.

13. Gaston CL, Grimer RJ, Parry M, et al: Current status and unanswered questions on the use of Denosumab in giant cell tumor of bone. *Clin Sarcoma Res* 2016;6(1):15.

The authors provide an update on the state-of-the-art use of denosumab in the management of giant cell tumors.

14. Girolami I, Mancini I, Simoni A, et al: Denosumab treated giant cell tumour of bone: A morphological, immunohistochemical and molecular analysis of a series. *J Clin Pathol* 2016;69(3):240-247.

    This retrospective study analyzes the molecular effects of denosumab on giant cell tumors by using immunohistochemistry for evaluating protein expression.

15. Watanabe N, Matsumoto S, Shimoji T, et al: Early evaluation of the therapeutic effect of denosumab on tartrate-resistant acid phosphatase 5b expression in a giant cell tumor of bone: A case report. *BMC Res Notes* 2014;7:608.

    The authors discuss how denosumab, working through the RANKL receptor, affects giant cell function via the tartrate-resistant acid phosphatase enzyme.

16. Bjornsson J, Wold LE, Ebersold MJ, Laws ER: Chordoma of the mobile spine: A clinicopathologic analysis of 40 patients. *Cancer* 1993;71(3):735-740.

17. DeLaney TF, Chen GT, Mauceri TC, et al: Intraoperative dural irradiation by customized 192iridium and 90yttrium brachytherapy plaques. *Int J Radiat Oncol Biol Phys* 2003;57(1):239-245.

18. Folkert MR, Bilsky MH, Cohen GN, et al: Intraoperative 32P high-dose rate brachytherapy of the dura for recurrent primary and metastatic intracranial and spinal tumors. *Neurosurgery* 2012;71(5):1003-1010, discussion 1010-1011.

    This retrospective study outlines the role of brachytherapy using P32 in plaques placed on the dura during tumor excision.

19. Imai R, Kamada T, Araki N; Working Group for Bone and Soft Tissue Sarcomas: Carbon ion radiation therapy for unresectable sacral chordoma: An analysis of 188 cases. *Int J Radiat Oncol Biol Phys* 2016;95(1):322-327.

    This large study outlines the local control of sacral chordomas using carbon ion therapy alone.

20. Fuchs B, Dickey ID, Yaszemski MJ, Inwards CY, Sim FH: Operative management of sacral chordoma. *J Bone Joint Surg Am* 2005;87(10):2211-2216.

21. Matsumoto K, Imai R, Kamada T, et al; Working Group for Bone and Soft Tissue Sarcomas: Impact of carbon ion radiotherapy for primary spinal sarcoma. *Cancer* 2013;119(19):3496-3503.

    The oncologic outcomes in patients with spinal sarcomas treated with carbon ion therapy are explored in this retrospective study.

22. Matsumoto T, Imagama S, Ito Z, et al: Total spondylectomy following carbon ion radiotherapy to treat chordoma of the mobile spine. *Bone Joint J* 2013;95-B(10):1392-1395.

This case report describes the combination of en bloc resection with carbon ion therapy in tumors of the mobile spine.

23. DeLaney TF, Liebsch NJ, Pedlow FX, et al: Long-term results of phase II study of high dose photon/proton radiotherapy in the management of spine chordomas, chondrosarcomas, and other sarcomas. *J Surg Oncol* 2014;110(2):115-122.

    This phase II study reports on the oncologic outcomes of patients with sarcomas of the spine treated with high-dose proton-based radiation. Some of the patients were treated with radiation alone, and others were treated with various forms of oncologic resection.

24. Rotondo RL, Folkert W, Liebsch NJ, et al: High-dose proton-based radiation therapy in the management of spine chordomas: Outcomes and clinicopathological prognostic factors. *J Neurosurg Spine* 2015;23(6):788-797.

    This retrospective study from Massachusetts General Hospital reports on a large series of chordomas treated with high-dose radiation and surgery. The report highlights the role of preoperative versus postoperative radiation.

25. Chen YL, Liebsch N, Kobayashi W, et al: Definitive high-dose photon/proton radiotherapy for unresected mobile spine and sacral chordomas. *Spine (Phila Pa 1976)* 2013;38(15):E930-E936.

    This is the largest published study that used radiation alone to treat chordomas. A proton-based radiation protocol

showed promise for good local control in short-term to midterm follow-ups.

26. Osler P, Bredella MA, Hess KA, et al: Sacral insufficiency fractures are common after high-dose radiation for sacral chordomas treated with or without surgery. *Clin Orthop Relat Res* 2016;474(3):766-772.

    This retrospective study highlights the effect of high-dose proton radiation on bone strength. Level of evidence: III.

27. Phukan R, Herzog T, Boland PJ, et al: How does the level of sacral resection for primary malignant bone tumors affect physical and mental health, pain, mobility, incontinence, and sexual function? *Clin Orthop Relat Res* 2016;474(3):687-696.

    This multicenter study reports on functional outcomes for patients treated with sacrectomy. Level of evidence: III.

28. Schoenfeld AJ, Koplin SA, Garcia R, et al: Monostotic fibrous dysplasia of the spine: A report of seven cases. *J Bone Joint Surg Am* 2010;92(4):984-988.

29. Schoenfeld AJ, Hornicek FJ, Pedlow FX, et al: Chondrosarcoma of the mobile spine: A review of 21 cases treated at a single center. *Spine (Phila Pa 1976)* 2012;37(2):119-126.

    This retrospective study highlights the importance of en bloc resection in the management of chondrosarcoma of the mobile spine.

Chapter 34

Intradural Spine Lesions

Daniel K. Resnick, MD, MS   Darnell T. Josiah, MD, MS

7: Neoplastic and Inflammatory Conditions

Abstract

Primary spinal cord tumors are uncommon but have the potential to cause substantial morbidity. The location of the tumor and the patient's symptoms and age are important determinants of outcome. MRI is paramount for making a diagnosis and helps to delineate the compartment (eg, extradural, intradural, or intramedullary) that the tumor occupies. Meticulous surgical technique along with intraoperative neuromonitoring are important for minimizing postoperative neurologic deficits.

Keywords: astrocytoma; ependymoma; hemangioma; intradural; meningioma; neurofibroma; schwannoma

Introduction

Primary spinal cord tumors account for 2% to 4% of all primary tumors of the central nervous system. Most primary spine tumors are benign in nature. An analysis of 11,712 incidences identified over a 4-year period determined that 22% of primary tumors were malignant.[1] Spinal cord tumors are classified based on their anatomic location as extradural, intradural extramedullary, or intradural intramedullary. Extradural tumors usually are metastatic. These extradural lesions commonly arise in the vertebral bodies, and they can cause spinal cord compression as they grow or, infrequently, by

---

intradural invasion. Intradural extramedullary tumors account for approximately two-thirds of primary spinal tumors.[1] These tumors arise within the dura mater but outside the spinal cord itself. Meningiomas account for 50% of the incidences, and schwannomas and neurofibromas each account for 25%. Intradural intramedullary tumors arise within the spinal cord parenchyma itself, and most are glial tumors. Ependymoma is the most common intradural intramedullary tumor. Ependymomas can occur anywhere along the spinal cord; more than half are in the lumbosacral spinal cord, and the remainder are in the cervical or thoracic spinal cord. Astrocytoma, the second most common type of intradural intramedullary tumor, also can occur throughout the spinal cord. Other primary intradural intramedullary tumors are hemangioblastoma, lymphoma, and melanoma. Although rare, primary intramedullary spinal melanoma has been reported.

Intradural Extramedullary Tumors

Meningiomas

Meningiomas are dura-based tumors that arise from arachnoid cap cells at any place along the neuraxis. Spinal meningiomas account for 10% of all central nervous system meningiomas. Approximately 80% occur in the thoracic region, 15% in the cervical region, and 5% in the lumbosacral region. Meningiomas are more common in women than in men.[2] Usually meningiomas are slow-growing, low-grade tumors (World Health Organization [WHO] grade I), but some are invasive and can erode or remodel the bone.[3] Neurofibromatosis type 2 and prior exposure to ionizing radiation are risk factors. Many patients have back pain (70%), motor deficits (60%), sensory changes (40%), or incontinence (40%).[4] Asymptomatic lesions often are incidentally found on imaging studies related to a degenerative or traumatic pathology.[5-7] Meningiomas contain areas of increased cellularity or vascularity, xanthomatous components, and, occasionally, areas of hemorrhage. On MRI examination, a meningioma appears as a solid, well-circumscribed tumor with dural attachment. The lesion is isointense to hypointense on T1-weighted sequences and slightly hyperintense

---

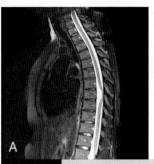 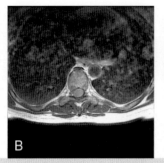 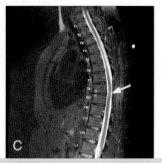 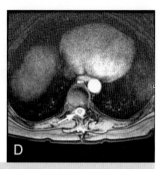

Figure 1 T2-weighted midsagittal (**A**) and T1-weighted contrast-enhanced axial (**B**) MRI sequences show midthoracic meningioma in a 45-year-old woman. The typical ventral location of the tumor and its homogeneous enhancement can be seen. The patient was treated with a wide laminectomy and microsurgical excision; the dural attachment was cauterized and scraped. The patient awoke without neurologic deficit. Postoperative T2-weighted midsagittal (**C**) and T2-weighted axial (**D**) MRI sequences show the complete resection postoperatively. The arrows indicate the prior site of the dural attachment. MRI at the 5-year follow-up showed no recurrence.

on T2-weighted or fluid-attenuated inversion recovery (FLAIR) sequences. Meningiomas are intensely enhanced with the use of contrast[8] (**Figure 1**).

An asymptomatic patient usually is followed with serial MRI. Surgical resection is the treatment of choice for a patient with a symptomatic lesion, and complete resection can be curative. The recurrence rate after complete resection was reported as 3% or 6% at 5 or 10 years, respectively.[9] Resection of the involved dura should be done if safe. Often the tumor arises from ventral or ventrolateral dura, which cannot be resected because of the high risk of cerebrospinal fluid leakage; cautery and curettage to remove all visible tumor usually is sufficient, however. Fractionated radiation therapy or stereotactic radiosurgery can be used after a subtotal resection or a recurrence. It is acceptable to sacrifice thoracic spinal roots to obtain a complete resection, but cervical and lumbar nerve roots must be preserved whenever possible.[5,9]

Meningiomas typically arise from the ventral or ventrolateral dura, and a wide exposure is required to avoid undue retraction of the spinal cord. Motor- and somatosensory-evoked potentials are used intraoperatively to detect a potential spinal cord injury. When an adequate surgical exposure has been achieved for resecting the tumor, the first priority is to eliminate the blood supply by amputating the tumor from its dural base. The tumor then can be further dissected, mobilized, and removed in a piecemeal fashion.

Schwannomas

Schwannomas are nerve sheath tumors that arise from the dorsal nerve root and generally are benign. Most schwannomas are slow growing and do not cause symptoms until they occupy a substantial volume. Patients typically report sensory symptoms such as paresthesias. Some asymptomatic schwannomas are found incidentally on imaging studies. Patients typically are in the fourth to sixth decade of life; however, schwannoma sometimes occurs with neurofibromatosis type 2, regardless of patient age. Schwannomas are composed of spindle cells arranged in short, intersecting fascicles. Abundant nuclear palisading results in the formation of Verocay bodies.[10] The two histologic patterns of Verocay bodies are Antoni A, in which there are compact areas of spindle cells with pink cytoplasm, and Antoni B, in which cells with a vacuolated, clear cytoplasm have a high lipid content.[2] On MRI, a schwannoma appears as a solid tumor in the dorsal aspect of the sensory root (**Figure 2**). There may be displacement of the spinal cord. These tumors are isointense on T1-weighted sequences and hyperintense on T2-weighted or FLAIR sequences. Contrast enhancement ranges from intensely homogenous to heterogeneous in the presence of intratumoral cysts, hemorrhage, or necrosis. Forty-seven percent of schwannomas are in the cervical spine, 22% are in the thoracic spine, 7% are in the conus medullaris, and 24% are in the cauda equina.[11]

Because of the benign nature of a schwannoma, asymptomatic patients can be followed with serial MRI. Patients with a large, symptomatic, or enlarging lesion should undergo a maximal safe resection. Gross total resection often is curative, but because almost all schwannomas are benign and slow growing, it is important to avoid creating a neurologic deficit. After partial resection of a symptomatic lesion, fractionated radiation therapy and stereotactic radiosurgery have been used.[12] Stimulus-evoked electromyography (EMG) is quite useful during surgery. The tumors arise from the nerve root ensheathing cells, and often they can be peeled away from the root to preserve neurologic function. Stimulus-evoked EMG can be used to identify the involved nerve root and can serve as a guide in determining whether it is safe to sacrifice involved fascicles. Typically, all regional muscle groups

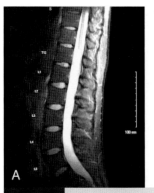
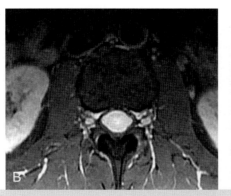
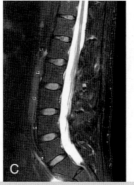
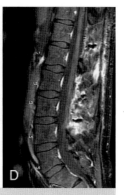

Figure 2 A 34-year-old man with sciatica had a completely normal physical examination. T2-weighted midsagittal MRI sequence (**A**) and T1-weighted contrast-enhanced axial MRI sequence at the T12 level (**B**) showed three discrete schwannomas attached to the roots of the cauda equina. Homogeneous enhancement with contrast is typical for benign nerve sheath tumors such as schwannomas. Postoperative T2-weighted midsagittal MRI sequence (**C**) and T1-weighted contrast-enhanced midsagittal MRI sequence (**D**) after complete microsurgical resection of the schwannomas. Preservation of all nerve roots was possible. The patient remained neurologically intact, with mild neuropathic pain in the sole of his right foot, probably resulting from root irritation caused by resection of the most caudal tumor. At 18-month follow-up, the patient remained disease free. The patient will undergo 5-year MRI follow-up.

are monitored intraoperatively, as well as bladder pressure and anal sphincters if the cauda equina region is involved. Electrodes are placed in the external anal sphincter and spontaneous EMG is monitored.[13]

Neurofibromas

Neurofibromas are benign tumors that arise from peripheral sensory nerves. The two types of neurofibromas are solitary and plexiform. Unlike a schwannoma, a neurofibroma encases the nerve roots and often cannot be resected without sacrificing the parent nerve root. Patients with neurofibromatosis type 1 may have multiple spinal cord neurofibromas that increase in size and number with age. Patients may have spontaneous pain and dysesthesias. Patients with neurofibromatosis type 1 should be followed with serial MRI because of the risk of malignant transformation. The incidence of such a transformation is 5% in patients with neurofibromatosis type 1 compared with 0.001% in the general population.[14] Solitary neurofibromas histologically are discrete, fusiform, or in globular nodules. Plexiform lesions have redundant loops of nerve fiber bundles interspersed with tumor cells in a disorganized pattern. Neurofibromas appear on MRI as round or fusiform lesions that are isointense on T1-weighted sequences and hyperintense on T2-weighted or FLAIR sequences, and they are intensely enhanced with contrast.[8] Patients with neurofibromatosis type 1 often have multiple tumors.

Patients who are symptomatic or have enlarging neurofibromas should undergo surgical resection. Complete resection of a solitary lesion often can be achieved without neurologic deficits. A complete resection of plexiform neurofibromas is challenging to obtain. These lesions may undergo transformation into malignant peripheral nerve sheath tumor. Radiation therapy is not recommended for benign neurofibromas because it can lead to malignant degeneration for patients with neurofibromatosis type 1. Chemotherapy generally is used only for malignant peripheral nerve sheath tumors.[15] Unlike schwannomas, these tumors cannot be freed from the parent nerve roots. Stimulus-evoked EMG is essential for determining whether the root has an important motor or other somatic (bladder or sphincter) function. If the root has no such function, it can be sacrificed to allow complete tumor removal. If the involved root has motor or somatic function, however, every effort is made to spare as many uninvolved fascicles as possible, and a complete resection may not be possible.

Intradural Intramedullary Tumors

Ependymomas

Ependymoma is the most common intradural intramedullary tumor in adults. The peak incidence is at age 30 to 40 years. The two types of ependymoma are cellular (WHO grades II and III) and myxopapillary (WHO grade I). Cellular ependymoma arises from the central canal of the cervical and thoracic spinal cord. Myxopapillary ependymoma arises from the filum terminale and almost always occurs at the conus medullaris.[4,16]

Cellular ependymoma has an indolent course. Patients often have localized pain for months to years with no other symptoms. The neurologic deficits can include lower extremity spasticity and sensory alterations in pain

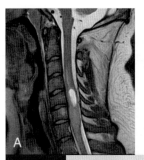 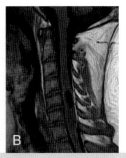 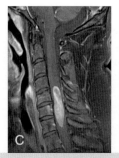 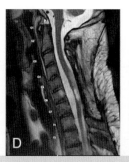 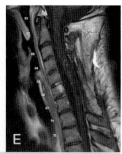

Figure 3   Magnetic resonance images from a 31-year-old man whose initial symptom was ataxia. T2-weighted (**A**), T1-weighted (**B**), and T1-weighted contrast-enhanced (**C**) MRI sequences show a discrete focal intramedullary tumor with the characteristic cystic components of a cellular ependymoma. The patient was treated with laminectomy. At his 5-year follow-up, T2-weighted MRI sequence (**D**) shows persistent syrinx and T1-weighted contrast-enhanced MRI sequence (**E**) shows no residual or recurrent lesion.

perception and temperature sensation secondary to disruption of the spinothalamic tracts by the ependymoma. The ependymoma grows symmetrically, causing the spinal cord to expand, sometimes over several segments, and occasionally with syrinx formation.[16] Cellular ependymomas most often are low grade, but anaplastic ependymoma, a malignant subtype (WHO grade III), can occur. The ependymoma appears on MRI as a focal expansion of the spinal cord that is isointense or hypointense on T1-weighted sequences and hyperintense on T2-weighted or FLAIR sequences. The contrast enhancement pattern is heterogeneous and often reveals cystic changes and a syrinx[8] (**Figure 3**). Local control rates after surgical resection are 90% to 100%; total or near-total resection usually can be achieved without causing further neurologic deficits.[16] Intraoperative monitoring of somatosensory- and motor-evoked potentials often is used to achieve a complete resection.[17] External beam radiation therapy at a 45- to 54-Gy dosage is indicated after a subtotal resection of a WHO grade II ependymoma or a WHO grade III malignant ependymoma. At 15 years after surgery, the overall progression-free survival rate was 35% and the overall survival was 75%.[18,19] Multivariate analyses supported the importance of complete resection but did not find adjuvant radiation therapy to be beneficial.[19] Chemotherapy has no current role in treating recurrent or metastatic ependymomas.

Cellular ependymomas usually can be completely resected (**Figure 4**). The resection often is aided by the presence of syrinx cavities above and below the tumor. Usually there is a distinct margin between the tumor and the spinal cord. A midline myelotomy most often exposes the tumor without causing substantial postoperative deficit, and the rostral and caudal margins of the tumor can be readily identified. A piecemeal resection technique and rolling of the capsule into the resection cavity often allow complete resection to be achieved. Monitoring of

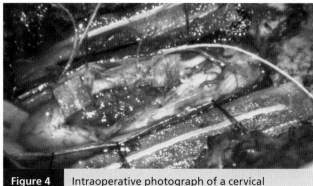

Figure 4   Intraoperative photograph of a cervical ependymoma resection in a 42-year-old woman. The midline myelotomy has been completed, and brownish/tan tumor can be seen compared with the yellow/white spinal cord.

somatosensory- and motor-evoked potentials is common during resection, but all visible tumor should be resected whenever possible.

Myxopapillary ependymomas are slow-growing glial tumors that are biologically different from other ependymomas (**Figure 5**). These tumors typically arise in the lumbosacral spinal cord and filum terminale. Young adult men most often are affected; the median age range at diagnosis is 35 to 37 years.[20] The patient often has low back pain, with or without radicular symptoms. Because myxopapillary ependymomas have a propensity to metastasize along the neuraxis, a complete brain and spine MRI should be done.[20] On MRI, these lesions are expansile in nature; they are hypointense or isointense on T1-weighted sequences and hyperintense on T2-weighted or FLAIR sequences. They are contrast enhancing, and hemosiderin staining may be seen on gradient echo or T2* sequences. Myxopapillary ependymomas initially are treated with surgical resection. Gross total resection often is curative, although local recurrence or leptomeningeal dissemination can occur as long as 20 years after the index procedure. Postoperative radiation therapy is associated with improved local control and progression-free survival.[20,21] These tumors are highly variable in their characteristics and the difficulty of surgical management. Tumors arising from the phylum terminale can be easily resected with minimal morbidity. Stimulus-evoked EMG is helpful for confirming the identity of the filum before resectioning. A tumor arising from the conus medullaris or filling the lumbar cistern is much more difficult to treat than a tumor arising from the phylum terminale; debulking followed by expansile duraplasty may be the best option. Postoperative radiation therapy may help delay progression of an incompletely resected lesion but is not curative.

Astrocytomas

Astrocytomas are tumors that arise from astrocytes, which are the supportive cells of the central nervous system, and account for approximately 40% of intramedullary tumors. Approximately 50% of spinal cord astrocytomas are pilocytic, and 50% are infiltrative. Pilocytic astrocytomas are well circumscribed, whereas diffuse fibrillary astrocytomas appear as nonencapsulated lesions.[22]

Patients with an intradural intramedullary tumor usually have pain and a combination of segmental sensory-level and upper motor neuron signs. A syrinx with altered pain and temperature sensation as well as motor neuron dysfunction with myelopathy may be present. Histologic analysis is the most important prognostic tool. A high-grade spinal cord glioma, although less common than a low-grade pilocytic astrocytoma, is associated with a poor survival rate.[4,23] On MRI, astrocytomas appear as a fusiform expansion of the spinal cord, and they may have a cystic component. A syrinx is seen in approximately 40% of astrocytomas.[8] These lesions are isointense to hypointense on T1-weighted sequences and hyperintense on T2-weighted or FLAIR sequences. Their degree of contrast enhancement is variable (**Figure 6**).

The initial treatment of an astrocytoma consists of a maximal safe surgical resection or a biopsy for tissue diagnosis followed by observation or external beam radiation therapy. Total or near-total resection of a pilocytic astrocytoma often is possible. Intraoperative monitoring of motor-evoked potentials can be helpful in determining the aggressiveness of a resection. For diffuse fibrillary lesions in which the tissue planes are not clear, resection usually is not possible, and an aggressive attempt at debulking risks severe neurologic injury.[23] The primary determinants of outcome for a patient with astrocytoma are neurologic functional status at the initial clinical

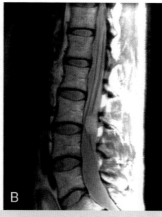

Figure 5 Images from a 30-year-old man whose initial symptom was radiculopathy. T1-weighted contrast-enhanced midsagittal MRI sequence (**A**) and T1-weighted midsagittal MRI sequence (**B**) show a focal mass at the junction of the conus medullaris and cauda equina, which is suggestive of a myxopapillary ependymoma. Because of the reluctance to resect eloquent tissue (as defined by intraoperative stimulus-evoked EMG), a limited resection was performed. The tumor recurred 5 years later, and the patient underwent tumor debulking followed by radiation therapy.

visit, tumor histology, and the extent of surgical resection. Radiation therapy is indicated in the presence of high-grade histology of biopsied tumors and progressive lesions. The use of postoperative radiation therapy has improved the survival rate for patients with diffuse fibrillary astrocytomas.[4,23]

Astrocytomas are extremely difficult tumors to treat. Complete resection is impossible unless the tumor is low grade and well circumscribed, and even an intralesional resection can lead to a neurologic deficit. The use of intraoperative motor-evoked potentials, frozen section pathology, and common sense leads to a maximal safe resection. An expansile duraplasty may be done if the tumor has expanded the cord.

Hemangioblastomas

Hemangioblastomas are the third most common form of intradural intramedullary tumors. Most often these vascular lesions occur as a solitary tumor. Ten percent to 30% of patients with hemangioblastoma have von Hippel-Lindau syndrome.[24] Most hemangioblastomas arise from the dorsal aspect of the spinal cord. More men than women are affected, most often in the fourth decade of life. Sensory disturbance symptoms are common, and the patient also may have proprioceptive deficits, long tract signs, or radicular symptoms. Subarachnoid or intramedullary hemorrhage occurs infrequently. On MRI sequences, hemangioblastomas appear as homogeneously

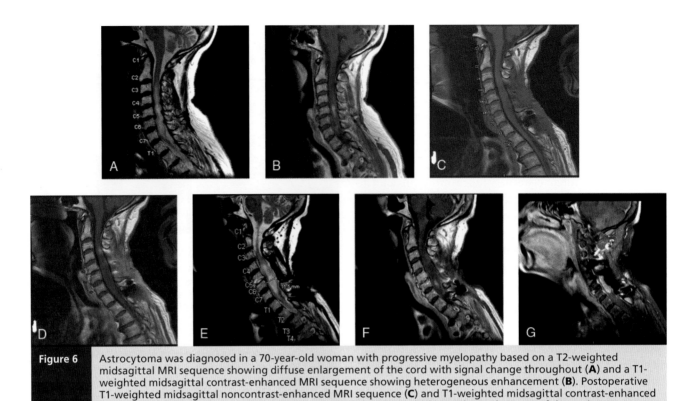

Figure 6 Astrocytoma was diagnosed in a 70-year-old woman with progressive myelopathy based on a T2-weighted midsagittal MRI sequence showing diffuse enlargement of the cord with signal change throughout (**A**) and a T1-weighted midsagittal contrast-enhanced MRI sequence showing heterogeneous enhancement (**B**). Postoperative T1-weighted midsagittal noncontrast-enhanced MRI sequence (**C**) and T1-weighted midsagittal contrast-enhanced MRI sequence (**D**) after laminectomy and expansile duraplasty, which was chosen because of the patient's advanced age. Although the patient's clinical course was stable for several months, T2-weighted midsagittal MRI sequence (**E**), T1-weighted midsagittal noncontrast-enhanced MRI sequence (**F**), and T1-weighted midsagittal noncontrast-enhanced MRI sequence (**G**) taken several months postoperatively revealed continuing expansion of the cord and increased enhancement. The disease progressed and led to the patient's death. Postmortem evaluation confirmed the diagnosis of diffuse astrocytoma.

enhancing hypervascular nodules that may be associated with a cyst or syrinx as well as cord edema. Hemangioblastomas are differentiated on MRI from ependymomas by vascular flow voids and are differentiated from a spinal cord vascular malformation by association with a syrinx.[8,25]

Surgical resection is the mainstay of treatment. Complete resection is achievable because the lesions have well-demarcated margins. Preoperative embolization can be done to reduce excessive intraoperative bleeding, which can lead to subtotal resection.[25,26] Serial MRI to detect new lesions should be performed in patients with von Hippel-Lindau disease. Stereotactic radiosurgery is an option for patients with an unresectable or recurrent hemangioblastoma.[27] These well-circumscribed lesions lend themselves to microsurgical resection. Access to the tumor usually is accomplished through the midline raphe or nerve root entry zone. Tumors with exophytic components are approached through the exophytic portion.

Primary Central Nervous System Lymphomas

Primary lymphoma appears rarely as an isolated intradural intramedullary lesion. On magnetic resonance images, the appearance of these lesions is multifocal with homogenous contrast enhancement. On diffusion-weighted imaging, the lesions often have restriction secondary to the high tumor cell density. A complete imaging evaluation of the neuraxis and histologic analysis of cerebrospinal fluid obtained through lumbar puncture are required. In rare incidences biopsy is required to establish a histologic diagnosis. The treatment is nonsurgical and often consists of methotrexate chemotherapy.[28]

Melanomas

A melanoma can arise in an isolated fashion in the intramedullary spinal cord with characteristics similar to those of other intradural intramedullary lesions. Primary melanoma of the spinal cord is a very rare diagnosis but is thought to arise from melanoblasts derived from neural crest cells early in development and are found in normal leptomeninges.[29] Intratumoral hemorrhages are common and may be mistaken for a cavernous malformation. Surgical resection allows tissue diagnosis but rarely is complete. Postoperative radiation therapy often is required.[30]

Summary

Recognizing the signs and symptoms in patients with primary spinal cord tumors will facilitate early diagnosis and treatment that can potentially limit neurologic deficits. The principal treatment of primary spinal cord tumors is surgical resection. Predictors of outcome include the patient's prior functional status, the tumor type, and the extent of the surgical resection.

Key Study Points

- Spinal cord tumors are rare and affect a small number of patients, but they may cause substantial pain and limb dysfunction and considerable morbidity. A prompt and accurate diagnosis is important.

- Well-circumscribed tumors have a better chance of complete surgical resection compared with diffuse, infiltrative tumors.

- The use of intraoperative neuromonitoring with spontaneous and stimulus-evoked EMG is vital for minimizing the risk of postoperative neurologic deficits.

Annotated References

1. Duong LM, McCarthy BJ, McLendon RE, et al: Descriptive epidemiology of malignant and nonmalignant primary spinal cord, spinal meninges, and cauda equina tumors: United States, 2004-2007. *Cancer* 2012;118(17):4220-4227.

   This large, population-based study provides new insights into the descriptive epidemiology of primary spinal cord tumors, spinal meninges, and cauda equina tumors with in-depth analyses of the incidence of these tumors in the United States.

2. Kernohan JW, Sayre GP: Tumors of the central nervous system, in *Atlas of Tumor Pathology, Fascicle 35*. Washington, DC, Armed Forces Institute of Pathology, 1952.

3. Lee JW, Lee IS, Choi KU, et al: CT and MRI findings of calcified spinal meningiomas: Correlation with pathological findings. *Skeletal Radiol* 2010;39(4):345-352.

4. Raco A, Esposito V, Lenzi J, Piccirilli M, Delfini R, Cantore G: Long-term follow-up of intramedullary spinal cord tumors: A series of 202 cases. *Neurosurgery* 2005;56(5):972-981, discussion 972-981.

5. Gezen F, Kahraman S, Canakci Z, Bedük A: Review of 36 cases of spinal cord meningioma. *Spine (Phila Pa 1976)* 2000;25(6):727-731.

6. Peker S, Cerçi A, Ozgen S, Isik N, Kalelioglu M, Pamir MN: Spinal meningiomas: Evaluation of 41 patients. *J Neurosurg Sci* 2005;49(1):7-11.

7. Solero CL, Fornari M, Giombini S, et al: Spinal meningiomas: Review of 174 operated cases. *Neurosurgery* 1989;25(2):153-160.

8. Abul-Kasim K, Thurnher MM, McKeever P, Sundgren PC: Intradural spinal tumors: Current classification and MRI features. *Neuroradiology* 2008;50(4):301-314.

9. Ryu SI, Chang SD, Kim DH, et al: Image-guided hypo-fractionated stereotactic radiosurgery to spinal lesions. *Neurosurgery* 2001;49(4):838-846.

10. Louis DN, Ohgaki H, Wiestler OD, Cavenee WK, eds: Pathology and genetics of tumours of the nervous system, in *World Health Organization Classification of Tumours of the Nervous System, Editorial and Consensus Conference Working Group*. Lyon, France, IARC Press, 2007.

11. Jinnai T, Koyama T: Clinical characteristics of spinal nerve sheath tumors: Analysis of 149 cases. *Neurosurgery* 2005;56(3):510-515, discussion 510-515.

12. Sachdev S, Dodd RL, Chang SD, et al: Stereotactic radiosurgery yields long-term control for benign intradural, extramedullary spinal tumors. *Neurosurgery* 2011;69(3):533-539, discussion 539.

    This study from Stanford University Medical Center examines the use of stereotactic radiosurgery as a viable alternative to microsurgical resection. Results demonstrated safe and efficacious long-term control of benign intradural extramedullary spinal tumors and a low rate of complications.

13. Krassioukov AV, Sarjeant R, Arkia H, Fehlings MG: Multimodality intraoperative monitoring during complex lumbosacral procedures: Indications, techniques, and long-term follow-up review of 61 consecutive cases. *J Neurosurg Spine* 2004;1(3):243-253.

14. Stadler JA III, Qadri U, Tang JA, et al: Malignant peripheral nerve sheath tumors of the spine: A SEER database analysis. *J Clin Neurosci* 2014;21(7):1106-1111.

    This study provides a population-based analysis using the Surveillance, Epidemiology, and End Results database, which focuses on patient characteristics and treatments. Surgery is associated with improved survival, whereas radiation therapy is associated with decreased survival in patients with malignant peripheral nerve sheath tumor of the spine.

15. Evans DG, Birch JM, Ramsden RT, Sharif S, Baser ME: Malignant transformation and new primary tumours after therapeutic radiation for benign disease: Substantial risks in certain tumour prone syndromes. *J Med Genet* 2006;43(4):289-294.

16. McCormick PC, Torres R, Post KD, Stein BM: Intramedullary ependymoma of the spinal cord. *J Neurosurg* 1990;72(4):523-532.

17. Quinones-Hinojosa A, Gulati M, Lyon R, Gupta N, Yingling C: Spinal cord mapping as an adjunct for resection of intramedullary tumors: Surgical technique with case illustrations. *Neurosurgery* 2002;51(5):1199-1206, discussion 1206-1207.

18. Isaacson SR: Radiation therapy and the management of intramedullary spinal cord tumors. *J Neurooncol* 2000;47(3):231-238.

19. Lee SH, Chung CK, Kim CH, et al: Long-term outcomes of surgical resection with or without adjuvant radiation therapy for treatment of spinal ependymoma: A retrospective multicenter study by the Korea Spinal Oncology Research Group. *Neuro Oncol* 2013;15(7):921-929.

    Examination results from 88 patients with spinal cord ependymomas showed that gross total removal alone is a good treatment strategy. Early diagnosis and surgery are important to obtain good functional outcomes. Subtotal resection plus radiation therapy for intramedullary lesions appears to offer no advantages over gross total removal.

20. Pica A, Miller R, Villà S, et al: The results of surgery, with or without radiotherapy, for primary spinal myxopapillary ependymoma: A retrospective study from the rare cancer network. *Int J Radiat Oncol Biol Phys* 2009;74(4):1114-1120.

21. Weber DC, Wang Y, Miller R, et al: Long-term outcome of patients with spinal myxopapillary ependymoma: Treatment results from the MD Anderson Cancer Center and institutions from the Rare Cancer Network. *Neuro Oncol* 2015;17(4):588-595.

    Myxopapillary ependymomas and long-term treatment outcomes are described. In a comparison of surgery alone and surgery plus radiation therapy, the authors found that younger patients and patients who are not treated initially with adjuvant radiation therapy or who do not undergo gross total resection are significantly more likely to have tumor recurrence or progression.

22. Minehan KJ, Brown PD, Scheithauer BW, Krauss WE, Wright MP: Prognosis and treatment of spinal cord astrocytoma. *Int J Radiat Oncol Biol Phys* 2009;73(3):727-733.

23. Innocenzi G, Salvati M, Cervoni L, Delfini R, Cantore G: Prognostic factors in intramedullary astrocytomas. *Clin Neurol Neurosurg* 1997;99(1):1-5.

24. Lonser RR, Weil RJ, Wanebo JE, DeVroom HL, Oldfield EH: Surgical management of spinal cord hemangioblastomas in patients with von Hippel-Lindau disease. *J Neurosurg* 2003;98(1):106-116.

25. Lee DK, Choe WJ, Chung CK, Kim HJ: Spinal cord hemangioblastoma: Surgical strategy and clinical outcome. *J Neurooncol* 2003;61(1):27-34.

26. Eskridge JM, McAuliffe W, Harris B, Kim DK, Scott J, Winn HR: Preoperative endovascular embolization of craniospinal hemangioblastomas. *AJNR Am J Neuroradiol* 1996;17(3):525-531.

27. Ryu SI, Kim DH, Chang SD: Stereotactic radiosurgery for hemangiomas and ependymomas of the spinal cord. *Neurosurg Focus* 2003;15(5):E10.

28. Abrey LE, Yahalom J, DeAngelis LM: Treatment for primary CNS lymphoma: The next step. *J Clin Oncol* 2000;18(17):3144-3150.

29. Fuld AD, Speck ME, Harris BT, et al: Primary melanoma of the spinal cord: A case report, molecular footprint, and review of the literature. *J Clin Oncol* 2011;29(17):e499-e502.

    This article presents a rare case of primary melanoma and details the molecular analysis performed on the pathologic specimen. The origins of primary spinal cord melanoma are discussed.

30. Farrokh D, Fransen P, Faverly D: MR findings of a primary intramedullary malignant melanoma: Case report and literature review. *AJNR Am J Neuroradiol* 2001;22(10):1864-1866.

7: Neoplastic and Inflammatory Conditions

Chapter 35
Spine Infections

Norman B. Chutkan, MD, FACS   Haitao Zhou, MD

Abstract

Infections of the spine manifest as a variety of conditions including pyogenic vertebral osteomyelitis, spondylodiscitis, nonpyogenic granulomatous lesions, epidural abscesses, and postoperative infections. Most patients receive antibiotics, which are combined with surgical intervention in selected cases. In patients with neurologic deficits or substantial spinal cord compression, expedited surgical decompression may be warranted. Surgical reconstruction also may be necessary if substantial associated instability or deformity exists.

Keywords: epidural abscess; granulomatous osteomyelitis; nonpyogenic; pyogenic vertebral osteomyelitis; spondylodiscitis

Introduction

Infections of the spine encompass a variety of conditions ranging from osteomyelitis of the vertebral body, discitis, and granulomatous lesions to abscess formation within the spinal canal. These conditions can exist in isolation or, frequently, in combination with each other.

Vertebral osteomyelitis is an infection of the vertebral body, end plate, intervertebral disk, and/or associated structures. Some authors believe that vertebral osteomyelitis and discitis represent points on the spectrum of the same disease. Vertebral osteomyelitis is also termed spinal osteomyelitis, spondylodiscitis, septic discitis, or disk space infection. Two types of vertebral osteomyelitis are pyogenic osteomyelitis, which is more common in developed countries, and nonpyogenic vertebral osteomyelitis, which is more common in developing countries. Vertebral osteomyelitis also can be classified as acute (occurring within several days to weeks) or chronic (occurring over several weeks to months). Common etiologic bacteria in pyogenic osteomyelitis include *Staphylococcus*, *Escherichia coli*, and *Propionibacterium acnes*. Nonpyogenic vertebral osteomyelitis, also called granulomatous vertebral osteomyelitis, is commonly caused by *Mycobacterium* species, *Nocardia*, *Brucella*, *Actinomyces*, and fungi. These organisms induce a granulomatous immune response, often resulting in progressive spinal column destruction. Spinal epidural abscess is a rare but potentially life-threatening condition defined by a collection of purulent material within the spinal epidural space.

Pyogenic Vertebral Osteomyelitis

Pyogenic vertebral osteomyelitis (PVO) is caused by a bacterial infection of the vertebral bodies that can extend into the adjacent intervertebral disk spaces or can originate in a disk space and spread to vertebral bodies. Three major pathways exist for bacteria to cause PVO: hematogenous seeding, direct inoculation, and rarely, by means of adjacent tissue infection.

Most cases of hematogenous seeding are thought to result from slow blood flow in the end arteriole system near the vertebral end plate or spread from the pelvic venous plexus via the perivertebral venous system. Spinal procedures such as lumbar puncture, epidural steroid injection, diskography, or surgery can inadvertently introduce bacteria into the vertebral body, disk space, or adjacent structures by means of direct inoculation. Infections from adjacent soft tissue include infections that arise from retropharyngeal abscesses or psoas abscesses.

Dr. Chutkan or an immediate family member has received royalties from Globus Medical and serves as a board member, owner, officer, or committee member of the American Academy of Orthopaedic Surgeons, the North American Spine Society, the American Orthopaedic Association, and AO Spine North America. Neither Dr. Zhou nor any immediate family member has received anything of value from or has stock or stock options held in a commercial company or institution related directly or indirectly to the subject of this chapter

Epidemiology and Microbiology

The annual incidence of PVO has been estimated at 2.4 cases per 100,000.[1] The incidence increases with age: from 0.3 per 100,000 in patients younger than 20 years to 6.5 per 100,000 in patients older than 70 years. The overall incidence is likely increasing because of a combination of an aging population and increased use of diagnostic tools with high sensitivity such as MRI.[2] The most common microorganisms that cause PVO are *S aureus* followed by *E coli* and coagulase-negative staphylococci and *P acnes*.[3] Based on clinical series published in the past 5 years, 50% to 60% of cases involved the lumbar spine, 20% involved the cervical spine, and 20% to 30% involved the thoracic spine.[4,5]

Clinical Features

Almost 90% of patients with vertebral osteomyelitis have site-specific pain associated with paraspinal muscle spasm.[6] Fever, chills, and malaise occur in approximately one-half of patients. A detailed medical history is necessary to identify risk factors for vertebral osteomyelitis. Risk factors include diabetes mellitus, end-stage renal disease, intravenous drug use, malignancy, endocarditis, prior surgical procedure, a history of organ transplantation, and immunosuppression. A thorough clinical examination is critical to identify any neurologic deficits, which occur in 15% to 35% of patients.[7,8] Worsening neurologic status can determine the urgency of surgical treatment. It also is essential to determine a neurologic status baseline for comparison during treatment and the ongoing follow-up period. Routine laboratory analysis, including complete blood cell count, erythrocyte sedimentation rate (ESR), and C-reactive protein (CRP) level, also are important for making a diagnosis and follow-up comparisons. The white blood cell count is normal in approximately 50% of patients with vertebral osteomyelitis; however, the CRP level and ESR are elevated in most patients. Although both are routinely monitored to determine the effectiveness of treatment, the CRP level has a shorter normalization time than the ESR; therefore, the CRP level responds more quickly to treatment and is more useful for evaluating the response to treatment. Blood culture results are also important, particularly when the patient is febrile. In more than 50% of patients, blood culture results identify the pathogen. In the absence of positive blood culture results, CT-guided biopsy may be indicated. In several studies, CT-guided biopsy successfully identified the offending organism in up to 70% of patients.[9-11] In patients already undergoing antibiotic treatment, this sensitivity diminished to 10% to 20%. Spine surgeons, emergency department physicians, internal medicine physicians, and hospitalists must combine efforts to ensure that antibiotics are not started until culture specimens have been obtained. If the patient requires surgical intervention, an open biopsy and culture is recommended. Open biopsies have a significantly higher rate of positive culture results than do percutaneous biopsies. Polymerase chain reaction assay from percutaneous biopsy tissue is more sensitive than a conventional culture, although it does not allow susceptibility testing.[12]

MRI is the study of choice when vertebral osteomyelitis is suspected. MRI without contrast enhancement will show high T2-weighted and low T1-weighted signal intensity in the affected disk space. MRI studies obtained following contrast enhancement often show lesion enhancement and help determine the extent of involvement. MRI also can demonstrate the presence of an epidural abscess. Because MRI findings do not reflect the pace of clinical improvement, serial MRI is of limited use in following the progress of treatment. Given that up to 47% patients have other often noncontiguous lesions, complete radiographic evaluation of the spine is recommended.[4,6,13]

Plain radiographic findings are normally not seen until after approximately 30% of bony destruction has occurred, which can take several weeks. Plain radiographic imaging findings, especially obtained while weight bearing, are important in the evaluation of overall alignment, mechanical stability, and any associated spinal deformity. Plain radiographs are also useful for follow-up after both surgical and nonsurgical treatment.

CT can identify bony destruction earlier than plain radiographic imaging; however, compared with MRI, the use of CT can result in a delayed diagnosis. CT is useful in the evaluation of the integrity of the bony structures and the extent of bony involvement and for preoperative planning.

Echocardiography is recommended to evaluate for endocarditis, especially in patients who do not respond to medical management. Up to 30% of all patients with hematogenous spinal infection have concomitant bacterial endocarditis.[14] A valve replacement procedure may be necessary to prevent recurrent seeding, depending on the extent of the endocarditis.

Treatment Options

After the diagnosis is made, medical treatment with antibiotics is indicated, irrespective of surgical treatment. A consultation with an infectious disease specialist can help with the selection, dosing, and duration of antibiotic treatment. Broad-spectrum empirical antibiotics should be started initially and switched to antibiotics specific to the culture results when sensitivities have been finalized. If the culture results are negative, continued use of broad-spectrum antibiotics is recommended.

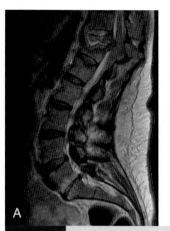 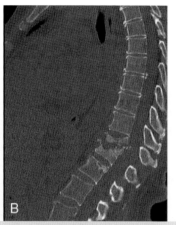 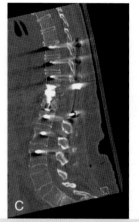 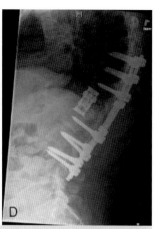

Figure 1 Images from a 51-year-old woman with a history of intravenous drug abuse and diabetes mellitus who presented with increasing mid back pain and weakness in her left lower extremity. The patient underwent posterior-only T11-12 corpectomy and posterior fusion of T8 through L3. **A,** T2-weighted lumbar magnetic resonance image shows spondylodiscitis at the T11-T12 level with focal kyphotic deformity. **B,** Reconstructed sagittal thoracolumbar spine CT shows partial destruction of the vertebral bodies at the T11-T12 level. **C,** Reconstructed sagittal CT obtained following corpectomy at T11-T12 level and posterior fixation from T8 through L3. **D,** Lateral radiograph obtained 1 month postoperatively shows correction of focal kyphotic deformity.

Some reports suggest that culture results may not be critical to the prognosis. A 2011 study reported that patients with positive culture results have long-term results similar to those with negative cultures.[7]

The duration of antibiotic treatment is controversial. One report shows that shorter periods (up to 8 weeks) of intravenous antibiotic treatment are associated with a higher relapse rate for methicillin-resistant *S aureus* and gram-negative bacteria.[15] The only randomized controlled trial examining the duration of antibiotics treatment of vertebral osteomyelitis reported similar success rates for patients receiving antibiotics for 6 weeks and for 12 weeks.[16]

Bracing can help limit motion and control pain in patients undergoing nonsurgical treatment for vertebral osteomyelitis. Surgery is indicated for patients who are refractory to antibiotic treatment or those in whom neurologic deficits, spinal instability, or deformity develop. The presence of an epidural abscess is also a relative indication for surgical intervention, depending on the location and extent of the abscess. The purpose of surgical treatment is to débride devitalized and infected tissue, decompress the neural elements, and restore spinal alignment and stability. Controversy exists in the timing of surgical intervention, surgical approach, use of instrumentation, and the types of grafts to be used. No consensus exists on the timing of surgical treatment. Early intervention is recommended in patients with neurologic deficits and potential neurologic involvement, such as epidural abscess and progressive deformity. Most spine surgeons believe that instrumentation in patients

with PVO does not increase the recurrence rate or rate of treatment failure following appropriate surgical débridement. A 2014 study reported on 118 patients treated with and without instrumentation and showed no increase in failure rate with the use of instrumentation.[17] In addition, a small retrospective comparison study showed no difference in outcomes for patients who underwent anterior débridement and fixation versus anterior débridement and posterior fixation.[18]

An anterior approach often is used for infections involving the vertebral body and disk and is frequently combined with anterior or posterior instrumentation. Recently, minimally invasive techniques using specialized retractors have allowed access to the anterior spine with reduced morbidity.[19] Percutaneous posterior fixation combined with anterior débridement and grafting also has become more common. Débridement and fixation by means of a posterior-only approach also has been reported.[20] Small case series that described anterior reconstruction and posterior instrumentation performed via a single posterior approach for PVO reported that such an approach is safe and effective for thoracic or lumbar vertebral osteomyelitis and is less invasive, resulting in faster recovery.[21,22] A 2014 study published findings that posterior fixation without débridement, in combination with aggressive antibiotic treatment, was successful in management of spinal infections.[23] Because the posterior approach is familiar to most spine surgeons, the trend is increasing toward management of thoracic and lumbar spondylodiscitis via posterior-only approaches[24] (**Figure 1**).

7: Neoplastic and Inflammatory Conditions

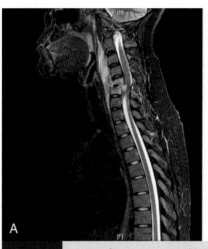
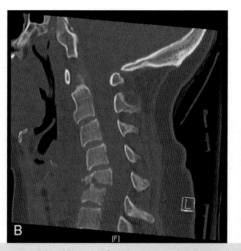
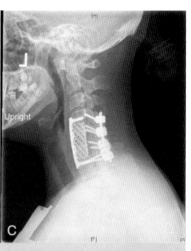

Figure 2 Images from a 25-year-old woman with a history of intravenous drug abuse who presented with increasing neck pain and right upper extremity weakness and numbness lasting 1 month. **A,** Preoperative T2-weighted sagittal cervical spine MRI shows a retropharyngeal abscess with C5-C6 spondylodiscitis and epidural abscess and spinal cord compression. **B,** Preoperative sagittal cervical spine CT image shows bony destruction of C5 and C6. **C,** Lateral radiograph obtained 3 months postoperatively demonstrates C5-C6 corpectomy and C4 through C7 anterior and posterior fixation and fusion with titanium mesh cage. Overall cervical alignment is maintained.

Cervical spondylodiscitis is relatively rare compared with thoracic or lumbar vertebral osteomyelitis. For cervical spondylodiscitis, approximately 40% of patients presented with neurologic deficits and 40% with septicemia. Up to 80% of patients had epidural abscesses and 10% died.[13] Increasingly, cervical spondylodiscitis has been safely addressed through combined anterior and posterior procedures.[25] Case series results also suggest that percutaneous endoscopic lavage and drainage can provide good control of the infection[26,27] (**Figure 2**).

Granulomatous Vertebral Osteomyelitis

Granulomatous vertebral osteomyelitis, or nonpyogenic vertebral osteomyelitis, is characterized by a spinal infection resulting in the formation of granuloma. Causative organisms can include bacteria such as *Mycobacterium tuberculosis*, fungi, or other parasites. Overall, nonpyogenic vertebral osteomyelitis is more prevalent in developing countries and most frequently related to *M tuberculosis* infection.

Pathophysiology

Spinal involvement by *M tuberculosis* most commonly occurs secondary to pulmonary tuberculosis. Direct spread from the genitourinary system or adjacent tissue also is possible. Three patterns of spinal involvement have been described: anterior, peridiskal, and central. Peridiskal involvement is the most common; it involves the metaphyseal portion of the vertebral bodies and can spread to adjacent levels. Disk tissue is spared in most cases, which helps distinguish *M tuberculosis* from PVO. This pattern also can cause collapse of the vertebral body, resulting in instability and late deformity. Central involvement, in the center of the vertebral body, is sometimes difficult to differentiate from a metastatic lesion. Anterior involvement originates between the anterior longitudinal ligament and the vertebral body. It can spread in both caudal and cephalad directions and causes scalloping of the anterior aspect of vertebral bodies and elevation of the anterior longitudinal ligament.

Epidemiology

Microorganisms that can cause granulomatous vertebral osteomyelitis include *Mycobacterium* species, *Brucella*, fungi, *Actinomyces*, and *Nocardia*. Incidence of this disease has been increasing, likely secondary to an increase in the number of immunocompromised patients such as those with AIDS, those on immunosuppression therapy after transplantation, and those undergoing chemotherapy for cancer.[28] The thoracic spine is the most common location for tuberculous spondylodiscitis.

Clinical Features

As with PVO, granulomatous vertebral osteomyelitis most often presents with back pain secondary to loss of structural integrity. Patients with granulomatous vertebral osteomyelitis tend to have more systemic symptoms such as malaise, night sweats, and weight loss. Pain is usually the most common symptom. Fever is seen less often with granulomatous vertebral osteomyelitis than PVO. Neurologic involvement can present as radiculopathy, myelopathy, or cauda equina syndrome. Paraplegia from tuberculosis is also known as Pott paraplegia.

A detailed history is important to identify risk factors for patients with suspected granulomatous vertebral osteomyelitis. Laboratory studies include white blood cell count, ESR, and CRP level as well as purified protein derivative test. Interpretation of this test is difficult in some patients, particularly those from developing countries who have been vaccinated against tuberculosis and those who are severely immunocompromised and whose immune response is insufficient. Blood interferon-γ release assay is a more sensitive test and provides a result within 24 hours.

Plain radiographs of the thoracolumbar spine and chest are indicated for initial radiographic evaluation. In a typical spinal tuberculosis infection, the disk is spared. MRI is frequently used for confirmation. Well-defined, thin-walled intraspinal or paraspinal abscesses on T1-weighted fat-suppressed contrast-enhanced sequences are typical MRI findings that differentiate tuberculous spondylitis from pyogenic spondylodiscitis. One study found increased vertebral collapse in HIV-negative patients.[29] CT is useful in the evaluation of the extent of bony destruction and for preoperative planning.

Treatment

As with pyogenic spondylodiscitis, medical treatment is most effective for tuberculous spondylitis.[30] No consensus exists on the length of antituberculosis treatment, which varies from 6 to 24 months.[31,32] Surgical intervention is indicated when an open biopsy is needed to confirm the diagnosis, with spinal instability, with substantial spinal cord compression despite medical treatment, or with deteriorating neurologic status. Historically, surgery has been performed via an anterior approach for débridement and grafting because tuberculous spondylitis is typically ventral in location. Posterior instrumented fusion is usually performed after the anterior procedure either concurrently or as a staged procedure. Several studies have reported on posterior-only approaches for anterior débridement and circumferential reconstruction using costotransversectomy or an extracavitary approach.[32-35] Some reports suggest that a posterior-only approach may result in better kyphosis correction and maintenance of correction.[36,37] The posterior-only approach also has been associated with better overall clinical outcomes. Since 2002, posterior-only vertebral column resection has become common in the treatment of angular kyphotic deformity resulting from tuberculosis.[37,38] Angular kyphotic deformity is a serious consequence of tuberculous spondylitis. It can result in neurologic deficits, sagittal imbalance, or cardiopulmonary restriction. Posterior vertebral column resection can correct the deformity, restore alignment, and decompress the neural elements; however, it is associated with high complication rates.[39] A minimally invasive procedure using specialized retractors and percutaneous fixation for débridement and stabilization of spinal infections also has become common.[40,41,42]

Prognosis

Most patients with tuberculous spinal infection have a good prognosis, with up to 95% of patients responsive to medical treatment, with pain relief and improved neurologic status.[43] Even among patients with myelopathy, almost 90% can benefit from combined medical and surgical treatment.[43]

Epidural Abscess

Epidemiology

Spinal epidural abscess is a rare, challenging condition with potentially devastating consequences. The incidence of spinal epidural abscess has been increasing over the past several decades because of an aging population, intravenous drug use, and possibly, improved diagnosis with the widespread use of MRI.[44]

Pathogenesis

Approximately 80% of patients with spinal epidural abscess have one or more risk factors including diabetes mellitus, intravenous drug use, end-stage renal disease, or some form of immunocompromise.[45] Approximately 50% of these abscesses are thought to result from hematogenous spread. Although direct spread accounted for approximately one-third of cases, the source of the infection could not be identified in the remaining cases.

In 2012, there was a large outbreak of fungal infections including spinal epidural abscesses caused by contaminated injections of methylprednisolone.[46] Methicillin-resistant *S aureus* was seen in 15% to 40% patients. Other etiologies include methicillin-sensitive *S aureus*, *E coli*, and *Pseudomonas aeruginosa*. Anaerobic bacteria, fungi, and parasites also have been reported.[47] Different reports cite the thoracic or lumbar spine as the most common site of spinal epidural abscess. In most instances, the abscess is located dorsal to the spinal cord;[25,45] however, the abscess was circumferential in approximately 23% of cases. In addition, the spinal epidural abscess commonly involves more than one location. Ventrally located epidural abscesses are more likely associated with spondylodiscitis. The exact mechanism of how an epidural abscess causes neurologic deficits is still controversial. Most plausibly, a combination of direct mechanical compression and vascular compromise and ischemia, with or without inflammation of the blood vessels, likely results in spinal cord injury.

Clinical Features

Clinically, patients with spinal epidural abscess can present with a variety of symptoms that range from simple back or neck pain to complete paralysis. Only a small percentage of patients present with the classic clinical triad of back pain, fever, and neurologic deficits. Almost all patients have site-specific pain and 50% of patients present with fever or weakness.[45,48] Based on previously published reports, the four stages of spinal epidural abscess are stage 1, site-specific back pain; stage 2, nerve root pain; stage 3, motor weakness; and stage 4, paralysis. Frequently, spinal epidural abscesses extend over three to four vertebrae. Involvement of the whole spine is termed holospinal epidural abscess.

Diagnosis

A through history and physical examination are critical in the evaluation of a patient suspected of having an epidural abscess. Most patients present with site-specific back or neck pain; however, only 50% of patients will be febrile and fewer than 50% of patients have neurologic deficits. ESR and CRP levels are elevated in most patients, but these findings are nonspecific. It is important to obtain baseline ESR and CRP levels to monitor the effectiveness of treatment.

MRI is the study of choice for diagnosis. MRI enhanced with gadolinium contrast has a sensitivity of greater than 90% for the detection of abscess. For patients unable to undergo MRI, CT myelography is sensitive but also invasive. MRI with gadolinium contrast can show a liquid abscess with peripheral enhancement on T1-weighted images. For phlegmonous infection without a liquid abscess, MRI usually shows homogeneous enhancement of the abnormal area without a substantial collection of pus. Plain radiography and CT are useful in determining overall alignment, stability, and the extent of bony destruction. Noncontiguous spinal epidural abscess lesions are common and have been reported to occur in up to 10% of patients with spinal epidural abscesses.[49] A 2015 study reported that a delay in presentation, a concomitant area of infection outside the spinal and paraspinal regions, and an ESR greater than 95 mm/h at presentation are predictors of noncontiguous involvement.[49] When all three predictors were present, 73% of the patients were found to have a skip lesion.

Treatment

In most retrospective studies, the mainstay of treatment is surgical decompression and débridement combined with antibiotics.[13] The selection of antibiotic is based on blood culture results or cultures obtained during surgical débridement. Initial broad-spectrum antibiotic coverage is recommended until the culture results have been obtained. After the results have been finalized, the antibiotic regimen can be modified toward the specific organism. Case series have also described nonsurgical treatment of spinal epidural abscesses.[50,51]

A 2014 study proposed that patients who cannot undergo surgery, those who sustained a complete spinal cord injury more than 48 hours previously with low clinical or radiographic concern for an ascending lesion, or patients who are neurologically stable and lack risk factors for failure of medical management can be initially treated with antibiotics alone and close clinical monitoring.[52] Another study reported that treatment was unsuccessful for 41% of patients treated with antibiotics alone, and a decrease occurred in the motor scores of these patients.[45] Final motor scores were still lower than the presenting motor score after delayed surgical treatment, although some improvement in the motor score occurred after the surgical intervention. Risk factors for failed nonsurgical treatment include diabetes mellitus, CRP level greater than 115 mg/L, white blood cell count greater than 12.5×10^9/L, and positive blood cultures.

Early surgical evacuation has been advocated since 1948.[53] Spinal epidural abscesses are treated as a relative emergency in most institutions. No randomized clinical studies have been published on the timing of surgery; however, the consensus seems to be that if the decision is made for surgical intervention, it should be performed as expeditiously as possible.

Prognosis

The mortality rate from spinal epidural abscess has decreased substantially with advances in antibiotic treatment and the widespread availability of MRI. The current mortality rate is approximately 10% compared with more than 30% during the 1950s.[54,55] The single most important predictor of final neurologic outcome is the patient's neurologic status immediately before surgery. The mortality rate remains elevated during the first year following spinal epidural abscess but decreases to almost that of the reference population over time.[56]

Iatrogenic Infections

Postoperative infections usually result from direct inoculation during the index procedure or from hematogenous seeding. The incidence of postoperative infection varies greatly, with increased rates associated with the use of instrumentation, multiple levels, prolonged surgical time, open procedures, and medical comorbidities such as diabetes mellitus.[57] The use of perioperative antibiotics for no more than 24 hours after surgery has been shown to reduce the rate of postoperative infections.[58]

A high index of suspicion and early, aggressive intervention is required for successful management of postoperative infection. Antibiotic treatment alone is rarely successful, and surgical débridement is frequently necessary. Débridement should proceed systematically from superficial layers to deep layers with cultures obtained at each layer. All necrotic tissues should be thoroughly excised. Management of bone graft in this situation is controversial. Most authors recommend removal of any loose graft material. Well-fixed instrumentation usually can be retained; however, loose hardware may require removal. Infected interbody polyether ether ketone cages are a particular challenge and frequently require removal to eradicate infection. Recently, several reports suggest that placement of vancomycin powder directly into the surgical wound significantly reduces the rate of postoperative infection.[59,60]

Summary

Spinal infections can include various conditions such as osteomyelitis of the vertebral bodies, discitis, granulomatous lesions, abscess formation within the spinal canal, or some combination. Treatment usually includes a combination of surgical intervention and antibiotics; however, selected cases can be treated with antibiotics alone with close monitoring. Irrespective of the underlying condition, the goals of surgical intervention are the same: débridement and excision of all infected and necrotic tissue, decompression of neural elements when necessary, and restoration of alignment and stability to the spinal column. Less-invasive surgical techniques are becoming more common in the surgical treatment of these patients and are associated with potentially less morbidity, faster recovery, and improved outcomes. However, these procedures should not override achieving the goals of surgery.

Key Study Points

- In most spine infections, surgical intervention is indicated for failure of antibiotic management, substantial instability or deformity, and substantial neural compression with or without neurologic deficits.
- Epidural abscesses frequently require emergent decompression. Neurologic deficits can result from a combination of ischemia and direct compression.
- Postoperative infections usually require aggressive surgical intervention in combination with antibiotics.

Annotated References

1. Grammatico L, Baron S, Rusch E, et al: Epidemiology of vertebral osteomyelitis (VO) in France: Analysis of hospital-discharge data 2002-2003. *Epidemiol Infect* 2008;136(5):653-660.

2. Kehrer M, Pedersen C, Jensen TG, Lassen AT: Increasing incidence of pyogenic spondylodiscitis: A 14-year population-based study. *J Infect* 2014;68(4):313-320.

   The incidence of osteomyelitis is increasing, but whether the increase is real or caused by improved diagnostic methods remains unknown.

3. Zimmerli W: Clinical practice: Vertebral osteomyelitis. *N Engl J Med* 2010;362(11):1022-1029.

4. Shiban E, Janssen I, Wostrack M, et al: A retrospective study of 113 consecutive cases of surgically treated spondylodiscitis patients: A single-center experience. *Acta Neurochir (Wien)* 2014;156(6):1189-1196.

   This retrospective study from one institution showed that a staged surgical approach and a short 1- to 2-week period of intravenous antibiotics followed by 3 months of oral antibiotics is effective.

5. Connor DE Jr, Chittiboina P, Caldito G, Nanda A: Comparison of operative and nonoperative management of spinal epidural abscess: A retrospective review of clinical and laboratory predictors of neurological outcome. *J Neurosurg Spine* 2013;19(1):119-127.

   The authors of this retrospective study from one institution concluded that immediate surgical decompression combined with appropriate antibiotic treatment is supported for patients with focal neurologic deficits.

6. Mylona E, Samarkos M, Kakalou E, Fanourgiakis P, Skoutelis A: Pyogenic vertebral osteomyelitis: A systematic review of clinical characteristics. *Semin Arthritis Rheum* 2009;39(1):10-17.

7. Lora-Tamayo J, Euba G, Narváez JA, et al: Changing trends in the epidemiology of pyogenic vertebral osteomyelitis: The impact of cases with no microbiologic diagnosis. *Semin Arthritis Rheum* 2011;41(2):247-255.

   The increase in the incidence of PVO and the detection of less infectious microorganisms in patients with microbiotically confirmed PVO indicate a possible epidemiologic change in this disorder.

8. Loibl M, Stoyanov L, Doenitz C, et al: Outcome-related co-factors in 105 cases of vertebral osteomyelitis in a tertiary care hospital. *Infection* 2014;42(3):503-510.

   This retrospective study presents demographic data and clinical features of vertebral osteomyelitis.

9. Gasbarrini A, Boriani L, Salvadori C, et al: Biopsy for suspected spondylodiscitis. *Eur Rev Med Pharmacol Sci* 2012;16(suppl 2):26-34.

The authors of this study demonstrated that CT-guided biopsy is the mainstay in making a diagnosis for spine lesions of unknown etiology.

10. Spira D, Germann T, Lehner B, et al: CT-guided biopsy in suspected spondylodiscitis: The association of paravertebral inflammation with microbial pathogen detection. *PLoS One* 2016;11(1):e0146399.

 The authors of this study demonstrated that inflammatory infiltration of the paravertebral space indicated successful pathogen detection by using CT-guided biopsy.

11. Pupaibool J, Vasoo S, Erwin PJ, Murad MH, Berbari EF: The utility of image-guided percutaneous needle aspiration biopsy for the diagnosis of spontaneous vertebral osteomyelitis: A systematic review and meta-analysis. *Spine J* 2015;15(1):122-131.

 This systematic review and meta-analysis concluded that image-guided spinal biopsy is highly specific and performs well in the prediction of spontaneous vertebral osteomyelitis but has moderate accuracy for ruling out this diagnosis.

12. Choi SH, Sung H, Kim SH, et al: Usefulness of a direct 16S rRNA gene PCR assay of percutaneous biopsies or aspirates for etiological diagnosis of vertebral osteomyelitis. *Diagn Microbiol Infect Dis* 2014;78(1):75-78.

 This prospective study reported that a 16S rDNA polymerase chain reaction assay with sequencing was more sensitive than routine culture for the etiologic diagnosis of vertebral osteomyelitis.

13. Shousha M, Boehm H: Surgical treatment of cervical spondylodiscitis: A review of 30 consecutive patients. *Spine (Phila Pa 1976)* 2012;37(1):E30-E36.

 The authors of this study reviewed 30 consecutive patients with cervical osteomyelitis and concluded that radical surgical débridement and appropriate antibiotic treatment provide a reliable approach to achieve complete healing of inflammation. Whole-spine MRI is recommended.

14. Cornett CA, Vincent SA, Crow J, Hewlett A: Bacterial spine infections in adults: evaluation and management. *J Am Acad Orthop Surg* 2016;24(1):11-18.

 This review article reports on spinal infection.

15. Park KH, Chong YP, Kim SH, et al: Clinical characteristics and therapeutic outcomes of hematogenous vertebral osteomyelitis caused by methicillin-resistant Staphylococcus aureus. *J Infect* 2013;67(6):556-564.

 This cohort study showed that antibiotic treatment of methicillin-resistant *S aureus* hematogenous vertebral osteomyelitis of at least 8 weeks is associated with less relapse.

16. Bernard L, Dinh A, Ghout I, et al; Duration of Treatment for Spondylodiscitis (DTS) study group: Antibiotic treatment for 6 weeks versus 12 weeks in patients with pyogenic vertebral osteomyelitis: An open-label, non-inferiority, randomised, controlled trial. *Lancet* 2015;385(9971):875-882.

 This open-label noninferiority randomized controlled trial compared 6 and 12 weeks of antibiotic treatment of vertebral osteomyelitis and concluded that 6 weeks of antibiotic treatment is not inferior to 12 weeks of antibiotic treatment.

17. Bydon M, De la Garza-Ramos R, Macki M, et al: Spinal instrumentation in patients with primary spinal infections does not lead to greater recurrent infection rates: An analysis of 118 cases. *World Neurosurg* 2014;82(6):e807-e814.

 A cohort study showed that instrumentation in patients with spinal infection did not increase the revision rate compared with patients who underwent decompression without instrumentation.

18. Si M, Yang ZP, Li ZF, Yang Q, Li JM: Anterior versus posterior fixation for the treatment of lumbar pyogenic vertebral osteomyelitis. *Orthopedics* 2013;36(6):831-836.

 This comparison study concluded that both anterior and posterior fixation had satisfactory outcomes and were reliable and safe treatments for PVO of the lumbar spine.

19. Verdú-López F, Vanaclocha-Vanaclocha V, Gozalbes-Esterelles L, Sánchez-Pardo M: Minimally invasive spine surgery in spinal infections. *J Neurosurg Sci* 2014;58(2):45-56.

 The use of minimally invasive surgical techniques to manage spine infections is discussed. The authors conclude that these techniques are safe and effective and can have beneficial effects on morbidity and allow faster patient recovery.

20. Zhang L, Cai WH, Huang B, Chen LW, Zhang N, Ni B: Single-stage posterior debridement and single-level instrumented fusion for spontaneous infectious spondylodiscitis of the lumbar spine. *Acta Orthop Belg* 2011;77(6):816-822.

 Ten adults with infectious spondylodiscitis of the lumbar spine were treated with posterior débridement and instrumented fusion. At 10 months, solid fusion was achieved in all 10 patients. No recurrence of infection was reported.

21. Gorensek M, Kosak R, Travnik L, Vengust R: Posterior instrumentation, anterior column reconstruction with single posterior approach for treatment of pyogenic osteomyelitis of thoracic and lumbar spine. *Eur Spine J* 2013;22(3):633-641.

 This case series reported that posterior-only débridement and reconstruction was a safe alternative treatment for patients with PVO of the thoracic and lumbar spine.

22. Skovrlj B, Guzman JZ, Caridi J, Cho SK: Posterior-only circumferential decompression and reconstruction in the surgical management of lumbar vertebral osteomyelitis. *Global Spine J* 2016;6(1):e35-e40.

 This study discusses the posterior-only approach with anterior débridement and posterior fixation for lumbar vertebral osteomyelitis without sacrificing the segmental nerve root.

23. Mohamed AS, Yoo J, Hart R, et al: Posterior fixation without debridement for vertebral body osteomyelitis and discitis. *Neurosurg Focus* 2014;37(2):E6.

This case series reported on patients with vertebral osteomyelitis who underwent treatment with posterior fixation and antibiotic treatment.

24. Dreimann M, Viezens L, Hoffmann M, Eicker SO: Retrospective feasibility analysis of modified posterior partial vertebrectomy with 360-degree decompression in destructive thoracic spondylodiscitis. *Acta Neurochir (Wien)* 2015;157(9):1611-1618.

The authors report that modified costotransversectomy achieved good clinical outcomes in a series of patients with thoracic spondylodiscitis.

25. Ghobrial GM, Viereck MJ, Margiotta PJ, et al: Surgical management in 40 consecutive patients with cervical spinal epidural abscesses: Shifting toward circumferential treatment. *Spine (Phila Pa 1976)* 2015;40(17):E949-E953.

This study demonstrated that the shift to staged anterior decompression and posterior stabilization in patients with cervical spine epidural abscesses did not increase the perioperative complication rate. Level of evidence: III.

26. Yang SC, Chen WJ, Chen HS, Kao YH, Yu SW, Tu YK: Extended indications of percutaneous endoscopic lavage and drainage for the treatment of lumbar infectious spondylitis. *Eur Spine J* 2014;23(4):846-853.

This study reported on percutaneous endoscopic lavage and drainage performed to obtain specimens to guide antibiotic treatment and relieve symptoms.

27. Fu TS, Chen LH, Chen WJ: Minimally invasive percutaneous endoscopic discectomy and drainage for infectious spondylodiscitis. *Biomed J* 2013;36(4):168-174.

This article discusses percutaneous endoscopic lavage and débridement in patients with infectious spondylodiscitis. It was found to be an effective alternative management method that was particularly useful in patients with serious comorbidities or those with spine infections in early stages.

28. Kilborn T, Janse van Rensburg P, Candy S: Pediatric and adult spinal tuberculosis: Imaging and pathophysiology. *Neuroimaging Clin N Am* 2015;25(2):209-231.

This review article discusses adult and pediatric spinal tuberculosis.

29. Anley CM, Brandt AD, Dunn R: Magnetic resonance imaging findings in spinal tuberculosis: Comparison of HIV positive and negative patients. *Indian J Orthop* 2012;46(2):186-190.

A discussion of MRI findings in patients with HIV and tuberculosis is presented.

30. Rajasekaran S, Khandelwal G: Drug therapy in spinal tuberculosis. *Eur Spine J* 2013;22(suppl 4):587-593.

Patients with uncomplicated tuberculosis of the spine usually can be successfully treated with drug therapy. Treatment is more challenging in patients with multidrug-resistant spinal tuberculosis or those who are HIV-positive. Patient compliance with the drug regimen is vital.

31. *WHO Treatment Guidelines for Drug-Resistant Tuberculosis: 2016 Update.* Geneva, Switzerland, World Health Organization, 2016.

32. Pang X, Wu P, Shen X, Li D, Luo C, Wang X: One-stage posterior transforaminal lumbar debridement, 360° interbody fusion, and posterior instrumentation in treating lumbosacral spinal tuberculosis. *Arch Orthop Trauma Surg* 2013;133(8):1033-1039.

This retrospective study reported on one-stage posterior débridement and fixation in combination with medical treatment of lumbosacral tuberculosis infection. The authors reported effective pain relief, improved neurologic function, and the achievement of spine stability.

33. Zeng H, Zhang P, Shen X, et al: One-stage posterior-only approach in surgical treatment of single-segment thoracic spinal tuberculosis with neurological deficits in adults: A retrospective study of 34 cases. *BMC Musculoskelet Disord* 2015;16:186.

This retrospective study reported on one-stage posterior-only transpedicular débridement and fusion for patients with thoracic spinal tuberculosis and neurologic deficits. Satisfactory healing was achieved.

34. Zhang HQ, Li JS, Zhao SS, et al: Surgical management for thoracic spinal tuberculosis in the elderly: Posterior only versus combined posterior and anterior approaches. *Arch Orthop Trauma Surg* 2012;132(12):1717-1723.

This retrospective cohort study compared posterior-only with a combined posterior-anterior approach for thoracic spinal tuberculosis in elderly patients and reported that the posterior-only procedure had better clinical outcomes.

35. Garg B, Kandwal P, Nagaraja UB, Goswami A, Jayaswal A: Anterior versus posterior procedure for surgical treatment of thoracolumbar tuberculosis: A retrospective analysis. *Indian J Orthop* 2012;46(2):165-170.

This retrospective study compared anterior and posterior approaches for thoracic spinal tuberculosis treatment.

36. Ma YZ, Cui X, Li HW, Chen X, Cai XJ, Bai YB: Outcomes of anterior and posterior instrumentation under different surgical procedures for treating thoracic and lumbar spinal tuberculosis in adults. *Int Orthop* 2012;36(2):299-305.

The authors of this study followed 217 patients who underwent either anterior or posterior procedures for thoracic and lumbar spinal tuberculosis and compared the clinical outcomes.

37. Lü G, Wang B, Li Y, Li L, Zhang H, Cheng I: Posterior vertebral column resection and intraoperative manual traction to correct severe post-tubercular rigid spinal deformities incurred during childhood: Minimum 2-year follow-up. *Eur Spine J* 2015;24(3):586-593.

In this retrospective study, 11 patients underwent posterior vertebral column resection for the correction of posttubercular spinal deformity. Use of this procedure along with intraoperative manual traction was found to be effective in the management of posttubercular spinal deformity. Neurologic complications are possible.

38. Zhang HQ, Li JS, Liu SH, et al: The use of posterior vertebral column resection in the management of severe post-tuberculous kyphosis: A retrospective study and literature review. *Arch Orthop Trauma Surg* 2013;133(9):1211-1218.

Fifteen patients were treated with vertebral column resection for posttubercular kyphotic deformity. This procedure can be safe and effective when performed by an experienced surgeon.

39. Kim SS, Cho BC, Kim JH, et al: Complications of posterior vertebral resection for spinal deformity. *Asian Spine J* 2012;6(4):257-265.

In this retrospective study, 233 patients underwent posterior vertebral resection for spinal deformity. Clinical outcomes and complications are discussed.

40. Kapoor S, Kapoor S, Agrawal M, Aggarwal P, Jain BK Jr: Thoracoscopic decompression in Pott's spine and its long-term follow-up. *Int Orthop* 2012;36(2):331-337.

In this retrospective long-term follow-up study, 30 patients underwent video-assisted thoracoscopic surgery for treatment of dorsal spine tuberculosis.

41. Lü G, Wang B, Li J, Liu W, Cheng I: Anterior debridement and reconstruction via thoracoscopy-assisted mini-open approach for the treatment of thoracic spinal tuberculosis: Minimum 5-year follow-up. *Eur Spine J* 2012;21(3):463-469.

This retrospective long-term follow-up study reported on anterior débridement and reconstruction via a thoracoscopy-assisted mini-open approach for thoracic tuberculosis.

42. Ito M, Sudo H, Abumi K, et al: Minimally invasive surgical treatment for tuberculous spondylodiscitis. *Minim Invasive Neurosurg* 2009;52(5-6):250-253.

43. Tuli SM: Historical aspects of Pott's disease (spinal tuberculosis) management. *Eur Spine J* 2013;22(suppl 4):529-538.

The author discusses spinal tuberculosis in this review article.

44. Darouiche RO: Spinal epidural abscess. *N Engl J Med* 2006;355(19):2012-2020.

45. Patel AR, Alton TB, Bransford RJ, Lee MJ, Bellabarba CB, Chapman JR: Spinal epidural abscesses: Risk factors, medical versus surgical management, a retrospective review of 128 cases. *Spine J* 2014;14(2):326-330.

In this retrospective study, 128 patients who underwent early surgery for spinal epidural abscesses had improved neurologic outcomes. Risk factors were identified for failed nonsurgical treatment.

46. Smith RM, Schaefer MK, Kainer MA, et al; Multistate Fungal Infection Outbreak Response Team: Fungal infections associated with contaminated methylprednisolone injections. *N Engl J Med* 2013;369(17):1598-1609.

The authors report on the outbreak of fungal infection from contaminated methylprednisolone acetate injections.

47. Hawkins M, Bolton M: Pediatric spinal epidural abscess: A 9-year institutional review and review of the literature. *Pediatrics* 2013;132(6):e1680-e1685.

This retrospective study reported on nine pediatric patients with spinal epidural abscess.

48. Adogwa O, Karikari IO, Carr KR, et al: Spontaneous spinal epidural abscess in patients 50 years of age and older: A 15-year institutional perspective and review of the literature. Clinical article. *J Neurosurg Spine* 2014;20(3):344-349.

This retrospective study demonstrated that patients older than 50 years with spinal epidural abscess did not benefit from early surgical decompression.

49. Ju KL, Kim SD, Melikian R, Bono CM, Harris MB: Predicting patients with concurrent noncontiguous spinal epidural abscess lesions. *Spine J* 2015;15(1):95-101.

This retrospective cohort study identified risk factors for patients to have concurrent noncontiguous spinal epidural abscess.

50. Grieve JP, Ashwood N, O'Neill KS, Moore AJ: A retrospective study of surgical and conservative treatment for spinal extradural abscess. *Eur Spine J* 2000;9(1):67-71.

51. Kim SD, Melikian R, Ju KL, et al: Independent predictors of failure of nonoperative management of spinal epidural abscesses. *Spine J* 2014;14(8):1673-1679.

Risk factors for failure of nonsurgical management of spinal epidural abscesses include diabetes in a patient older than 65 years, infection with methicillin-resistant *S aureus*, and neurologic compromise.

52. Tuchman A, Pham M, Hsieh PC: The indications and timing for operative management of spinal epidural abscess: Literature review and treatment algorithm. *Neurosurg Focus* 2014;37(2):E8.

This literature review of 28 case series with a minimum of 30 patients each presented an algorithm for selecting patients who may be safe candidates for nonsurgical management of spinal epidural abscess.

53. Heusner AP: Nontuberculous spinal epidural infections. *N Engl J Med* 1948;239(23):845-854.

54. Lu CH, Chang WN, Lui CC, Lee PY, Chang HW: Adult spinal epidural abscess: Clinical features and prognostic factors. *Clin Neurol Neurosurg* 2002;104(4):306-310.

55. Reihsaus E, Waldbaur H, Seeling W: Spinal epidural abscess: A meta-analysis of 915 patients. *Neurosurg Rev* 2000;23(4):175-204, discussion 205.

56. Kehrer M, Pedersen C, Jensen TG, Hallas J, Lassen AT: Increased short- and long-term mortality among patients with infectious spondylodiscitis compared with a reference population. *Spine J* 2015;15(6):1233-1240.

This case cohort study compared mortality rates in patients with infectious spondylodiscitis with a reference population based on data from Funen County, Denmark.

57. Parchi PD, Evangelisti G, Andreani L, et al: Postoperative spine infections. *Orthop Rev (Pavia)* 2015;7(3):5900.

This review article provides information about the latest achievements in prevention, diagnosis, microbiology, and treatment of postoperative spinal wound infections. Information on risk factors also is presented.

58. Rubinstein E, Findler G, Amit P, Shaked I: Perioperative prophylactic cephazolin in spinal surgery: A double-blind placebo-controlled trial. *J Bone Joint Surg Br* 1994;76(1):99-102.

59. Schroeder JE, Girardi FP, Sandhu H, Weinstein J, Cammisa FP, Sama A: The use of local vancomycin powder in degenerative spine surgery. *Eur Spine J* 2016;25(4):1029-1033.

The authors report on the local placement of vancomycin powder in surgical spine wounds prior to fascial closing. Vancomycin was used in 1,224 cases, and 2,253 cases did not use vancomycin. The rate of deep wound infections and the need for irrigation and débridement procedures decreased in patients treated with vancomycin compared with those whose wounds were not treated with vancomycin.

60. Dennis HH, Wei DT, Darren KZ, et al: Is intraoperative local vancomycin powder the answer to surgical site infections in spine surgery? *Spine (Phila Pa 1976)* 2016; May 23 [Epub ahead of print].

This retrospective cohort study of all patients who underwent instrumented spine surgery at a single institution compared surgical site infections in wounds treated with vancomycin power and those not treated with vancomycin powder. The authors concluded the local use of vancomycin powder decreased the infection rate.

Chapter 36

Inflammatory Arthritides

Peter G. Passias, MD   Gregory W. Poorman, BA   M. Burhan Janjua, MD   Samantha R. Horn, BA

7: Neoplastic and Inflammatory Conditions

Abstract

Inflammatory arthritides are the seronegative spondyloarthropathies and rheumatoid arthritis. The joints, bones, ligaments, tendons, and synovial tissues of the the spine are affected by these disorders. Rheumatoid arthritis frequently affects the cervical spine. Early medical intervention can prevent disease progression, which can result in spinal instability. Other spondyloarthropathies similarly respond to medical management; however, fracture and deformity can develop in patients with advanced disease.

Keywords: ankylosing spondylitis; inflammatory arthritides; rheumatoid arthritis

Introduction

Inflammatory arthritides are categorized separately from osteoarthritis, which is the most common form of spinal arthritis. These entities represent systemic autoimmune diseases that induce the body to form antibodies that attack multiple body systems, including the spine. Inflammatory arthritides affect joints, bones, ligaments, tendons, and synovial tissues throughout the skeleton.

Most inflammatory arthritides of the spine exhibit characteristic targets. For example, rheumatoid arthritis (RA) specifically targets the upper cervical spine, which

Dr. Passias or an immediate family member serves as a paid consultant to Zimmer; serves as an unpaid consultant to Medicrea; and has received research or institutional support from the Cervical Scoliosis Research Society. None of the following authors or any immediate family member has received anything of value from or has stock or stock options held in a commercial company or institution related directly or indirectly to the subject of this chapter: Mr. Poorman, Dr. Janjua, and Ms. Horn.

results in synovial inflammation and, later, diffuse joint destruction. Ankylosing spondylitis characteristically targets the sacroiliac joints and anterior longitudinal ligament.

Other inflammatory arthritides include psoriatic arthritis, reactive arthritis, gout, polymyalgia rheumatica, and enteropathic arthritis. Diffuse idiopathic skeletal hyperostosis (DISH), which is a noninflammatory osteoarthritis variant that causes spinal ankylosis, is similar to the inflammatory arthritides.

Recognizing the features that differentiate these conditions is essential for tailoring a treatment plan. Recently, systemic treatment of these diseases has advanced markedly. However, surgical intervention is still frequently indicated to address compression of neural elements, spinal instability, and spinal deformity.

Rheumatoid Arthritis

Epidemiology

RA is a chronic, systemic, and progressive autoimmune disorder that affects approximately 0.5% to 1% of the US population and more than 1.3 million adults.[1-10] RA is approximately two to three times more common in women than men. This disorder may present at any age, but most commonly occurs between the ages of 40 and 60 years. Combinations of early aggressive treatments, including disease-modifying antirheumatic drugs (DMARDs) and biologic agents, have markedly decreased the rate of cervical spine surgery for RA.

In order of frequency, RA manifestations in the cervical spine are atlantoaxial subluxation, subaxial subluxation, and cranial settling (also known as basilar impression or invagination, atlantoaxial impaction, or superior migration of the odontoid). The current literature suggests a 25% to 88% prevalence of any type of cervical spine involvement in patients with RA. Neurologic symptoms severe enough to require surgical consultation develop in only 7% to 34% of these patients. The prevalence of involvement of the atlantoaxial spine is approximately 19% to 70%, with or without the involvement of the craniocervical junction.[8] Subaxial cervical spine involvement has been reported in 7% to 88% of patients with RA, usually occurs at multiple levels, and causes spinal canal stenosis.[11] Synovitis-induced erosive changes in the cervical spine frequently occur in patients with active peripheral RA. The lumbar spine is rarely involved.

Microbiology

The pathogenesis of RA is characterized by inflammation in the synovium and synovial fluid. A complex interplay between the adaptive and innate immune systems results in an erosive and hypertrophic synovitis, often described as pannus. Dendritic cells, mast cells, macrophages, and neutrophils all play an important role. T and B cells produce cytokines and autoantibodies in response to currently unknown antigens expressed on synovial cells. The synovium of patients with RA has an increased number of CD4+ T antibodies. T cell– and B cell–associated phosphoinositide-3-kinases delta and gamma recruit neutrophils and mast cells. Production of tumor necrosis factor-alpha (TNF-α) and interleukin-1 attracts more lymphocytes and neutrophils in a positive feedback cascade. Synovial cells release procollagenase, progelatinase, and other metalloproteinases, which promote destruction of the synovium, cartilage, bone, joint, and the surrounding tissue.

Etiology of Spine Instability

Atlantoaxial instability begins with erosive pannus formation at the C1-C2 joints, bone destruction, and subsequent laxity of the transverse atlantal ligament. This ligament restrains the dens in the anterior atlantoaxial joint. The loss of integrity of the transverse atlantal ligament results in the anterior translation of the patient's head and C1 on the dens.

The normal anterior atlantodental interval is less than 3 mm. In patients with atlantoaxial instability, this value increases and the value of the posterior atlantodental interval decreases, which increases the risk of compression of the upper segment of the cervical spinal cord. Posterior or lateral subluxation is rare, and usually occurs secondary to a rotational or a traction injury resulting in fractures of the axial spine.

Subaxial subluxation, from autoimmune destruction of the facet joints, is seen in approximately 7% to 29% of patients with RA. Subluxation is defined as 3.5 mm or more of translation, or more than 11° of angular instability. Multiple levels of the cervical spine may be involved, leading to a "staircase" deformity (**Figure 1**).

Cranial migration (also known as atlantoaxial impaction or basilar invagination) may occur when there is a high degree of destruction of the occipitoatlantal condyles and/or the atlantoaxial facet joint; however, it usually

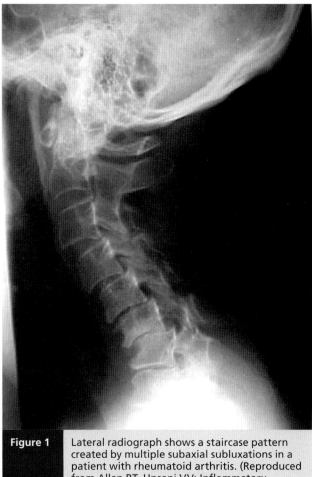

Figure 1   Lateral radiograph shows a staircase pattern created by multiple subaxial subluxations in a patient with rheumatoid arthritis. (Reproduced from Allen RT, Upsani VV: Inflammatory arthritides of the spine, in Rao RD, Smuck M, eds: *Orthopaedic Knowledge Update: Spine 4*. Rosemont, IL, American Academy of Orthopaedic Surgeons, 2012, pp 549-563.)

results from C1 lateral mass destruction. The cranium may settle caudally, concurrent with pannus development, and ventral brain stem compression may occur via pannus formation around the dens. Asymmetric bone loss from the occipital condyles and C1 lateral masses may contribute to a torticollis deformity.

Clinical Presentation

Physical Evaluation

Clinical manifestations of cervical disease in RA are varied. Neck pain is the most common presentation, with subtle and progressive instability as the underlying pathophysiology. Joint arthropathy, muscle wasting, decreased range of motion, neurologic symptoms, and altered mental status may be present. However, because 33% to 50% of all RA patients with cervical instability are asymptomatic, it is crucial to determine if there is cervical involvement in the early stages of RA. Early recognition of cervical symptomology and intervention with medication may spare the cervical spine and slow disease progression.[12]

Pain is common in patients with RA of the cervical spine. In patients with atlantoaxial subluxation, the C2 spinous process may become prominent with neck flexion. Asymmetric destruction of the lateral atlantoaxial joints can induce the head to be held downward with a lateral tilt. Instability may cause secondary impingement of the greater and/or lesser occipital nerves (medial divisions of dorsal rami of C2 and C3 nerve roots, respectively), resulting in occipital headaches. In addition, C2 nerve claudication may cause pain in the face, ear, or mastoid. Patients with C1-C2 instability may report symptoms of vertigo, syncope, nystagmus, dysarthria, sleep apnea, swallowing difficulty, or facial paresthesia. Instability in the subaxial cervical spine may result in more caudal neck pain. The radiation of pain to the clavicles from C3-C4 or the scapulae from C5-C6 or C6-C7 is often described.

Neurologic Symptoms

Given the morbidity and mortality associated with upper cervical instability in patients with RA, it is important to perform a careful assessment for myelopathy. Muscle weakness, atrophy, numbness, tingling or paresthesia, bowel or bladder incontinence, hyperreflexia, loss of proprioception, and/or gait instability may indicate myelopathy. Neurologic abnormalities occur in approximately 10% of patients with RA who have cervical involvement. Because RA frequently affects the metacarpophalangeal joints, progressive neurologic deficits may be falsely attributed to direct hand involvement, which can result in a disastrous delay in the diagnosis of myelopathy.

Laboratory Findings

Rheumatoid factor antibodies are present in 80% of patients with RA, and antinuclear antibodies are present in 30%. Inflammatory markers include an elevated erythrocyte sedimentation rate, C-reactive protein level, and serum globulin level. The C-reactive protein level has been shown to predict the risk of joint deterioration and should be monitored. Because of the low specificity of rheumatoid factor antibodies, the anticyclic citrullinated peptide (anti-CCP) and antimutated citrullinated vimentin assay (anti-MCV) serologic tests have been developed. These widely used tests have high diagnostic sensitivity and specificity and have important predictive and prognostic value in RA. However, the diagnostic use of the anti-MCV test is somewhat different from that of the anti-CCP test. The anti-MCV test is especially useful in the diagnosis of RA in patients with rheumatoid factor who are anti-CCP2 seronegative. Interestingly, patients who are seronegative for rheumatoid factor but positive for anti-CCP antibodies have increased radiographic progression and poorer functional outcomes than other patients with RA. Recently, a serologic point-of-care test for early detection of RA has been developed.[13]

Radiographic Findings

A high prevalence of asymptomatic cervical instability exists in patients with RA. Assessment with plain radiography, even in asymptomatic patients with RA, should include standard AP, PA, lateral, lateral flexion-extension, and open-mouth views, although CT has somewhat eliminated the need for open-mouth radiographic views.[14] The lateral displacement of atlas over axis by more than 2 mm in the open-mouth view has been reported as lateral subluxation. Because instability may be missed on static lateral projections, flexion-extension views are important.

Several sagittal parameters and measurements are helpful in identifying and quantifying the presence and severity of disease. Anterior and posterior atlantodental intervals should be routinely measured. The anterior atlantodental interval is the distance from the posterior margin of the anterior arch of C1 to the anterior margin of the dens process of the axis vertebra. The normal atlantodental interval is 2.5 mm or less in adult women and 3.0 mm in adult men. Surgery has been recommended in patients with an anterior atlantodental interval greater than 6 to 10 mm. The posterior atlantodental interval, measured from the posterior margin of the dens to the anterior margin of the posterior arch of C1 (anterior-posterior diameter of the bony canal), is a more reliable indicator for neurologic compromise and correlates with the presence and severity of paralysis. Posterior atlantodental interval values less than 13 mm or 14 mm are considered an indication for surgery.

Open-mouth radiographic views should be evaluated for odontoid erosion and narrowed occipitoatlantal and atlantoaxial joints. Multidetector computed tomography, which uses two-dimensional acquisition of multiple images, can greatly enhance bone imaging details.

Bony erosion is the most important factor in the development of subluxation. Bony erosion may lead to an underestimation of the extent of vertical migration of the cervical cord with medullary kinking or ventral brain stem compression. Cranial migration is best diagnosed with a combination of the Clark station, the Ranawat criterion, and the Redlund-Johnell criterion (**Table 1**).

A diagnosis of subaxial subluxation is made when the listhesis exceeds 3.5 to 4 mm. Recently, reduction of the spinal canal diameter to less than 13 to 14 mm has been proposed as an alternative definition for subaxial subluxation.[10]

Table 1		
The Clark Station, Ranawat Criterion, and Redlund-Johnell Criterion in Diagnostic Cutoffs for Surgical Indications of Rheumatoid Arthritis		
	Description	**Diagnostic Cutoff**
Clark station	In the sagittal plane, divide the odontoid process into three equal parts (stations), and determine the level at which the anterior arch of C1 falls	Station I: anterior arch of C1 falls at the superior third (normal) Station II: anterior arch of C1 falls at middle third (mild) Station III: anterior arch of C1 falls at inferior third (severe)
Ranawat criterion	Distance between the center of the C2 pedicle and the transverse axis of C1 measured along the axis of the odontoid process	Measurements less than 15 mm in males or 13 mm in females are indicative of myelopathy
Redlund-Johnell criterion	Distance between the inferior margin of the C2 vertebral body and a line drawn from the posterior tip of the hard palate to the caudal cortical margin of the foramen magnum (McGregor Line)	Measurements less than 34 mm in males or 29 mm in females are indicative of cranial migration

In patients with neurologic symptoms, plain radiography may not demonstrate the effect of pannus formation on neural structures; CT and/or MRI may be necessary to detect these changes. MRI can be used to detect cervical involvement before the development of bony erosion by allowing evaluation of periodontoid synovial spaces. Enhancement of periodontoid synovial spaces may indicate inflammatory synovitis and marrow edema.

Natural History

Without treatment, RA of the spine can be associated with progressive disability resulting from atlantoaxial dislocation along with the risk of sudden death caused by cord or brain stem compression.[15] However, there is wide variation in the prevalence of atlantoaxial subluxation in patients with RA. For example, a general population survey reported a 5.3% incidence of RA in 1,478 cervical radiographs.[16] Of those showing RA, only 6.4% showed signs of subluxation. In 241 patients with RA, the mean time from diagnosis of RA to findings of subluxation was 3.9 years.[17] After subluxation develops, the patient's prognosis is severely altered. A 7-year survival probability of zero was reported in a study of 21 patients with myelopathy secondary to atlantoaxial subluxation who had refused surgical treatment.[18]

Advances in Nonsurgical Management

Nonsurgical management of RA is possible with physical therapy and medication. Close follow-up is needed to accurately monitor disease progression. Soft or rigid collars also may be used. Although soft collars cannot protect against spinal instability, they may provide comfort for the patient. Rigid collars are offered to patients with known spinal instability, but there is no evidence that they reduce neurologic progression or prevent further subluxation. Because temporomandibular joint involvement is common in patients with RA, rigid collars are often poorly tolerated.

DMARDs are increasingly being used to slow disease progression. For patients classified as having early adult RA, the American College of Rheumatology recommends double or triple DMARD therapy (methotrexate preferred; others drugs include hydroxychloroquine, leflunomide, and sulfasalazine) if disease activity is low and the patient has not previously had DMARD therapy.[9] If disease activity remains moderate or high despite the administration of DMARDs, a TNF inhibitor (adalimumab, certolizumab pegol, etanercept, golimumab, or infliximab) or a non-TNF biologic (abatacept, rituximab, or tocilizumab) should be added. In patients with established RA, similar initial attempts should be made with DMARD therapy first, then the addition of a TNF inhibitor, non-TNF biologic, or tofacitinib. If disease activity remains moderate or high despite intervention, adding one or two DMARDs may be beneficial.

Surgical Management

Surgical intervention is indicated for patients with persistent axial or radicular pain, progressive neurologic deficit or myelopathy, or instability. Surgical stabilization should be considered in the absence of symptoms if the following radiographic criteria are met: an atlantodental interval of 6 mm or more, a posterior atlantodental interval less than 13 mm, or proximal odontoid migration of the rostral to the McGregor line of at least 5 mm as identified by the Clark station, Redlund-Johnell criterion, and Ranawat criterion. Myelopathy should be corrected before reaching Ranawat grade III (objective weakness with long tract signs). The cervicomedullary angle, which is measured on sagittal MRI or CT myelography, is formed by the intersection of lines drawn along the clivus and the anterior aspect of the cervical cord (posterior aspect of the dens). This angle is useful in predicting neurologic compression. The cervicomedullary angle in normal individuals ranges from 135° to 175°, compared with less than 135° in patients with signs of cord compression or myelopathy.[19]

Specific Procedures

The natural course of RA of the cervical spine can include occipitoatlantal or atlantoaxial instability resulting from laxity or incompetence of the craniocervical ligaments, disruption of the transverse ligament of the axis, and/or the development of a periodontoid mass. These manifestations can result in irreducible atlantoaxial kyphosis. Moreover, cranial settling or superior migration of odontoid accompanied by subaxial subluxation also can occur.

Atlantoaxial instability is typically treated with posterior C1-C2 fusion. Historically, semirigid wiring techniques were commonly performed. More rigid techniques, such as Magerl C1-C2 transarticular screw fixation, later evolved. More recently, the Goel-Harms technique using posterior C1 lateral mass screws and C2 pedicle or pars screws has become popular because of technical difficulties (such as positioning) associated with the Magerl technique along with the high frequency of anatomic contraindications.[20] In the Goel-Harms technique, C2 translaminar crossing screws or unilateral fixation with pars or pedicle screws can secure the construct.[21]

In a progressive and irreducible atlantoaxial kyphosis, fixation can be achieved using anterior plating in combination with posterior wire fusion;[20,22] however, posterior C1-C2 instrumented fusion is the preferred treatment. In lieu of an impending dorsal compression, a C1 laminectomy also may be necessary and is aided by occipitocervical fusion. Occipital plating and cervical screws may alleviate progressive dorsal compression caused by ventral kinking of the upper cervical cord and an increased cervicomedullary angle. Normal alignment and a normal cervicomedullary angle in flexion and extension obviates the need for occipitocervical fusion; however, patients with occipitoatlantal instability and an increased cervicomedullary angle, even without C1-C2 involvement, are treated with occipitocervical fusion.

In patients with severe cranial settling or superior migration of the odontoid, symptoms are caused by ventral compression and/or kinking at the cervicomedullary junction. In addition to ventral symptomatology, determining the cervicomedullary angle also aids in radiographic assessment. However, early superior migration of the odontoid can be treated with C1-C2 fusion. Progressive superior migration of the odontoid without significant ventral compression and a normal cervicomedullary angle is treated with suboccipital craniotomy and C1 laminectomy. Neuronavigation-assisted transnasal resection of the odontoid process is an option if symptoms of ventral compression caused by periodontoid pannus persist and the cervicomedullary angle fails to improve (even after occipitocervical fusion).

It is common for subaxial subluxation to develop after C1-C2 fusions in patients with RA. One study reported that subaxial subluxation developed in 39% of patients after C1-C2 fusion.[21] Subaxial subluxation with signs of compression and/or myelopathy can be treated with laminectomy and instrumented fusion. Traditionally, the level to be addressed depends entirely on the degree of compression in the corresponding segments of the cervical spine. Placement of polyaxial lateral mass screws with a rod construct is routinely performed.[23]

Outcomes

RA and the various medications used to treat it affect bone mineral density.[24] Bone loss also occurs as a result of systemic inflammation and impaired mobility, and a substantial portion of patients with RA are older women with osteopenia or osteoporosis. Bone loss may adversely affect fusion rates and increase the risk of implant failure. Patients with RA have been shown to have a higher incidence of infection after surgery because of the immunosuppressive effect of DMARDs.[25] In addition, patients with more severe RA may have lower limb disease, and the associated impaired mobility may inhibit postoperative rehabilitation. Patients with RA also may have cardiovascular and pulmonary comorbidities that increased the risk of atrial fibrillation, stroke, and/or hypertension. Negative cardiovascular effects can be mitigated by TNF inhibitors, DMARDs, and steroids.[26]

An increased posterior atlantodental interval was the strongest predictor for postoperative neurologic improvement after surgical intervention for RA.[27] One study reported that patients with a lower preoperative Ranawat classification had a much lower 10-year mortality.[28] After surgical intervention, 96% of class I patients showed no deterioration in neurologic status, and patients in class II and III improved to class I and II, respectively.

7: Neoplastic and Inflammatory Conditions

Ankylosing Spondylitis

Epidemiology

Ankylosing spondylitis affects 1% to 2% of the Caucasian population and is the most common seronegative (no rheumatoid factor) spondyloarthropathy.[29] Other seronegative spondyloarthropathies include reactive arthritis, psoriatic arthritis, and enteropathic arthritis. Four times as many men as women are affected by ankylosing spondylitis, which is most commonly diagnosed between the second and third decade of life. Although the histocompatibility complex antigen HLA-B27 is found in 90% of patients with ankylosing spondylitis, only 10% of individuals who are positive for the HLA-B27 antigen have this condition. If a diagnosis is made before the patient is 16 years of age, the condition is classified as juvenile ankylosing spondylitis.

In at least one-third of patients with ankylosing spondylitis, the disease will progress to cause severe disability.[30] Because ankylosing spondylitis often starts at an early age, the lifetime economic burden of this disease can be high. Improved disease-modifying treatments, diagnostic tools, and validated outcome measures recently have become available.

Pathophysiology

Ankylosing spondylitis can be distinguished from other spondyloarthropathies by the universal involvement of the sacroiliac joint. Sacroiliac joint changes form the basis for the modified New York criteria for the classification of ankylosing spondylitis.[29,30]

Unlike RA, which causes synovitis, ankylosing spondylitis causes enthesitis, which typically involves the fibrocartilaginous entheses and enthesis-like structures.[31,32] HLA-B27 is the most robust genetic marker associated with ankylosing spondylitis; however, its involvement in pathogenesis has not been well defined. It is postulated that certain alleles or subtypes of HLA-B27 bind peptides of self-origin and present them to CD8+ T cells. The principle of molecular mimicry is proposed as a mechanism by which antibodies directed against foreign antigens in a bacterial infection are cross-reactive with HLA-B27. Other than homology between certain HLA-B27 alleles with bacterial antigens, several other mechanisms of action involving HLA-B27, CD4+ T cells, and CD8+ T cells have been proposed to explain ileal inflammation and enthesitis.

Clinical Presentation

Signs and Symptoms

Patients typically have inflammatory low back pain.[33-37] Symptoms may be mild initially, and patients may not be able to accurately identify when their pain started. Inflammatory back pain can be differentiated by the following properties: pain that is worse in the morning or after long periods of inactivity and is improved by exercise and movement. In addition, patients may report pain that is not relieved with rest or lying down, and difficulty sleeping may occur. Pain in the gluteal region may indicate sacroiliac involvement. The compression of the L5 nerve secondary to sacroiliitis can result in radiation of pain to the legs.

Approximately 70% of patients with ankylosing spondylitis report neck pain. In one study of 571 patients with ankylosing spondylitis, radiographic evidence of cervical spine involvement was identified in more than 50% of the patients. Cervical involvement was found to be a function of disease progression, with 20% of the patients having radiographic involvement after 5 years and 70% after 20 years.[38]

Physical Examination

A diagnosis of ankylosing spondylitis should be based on the physical evaluation and radiographic evidence of disease[39] (**Figure 2**) and (**Table 2**). The New York criteria are universally used when making a diagnosis. Ankylosis of the spine in kyphosis and flexion deformity of the hips may contribute to sagittal deformity. The Schober test evaluates anterior spinal flexion, which is often severely impaired in patients with ankylosing spondylitis. Chest expansion also is limited and is typically measured at the fourth intercostal space.

Radiographic Findings

Radiographic features of ankylosing spondylitis may take years to develop, which can limit the ability of clinicians to make an early definitive diagnosis. Osteitis with erosion of the anterior and superior surfaces causes "squaring" of the vertebral bodies. Ossification of the spinal ligaments between the intervertebral disks results in syndesmophytes, giving the appearance of "bamboo spine" in more advanced cases. CT and MRI demonstrate higher sensitivity in early stages of the disease. MRI of peripheral joints also may aid in the diagnosis of early RA, and more than 20% of patients with ankylosing spondylitis present with peripheral arthritis.[40] The hips, shoulders, and larger joints of the legs are most frequently affected. MRI will show joint space narrowing, bony erosion, and synovitis.

Laboratory Findings

Laboratory findings cannot be used to make a definitively diagnosis of ankylosing spondylitis; however, systemic inflammation accompanies the disease. Levels of C-reactive protein, rheumatoid factor, and antinuclear

Table 2

Indications of Ankylosing Spondylitis

Criterion	Indication
Radiographic	Bilateral sacroiliitis grade ≥II or unilateral sacroiliitis grade III to IV
Clinical	Low back pain and stiffness of at least 3 months' duration improved by exercise and not relieved by rest
	Limitation of motion of the lumbar spine in both the sagittal and the frontal planes
	Limitation of chest expansion relative to values normal for age and sex

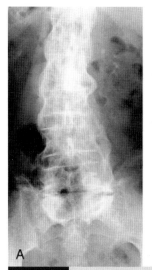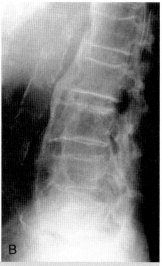

Figure 2 AP (**A**) and lateral (**B**) radiographs of the lumbar spine in a patient with ankylosing spondylitis. This patient presented to the emergency department with increasing back pain after a motor vehicle collision. Careful review of the radiographs shows a cleft in the fusion mass at L5-S1. A bone scan confirmed increased activity at this level, which is indicative of a new fracture. (Reproduced from Fischgrund JS: Surgical care of the arthritides of the spine, in Fardon DF, Garfin SR, Abitbol JJ, Boden SD, Herkowitz HN, Mayer TG, eds: *Orthopaedic Knowledge Update Spine 2*. Rosemont, IL, American Academy of Orthopaedic Surgeons, 2002, pp 393-400.)

antibodies have no correlation with disease activity. HLA-B27 testing is particularly useful in African and Japanese patients because the prevalence of the antigen is low in those populations when ankylosing spondylitis is not present.

Nonsurgical Management

In 2015, the American College of Rheumatology published guidelines and recommendations for the management of ankylosing spondylitis.[9] NSAIDs are recommended for patients with active disease; if NSAID use is unsuccessful, a TNF inhibitor should be given. If inflammatory bowel disease also is present, TNF inhibitor monoclonal antibodies should be given rather than etanercept. Glucocorticoids should not be used. Physical therapy also is recommended.

Traumatic Management

Longer lever arms in the ankylosed spine increase the risk of spine fracture.[41] The risk of neurologic injury after these fractures is compounded by ossification of elastic soft tissues and supportive elements. Epidural hematoma also can cause neurologic injury. Most fractures in patients with ankylosing spondylitis result from low-energy trauma. Fractures most frequently occur through the disk space and are particularly common in the cervical spine.

In traumatic fracture, low-weight traction devices may facilitate fracture reduction and prevent further neurologic injury. Usually, the nonsurgical treatment of fracture associated with ankylosing spondylitis begins with cervical traction and is followed by immobilization in a hard collar. Definitive management with a brace may be used if the fracture is stable (absence of fracture-dislocation through the disk space and/or absence of radiographic evidence of cord compression) and is not accompanied by a neurologic deficit.

Surgical fixation with or without decompression may be used, depending on neurologic status or the presence of a hematoma. In most patients, a posterior approach using multilevel transpedicular instrumentation is recommended. High rates of complications have been reported, including implant failure, deformity progression, and further neurologic decline.

Management of Spine Deformity

Deformity in patients with ankylosing spondylitis results from progressive erosion, ossification, and fusion of the vertebral joints and intervertebral disk spaces.[42] This deformity results in progressive flexion of the cervical, thoracic, and lumbar spine. Thoracic kyphosis develops as a patient tries to unload the loaded spondylitic facet joints, and autofusion results in abnormal sagittal alignment. Anterior displacement of the patient's center of gravity increases kyphotic moment and deformity progresses. This deformity of the spine can cause severe disability. For example, a fixed cervical spine may result in difficulty maintaining a horizontal gaze, swallowing, and carrying out tasks related to personal hygiene.

Table 3

Factors Differentiating Ankylosing Spondylitis and Diffuse Idiopathic Skeletal Hyperostosis (DISH)

Factor	Ankylosing Spondylitis	DISH
Age at onset	<40 years	>50 years
Pain	Common	Unusual
Sacroiliac joint erosion	Common	Absent
Synovial sacroiliac joint obliteration	Common	Unusual
Apophyseal joint obliteration	Common	Absent
Anterior longitudinal ligament ossification	Unusual	Common

The goal of surgical correction is to halt the progression of sagittal deformity and restore horizontal gaze. Primary lumbar and thoracic deformities may be treated with multilevel osteotomies and fixation of the spine. Various osteotomy techniques increase correction as the osteotomy site progresses caudally. A three-column osteotomy or vertebral column resection may be used at a caudal lumbar level to attain maximum sagittal correction. More importantly, cervicothoracic deformities are typically addressed at the C7-T1 junction because of nerve root mobility, a large canal diameter, and extraosseous vertebral arteries.

Diffuse Idiopathic Skeletal Hyperostosis

DISH, also known as Forestier disease, is a noninflammatory disease characterized by ossification of the longitudinal ligaments (especially the anterior longitudinal ligament) and entheses. DISH is diagnosed when flowing mantles of ossification of the anterior longitudinal ligament are identified on spine radiographs across at least four consecutive levels.[43] Ossification of the anterior longitudinal ligaments of the spine produces a tortuous paravertebral mass anterior to and distinct (at least radiographically) from the vertebral bodies grossly, giving the appearance of candle wax dripping down the spine. Various clinical and radiographic criteria distinguish DISH from ankylosing spondylitis (**Table 3**).

The prevalence of DISH ranges from 2.9% in the Korean population to 25% in a specific population of American Caucasian males.[44,45] Because the prevalence of DISH increases with age, the number of individuals with this disease is expected to increase in coming decades because of the growing aging population. DISH predisposes patients to low-energy fractures of the spine resulting from pathomechanics analogous to those seen in ankylosing spondylitis[46] (**Table 3**).

Psoriatic Arthritis

Twenty-three percent of patients with psoriatic arthritis have spinal involvement.[47] Up to 50% of patients have inflammation in the axial skeleton that causes inflammatory back pain and radiographic changes, including unilateral or bilateral sacroiliitis. These changes are less well understood in psoriatic arthritis than in ankylosing spondylitis. Because psoriatic arthritis usually affects only one side of the body, this may aid in the initial diagnosis. Radiographic changes include erosion, sclerosis, and ankylosis at the sacroiliac joint. The prevalence of surface antigen HLA-B27 is much lower in psoriatic arthritis (only 40% to 50%) than in ankylosing spondylitis.[48]

The goal of treatment is to control inflammation. Medications include immunosuppressive drugs, anti-inflammatory drugs, and TNF-α inhibitors.

Reactive Arthritis

Reactive arthritis is an aseptic inflammatory reaction to certain bacterial infections. Inflammation in the peripheral joints and lumbar spine may occur. Cervical spine involvement is rare. The HLA-B27 antigen is present in 60% to 80% of patients with reactive arthritis.

Treatment includes sulfasalazine to decrease joint pain and swelling. Oral corticosteroids and immunosuppressive drugs such as those used in RA can be beneficial.

Enteropathic Arthritis

Enteropathic arthritis is associated with inflammatory bowel disease such as Crohn disease or ulcerative colitis and typically follows the activity of the bowel disease. Axial enteropathic arthritis, however, is usually independent of bowel inflammatory disease. Approximately 70% of affected patients are HLA-B27 positive. Management is similar to that of ankylosing spondylitis, and use of TNF-α inhibitors may alleviate symptoms.

Gout

Gout is characterized by urate deposits in soft tissue.[49] Although more typical in the peripheral joints, gout may infrequently affect the spine and sacroiliac joints. Patients without concurrent neurologic deficits can be treated with NSAIDs and steroids to control pain. A urate-reducing agent, such as probenecid, allopurinol, or rasburicase, should be administered.

Polymyalgia Rheumatica

Polymyalgia rheumatica typically manifests in patients older than 50 years as an inflammatory disease primarily affecting the shoulder and/or pelvis.[50] The disease is more common among northern Europeans, which may indicate a genetic predisposition. Seasonal variations in the incidence of polymyalgia rheumatica suggest an infectious agent. Polymyalgia rheumatica is associated with the HLA-DR4 haplotype. A high level of interleukin-6 is associated with increased disease activity. Many investigators believe that nonerosive synovitis and tenosynovitis are responsible for many symptoms of this disease. A diagnosis typically is made after at least 1 month of morning stiffness in the shoulder or pelvic girdle. Several diagnostic criteria exist for polymyalgia rheumatica. One set of diagnostic criteria is age at onset of 50 years or older; an erythrocyte sedimentation rate of 40 mm/h or greater; pain persisting for 1 month or more and involving two of the following areas: neck, shoulders, and pelvic girdle; absence of other diseases capable of causing the same musculoskeletal symptoms; morning stiffness lasting 1 hour or more; and rapid response to prednisone (≤20 mg).[51] One-third of patients report concurrent low-grade fever, loss of appetite, and weight loss.

Treatment regimens may include NSAIDs for mild cases. Glucocorticoid therapy may be administered in those with moderate to severe disease. Typically, the prognosis is excellent; however, exacerbations may occur if steroid use is tapered too rapidly. Relapse is common.

Summary

Inflammatory arthritides of the spine include RA and the seronegative spondyloarthropathies, such as ankylosing spondylitis. Inflammation in the synovial tissue, joints, and ligaments results in patterns of joint destruction unique to each disorder.

RA is the most common inflammatory arthritis and characteristically causes upper cervical instability. Ankylosing spondylitis is characterized by enthesitis, ossification, and sacroiliitis that results in a bamboo-type spine deformity. Pharmacologic treatment, including DMARDs, corticosteroids, and immune-system modulators (such as TNF-α and interleukin-1 inhibitors), has improved markedly over the past two decades.

Despite improvements in nonsurgical management, surgical intervention is still occasionally required in the presence of spinal cord compression, spine instability, or progressive deformity.

Key Study Points

- Inflammatory arthritides, including RA, are typically managed initially with DMARDs followed by TNF inhibitors or other biologics in patients with persistent symptoms.
- First-line intervention for seronegative spondyloarthropathies such as ankylosing spondylitis should be NSAIDs followed by TNF inhibitors for chronic symptoms.
- Surgical intervention for inflammatory arthritides is occasionally required in the presence of spinal cord compression, spine instability, or progressive deformity.

Annotated References

1. Stein BE, Hassanzadeh H, Jain A, Lemma MA, Cohen DB, Kebaish KM: Changing trends in cervical spine fusions in patients with rheumatoid arthritis. *Spine (Phila Pa 1976)* 2014;39(15):1178-1182.

   Treatment for RA has changed substantially with the introduction of DMARDs. Although the total number of cervical fusions for RA increased from 1992 through 2008, any individual patient with RA is significantly less likely to undergo cervical surgical procedures compared with those in the general population. Level of evidence: II.

2. Bodur H, Ataman S, Akbulut L, et al: Characteristics and medical management of patients with rheumatoid arthritis and ankylosing spondylitis. *Clin Rheumatol* 2008;27(9):1119-1125.

3. Coates LC, FitzGerald O, Helliwell PS, Paul C: Psoriasis, psoriatic arthritis, and rheumatoid arthritis: Is all inflammation the same? *Semin Arthritis Rheum* 2016;46(3):291-304.

   Psoriasis, psoriatic arthritis, and RA all cause dysfunction in different constituents of the immune system, which result in varying clinical features. Comorbidities, including cardiovascular disease, malignancies, and nonalcoholic fatty liver disease, are increased.

4. Calabrò A, Caterino AL, Elefante E, et al: One year in review 2016: Novelties in the treatment of rheumatoid arthritis. *Clin Exp Rheumatol* 2016;34(3):357-372.

A review of the most relevant studies published on treatment for RA in 2016 is presented.

5. Gillick JL, Wainwright J, Das K: Rheumatoid arthritis and the cervical spine: A review on the role of surgery. *Int J Rheumatol* 2015;2015:252456.

Atlantoaxial instability, cranial settling, and subaxial subluxation may require surgical intervention. The use of DMARDs has resulted in fewer patients presenting with the manifestations of RA in the cervical spine. If DMARD use is unsuccessful, improved surgical techniques are available.

6. Joaquim AF, Appenzeller S: Cervical spine involvement in rheumatoid arthritis: A systematic review. *Autoimmun Rev* 2014;13(12):1195-1202.

This current literature review reports that uncontrolled RA is the main risk factor in the development of spinal instability. However, treatment with DMARDs may prevent the development of spinal instability.

7. Joaquim AF, Appenzeller S: Neuropsychiatric manifestations in rheumatoid arthritis. *Autoimmun Rev* 2015;14(12):1116-1122.

Common neuropsychiatric manifestations of RA include depression, cognitive dysfunction, behavior changes, spinal cord compression, and peripheral nerve involvement. Clinicians must be aware of neuropsychiatric manifestations so that an appropriate diagnosis can be made.

8. Narváez J, Narváez JA, Serrallonga M, et al: Subaxial cervical spine involvement in symptomatic rheumatoid arthritis patients: Comparison with cervical spondylosis. *Semin Arthritis Rheum* 2015;45(1):9-17.

Subaxial stenosis is a consequence of both inflammatory processes and mechanical and degenerative changes. Although subaxial stenosis is not usually related to the symptoms of myelopathy, both disorders occur together at a high frequency.

9. Singh JA, Saag KG, Bridges SL Jr, et al: 2015 American College of Rheumatology guideline for the treatment of rheumatoid arthritis. *Arthritis Rheumatol* 2016;68(1):1-26.

This guideline provides tools for clinicians and patients regarding pharmacologic treatments for RA.

10. Wasserman BR, Moskovich R, Razi AE: Rheumatoid arthritis of the cervical spine: Clinical considerations. *Bull NYU Hosp Jt Dis* 2011;69(2):136-148.

A careful patient history is crucial in identifying the symptoms of RA. Radiographs and an extensive physical examination are necessary.

11. Kroft LJ, Reijnierse M, Kloppenburg M, Verbist BM, Bloem JL, van Buchem MA: Rheumatoid arthritis: Epidural enhancement as an underestimated cause of subaxial cervical spinal stenosis. *Radiology* 2004;231(1):57-63.

12. Neva MH, Häkkinen A, Mäkinen H, Hannonen P, Kauppi M, Sokka T: High prevalence of asymptomatic cervical spine subluxation in patients with rheumatoid arthritis waiting for orthopaedic surgery. *Ann Rheum Dis* 2006;65(7):884-888.

13. Rojanasantikul P, Pattrapornpisut P, Anuruckparadorn K, Katchamart W: The performance of a point of care test for detection of anti-mutated citrullinated vimentin and rheumatoid factor in early rheumatoid arthritis. *Clin Rheumatol* 2014;33(7):919-923.

The authors report that a point-of-care test for the detection of anti-MCV in early RA yielded high specificity.

14. Burry HC, Tweed JM, Robinson RG, Howes R: Lateral subluxation of the atlanto-axial joint in rheumatoid arthritis. *Ann Rheum Dis* 1978;37(6):525-528.

15. Mikulowski P, Wollheim FA, Rotmil P, Olsen I: Sudden death in rheumatoid arthritis with atlanto-axial dislocation. *Acta Med Scand* 1975;198(6):445-451.

16. Sharp J, Purser DW: Spontaneous atlanto-axial dislocation in ankylosing spondylitis and rheumatoid arthritis. *Ann Rheum Dis* 1961;20(1):47-77.

17. Riise T, Jacobsen BK, Gran JT: High mortality in patients with rheumatoid arthritis and atlantoaxial subluxation. *J Rheumatol* 2001;28(11):2425-2429.

18. Sunahara N, Matsunaga S, Mori T, Ijiri K, Sakou T: Clinical course of conservatively managed rheumatoid arthritis patients with myelopathy. *Spine (Phila Pa 1976)* 1997;22(22):2603-2607, discussion 2608.

19. Bundschuh C, Modic MT, Kearney F, Morris R, Deal C: Rheumatoid arthritis of the cervical spine: Surface-coil MR imaging. *AJR Am J Roentgenol* 1988;151(1):181-187.

20. Harms J, Melcher RP: Posterior C1-C2 fusion with polyaxial screw and rod fixation. *Spine (Phila Pa 1976)* 2001;26(22):2467-2471.

21. Clarke MJ, Cohen-Gadol AA, Ebersold MJ, Cabanela ME: Long-term incidence of subaxial cervical spine instability following cervical arthrodesis surgery in patients with rheumatoid arthritis. *Surg Neurol* 2006;66(2):136-140, discussion 140.

22. Brooks AL, Jenkins EB: Atlanto-axial arthrodesis by the wedge compression method. *J Bone Joint Surg Am* 1978;60(3):279-284.

23. Xu R, Haman SP, Ebraheim NA, Yeasting RA: The anatomic relation of lateral mass screws to the spinal nerves: A

comparison of the Magerl, Anderson, and An techniques. *Spine (Phila Pa 1976)* 1999;24(19):2057-2061.

24. van der Goes MC, Jacobs JW, Bijlsma JW: The value of glucocorticoid co-therapy in different rheumatic diseases: Positive and adverse effects. *Arthritis Res Ther* 2014;16(suppl 2):S2.

    Glucocorticoid steroids play a pivotal role in the management of inflammatory rheumatic diseases. Multiple indications exist that adverse effects correlate with longer use of glucocorticoids and higher dosages.

25. Dixon WG, Suissa S, Hudson M: The association between systemic glucocorticoid therapy and the risk of infection in patients with rheumatoid arthritis: Systematic review and meta-analyses. *Arthritis Res Ther* 2011;13(4):R139.

    Observational studies suggest an increased risk of infection with glucocorticoid therapy, whereas randomized controlled trials suggest no increased risk. Clinicians should remain vigilant for infection in patients with RA who are being treated with glucocorticoid therapy.

26. Roubille C, Richer V, Starnino T, et al: The effects of tumour necrosis factor inhibitors, methotrexate, non-steroidal anti-inflammatory drugs and corticosteroids on cardiovascular events in rheumatoid arthritis, psoriasis and psoriatic arthritis: A systematic review and meta-analysis. *Ann Rheum Dis* 2015;74(3):480-489.

    A meta-analysis, which included 34 studies, concluded that there is a reduced risk of cardiovascular events in patients with RA or psoriasis who are treated with a TNF inhibitor. The use of corticosteroids increases the risk of cardiovascular events.

27. Boden SD, Dodge LD, Bohlman HH, Rechtine GR: Rheumatoid arthritis of the cervical spine: A long-term analysis with predictors of paralysis and recovery. *J Bone Joint Surg Am* 1993;75(9):1282-1297.

28. Wolf BS, Khilnani M, Malis L: The sagittal diameter of the bony cervical spinal canal and its significance in cervical spondylosis. *J Mt Sinai Hosp N Y* 1956;23(3):283-292.

29. Mansour M, Cheema GS, Naguwa SM, et al: Ankylosing spondylitis: A contemporary perspective on diagnosis and treatment. *Semin Arthritis Rheum* 2007;36(4):210-223.

30. Ozgocmen S, Akgul O, Altay Z, et al; Anatolian Group for the Assessment in Rheumatic Diseases: Expert opinion and key recommendations for the physical therapy and rehabilitation of patients with ankylosing spondylitis. *Int J Rheum Dis* 2012;15(3):229-238.

    Physiotherapy, including physical therapy and rehabilitation, is an integral part of the management of ankylosing spondylitis.

31. Kim TH, Uhm WS, Inman RD: Pathogenesis of ankylosing spondylitis and reactive arthritis. *Curr Opin Rheumatol* 2005;17(4):400-405.

32. Braun J, Baraliakos X: Treatment of ankylosing spondylitis and other spondyloarthritides. *Curr Opin Rheumatol* 2009;21(4):324-334.

33. Arun R, Dabke HV, Mehdian H: Comparison of three types of lumbar osteotomy for ankylosing spondylitis: A case series and evolution of a safe technique for instrumented reduction. *Eur Spine J* 2011;20(12):2252-2260.

    Better radiographic correction is obtained using a pedicle subtraction closing wedge osteotomy and a polysegmental posterior lumbar wedge osteotomy compared with a Smith-Peterson open wedge osteotomy.

34. Bhan S, Eachempati KK, Malhotra R: Primary cementless total hip arthroplasty for bony ankylosis in patients with ankylosing spondylitis. *J Arthroplasty* 2008;23(6):859-866.

35. Koivikko MP, Koskinen SK: MRI of cervical spine injuries complicating ankylosing spondylitis. *Skeletal Radiol* 2008;37(9):813-819.

36. Olerud C, Frost A, Bring J: Spinal fractures in patients with ankylosing spondylitis. *Eur Spine J* 1996;5(1):51-55.

37. Whang PG, Goldberg G, Lawrence JP, et al: The management of spinal injuries in patients with ankylosing spondylitis or diffuse idiopathic skeletal hyperostosis: A comparison of treatment methods and clinical outcomes. *J Spinal Disord Tech* 2009;22(2):77-85.

38. El Maghraoui A, Bensabbah R, Bahiri R, Bezza A, Guedira N, Hajjaj-Hassouni N: Cervical spine involvement in ankylosing spondylitis. *Clin Rheumatol* 2003;22(2):94-98.

39. Ward MM, Deodhar A, Akl EA, et al: American College of Rheumatology/Spondylitis Association of America/Spondyloarthritis Research and Treatment Network 2015 recommendations for the treatment of ankylosing spondylitis and nonradiographic axial spondyloarthritis. *Arthritis Rheumatol* 2016;68(2):282-298.

    Recommendations are made for managing ankylosing spondyloarthritis. The use of NSAIDs and TNF inhibitors is strongly endorsed, and recommendations are made against the use of glucocorticoids, physical therapy, and hip arthroplasty.

40. Jung Y-O, Kim I, Kim S, et al: Clinical and radiographic features of adult-onset ankylosing spondylitis in Korean patients: Comparisons between males and females. *J Korean Med Sci* 2010;25(4):532-535.

41. Westerveld LA, Verlaan JJ, Oner FC: Spinal fractures in patients with ankylosing spinal disorders: A systematic review of the literature on treatment, neurological status and complications. *Eur Spine J* 2009;18(2):145-156.

42. Hoh DJ, Khoueir P, Wang MY: Management of cervical deformity in ankylosing spondylitis. *Neurosurg Focus* 2008;24(1):E9.

7: Neoplastic and Inflammatory Conditions

43. Resnick D, Shaul SR, Robins JM: Diffuse idiopathic skeletal hyperostosis (DISH): Forestier's disease with extraspinal manifestations. *Radiology* 1975;115(3):513-524.

44. Verlaan JJ, Oner FC, Maat GJ: Diffuse idiopathic skeletal hyperostosis in ancient clergymen. *Eur Spine J* 2007;16(8):1129-1135.

45. Weinfeld RM, Olson PN, Maki DD, Griffiths HJ: The prevalence of diffuse idiopathic skeletal hyperostosis (DISH) in two large American Midwest metropolitan hospital populations. *Skeletal Radiol* 1997;26(4):222-225.

46. Paley D, Schwartz M, Cooper P, Harris WR, Levine AM: Fractures of the spine in diffuse idiopathic skeletal hyperostosis. *Clin Orthop Relat Res* 1991;267:22-32.

47. Baraliakos X, Coates LC, Braun J: The involvement of the spine in psoriatic arthritis. *Clin Exp Rheumatol* 2015;33(5suppl 93):S31-S35.

This review gives an overview of the existing evidence pertaining to the clinical and imaging presentation and therapeutic consequences of psoriatic arthritis.

48. Gladman DD, Antoni C, Mease P, Clegg DO, Nash P: Psoriatic arthritis: Epidemiology, clinical features, course, and outcome. *Ann Rheum Dis* 2005;64(suppl 2):ii14-ii17.

49. Jajić I: Gout in the spine and sacro-iliac joints: Radiological manifestations. *Skeletal Radiol* 1982;8(3):209-212.

50. Soubrier M, Dubost JJ, Ristori JM: Polymyalgia rheumatica: Diagnosis and treatment. *Joint Bone Spine* 2006;73(6):599-605.

51. Healey LA: Long-term follow-up of polymyalgia rheumatica: Evidence for synovitis. *Semin Arthritis Rheum* 1984;13(4):322-328.

Special Populations in Spine Care

SECTION EDITOR:

Andrew J. Schoenfeld, MD

Chapter 37

Clinical Outcome Measures for Spine

Donna D. Ohnmeiss, DrMed

Abstract

Focus is increasing on the need for evidence supporting the most effective and cost-effective treatment pathways in spine care. Outcome assessments are at the core of this evidence. In the spine, many outcome assessments have been introduced, and using all of them is not feasible. Intuitively, condition-specific instruments appear preferable and perhaps more sensitive to changes in condition over time. However, general health assessments are important when comparing the cost-effectiveness of various spine care interventions with other health conditions. The surgeon should understand the preferred characteristics of assessments, the more commonly used disease-specific and general health tools, and the potential use of registries and electronically administered questionnaires.

Keywords: back pain; outcome assessment; patient-completed questionnaire; neck pain

Introduction

The increased focus on spine care outcomes has been accompanied by an expansion of the types of data needed, including cost-effectiveness, quality-adjusted life-year (QALY), and similar calculations. Numerous outcome assessments are available for the evaluation of spine patients, and all have disadvantages, particularly considering the wide spectrum of patients seeking care for spinal problems. Most recently, demand has increased for patient-centered assessments such as the assessment of satisfaction with care. The ongoing advancements in

Dr. Ohnmeiss serves as a board member, officer, or committee member of the International Society for Advancement of Spine Surgery and the North American Spine Society.

technology and patients' increasing comfort with using these technologies have resulted in a broad move from paper to electronic data collection.

Properties of Outcome Assessments

From a practical standpoint, an outcome assessment should be relatively short, have wording that is easily understood, be inexpensive to administer, and appear meaningful to patients. This enables patients to complete the assessment as accurately as possible and for clinicians and researchers to use it on a wide scale. From a psychometric perspective, validity and reproducibility are important for the scientific interpretation of the data collected from such evaluations.

An international group of spine care providers and researchers working with the International Consortium of Health Outcome Measures recommended a core set of outcome assessments to be used for patients with low back pain.[1] The core set included numerical rating scale (NRS) scores for assessing back and leg pain (specifying average pain over the past week), Oswestry Disability Index (ODI), EuroQol Five Dimensions questionnaire (EQ-5D; EuroQol Group) level 3 (3L) as a general health assessment, work status, analgesic use, and treatment-related complications. It was recommended that the assessments be conducted before treatment and at 6, 12, and 24 months after initiating treatment, with optional follow-up at 3 months and 5 years. The core set also included general demographic and other factors that could be used to help stratify patients by general health conditions and history of back pain. Journal publishers and reviewers should require a description of the questionnaires used or include a sample as an appendix, which would help readers and those performing meta-analyses or systematic reviews to interpret the results in the context of other studies.

One study investigated the consistency of change from preoperative to 1-year postoperatively among commonly used outcome assessments (ODI, Medical Outcomes Study 36-Item Short Form [SF-36], NRS pain scales, and satisfaction) in a lumbar spine surgery population:[2] 40.5% of patients reported consistent outcome changes on all four measures. The results could have several implications. Intuitively, a high level of consistency between outcome assessments is preferred to ensure that changes in symptoms are evaluated adequately. Lack of consistency suggests the assessments may be measuring different aspects of the patient's condition and raises greater concerns over the reliability of the assessments. From a practical clinical perspective, the lack of consistency between assessments in the same group of patients makes it more challenging to interpret the effectiveness of the treatment provided.

Outcome assessments were originally used to describe the results of various treatments. Currently, outcomes assessments play a critical role in cost-effectiveness assessments, including QALYs and incremental cost-effectiveness ratios. One challenge is the inconsistency of results seen from various questionnaires in the same patient population.[2] This inconsistency can substantially affect the results of cost-effectiveness studies. One study compared lumbar total disk arthroplasty (TDA) with multidisciplinary rehabilitation and reported that TDA was cost-effective based on EQ-5D scores, but was not cost-effective if the Medical Outcomes Study 6-Item Short Form (SF-6) was used in the calculations.[3] Such findings highlight the need for caution in interpreting results and the challenge in deriving meaningful conclusions.

Psychometric Validity

One challenge in questionnaire design and validity evaluation is that no definitive gold standard exists against which to assess the questionnaire. Most assessments measure pain and self-reported function; both items can be affected by multiple factors, including a wide variety of psychosocial factors and secondary gains. One of the basic properties is reproducibility. Otherwise, changes in responses over time may not reflect a true change in the condition being studied. The concept of questionnaire validity includes ensuring that measures reflect the patient's condition and are sensitive to changes in the condition, including both improvement and worsening of the patient's symptoms. In the absence of a gold standard, the validity of most questionnaires is evaluated by determining if they correlate well with existing questionnaires and/or appear to provide greater sensitivity to changes in patient condition.

Minimal Clinically Important Difference

The concept of the minimal clinically important difference (MCID) has been present in spine literature for more than a decade.[4] However, although widely used, the application and interpretation of MCID values have been questioned.[5] Using MCID or similar criteria allows investigators to classify whether a patient has or does not have a successful outcome. Several methods have been used such as requiring a minimum change in scores or reaching a certain value for treatment to be considered a success. However, these values may need to be refined for different populations. For example, it may not be realistic for a 70-year-old patient with hip and/or knee problems undergoing treatment for stenosis to be expected to have the same improvement as a 30-year-old patient undergoing treatment for a herniated disk with no other health problems. MCID cited criticisms include the variation of values with the methods of calculation, the absence of a cost component, and the reliance on a baseline value.[5] Although cost is important, collecting meaningful cost data is difficult. Mandating cost as a component of MCID would greatly limit the usefulness of these values and likely exceeds the original intent of the MCID, which was to determine a clinically relevant change, not its cost-effectiveness.[6]

Spine-Specific Assessments

Many outcome assessments specific to the spine are used, and most have been designed to determine changes in patient symptoms after treatment. These assessments generally are designed for back or neck pain. Some assessments have been designed for specific diagnoses: the Scoliosis Research Society assessment is designed to assess patients with spinal deformity and has questions specifically applicable to that population that are not likely to be relevant, such as questions about appearance, to most degenerative spine conditions. A brief overview of commonly used outcome assessments in spine is provided in **Table 1**.

The potential for a floor or a ceiling effect is another consideration in questionnaire use. A floor effect includes sensitivity to changes in scores or may not adequately reflect low levels of conditions. For example, on the ODI, if the group mean score is 20 on a 0 to 100 scale prior to treatment, it may be difficult to demonstrate a significant improvement after treatment or interpret functional compromise in the group. Some studies use a minimal score on assessments to avoid a potential floor effect. Similarly, if many patients score at the upper end of the range of possible scores on an evaluation, there may be a

Table 1

Summary of Content and Scoring for Commonly Used Outcome Assessment Instruments

Instrument	Content and Scoring	Number of Items and Response Options	Estimated Completion Time (min)
ODI	Pain intensity, personal care, lifting, walking, sitting, standing, sleeping, sex life, social life, traveling; overall score 0-100.	10 items, 6 response options per item	5
NDI	Pain intensity, personal care, lifting, reading, headache, concentration, work, driving, sleeping, recreation; overall score 0-100 (typically used; originally described version had overall score of 0-50)	10 items, 6 response options per item	5
VAS or NRS	Pain intensity, generally asks about 2 to 4 body regions such as neck, arms, lower back, legs	2 to 4 body regions, each scored on 0-10 scale	<3
Pain drawing	Page sized outlines of the front and back of the human body on which patients are instructed to use various symbols representing different sensation to indicate where each sensation is felt	Multiple scoring methods available	<3
Satisfaction	No generally accepted questionnaire used in spine research	NA	NA
SF-36	36-item general health questionnaire that is generally reported in the PCS and MCS composites	36 items, varying number of response options	<10
EQ-5D	Mobility, self-care, usual activities, pain/discomfort, anxiety/depression; overall scores range from 0-1	5 items with 5 response options for each item	<3

EQ-5D = EuroQol Five Dimensions questionnaire, MCS = mental component summary, NA = not applicable, NDI = Neck Disability Index, NRS = numerical rating scale, ODI = Oswestry Disability Index, PCS = physical component summary, SF-36 = Medical Outcomes Study 36-Item Short Form, VAS = visual analog scale.

ceiling effect because their condition may be too severe to be appropriately evaluated by that particular instrument. This effect also can compromise the instrument's sensitivity and ability to adequately reflect change in a patient's condition.

Oswestry Disability Index

One of the most well-investigated, widely used outcome assessments for back pain is the ODI,[7] which is composed of 10 items that assess various aspects of back pain. The ODI is easy to administer and score. Each item is measured on a scale from 0 to 5. The total score is divided by 50 to generate a percentage disability score; lower scores indicate a lower level of disability. Revisions have been developed, and the version currently used is v2.1a.[8,9]

Several "rogue" versions of the ODI have been used in various studies.[8] Some modifications have included changing the wording on some items or replacing an item altogether. Such modifications can alter the reliability and validity of the tool. One modified version of the ODI

exchanged the question about sexual activity with an item asking patients to rate their symptoms compared with their past status. Careful analysis of the psychometric properties of this version verified that the questions did not belong with the other items on the ODI and measured a different underlying construct.[10]

In most outcome studies using the ODI, the mean scores before and after treatment are compared for one or more groups of patients. More recent efforts have been made to determine the percentage of patients with a clinically meaningful change in ODI scores. This metric has often been used to determine if the patient has had a successful treatment outcome. Although commonly used, little information is available on what value should be used to determine a successful outcome based on the ODI score. One of the first articles on the MCID reported that a change of 10 points in the total ODI score represented a clinically relevant change.[4] The measure most commonly used in FDA-regulated trials requires an improvement of at least 15 points in the ODI score.[11,12] In the setting of spondylolisthesis, a change of 22 points in ODI score was recently determined to be clinically important.[13] In addition to the minimal change to be classified as successful treatment, requiring a specific maximal score also has been considered to classify a patient as having a successful outcome. Based on recent registry data of surgery for lumbar degenerative conditions, it was suggested that a value of 22 or less on the ODI during postoperative assessment be considered a beneficial response to surgery.[14] This corresponds well with the value of 20 or less in the original description of the ODI that was considered essentially normal.[7] However, it can be argued that this value is too low, considering that many patients have a preoperative score greater than 60 and the MCID is generally considered a reduction of at least 15 points. Therefore, the question arises as to whether surgery can be considered successful only if the patient is somewhat restored to an approximately healthy state.

Neck Disability Index

The Neck Disability Index (NDI) was patterned after the ODI and designed for use in patients with neck pain. In contrast to the ODI, multiple modified versions of the NDI are not used. In a study of instruments used in a spine surgery registry, the NDI was found to be the most valid and responsive measure.[15] As with the ODI, in most studies, the NDI is used to determine treatment outcome by comparing mean scores before and after intervention and/or mean scores between treatment groups to determine if any differences exist between groups. In addition, as with the ODI, a 15-point change is commonly used in FDA-regulated trials to classify a patient as having achieved a clinically important change following treatment.[16,17] Other studies have used a minimum 30-point improvement from baseline to determine success using the NDI.[18]

Visual Analog Scales and NRS

The most common reason for patients to seek spine care is the presence of back, neck, or radicular pain. Therefore, assessing pain intensity is valuable in measuring treatment outcome. One of the most commonly used methods to record a patient's pain level has been the visual analog scale (VAS). The VAS is generally 10 cm long with the end points labeled "no pain" and "worst possible pain." The patient is asked to place a mark on the line to indicate his or her pain severity. To date, no standardized instructions are provided to patients who complete the questionnaire. Variations include qualifiers such as "on average," "over the past week," and separating left and right leg pain to different scales.

The VAS is differentiated from the NRS in that the VAS is an analog scale, generally with 101 possible values, whereas the NRS has 11 discrete values ranging from 0 to 10. The NRS may have the same problem as the VAS with respect to the variation in instructions provided to patients.

The VAS may be more sensitive than the NRS, but challenges exist with reliably reproducing or printing the 10-cm line length or displaying it well on a screen. The NRS may be less sensitive because it has fewer possible values.

Pain Drawings

Pain drawings provide an easily administered means for patients to record the location of their symptoms. The drawings also have been found to be helpful in identifying back pain patients who may have a substantial psychologic component to their symptoms.[19] Multiple scoring methods have been described for use with pain drawings, and the method used may best be determined based on the goal of the evaluator.[20] Multiple methods of scoring pain drawings have been found to be reliable in patients with back pain.[21] One of the recent applications of pain drawings as a clinical outcome tool involved a computerized version of the drawings.[22]

Success Following Treatment

Although one of the most commonly asked questions about any spine intervention is "what is the success rate?" no standardized criteria exist to determine success. Also, what is considered success can vary widely based on an individual's problems, goals, and lifestyle. Many FDA-regulated trials have incorporated various combinations of patient-reported outcomes, and physical examination and radiographic findings, as well as the need for further medical intervention, into the definition of treatment success. However, the validity of this type of combined success rate has not yet been investigated. Of note, the relationship of the combined success criteria has not been studied relative to what a patient may consider success following surgical intervention.

Patient Satisfaction

Recently, a concerted effort has been made to include patient satisfaction as a measure of clinical outcome. This trend likely will continue because the United States government is focusing more on this aspect of patient care. Although intuitively this assessment seems useful, some problems exist in its application. No standardized, validated assessment exists for the satisfaction of clinical outcomes in the spine. Some instruments have used a VAS or a three- or five-point scale, which may be useful to some extent, but may not be specific enough to yield the type of information needed. Satisfaction can mean various things to different patients, encompassing everything from satisfaction with their clinical outcomes to issues that are more customer service–related than clinical, such as the attentiveness of the staff, hospital experience, and clinic wait time. Satisfaction scores also have been found to be lower among spine surgery patients who were classified as being distressed based on a psychologic questionnaire.[23] Another study among workers with low back pain found that they were more satisfied with care delivered by surgeons, chiropractors, or physical therapists than if treated by physicians who were not surgeons.[24] Greater satisfaction with the provider was associated with approximately a 25% reduction in claim duration. These workers were more concerned with the effectiveness of care than with bedside manner. With so many factors potentially affecting satisfaction, it can be challenging to adequately assess patient satisfaction with the medical outcome of care.

The Press Ganey survey has been used widely to evaluate patient satisfaction with healthcare encounters.[25] The questions appear to be related more to customer service aspects of care rather than satisfaction with the care received or the outcome achieved. Investigators have found that, among spine care patients, two factors related to greater satisfaction measured by the Press Ganey questionnaire were a lower pain score and feeling that the care provider spent more time with them.

In a study involving lumbar and cervical spine patients, satisfaction was not found to be highly related to improvement in general health status as assessed by the Medical Outcomes Study 12-Item Short Form (SF-12), spine-specific measure of the ODI or NDI, or readmission or morbidity rates.[26] Although satisfaction is important to assess, it was not considered a valid measure of the quality or effectiveness of spine surgery.

Other Spine-Specific Questionnaires

Several other outcome assessments have been introduced for use among patients with spinal conditions. All have advantages and disadvantages, and their development highlights the fact that no perfect, or near-perfect, outcome assessment likely exists for spinal disorders. Some assessments are for specific spinal conditions such as stenosis, spinal deformity, or trauma. A tradeoff is always present with use of these assessments in that although they may be preferred for the evaluation of a specific condition, the results may be more difficult to evaluate by other providers or be interpreted in the context of other conditions. The Zurich Claudication Questionnaire was designed to evaluate patients with spinal stenosis[27] and was found to

have good reliability. However, it is difficult to put the scores in the context of more common questionnaires such as the ODI when determining the effectiveness of treatment of different conditions or among patients with multiple diagnoses, including stenosis.

General Health Measures

Rationale for Use in Spine Conditions

General health measures are commonly used in a variety of health conditions. Originally, the apparent lack of relevance of these measures to patients with spine conditions resulted in resistance to their use. The use of general health measures is increasing in spine research at this time. The use of these measures helps compare the condition of spine patients and the results of their treatment with other disease states. This could facilitate increasing the appreciation for the severity of spine-related pain. Using SF-36 scores that assess physical function, it was found that patients with back pain had similar or worse scores than patients with congestive heart failure, lupus, cancer, or those with large joint arthritis undergoing hip or knee arthroplasty.[28] This type of study, which uses a standardized general health questionnaire, can be important in providing a context for interpreting the importance of back pain. It also provides the foundation of cost-effectiveness studies across multiple health problems. Increasing the awareness of the importance of back pain also can be of particular relevance in the context of the current lack of funding for spine research.[29]

Short Form Series

Among the most widely used general health questionnaires have been multiple versions of the Medical Outcomes Short Form. The original 36-item version (SF-36) was used to provide a general health assessment on eight subscales. However, the combined physical component score (PCS) and the mental component score have been the most commonly reported subscales. The questionnaire was originally developed for the Medical Outcome Study; shorter subsequent versions (SF-12 and SF-6) have been introduced.

Many FDA-regulated trials use the SF-36 or SF-12 as a general health measure,[11,16-18] which should facilitate comparisons of new technologies with existing spine outcome studies or with nonspinal interventions. For newer technologies such as cervical TDA, SF-36 scores were combined with cost data to create several scenarios investigating the long-term (7-year) cost-effectiveness of TDA compared with anterior cervical fusion for the treatment of symptomatic single-level disk degeneration.[30]

8: Special Populations in Spine Care

Similarly, although hip and knee arthroplasty are widely accepted procedures for the treatment of pain and compromised function resulting from osteoarthritis, surgery for the treatment of painful spinal osteoarthritis remains controversial. A Canadian study used the SF-36 to compare the incremental cost-utility ratio (ICUR) of spinal stenosis surgery with that of total hip and total knee arthroplasty and found similar results.[31] Using general health assessments in studies such as this may help communicate the effectiveness of spine surgery after unsuccessful nonsurgical care.

EQ-5D Series

The EQ-5D, an increasingly common general health assessment, originated in Europe, so its use was more widespread there before its introduction in the United States. This simple five-item questionnaire may be more palatable for patients than the SF-36, particularly for those who are asked to complete the measure on multiple occasions. As with the SF series, multiple versions of the EQ-5D exist. The currently recommended version is the EQ-5D-3L.[1] The questions cover five domains: mobility, self-care, usual activities, pain/discomfort, and anxiety/depression. The assessment generates a score ranging from 0 to 1; 0 represents death and 1 indicates perfect health.

A systematic review of general health assessments found that the EQ-5D showed good validity and responsiveness in patients with low back pain and was appropriate to use for cost analyses in this population.[32] However, EQ-5D was noted as adequate for detecting change among patients with less severe health status. In a study of patients with spondylolisthesis, compared with the SF-12, ODI, NRS for pain, and the Zung Depression Scale, the EQ-5D was the most valid and responsive measure of improvement following spine surgery.[33]

Patient-Reported Outcomes Measurement Information System

One of the newer general health questionnaires is the Patient-Reported Outcomes Measurement Information System (PROMIS), which was developed by the National Institutes of Health as a set of person-centered measures to evaluate physical, mental, and social health. It has been validated for a wide variety of health conditions. Although described as easy to use, some clinicians and researchers may find, at least initially, that sorting through more than 48 PROMIS forms for use with adult populations is rather cumbersome. This variety can initially appear daunting, but only three questionnaires comprise the core set often used with adults with spinal pain: those for physical health, mental health, and social health. The forms themselves appear to be easily administered after specific forms are selected for use. Currently, few reports exist on the use of PROMIS assessments in spine populations, but these will likely increase in the future.

Computer-adaptive testing has been described for use with the PROMIS instrument.[34] This form of item response theory provides the person completing the evaluation with questions based on answers to previous questions. The goals are to continually improve the questionnaire and add a greater level of individualization to the testing. Computer-adaptive testing requires a computing device for assessment responses. The use of computer-adaptive testing has not yet been well investigated in spine research. However, one study investigated the psychometric properties of the PROMIS Physical Function (PROMIS PF) administered using the computer-adaptive testing application in a population of more than 1,600 patients with back and/or leg pain. The PROMIS PF computer-adaptive testing had better ceiling and floor effects and required less time to complete than other measures, including the ODI and the SF-36 PCS.

Electronic Questionnaires

Interest has increased in the electronic administration of patient-completed outcome measures. Paperless administration has many potential advantages: the elimination of data entry time and entry-related errors, patients cannot select more than one response or write in qualifying comments, and assessments can be completed via portal rather than in person or by mailing forms to patients. In addition, the data may be available for real-time progress charting during the patient encounter.

Paperless testing offers challenges such as data security, Health Insurance Portability and Accountability Act compliance, and backing up of files. Also, other means need to be available for patients who are not comfortable using electronics. In a study of a large number of patients completing the SF-36 and/or the ODI on paper and electronically, the response rate and the missing data rate were both substantially lower among groups using the electronically administered forms.[35] The PROMIS PF computer-adaptive testing was reported to have better properties than the ODI or SF-36 PCS.[34] This type of computer-adaptive testing could represent an upcoming era in healthcare data collection. Of course, a plan should always be in place to treat patients who do not have, or prefer not to use, electronic entry. Most often, the patient can use paper forms available in the office and a staff member can enter the data later. However, as an increasing proportion of the population is using smartphones and tablets, this will likely become a more common format for data collection. Patient satisfaction with using a

8: Special Populations in Spine Care

mobile tablet for data collection in a spine clinic has been investigated and found to be acceptable.[36] Patients' use of smartphones and typing proficiency were independent predictors of acceptance of the system.

A 2010 study compared the validity of electronically administered questionnaires with that of traditional paper forms.[37] The electronic version was found to be valid and of further benefit, with 0% missing data; paper forms had 2.3% missing data for individual questions; and composite scores had 12% missing data.

Spine Registries

One of the greatest potential uses for electronic data collection is for a comprehensive spine registry. Multiple registries have been used in Europe for several years, but none have been used extensively in the United States. The North American Spine Society is piloting a registry that is designed for spine care providers, including both surgical and nonsurgical specialists. Use of such a registry should help to generate large amounts of data that can be used to identify trends in care, complications, help evaluate and compare outcomes of various treatments, allow providers to benchmark their outcomes against the cumulative values of other providers, standardize assessments, and facilitate future study design.

However, much of the reporting of outcomes, particularly for complications, depends on self-reporting by healthcare providers. This can easily be manipulated either intentionally or inadvertently. It is important to at least provide well-defined guidance to registry participants for which complications and reoperations should be entered into the registry. In one study using the same population of surgical patients, the reoperation rate varied substantially based only on the criteria used to classify patients as having undergone revision surgery or not.[38]

QALYs and Incremental Cost-effectiveness Ratios

The demand for demonstrable cost-effective care will continue in all areas of medicine, including spine. At the core of these potentially highly impactful measurements is the outcome assessments used in their calculations. Defining costs, collecting comprehensive cost data, and interpreting cost-effective data can be challenging, and no single widely accepted process exists.

One commonly used metric in the measure of cost-effectiveness is the QALY. One QALY is 1 year in perfect health, taking into account both the quality of life and the quantity of life. A value of 0 is death, and a value of 1 represents 1 year of life in perfect health. Questionnaires such as the SF-series and EQ-5D are often used

to determine QALYs because they provide measures of compromised health quality. In back pain studies, QALY is not typically used, but study duration is used. The duration component of spine surgery is important. The initial cost of spine surgery may be relatively high; however, if good outcomes are maintained during multiple-year follow-ups, costs decline per QALYs.

Incremental cost-effectiveness ratios can be used to compare the cost effectiveness of two treatments. This measure is the ratio between the difference in costs and the difference in effectiveness of the two interventions. The effectiveness is often calculated based on commonly used, patient-completed outcome assessments.

Special Considerations

Spine outcome assessments require continued development. The validity of the electronic administration of questionnaires that are currently recorded on paper needs to be determined. The increased interest in long-term follow-up, particularly for surgical intervention, is accompanied by an increasing need to collect data by means of mailings, electronic forms, and telephone calls. Patients can complete the same forms via mail that they would in the clinic. With increased use of electronic forms, it is feasible for patients to log in and complete questionnaires online. One study has reviewed data collection via telephone and found that VAS leg pain and back pain scores as well as ODI scores had similar values for both telephone and in-person completion.[39] Although these issues seem simple, the format of questionnaire administration can potentially affect patient responses, and it is important to consider this possibility.

A major challenge in standardizing outcome assessments or introducing new ones is the potential for losing a substantial amount of data collected to date. Changing the assessments used is difficult for clinicians and researchers after years of using a particular set.

Future Directions

Ongoing changes will likely occur in the use of outcome assessments in spine care, including greater reliance on electronic administration of questionnaires, which has already begun. The use of electronically administered questionnaires and registries will help to standardize the questionnaires used for outcomes to facilitate meta-analyses, comparison studies, and the determination of cost-effectiveness for various treatments. A movement toward more patient-centered outcomes is already occurring, as has been seen with increasing demands for patient satisfaction surveys. Increased assessment of patient expectations for treatment outcome and the evaluation of the extent to which those expectations were met may be tied to satisfaction. The use of computer-adaptive testing such as with PROMIS likely will increase with the potential to refine the responsiveness of questionnaires. Greater sensitivity and responsiveness may allow for studies to be performed with smaller sample sizes, reducing the cost of the study as well as the time to complete the work. However, it should be noted that, as the number of data points to be collected increases, the ability to collect them inherently declines. This decline was measured in a registry-based study that found the rate of completion when using four to five questionnaires was less than 50% of that using two to three questionnaires.[40]

Summary

Demand is increasing for evidence in spine care, the core of which is outcome measures. The demand for patient-centered outcomes also has contributed to the patient-level interpretation of existing questionnaires. Most studies report clinical outcomes as changes in mean scores on various outcome measures, with comparisons between scores before and after treatment or comparisons of scores between groups. Although helpful in comparing groups, these studies have not provided insight into how many patients had clinically significant improvement. Among providers, awareness is increasing of the need to collect outcomes data; however, trying to determine which instruments should be used can be somewhat overwhelming given the large number of instruments described in the literature.

In addition, better assessments are likely needed. Although good tools are available, they may not be applicable to the breadth of the population with spine conditions, which includes individuals of varying ages, occupations, recreational pursuits, and lifestyles. There also is an increasing preference for assessments that are more centered on the patient. Given the variety of questionnaires available for spine patients, all with their own advantages and disadvantages, it can be tempting to use many of them. Although using a blend of disease-specific and general health assessments is recommended, using too many different forms is not advised in the same group of patients.

One developing improvement in outcome data collection is electronic capture, which has improved data quality by reducing problems encountered with paper administration. Electronic administration likely will facilitate more patient-oriented outcome assessments to better reflect the patient's condition and improve the responsiveness of the assessment tools. This would not only improve the ability to compare changes in a patient's condition before and after intervention but also would facilitate comparing treatment outcomes across groups of patients. The greater responsiveness of questionnaires also likely will improve cost-effectiveness research. All of these efforts will produce more reliable evidence that can be used to guide patient care.

Key Study Points

- Data collection in patients with spine pain is a continually evolving process.
- A need exists for greater standardization of spine surgery outcome assessments, particularly the format and instructions provided to facilitate data pooling from multiple sources and also for more meaningful meta-analyses and other comprehensive reviews.
- The use of electronically administered outcome assessments will likely continue to improve data collection, including the use of registries to accumulate large numbers of patients, all completing the same assessments, for data analyses.

Annotated References

1. Clement RC, Welander A, Stowell C, et al: A proposed set of metrics for standardized outcome reporting in the management of low back pain. *Acta Orthop* 2015;86(5):523-533.

   A diverse international group of individuals with an interest in spine care outcomes collaborated to develop a suggested core set of outcome assessments to be used in spine research. The goal was achieved, and the suggested metrics are detailed in this article.

2. Copay AG, Martin MM, Subach BR, et al: Assessment of spine surgery outcomes: Inconsistency of change amongst outcome measurements. *Spine J* 2010;10(4):291-296.

3. Johnsen LG, Hellum C, Storheim K, et al; Norwegian Spine Study Group: Cost-effectiveness of total disc replacement versus multidisciplinary rehabilitation in patients with chronic low back pain: A Norwegian multicenter RCT. *Spine (Phila Pa 1976)* 2014;39(1):23-32.

   This review of motion-preserving technology found that cost-effectiveness can vary substantially based on which widely used general health assessment was used in the calculation. This report highlights the challenges in reporting and interpreting cost-effectiveness literature and how inconsistent the literature can be. Level of evidence: II.

4. Hägg O, Fritzell P, Nordwall A; Swedish Lumbar Spine Study Group: The clinical importance of changes in outcome scores after treatment for chronic low back pain. *Eur Spine J* 2003;12(1):12-20.

5. Zannikos S, Lee L, Smith HE: Minimum clinically important difference and substantial clinical benefit: Does one size fit all diagnoses and patients? *Semin Spine Surg* 2014;26(1):8-11.

    This study reviewed MCID values and some of the challenges in calculating and interpreting these values.

6. Guyer RD, Ohnmeiss DD: How to calculate the cost of spine care, in Rihn JA, Vaccaro AR, Albert TJ, eds: *Defining the Value of Spine Care*. New Delhi, India, Jaypee Brothers Medical Publishers, 2012, pp 109-118.

    Cost is an increasingly important component of spine research. This study describes multiple methods of considering costs and some of the barriers in performing optimal cost analyses.

7. Fairbank JC, Couper J, Davies JB, O'Brien JP: The Oswestry low back pain disability questionnaire. *Physiotherapy* 1980;66(8):271-273.

8. Fairbank JC: Use and abuse of Oswestry Disability Index. *Spine (Phila Pa 1976)* 2007;32(25):2787-2789.

9. Fairbank J: Oswestry Disability Index. Basic description. Available at: https://eprovide.mapi-trust.org/instruments/oswestry-disability-index. Accessed April 4, 2017.

10. Davidson M: Rasch analysis of three versions of the Oswestry Disability Questionnaire. *Man Ther* 2008;13(3):222-231.

11. Musacchio MJ, Lauryssen C, Davis RJ, et al: Evaluation of decompression and interlaminar stabilization compared with decompression and fusion for the treatment of lumbar spinal stenosis: 5-year follow-up of a prospective, randomized, controlled trial. *Int J Spine Surg* 2016;10:6.

    The 5-year outcomes of patients with lumbar stenosis treated with an interlaminar device to provide spinal stability without fusion were evaluated. One measure of success was the FDA criterion that the patient had greater than a 15-point improvement in his or her ODI score. Level of evidence: I.

12. Zigler JE, Delamarter RB: Five-year results of the prospective, randomized, multicenter, Food and Drug Administration investigational device exemption study of the ProDisc-L total disc replacement versus circumferential arthrodesis for the treatment of single-level degenerative disc disease. *J Neurosurg Spine* 2012;17(6):493-501.

    This study compared preoperative and postoperative outcomes using a predetermined value of a 15-point change in the ODI as a measure of the minimal improvement required for an outcome to be classified as successful.

13. Parker SL, McGirt MJ: Determination of the minimum improvement in pain, disability, and health state associated with cost-effectiveness: Introduction of the concept of minimum cost-effective difference. *Neurosurgery* 2015;76(suppl 1):S64-S70.

    This study investigated cost-effectiveness by determining the minimal amount of improvement needed on an outcome assessment for the treatment to be considered cost-effective.

14. van Hooff ML, Mannion AF, Staub LP, Ostelo RW, Fairbank JC: Determination of the Oswestry Disability Index score equivalent to a "satisfactory symptom state" in patients undergoing surgery for degenerative disorders of the lumbar spine-a Spine Tango registry-based study. *Spine J* 2016;16(10):1221-1230.

15. Godil SS, Parker SL, Zuckerman SL, Mendenhall SK, McGirt MJ: Accurately measuring the quality and effectiveness of cervical spine surgery in registry efforts: Determining the most valid and responsive instruments. *Spine J* 2015;15(6):1203-1209.

    Rather than requiring that a specific change in outcome scores be achieved, this study proposed determining a minimal value be achieved on an assessment for an outcome to be classified as successful.

16. Murrey D, Janssen M, Delamarter R, et al: Results of the prospective, randomized, controlled multicenter Food and Drug Administration investigational device exemption study of the ProDisc-C total disc replacement versus anterior discectomy and fusion for the treatment of 1-level symptomatic cervical disc disease. *Spine J* 2009;9(4):275-286.

17. Phillips FM, Lee JY, Geisler FH, et al: A prospective, randomized, controlled clinical investigation comparing PCM cervical disc arthroplasty with anterior cervical discectomy and fusion: 2-year results from the US FDA IDE clinical trial. *Spine (Phila Pa 1976)* 2013;38(15):E907-E918.

    This study required a minimum 15-point change in the NDI score for an outcome to be considered successful. Level of evidence: I.

18. Hisey MS, Zigler JE, Jackson R, et al: Prospective, randomized comparison of one-level Mobi-C Cervical Total Disc Replacement vs. anterior cervical discectomy and fusion: Results at 5-year follow-up. *Int J Spine Surg* 2016;10:10.

    This study required a 30-point NDI improvement to determine a successful outcome rather than a 15-point NDI improvement. Level of evidence: I.

19. Ransford AO, Cairns D, Mooney V: The pain drawing as an aid to the psychological evaluation of patients with low-back pain. *Spine* 1976;1(2):127-134.

20. Ohnmeiss DD: *Pain Drawings in the Evaluation of Lumbar Disc-Related Pain*. Stockholm, Sweden, Karolinska Institute, 2000.

8: Special Populations in Spine Care

21. Ohnmeiss DD: Repeatability of pain drawings in a low back pain population. *Spine (Phila Pa 1976)* 2000;25(8):980-988.

22. Huang P, Sengupta DK: How fast pain, numbness, and paresthesia resolves after lumbar nerve root decompression: A retrospective study of patient's self-reported computerized pain drawing. *Spine (Phila Pa 1976)* 2014;39(8):E529-E536.

    This study used an electronic version of the classic pain drawing to investigate the recovery pattern of various sensations after surgical decompression of lumbar nerve roots. Level of evidence: IV.

23. Abtahi AM, Brodke DS, Lawrence BD, Zhang C, Spiker WR: Association between patient-reported measures of psychological distress and patient satisfaction scores after spine surgery. *J Bone Joint Surg Am* 2015;97(10):824-828.

    This study reported that satisfaction scores can be substantially affected by factors other than the quality of care received, such as distress. Level of evidence: III.

24. Butler RJ, Johnson WG: Satisfaction with low back pain care. *Spine J* 2008;8(3):510-521.

25. Etier BE Jr, Orr SP, Antonetti J, Thomas SB, Theiss SM: Factors impacting Press Ganey patient satisfaction scores in orthopedic surgery spine clinic. *Spine J* 2016;16(11):1285-1289.

    Based on a satisfaction survey sometimes used in health care, greater satisfaction for patients undergoing spine surgery was related to lower pain scores and a feeling that a care provider spent more time with them. Level of evidence: IV.

26. Godil SS, Parker SL, Zuckerman SL, et al: Determining the quality and effectiveness of surgical spine care: Patient satisfaction is not a valid proxy. *Spine J* 2013;13(9):1006-1012.

    Although demand is increasing for the inclusion of patient satisfaction in outcome reporting, satisfaction was not related to commonly used outcome assessments, hospital readmission, or morbidity rates.

27. Stucki G, Daltroy L, Liang MH, Lipson SJ, Fossel AH, Katz JN: Measurement properties of a self-administered outcome measure in lumbar spinal stenosis. *Spine (Phila Pa 1976)* 1996;21(7):796-803.

28. Fanuele JC, Birkmeyer NJ, Abdu WA, Tosteson TD, Weinstein JN: The impact of spinal problems on the health status of patients: Have we underestimated the effect? *Spine (Phila Pa 1976)* 2000;25(12):1509-1514.

29. Hanna M: Funding research to achieve the Spine "10×25" goal. *Spine J* 2016;16(7):805-810.

    This comprehensive analysis reported on the cost of spine problems in the United States and the disproportionally low amount of research funding spent on spine disorders compared with various other conditions.

30. Radcliff K, Lerner J, Yang C, Bernard T, Zigler JE: Seven-year cost-effectiveness of ProDisc-C total disc replacement: Results from investigational device exemption and post-approval studies. *J Neurosurg Spine* 2016;24(5):760-768.

    This study used data from an FDA-regulated trial in which the SF-36 was used to perform a long-term cost-effectiveness study comparing TDA traditional fusion and found the new technology was more cost effective. This refutes traditional thought that new techniques are inherently more expensive.

31. Rampersaud YR, Tso P, Walker KR, et al: Comparative outcomes and cost-utility following surgical treatment of focal lumbar spinal stenosis compared with osteoarthritis of the hip or knee: Part 2. Estimated lifetime incremental cost-utility ratios. *Spine J* 2014;14(2):244-254.

    This study demonstrates how general health instruments can be used to investigate the cost-effectiveness of spine care in the context of other problems generally accepted as cost effective.

32. Finch AP, Dritsaki M, Jommi C: Generic preference-based measures for low back pain: Which of them should be used? *Spine (Phila Pa 1976)* 2016;41(6):E364-E374.

    This systematic review of general health assessments in back pain patients found that the EQ-5D had good responsiveness characteristics; however, it was not as responsive in patients with less severe conditions, possibly reflecting a floor effect.

33. Godil SS, Parker SL, Zuckerman SL, Mendenhall SK, Glassman SD, McGirt MJ: Accurately measuring the quality and effectiveness of lumbar surgery in registry efforts: Determining the most valid and responsive instruments. *Spine J* 2014;14(12):2885-2891.

    This study compared several disease-specific and general health assessments in back pain patients; it was determined that the EQ-5D was the most responsive to change in patients being treated for lumbar spondylolisthesis.

34. Papuga MO, Mesfin A, Molinari R, Rubery PT: Correlation of PROMIS physical function and pain CAT instruments with Oswestry Disability Index and Neck Disability Index in spine patients. *Spine (Phila Pa 1976)* 2016;41(14):1153-1159.

    This study introduces the use of computer-adaptive testing using PROMIS evaluations, which could represent the next step in refining outcome assessments in health care.

35. Hanscom B, Lurie JD, Homa K, Weinstein JN: Computerized questionnaires and the quality of survey data. *Spine (Phila Pa 1976)* 2002;27(16):1797-1801.

36. Kim CH, Chung CK, Choi Y, et al: The usefulness of a mobile device-based system for patient-reported outcomes in a spine outpatient clinic. *Spine J* 2016;16(7):843-850.

    A good rate of patient acceptance was found for using a mobile tablet to collect patient-completed questionnaires.

37. Frennered K, Hägg O, Wessberg P: Validity of a computer touch-screen questionnaire system in back patients. *Spine (Phila Pa 1976)* 2010;35(6):697-703.

38. Ohnmeiss DD, Guyer RD, Blumenthal SL, et al: Reoperation rates in lumbar spine surgery: Statistically significant differences exist in the same dataset when different definitions for reoperation are applied. *Spine J* 2016;16(10):S292.

    This study highlights the need for carefully worded and rigorously implemented definitions for data points such as reoperation in clinical studies. The reoperation rates varied substantially among the same patients based on the definitions applied.

39. Adogwa O, Elsamadicy AA, Cheng J, Bagley C: Assessing patient reported outcomes measures via phone interviews versus patient self-survey in the clinic: Are we measuring the same thing? *World Neurosurg* 2016;87:230-234.

    This study found that similar data values were collected using either telephone interview or having the patient complete the form in the clinic.

40. Morris S, Booth J, Hegarty J: Spine Tango registry data collection in a conservative spinal service: A feasibility study. *Eur Spine J* 2016;25(9):2984-2992.

    This study reported that the greater the number of evaluations administered, the greater the rate of data loss.

8: Special Populations in Spine Care

Chapter 38

Spine Injuries in Sports

Michael J. Vives, MD   Colin B. Harris, MD

Abstract

Spine injuries can occur in the athletic setting. Those who care for athletes should be familiar with injury prevention methods along with the on-field management of spine injuries and return-to-play considerations. The ability of an athlete to return to play depends on the pathoanatomy of the injury and the consequences of treatments. The risk for further injury is the primary consideration in the determination if an athlete can return to sports participation.

Keywords: athletic injuries; cervical fractures; return-to-play guidelines; team physicians

Introduction

Sports-related injuries are a common cause of accidental injury, accounting for approximately 5.3 million visits to healthcare providers annually.[1] Although spine injuries are less common than extremity injuries, spine injury is among the injuries most feared by athletes because of the potential for catastrophic disability. Such fears must be weighed against the benefits that sports and recreational activities provide, however. Participation in sports activities is important for physical health and overall well-being. Surgeons who provide spine care must

Dr. Vives or an immediate family member is a member of a speakers' bureau or has made paid presentations on behalf of Musculoskeletal Transplant Foundation; has stock or stock options held in Accelalox, NOC² Healthcare, and CreOsso; and serves as a board member, owner, officer, or committee member of the American Academy of Orthopaedic Surgeons and the North American Spine Society. Neither Dr. Harris nor any immediate family member has received anything of value from or has stock or stock options held in a commercial company or institution related directly or indirectly to the subject of this chapter.

understand the mechanisms and patterns of injury in sport-specific settings, on- and off-the-field management of such injury, and the steps involved in safe return to play.

Sport-Specific Epidemiology

Epidemiologic data on sports-related spine and spinal cord injuries varies by country. Spine injuries range from simple contusions and muscular strains to fractures with complete spinal cord injury. A recent systematic review evaluated data from 54 studies in 25 countries.[2] The six countries in which sports activity accounts for greater than 13% of traumatic spinal cord injury are Russia (33%), Fiji (32%), New Zealand (20%), Iceland (19%), France (16%), and Canada (13.1%). In the United States, approximately 12% of spinal cord injuries are related to sports and recreational activities. Worldwide, the sports associated with the highest risk for spinal cord injury are diving, skiing, rugby, horseback riding, and American football.

The popularity of American football, particularly at the collegiate and professional levels, makes spinal injuries in these settings newsworthy occurrences in the United States. Because most studies of football-related spine injuries have focused on severe injuries, the true frequency of the broad spectrum of spinal injuries is less well understood. The occurrence of football-related injuries of the axial skeleton or spine in the United States is estimated to be 60,000 to 300,000 annually.[3,4] In the National Football League, injuries are tracked by the training staff of each team and collated in a league-wide injury surveillance system. A 2012 study used this system to study spinal injuries over an 11-year period ending in 2010.[5] The 2,208 injuries to the spine or axial skeleton accounted for 7% of the total injuries reported; the cervical spine was involved in 44.7% of these injuries. Tackling and blocking were the most frequently reported mechanisms of injury. Tackling produced more cervical spine injuries (Figure 1), whereas blocking produced more lumbar spine injuries. Offensive linemen were the most likely to sustain a spinal injury, followed by defensive backs, defensive linemen, and linebackers. In a study of previous injuries

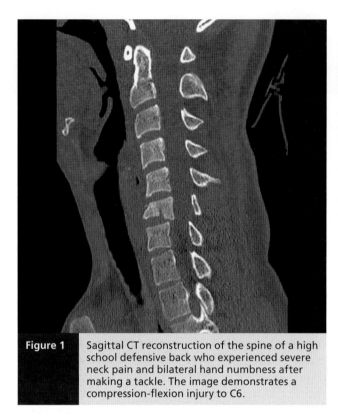

Figure 1   Sagittal CT reconstruction of the spine of a high school defensive back who experienced severe neck pain and bilateral hand numbness after making a tackle. The image demonstrates a compression-flexion injury to C6.

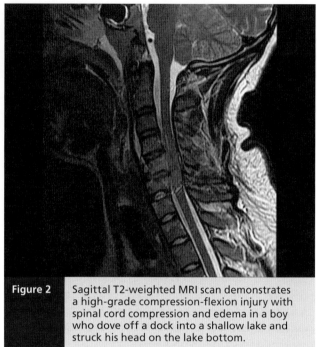

Figure 2   Sagittal T2-weighted MRI scan demonstrates a high-grade compression-flexion injury with spinal cord compression and edema in a boy who dove off a dock into a shallow lake and struck his head on the lake bottom.

incurred by participants in the National Football League Scouting Combine event, the incidence of so-called burners was second only to ankle sprain.[6] Incidence rates of catastrophic spinal injuries vary by level of play. One study reported rates of spinal injury per 100,000 athletes of 0.52 among high school athletes, 1.55 among college athletes, and 14 among professional athletes.[7]

Diving injuries, which account for 8.5% of spinal cord injuries in the United States, are the fourth leading cause of spinal cord injury overall.[8] The incidence of diving injuries is highest during the summer months, and young men are most commonly involved. Most injuries occur in unsupervised settings, as opposed to organized swimming or diving events. The typical circumstance is a headfirst dive into shallow water. With reversal of lordosis resulting from neck flexion, the normal capacity to dissipate an axial load is diminished. Compression-flexion and burst fractures are the most common injury patterns (**Figure 2**). The C5 level is thought to be the most commonly involved.[9] One study estimated that spine injuries account for 9% of all injuries sustained by hockey players.[10] Checking from behind and causing a player to be driven headfirst into the boards is the most frequently cited event resulting in spinal injury, with the injury typically involving the cervical region. The incidence of spinal injury is highest at the juvenile level, perhaps because of

underdeveloped axial musculature at a time when players are capable of increased speed and aggressiveness.[11] The annual incidence of spinal cord injury with paralysis in ice hockey is more than three times greater than that of American football.[12]

Rugby is not a high-profile sport in the United States, but it enjoys immense popularity elsewhere in the world. Although protective gear is not worn, the style of play is physical and spinal injuries are relatively common. Most cervical injuries incurred by rugby players take place during the scrum, which is a play that restarts the game after a stoppage.[13,14] In the scrum, the forward from each team organizes himself or herself in a formation to collide with the other forward, locking heads and shoulders and pushing to gain possession of the ball. Front-row players are placed at highest risk for hyperflexion injuries to the cervical spine as players behind the forwards push against each other. The subaxial levels of C4-C5 and C5-C6 are most commonly injured.

A wide range of spinal injuries result from skiing and snowboarding. One study determined that the chance of sustaining a spinal fracture was 0.009% per ski or snowboard day, with no clear difference between the two activities.[15] Another study performed at a tertiary trauma center in Switzerland evaluated 6 years of data gathered on injuries sustained while skiing or snowboarding.[16] The lumbar spine was most commonly involved, followed in order of incidence by the thoracic spine, cervical spine, and sacrum. Transverse and spinous process fractures were the most frequent type, followed by anterior thoracolumbar compression fractures and burst fractures, respectively. It appears that most spinal injuries among skiers and snowboarders are the result of simple falls (frequently experienced by beginners); however, another subset of spinal injuries occurs in more experienced alpine athletes, resulting from jumping maneuvers. Spinal cord injuries are most common at the cervical level, although snowboarding is associated with spinal cord injury at the thoracic and thoracolumbar levels as well.[17]

Gymnastics is associated with the rare but devastating risk for major cervical spine injuries. The risk is present even for skilled and experienced gymnasts because they attempt more complex maneuvers. Repeated hyperextension and rotation resulting in lumbar spondylolysis in gymnasts also is well described. A classic study examining the lumbar radiographs of 100 gymnasts found an 11% incidence of lumbar spondylolysis.[18] Cheerleading injuries are most commonly attributed to falls from an attempted basket toss or from the top of a pyramid formation. In a report from 2005, cheerleading injuries during practice, sideline performances, and competitions were found to account for approximately 50% of catastrophic spine injuries in female high school and collegiate athletes.[19]

Injury Prevention

Injury prevention in sports is multifaceted and ongoing. For high-speed and collision sports, protective equipment for the head and face may have had unintentional effects on the risk for spinal injuries. It has been suggested that the introduction of energy-absorbing helmets in the 1970s may have contributed to an increased rate of catastrophic cervical spine injuries in American football because it fostered use of the crown of the head during tackling, also known as spear tackling.[20] Similarly, the introduction of protective head and face gear in ice hockey in the 1980s was speculated to have resulted in an increase in spine injuries through promotion of more aggressive play.[21]

For American football players, properly fitted shoulder pads and so-called cowboy collars can limit cervical range of motion and redistribute loads to the shoulder girdle and trunk; however, these pieces of equipment cannot fully protect the cervical spine. As such, rule changes restricting potentially dangerous styles of play have been another important aspect of injury prevention.

Prohibiting checking from behind has likely contributed to a decreased incidence of severe spinal injuries in ice hockey. Rule changes to eliminate spear tackling in American football also have resulted in a notable reduction in the incidence of catastrophic cervical injuries. Beyond enforcement of penalties for such infractions

during games, proper coaching in safe techniques for tackling and checking at all levels of participation are necessary. Many sports-related injuries occur in unsupervised settings; thus, public awareness is another important component of injury prevention.[22] The slogan "Feet First! First Time!," promoted by the ThinkFirst National Injury Prevention Foundation, is an example of a broad-based effort aimed at decreasing risky behavior leading to diving-related cervical spine injury. Also, an American Academy of Pediatrics position statement recommends that pediatricians actively advise parents against trampoline use by children.[23]

On-the-Field Management

The key components of on-the-field management (preparation and establishment of a series of algorithms for the management of severe injuries) occur long before the game takes place. Proper equipment for immediate stabilization of an injured player must be available, including a rigid spine board and stretcher, cervical immobilization collars, tools to remove facemasks, supplemental oxygen and airway management devices, and cardiopulmonary resuscitative equipment.[24] Sideline physicians require the help of additional assistants who are familiar with the techniques to resuscitate, stabilize, and safely transfer injured players. Contingency plans should be in place for rapid transport to a predesignated hospital if needed.

The injured player who is unable to leave the field without assistance should initially be examined in place, if possible. The player can be log-rolled to the supine position using cervical spine precautions. Helmets and pads promote relative neutral alignment, so they should be left in place during this process. Management should use standard ABCDE (airway, breathing, circulation, disability, exposure) protocol, beginning with assessment of the airway, breathing, and circulation. For injured players with airway compromise, the facemask should be removed with proper tools or bolt cutters, if necessary. Depending on the mechanism of injury, the examining physician must maintain a high index of suspicion for spinal injury. A cervical collar should be applied and a rigid spine board used to transport the injured athlete from the field. The addition of bolsters along the sides of the head and manual splinting by a designated individual are precautions used to maintain neutral alignment during transport. Players who exit the playing field independently but who later notify the medical staff of a potential spinal injury should be examined on the sideline in a seated or supine position. For athletes whose symptoms and examination suggest a minor injury, monitoring their condition is sufficient.

Table 1

Summary of Sports-Related Injuries to the Cervical Spine

Injury	Mechanism of Injury	Prominent Symptoms	Treatment
Spinous process fracture	Avulsion from forceful contraction of trapezius/rhomboid muscles	Axial pain	Activity restriction, NSAIDs
Compression/burst fracture	Collision, diving injury, fall	Axial pain	External immobilization for low-grade injury, surgery for higher-grade injury
Facet subluxation/dislocation	Collision, diving injury, fall	Axial pain	Closed reduction and surgical stabilization
Acute spinal cord injury	Collision, diving injury	Axial pain, neurologic deficits	Urgent decompression and stabilization
Cervical cord neurapraxia	Collision, fall	Ranges from paresthesias in more than one extremity to transient quadriplegia	Resolves within 48 hours; exclude instability; evaluate for stenosis and disk herniation
Stingers	Forced lateral bending of the neck with depression of contralateral shoulder; axial load of a rotated or laterally bent cervical spine	Pain, paresthesias, weakness in a single upper extremity	Often resolves spontaneously (2 weeks for traction injuries); oral steroids for persistent symptoms; electrodiagnostic testing for refractory cases
Disk herniation	Axial load from collision, fall, forceful rotation, or lateral bending	Neck pain with or without radicular symptoms	NSAIDs; physical therapy; surgery for refractory cases or for cord compression in athletes who participate in contact sports
Ligamentous sprain, muscular strain	Aggressive bending or rotation forces	Axial pain, may manifest in a delayed manner over 24 hours	Exclude fracture/instability; ice, NSAIDs, and physical therapy

Cervical Injury

Fractures

A variety of cervical spine fractures occur in the athletic setting (**Table 1**). Spinous process fractures are relatively benign and often represent avulsion injuries resulting from forceful contraction of the trapezius and rhomboid muscles. Compression fractures can be caused by relatively low-energy mechanisms of injury as well. In higher-energy collisions, the position of the cervical spine and the direction of loading influence injury patterns. When the neck is in neutral alignment, the cervical spine is lordotic and energy inputs can be dissipated somewhat by the intervertebral disks and paraspinal muscles. Biomechanical analysis has suggested that with flexion of approximately

30°, the straightened cervical spine assumes the physical characteristics of a segmented column.[25] Axially applied force is directly transmitted to the spinal structures. When the threshold of vertical compression is reached, the cervical spine fails and buckles in a flexion mode with anterior column failure and possible facet subluxation or dislocation.[25]

Spinal Cord Injury

Acute spinal cord injury in the athletic setting typically occurs by the mechanisms previously described. If an injured player sustains an apparent or suspected spinal cord injury, the on-the-field management protocol previously described should be followed for initial treatment. Efforts to maintain oxygenation and blood pressure to maximize spinal cord perfusion should be initiated during transport to the hospital.[26] High-dose methylprednisolone use and induction of systemic hypothermia remain controversial. After initial resuscitation, the injured player should be transported to a tertiary referral trauma center where prompt reestablishment of spinal alignment and neurologic decompression can be performed via closed or open methods.

Cervical cord neurapraxia, also referred to as transient quadriparesis, can occur as a result of forced hyperflexion or hyperextension in a stenotic canal. Symptoms, which last from a few minutes to 48 hours, range from mild paresthesias in more than one extremity to transient quadriplegia. Neck pain is minimal to nonexistent in the absence of structural injury to the spinal column. Injured players who have these findings are immobilized until instability is excluded on imaging studies. Recurrence of cervical cord neurapraxia has been reported in up to 50% of cases, with the risk correlating to the extent of canal stenosis.[27] The risk of a later, sustained catastrophic spinal cord injury in athletes who sustain cervical cord neurapraxia has been debated, with at least one report of quadriplegia in an athlete who had previously experienced cervical cord neurapraxia.[27,28] Spear tackler's spine is diagnosed based on radiographic findings of reversal of lordosis, evidence of previous vertebral injury, and cervical stenosis in a football player who frequently uses the tackling technique involving leading with the head (spearing) (**Figure 3**).

Stingers

Stingers or burners are caused by neurapraxia of one or more ipsilateral cervical nerve roots or the brachial plexus, resulting in pain, paresthesias, and weakness in a single upper extremity. The player usually reports tingling and burning radiating from the neck into the arm. Physically immature athletes may sustain this injury by a combination of lateral bending of the neck and depression of the contralateral shoulder, resulting in traction to the upper cervical nerve roots or the brachial plexus trunk. Physically mature athletes can experience similar symptoms caused by axial loading of an extended, rotated, or laterally bent cervical spine causing neuroforaminal compression. This latter presentation is more common in athletes with preexisting degenerative changes and may result in more severe symptoms.

A stinger can be distinguished from cervical cord neurapraxia by its unilateral features and absence of long tract signs. Patients who have stingers resulting from a traction mechanism of injury typically have a negative Spurling test. If radiculopathy is suspected based on clinical features, advanced imaging studies can help confirm

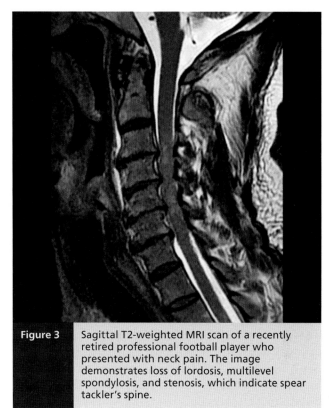

Figure 3 | Sagittal T2-weighted MRI scan of a recently retired professional football player who presented with neck pain. The image demonstrates loss of lordosis, multilevel spondylosis, and stenosis, which indicate spear tackler's spine.

the diagnosis. Traction-induced neurapraxias typically resolve within 2 weeks. An oral steroid taper may provide symptomatic relief. Persistent symptoms may suggest higher grade injury such as axonotmesis or neurotmesis. The use of electrodiagnostic studies and the involvement of a hand or microvascular specialist are helpful in these difficult cases.[29]

Disk Herniation

Although disk herniation resulting from degenerative changes in the spine is common in the general population, axial loading of the neck during sports activities may contribute to disk herniation in athletes. Disk herniation may result in isolated neck pain, or it may be accompanied by radicular symptoms. Athletes with persistent symptoms should be evaluated with MRI. The initial management of disk herniation in athletes is similar to that for the general population for management of axial pain and isolated root compression. Surgical treatment of patients with findings of cord compression and intrinsic signal changes on MRI has been favored, particularly in patients who play contact sports. Effacement of the spinal cord can be managed nonsurgically, but repeat imaging should be performed to exclude cord compression in symptomatically improved athletes before they return to sports activities.[30] Several factors should be considered in selecting an appropriate surgical procedure, including the location of the pathology (central versus foraminal), the number of levels involved, and the athlete's desire to return to the sport. Certain procedures may preclude a safe return to play; however, this consideration should not encourage the surgeon to perform a procedure with a decreased likelihood of clinical success.

Musculoligamentous Injuries

Muscular and ligamentous injuries are common sports-related injuries. Ligamentous sprain or muscular strain can occur after aggressive bending or rotational injuries to the neck. Pain may not be immediate; instead, it may manifest over the 24-hour period after injury. Tenderness is typically seen on palpation, and range of motion may be limited by patient guarding. Radiographs typically yield minimal findings such as loss of lordosis. CT or MRI may be necessary to exclude occult fracture or ligamentous injury. If necessary, a collar should be used until ligamentous injury is definitively ruled out. Treatment should focus on management of pain and inflammation with ice, NSAIDs, and muscle relaxants if necessary. Active range of motion and strengthening exercises can be initiated as pain improves. Formal physical therapy may be helpful if recovery does not progress quickly. Athletes should be asymptomatic and display normal strength and range of motion before resuming sports-related activities.

Return to Play

No major sporting association has adopted a policy specifically regarding return to play after cervical injury. The decision regarding return to play is complex because of the heterogeneity of the involved pathoanatomy. Although some guidelines on return to play have been offered (**Table 2**), no high-level evidence exists to support the recommendations.[31] The primary goal of deciding whether to clear a patient with cervical injury to return to play is to identify whether the athlete would be subject to increased risk of additional injury on return to sports-related activity. The basic prerequisites for return to play include normal strength, pain-free range of motion, spinal stability, and adequate canal space for the spinal cord.

The Torg ratio, or spinal canal diameter relative to vertebral body diameter, can be calculated based on measurements obtained from a lateral radiograph. The Torg ratio is helpful in determining whether an athlete has cervical stenosis. A value higher than 0.8 was previously used as a threshold for allowing an athlete to return to contact sports. Subsequent studies suggest that the Torg ratio may have inadequate predictive value for determining future injury. Currently, MRI assessment of functional stenosis is recommended to assess not only canal dimensions but also cord diameter and the amount of buffering cerebrospinal fluid.[32] Patients who experience a single episode of cervical cord neurapraxia and whose MRI findings indicate severe stenosis or patients who experience a recurrence of cervical cord neurapraxia should be precluded from returning to contact sports, irrespective of the degree of recovery. Athletes with mild or moderate stenosis and no findings of parenchymal injury, whose symptoms resolve quickly, may be considered relatively contraindicated to return to contact sports. The final decision regarding return to play should consider the degree of stenosis and the propensity for injury during the intended sports activity.

Athletes who undergo one- or two-level instrumented fusion of the subaxial spine and who demonstrate radiographically confirmed fusion are relatively contraindicated for return to play. These athletes must demonstrate full painless range of motion before return to play can be considered. Several studies have indicated that professional American football players and baseball players can return to their sport at or near their preoperative performance level.[33] One study, however, reported an increased risk of adjacent-segment disease above or below the fusion.[34] Fusion of three or more levels should preclude athletes from returning to contact sports. Occipitocervical and atlantoaxial fusion, whether postoperative or congenital (Klippel-Feil syndrome), also are considered absolute contraindications to return to contact sports.[35] Posterior cervical laminoforaminotomy may allow athletes to return to contact sports provided their inciting symptoms have resolved completely and they regain full strength and painless range of motion.[24] Currently, data are insufficient to offer guidelines on return to contact sports after cervical disk arthroplasty.

Thoracic and Lumbar Injuries

Thoracic Injury

Compared with injuries to the cervical and lumbar spine in athletes, thoracic spine injuries are relatively uncommon because of the increased biomechanical support provided by the ribs, sternum, and costal cartilage with associated ligamentous structures (**Table 3**). However, thoracic spine injuries tend to be missed and are associated with the potential for catastrophic outcomes if not identified and managed. The transitional cervicothoracic and thoracolumbar zones are especially vulnerable to unstable injury patterns.

Thoracic spine injuries can involve concomitant rib fractures, pneumothorax, or visceral injuries, and the Advanced Trauma Life Support protocol should always be observed in the acute setting. A complete neurologic examination is necessary, including assessment of motor

Table 2

Suggested Return-to-Play Criteria

Not Considered Contraindications	Relative Contraindications	Absolute Contraindications
Healed subaxial fracture	Healed upper cervical spine fractures	Healed subaxial fracture with deformity
Asymptomatic spinous process fracture	Three or more stingers	Cord compression after fracture
Single-level subaxial Klippel-Feil anomaly	Stinger with residual symptoms	C1-C2 instability
One or two stingers	Cervical cord neurapraxia with symptoms >24 hours	Continued cervical axial pain, decreased range of motion or neurologic deficit
Single episode of cervical cord neurapraxia	Two-level anterior cervical fusion	Multilevel Klippel-Feil anomaly
Laminoforaminotomy	Posterior thoracic fusions not crossing the cervicothoracic or thoracolumbar junction	Occipitocervical assimilation
Single-level subaxial cervical fusion	Posterolateral fusion for spondylolisthesis or degenerative disk disease	Ankylosing spondylitis
Single-level lumbar microdiskectomy	Multilevel lumbar microdiskectomies	Diffuse idiopathic skeletal hyperostosis
Direct pars repair for spondylolysis	Healed lumbar compression fractures	Cervical fusion at three or more levels
Single-level lumbar total disk arthroplasty		C1-C2 fusion
Single or multilevel lumbar laminectomy		Symptomatic cervical disk herniation
Healed lumbar spinous process, transverse process, and facet fractures		Multiple instances of cervical cord neurapraxia
		Cervical myelopathy
		Cervical laminectomy
		Spear tackler's spine
		Thoracic fusions crossing the cervicothoracic or thoracolumbar junctions
		Multilevel lumbar fusions
		Nonunion following single-level or multilevel lumbar fusion

and sensory function, rectal examination, assessment of deep tendon reflexes, and assessment for the bulbocavernosus reflex. Radiographic workup should include AP and lateral views of the thoracic spine in addition to a CT scan, which has replaced plain radiographs as a screening study in most trauma centers. Indications for MRI include any neurologic deficit and suspicion for ligamentous or soft-tissue injury, such as the presence of interspinous widening on a lateral radiograph or CT.

Musculoligamentous injuries occur as a result of overuse in sports such as rowing, golf, and throwing sports, but they also occur as a result of acute, higher-energy injuries. Symptom onset can be delayed as a result of inflammation, and management is almost always nonsurgical, consisting of rest, active and passive exercise, and NSAIDs. Injections can be useful in managing refractory injuries but are generally not indicated. Advanced imaging, including CT or MRI, may be necessary to rule

Table 3

Summary of Sports-Related Injuries to the Thoracolumbar Spine

Injury	Sports Mechanism	Prominent Symptoms	Treatment Recommendations
Thoracic or lumbar musculoligamentous	Overuse or acute strain	Back pain, muscle spasms	If symptomatic, NSAIDs, physical therapy
Thoracic disk herniation	Combined bending and torsional forces	Back pain, intercostal radiating pain, spinal cord injury, myelopathy	Initial rest, NSAIDs, injections, surgery for cord compression or myelopathy
Thoracic fracture	Axial load, distraction, direct blow	Back pain, spinal cord injury	Bracing for stable patterns, surgery for unstable (posterior ligamentous disruption, cord compression, kyphosis)
Lumbar fracture	Axial load, distraction, direct blow	Low back pain, nerve root injury, radicular pain, cauda equina syndrome	Bracing for stable injuries, surgery for unstable or neurologic deficits
Lumbar disk herniation	Combined flexion and compression	Low back pain, radicular pain, cauda equina syndrome	Initial rest, NSAIDs, exercise program. Surgery for refractory pain or progressive neurologic deficit
Lumbar spondylolysis	Repetitive extension and torsional bending	Low back pain, hamstring tightness, referred buttock or leg pain	Bracing and graduated exercise program, pars repair or fusion for refractory cases
Lumbar spondylolisthesis	Repetitive extension and torsional bending	Low back pain, hamstring tightness, radicular pain (L5 most common)	Physical therapy, bracing, fusion for progressive slip >50% or neurologic deficit, failure of nonsurgical treatment

out bony or ligamentous injuries, and return to play is based on resolution of symptoms. Thoracic disk herniations resulting from sports injuries are considerably less common than disk herniations in the cervical or lumbar spine,[36] and typically occur in the lower one-third of the thoracic spine.[37] MRI is diagnostic, and symptoms of disk herniation may include axial pain, radiculopathy (radiating to the anterior chest wall), and myelopathy as well as acute spinal cord injury. Most thoracic disk herniations respond well to nonsurgical management. Compression fractures, burst fractures, and fracture-dislocations in the thoracic spine secondary to sports injuries are uncommon. Management of these uncommon injuries is similar to that of injuries resulting from other mechanisms.

Lumbar Injury
Low Back Pain in Athletes
Low back pain is common in the general population, presenting in most adults at some point in their lifetime.[38] Although athletes are generally in better physical condition and possess greater flexibility than the general population, athletes place substantially greater loads on the lumbar spine, including repetitive flexion, extension, and axial loading.[39] Some studies also have shown a higher incidence of degenerative disk changes in elite athletes than in the general population, with L5-S1 being the most commonly affected level.[40]

Evaluation of low back pain in the athlete begins with a thorough history and physical examination to determine the source of the symptoms. Pain with extension often is associated with spondylolysis and posterior facet injuries, whereas pain with flexion is often discogenic. A thorough neurologic examination is required, and a history of any loss of bowel or bladder function should prompt urgent imaging to rule out compression of the cauda equina. Upright AP and lateral radiographs are obtained. MRI may be necessary if plain radiographs do not provide a specific diagnosis or if radicular pain or neurologic deficit is suspected. MRI is useful in the detection of a pars stress reaction in the absence of findings on plain radiography, and MRI has been recommended as a better initial study than CT because of the lack of ionizing radiation to the patient.[41]

In patients who have acute trauma resulting from higher-energy mechanisms of injury, CT is recommended to assess for fracture, anterolisthesis, or abnormalities in alignment. CT remains the best imaging modality for evaluating the bony detail of a pars defect or healing of the pars with nonsurgical management. If imaging studies are negative for underlying structural pathology, muscular or ligamentous strain is the likely cause of low back pain, and a brief course of rest and NSAIDs is indicated, followed by a short course of strengthening and flexibility exercises prior to return to play.

Fracture

Lumbar spine fractures in the athlete can be broadly characterized as minor fractures occurring with lower-energy trauma or repetitive activity, or as major fractures capable of causing substantial instability or neurologic deficit. Major fractures are rare. Fractures involving one column of the spine, such as isolated spinous process, transverse process, or vertebral body compression fractures, are generally stable and require symptomatic management only, including a brief period of rest, NSAIDs, muscle relaxants, and bracing. Return to play is guided by resolution of symptoms and a progressive rehabilitation program involving sport-specific activity and restoration of full painless range of motion. Major fractures, which occur primarily in collision sports such as skiing or snowboarding, include burst fractures, fracture-dislocations, and other potentially unstable three-column injuries. Isolated facet fractures are generally managed with a brace if the fracture is unilateral and no associated vertebral body fracture is present. Surgical management may prevent return to play at an elite level, but few data exist to guide treatment.

Spondylolysis and Spondylolisthesis

Spondylolysis, or defects of the pars interarticularis, is common in young athletes and has been reported in up to 47% of young athletes who have low back pain.[42] The most common sports associated with defects of the pars interarticularis are soccer, gymnastics, and football, with injury resulting from repetitive extension and twisting forces applied to the lumbar spine. Patients often experience low back pain that is worse with extension and that may be unilateral. Associated neurologic deficits are rare, unless a higher grade of spondylolisthesis is present, typically in the L5 distribution. Initial workup includes weight-bearing radiographs of the lumbar spine. Although oblique radiographic views were historically recommended to increase visualization of the pars, this practice has become less common because of the increased radiation and low sensitivity.[43] MRI has replaced CT as the initial advanced imaging modality of choice because of the lack of radiation to the athlete and the ability to detect pars edema (stress reaction) not visualized on initial plain radiographs or CT.[44]

Most pars defects are bilateral (85%) and are more likely than unilateral defects to progress to spondylolisthesis.[39] For most acute pars defects or stress reactions, nonsurgical management consisting of a full-time Boston brace for 8 to 12 weeks in addition to a graduated exercise program is sufficient. Surgery may be considered for athletes who have recurrent symptoms after bracing, pain lasting at least 6 months, pain that precludes return to sport, or progressive spondylolisthesis (greater than 50% slip). Pars repair with thorough débridement of the fibrous defect is appropriate if the associated disk is normal, and anterior or posterior fusion is considered in the presence of grade II or higher anterolisthesis or substantial disk degeneration. Return to play is possible at 6 to 12 months postoperatively, but patients should be counseled that lumbar fusion may be a career-ending treatment. Many surgeons allow return to noncontact sports only.

Lumbar Disk Herniation

Lumbar disk herniation is most common in athletes younger than 35 years and those who participate in sports with repetitive flexion and compression movements, such as football, wrestling, hockey, tennis, and golf. Patients commonly report prodromal low back pain followed by radicular pain that is sometimes accompanied by a neurologic deficit. Cauda equina syndrome is rare but should be ruled out. Signs of nerve root tension on examination should prompt imaging of the lumbar spine, including weight-bearing radiographs and MRI.

The overall prognosis of patients who have lumbar disk herniation is favorable, with one large study of 342 professional athletes reporting that athletes successfully returned to play 82% of the time.[45] Most athletes with lumbar disk herniation can be treated successfully with nonsurgical techniques consisting of early activity and core-strengthening protocols, with a gradual return to sport-specific activity. Epidural corticosteroid injections may help speed recovery; however, data to support this treatment are limited. Surgical management generally consists of laminotomy and disk fragment excision, although several studies have found approximately equivalent return-to-play rates after surgical management (mean, 80%) compared with nonsurgical management.[45,46] Minimally invasive surgical techniques are promising, because decreased manipulation of soft tissues may result in quicker recovery times in athletes. However, data regarding outcomes after minimally invasive surgery are lacking. Among elite athletes, time to recovery after lumbar diskectomy ranges from 3 to 9 months, with a mean 3 to 5 years of career length postoperatively.[47]

Return to Play After Thoracolumbar Injuries

In general, return to play after most lumbar spine injuries is dependent on resolution of symptoms, restoration of complete range of motion, and demonstration of sport-specific movements in a practice environment without experiencing recurrent symptoms. As previously noted, return-to-play rates for athletes undergoing surgical treatment of lumbar disk herniation are high and are comparable to those in athletes undergoing nonsurgical treatment. A successful return-to-play rate of 80% was reported in a study of adolescent athletes who underwent nonsurgical treatment for lumbar spondylolysis.[48] Four to 12 weeks of rest and immobilization is recommended.[49] Although return to play at the preinjury level 6 to 12 months postoperatively is possible,[50] return to contact sports is less predictable after fusion for spondylolysis and spondylolisthesis. In general, up to 12 months of rehabilitation may be required for select patients who are able to return to play after lumbar fusion.

Summary

Spine injuries in athletes can range from minor sprains and strains to catastrophic spinal cord injury. Team physicians and consultants should develop a comprehensive management protocol to address on-the-field injuries. The ability to return to play varies because of the heterogeneity of involved pathoanatomy and the consequences of necessary treatments. The risk for further injury after return to play should be the primary consideration in the decision-making process.

Key Study Points

- Team physicians should develop a checklist and a comprehensive algorithm for management of on-the-field spine injuries in advance of game day.
- Stingers and burners involve a unilateral upper extremity, and symptoms are usually self-limited. Symptoms involving more than one extremity suggest a more substantial neurapraxia of the cervical cord.
- The most common sports associated with lumbar spondylolysis are soccer, gymnastics, and football, as a result of the repetitive extension and twisting forces applied to the lumbar spine.
- Three-level cervical fusion, occipitocervical fusion, and atlantoaxial fusion are generally regarded as contraindications to return to contact sports.

Annotated References

1. Pleis JR, Ward BW, Lucas JW: Summary health statistics for U.S. adults: National Health Interview Survey, 2009. National Center for Health Statistics. Vital Health Stat 10(249). 2010. Available at: https://www.cdc.gov/nchs/data/series/sr_10/sr10_249.pdf. Accessed February 17, 2017.

2. Chan CW, Eng JJ, Tator CH, Krassioukov A; Spinal Cord Injury Research Evidence Team: Epidemiology of sport-related spinal cord injuries: A systematic review. J Spinal Cord Med 2016;39(3):255-264.

   This systematic review of the published worldwide literature reports on the epidemiology of sports-related spinal cord injury. Individual sports with the highest risk for spinal cord injury and the most common level of injury for various sports are reported.

3. Shankar PR, Fields SK, Collins CL, Dick RW, Comstock RD: Epidemiology of high school and collegiate football injuries in the United States, 2005–2006. Am J Sports Med 2007;35(8):1295-1303.

4. Dick R, Ferrara MS, Agel J, et al: Descriptive epidemiology of collegiate men's football injuries: National Collegiate Athletic Association injury surveillance system, 1988-1989 through 2003-2004. J Athl Train 2007;42(2):221-233.

5. Mall NA, Buchowski J, Zebala L, Brophy RH, Wright RW, Matava MJ: Spine and axial skeleton injuries in the National Football League. Am J Sports Med 2012;40(8):1755-1761.

   A retrospective analysis of 11 seasons of data from the National Football League injury surveillance database identifies characteristics of spinal injuries. Blocking and tackling were found to be the most frequent mechanisms of injury.

6. Brophy RH, Barnes R, Rodeo SA, Warren RF: Prevalence of musculoskeletal disorders at the NFL Combine: Trends from 1987 to 2000. *Med Sci Sports Exerc* 2007;39(1):22-27.

7. Cantu RC, Mueller FO: Catastrophic spine injuries in American football, 1977-2001. *Neurosurgery* 2003;53(2):358-362, discussion 362-363.

8. DeVivo MJ, Sekar P: Prevention of spinal cord injuries that occur in swimming pools. *Spinal Cord* 1997;35(8):509-515.

9. Amorim EC, Vetter H, Mascarenhas LB, Gomes EG, Carvalho JB, Gomes JF: Spine trauma due to diving: Main features and short-term neurological outcome. *Spinal Cord* 2011;49(2):206-210.

   This retrospective study of data collected at a Brazilian trauma center over a 15-year period found that 10.6% of patients sustained a spine injury as the result of diving; 32% had complete neurologic injuries.

10. Flik K, Lyman S, Marx RG: American collegiate men's ice hockey: An analysis of injuries. *Am J Sports Med* 2005;33(2):183-187.

11. Tator CH, Provvidenza C, Cassidy JD: Spinal injuries in Canadian ice hockey: An update to 2005. *Clin J Sport Med* 2009;19(6):451-456.

12. Banerjee R, Palumbo MA, Fadale PD: Catastrophic cervical spine injuries in the collision sport athlete: Part 1. Epidemiology, functional anatomy, and diagnosis. *Am J Sports Med* 2004;32(4):1077-1087.

13. Quarrie KL, Cantu RC, Chalmers DJ: Rugby union injuries to the cervical spine and spinal cord. *Sports Med* 2002;32(10):633-653.

14. Quarrie KL, Gianotti SM, Hopkins WG, Hume PA: Effect of nationwide injury prevention programme on serious spinal injuries in New Zealand rugby union: Ecological study. *BMJ* 2007;334(7604):1150-1153.

15. Gertzbein SD, Khoury D, Bullington A, St. John TA, Larson AI: Thoracic and lumbar fractures associated with skiing and snowboarding injuries according to the AO Comprehensive Classification. *Am J Sports Med* 2012;40(8):1750-1754.

    This retrospective study reports on thoracic and lumbar spinal injuries resulting from skiing or snowboarding seen at an alpine trauma center over a 5-year period. Compression fractures and fractures of the spinous or transverse processes were the most common injuries.

16. Franz T, Hasler RM, Benneker L, Zimmermann H, Siebenrock KA, Exadaktylos AK: Severe spinal injuries in alpine skiing and snowboarding: A 6-year review of a tertiary trauma centre for the Bernese Alps ski resorts, Switzerland. *Br J Sports Med* 2008;42(1):55-58.

17. Wakahara K, Matsumoto K, Sumi H, Sumi Y, Shimizu K: Traumatic spinal cord injuries from snowboarding. *Am J Sports Med* 2006;34(10):1670-1674.

18. Jackson DW, Wiltse LL, Cirincione RJ: Spondylolysis in the female gymnast. *Clin Orthop Relat Res* 1976;117:68-73.

19. Mueller FO, Cantu RC: *National Center for Catastrophic Sports Injury Research: Twenty-Third Annual Report. Fall 1982-Spring 2005*. Chapel Hill, NC, National Center for Catastrophic Sports Injury Research, 2005.

20. Torg JS, Quedenfeld TC, Burstein A, Spealman A, Nichols C III: National football head and neck injury registry: Report on cervical quadriplegia, 1971 to 1975. *Am J Sports Med* 1979;7(2):127-132.

21. Stuart MJ, Smith AM, Malo-Ortiguera SA, Fischer TL, Larson DR: A comparison of facial protection and the incidence of head, neck, and facial injuries in Junior A hockey players: A function of individual playing time. *Am J Sports Med* 2002;30(1):39-44.

22. Mattera CJ: Spinal trauma: New guidelines for assessment and management in the out-of-hospital environment. *J Emerg Nurs* 1998;24(6):523-534, quiz 535-538.

23. American Academy of Pediatrics, Committee on Injury and Poison Prevention and Committee on Sports Medicine and Fitness: Trampolines at home, school, and recreational centers. *Pediatrics* 1999;103(5 pt 1):1053-1056.

24. Kepler CK, Vaccaro AR: Injuries and abnormalities of the cervical spine and return to play criteria. *Clin Sports Med* 2012;31(3):499-508.

    Current thoughts on preparation and game-day management of sports-related spine injuries are presented in this review article, along with considerations for athletes returning to sports after injury.

25. Chao S, Pacella MJ, Torg JS: The pathomechanics, pathophysiology and prevention of cervical spinal cord and brachial plexus injuries in athletics. *Sports Med* 2010;40(1):59-75.

26. Ryken TC, Hurlbert RJ, Hadley MN, et al: The acute cardiopulmonary management of patients with cervical spinal cord injuries. *Neurosurgery* 2013;72(suppl 2):84-92.

    This study reviews medical evidence on the benefit of blood pressure management on neurologic outcomes after cervical spinal cord injury. For the first 7 days after injury, patients with cervical spine cord injury should be treated in an intensive care setting, and mean arterial pressures of 85 to 90 mm Hg should be maintained.

27. Torg JS, Naranja RJ Jr, Pavlov H, Galinat BJ, Warren R, Stine RA: The relationship of developmental narrowing of the cervical spinal canal to reversible and irreversible injury of the cervical spinal cord in football players. *J Bone Joint Surg Am* 1996;78(9):1308-1314.

8: Special Populations in Spine Care

28. Castro FP Jr: Stingers, cervical cord neurapraxia, and stenosis. *Clin Sports Med* 2003;22(3):483-492.

29. Olson DE, McBroom SA, Nelson BD, Broton MS, Pulling TJ, Olson DE: Unilateral cervical nerve injuries: Brachial plexopathies. *Curr Sports Med Rep* 2007;6(1):43-49.

30. Meredith DS, Jones KJ, Barnes R, Rodeo SA, Cammisa FP, Warren RF: Operative and nonoperative treatment of cervical disc herniation in National Football League athletes. *Am J Sports Med* 2013;41(9):2054-2058.

   The records kept by a single National Football League team and its consulting physicians over an 11-year period are reviewed to analyze the treatment outcomes of cervical disk herniations incurred by the athletes. Cord compression with signal changes was a consistent surgical indication. Level of evidence: IV.

31. Huang P, Anissipour A, McGee W, Lemak L: Return-to-play recommendations after cervical, thoracic, and lumbar spine injuries: A comprehensive review. *Sports Health* 2016;8(1):19-25.

   The authors present a review of the available literature regarding return-to-play guidelines after spine injuries. Although some general principles have wide agreement, specific guidelines have poor supporting evidence. Level of evidence: IV.

32. Bailes JE: Experience with cervical stenosis and temporary paralysis in athletes. *J Neurosurg Spine* 2005;2(1):11-16.

33. Molinari RW, Pagarigan K, Dettori JR, Molinari R Jr, Dehaven KE: Return to play in athletes receiving cervical surgery: A systematic review. *Global Spine J* 2016;6(1):89-96.

   A systematic review identified nine retrospective studies involving 175 athletes who underwent cervical spine surgery. Two studies reported on recreational athletes, and seven studies reported on professional athletes. Seventy-five percent of professional athletes returned to their sport postoperatively; most of these professional athletes were treated for disk herniation.

34. Maroon JC, Bost JW, Petraglia AL, et al: Outcomes after anterior cervical discectomy and fusion in professional athletes. *Neurosurgery* 2013;73(1):103-112, discussion 112.

   A single surgeon's experience with 15 professional athletes involved in contact sports who underwent single-level anterior cervical diskectomy and fusion is presented. Thirteen players returned to their sport at a mean of 6 months postoperatively.

35. Torg JS, Ramsey-Emrhein JA: Management guidelines for participation in collision activities with congenital, developmental, or postinjury lesions involving the cervical spine. *Clin J Sport Med* 1997;7(4):273-291.

36. Gray BL, Buchowski JM, Bumpass DB, Lehman RA Jr, Mall NA, Matava MJ: Disc herniations in the National Football League. *Spine (Phila Pa 1976)* 2013;38(38):1934-1938.

   This retrospective review of the National Football League surveillance database over a 12-year period was done to determine the incidence, location, and type of disk herniations in professional football players. Of 275 disk herniations, 76% were in the lumbar spine. Further characteristics of cervical, thoracic, and lumbar disk herniations were reviewed, focusing on mechanism of injury, player position, and lost playing time.

37. Vanichkachorn JS, Vaccaro AR: Thoracic disk disease: Diagnosis and treatment. *J Am Acad Orthop Surg* 2000;8(3):159-169.

38. Dreisinger TE, Nelson B: Management of back pain in athletes. *Sports Med* 1996;21(4):313-320.

39. Lawrence JP, Greene HS, Grauer JN: Back pain in athletes. *J Am Acad Orthop Surg* 2006;14(13):726-735.

40. Ong A, Anderson J, Roche J: A pilot study of the prevalence of lumbar disc degeneration in elite athletes with lower back pain at the Sydney 2000 Olympic Games. *Br J Sports Med* 2003;37(3):263-266.

41. Kobayashi A, Kobayashi T, Kato K, Higuchi H, Takagishi K: Diagnosis of radiographically occult lumbar spondylolysis in young athletes by magnetic resonance imaging. *Am J Sports Med* 2013;41(1):169-176.

   The authors of this prospective cohort study evaluated the use of MRI to identify early, active spondylolysis in adolescent athletes with low back pain and negative or inconclusive radiographic findings; 48.5% of these patients had positive MRI findings indicative of early spondylolysis. The authors concluded that MRI is effective and safe, and they recommend it as a first-line diagnostic study in this patient population. Level of evidence: III.

42. Micheli LJ, Wood R: Back pain in young athletes: Significant differences from adults in causes and patterns. *Arch Pediatr Adolesc Med* 1995;149(1):15-18.

43. Beck NA, Miller R, Baldwin K, et al: Do oblique views add value in the diagnosis of spondylolysis in adolescents? *J Bone Joint Surg Am* 2013;95(10):e65.

   This retrospective cohort study evaluated the radiographs of patients with L5 spondylolysis without spondylolisthesis and a control group of healthy subjects. No significant difference was found in sensitivity or specificity between four-view (with oblique views) and two-view (AP and lateral only) radiographs. The authors concluded that the increased radiation and cost of adding oblique images are not worthwhile.

44. Campbell RS, Grainger AJ, Hide IG, Papastefanou S, Greenough CG: Juvenile spondylolysis: A comparative analysis of CT, SPECT and MRI. *Skeletal Radiol* 2005;34(2):63-73.

45. Hsu WK, McCarthy KJ, Savage JW, et al: The Professional Athlete Spine Initiative: Outcomes after lumbar disc herniation in 342 elite professional athletes. *Spine J* 2011;11(3):180-186.

   A large, retrospective cohort study examines treatment outcomes of professional athletes who underwent non-surgical or surgical treatment for lumbar disk herniation. Only athletes who were followed for at least 2 years were included in the study. The study reports on return to play, length of professional athletic career after treatment, and sport-specific trends.

46. Hsu WK: Performance-based outcomes following lumbar discectomy in professional athletes in the National Football League. *Spine (Phila Pa 1976)* 2010;35(12):1247-1251.

47. Nair R, Kahlenberg CA, Hsu WK: Outcome of lumbar discectomy in elite athletes: The need for high-level evidence. *Clin Orthop Relat Res* 2015;473(6):1971-1977.

   The authors present a literature review of 66 years of data in MEDLINE and EMBASE evaluating outcomes in elite athletes undergoing lumbar diskectomy for lumbar disk herniation. The recovery period, percentage of baseline preoperative function, and career length after surgery are detailed and provide guidance for orthopaedic surgeons who care for this patient population.

48. d'Hemecourt PA, Zurakowski D, Kriemler S, Micheli LJ: Spondylolysis: Returning the athlete to sports participation with brace treatment. *Orthopedics* 2002;25(6):653-657.

49. Radcliff KE, Kalantar SB, Reitman CA: Surgical management of spondylolysis and spondylolisthesis in athletes: Indications and return to play. *Curr Sports Med Rep* 2009;8(1):35-40.

50. Cook RW, Hsu WK: Return to play after lumbar spine surgery. *Clin Sports Med* 2016;35(4):609-619.

   Sport-specific return-to-play recommendations are reviewed for athletes who underwent surgical treatment of lumbar disk herniation, degenerative disk disease, spondylolysis, and spondylolisthesis.

8: Special Populations in Spine Care

Chapter 39

Osteoporosis

Amandeep Bhalla, MD   Christopher M. Bono, MD

Abstract

Because of the growing aging population in the United States, osteoporosis and its implications in the management of spinal care is of increasing relevance for the medical community. Spinal fragility fractures attributable to osteoporosis are associated with substantial morbidity and mortality. To adequately educate patients about osteoporotic fracture prevention, it is incumbent on orthopaedic surgeons to understand treatment guidelines and pharmacologic options. Although nonsurgical management of vertebral compression fractures is the mainstay of treatment, cement augmentation procedures can be considered for patients hospitalized for pain and functional impairment. Low bone mineral density warrants unique technical considerations in degenerative and traumatic spinal surgeries.

Keywords: compression fracture; kyphoplasty; vertebroplasty

Introduction

Osteoporosis is characterized by low bone mineral density (BMD) in the setting of normal biochemical bone composition and microscopic structure. It is a metabolic imbalance favoring osteoclast activity and bone resorption over

Dr. Bono or an immediate family member has received nonincome support (such as equipment or services), commercially derived honoraria, or other non-research–related funding (such as paid travel) from United Healthcare and serves as a board member, owner, officer, or committee member of the American Academy of Orthopaedic Surgeons and the North American Spine Society. Neither Dr. Bhalla nor any immediate family member has received anything of value from or has stock or stock options held in a commercial company or institution related directly or indirectly to the subject of this chapter.

osteoblastic bone deposition. The disorder initially affects trabecular or cancellous bone, a predominant component of the vertebral body, predisposing this region to fragility fractures. The occurrence of an osteoporotic spine fracture is associated with an increased risk of mortality within 1 to 3 years after the fracture, which is similar to the risk engendered by a fragility hip fracture. Compression fractures also are frequently associated with progressive spinal deformity, chronic back pain, and decreased health-related quality of life.

The prevention of fractures includes patient counseling on the risks of osteoporosis and advising a diet that includes adequate calcium intake (1,000 mg/d for men aged 50 to 70 years; 1,200 mg/d for women aged 51 years and older and men aged 71 years and older), and adequate vitamin D intake (800 to 1,000 IU/d) for individuals aged 50 years and older. Weight-bearing and muscle-strengthening exercises improve balance and agility while decreasing the risk of falls and maintaining bone strength. The American Academy of Orthopaedic Surgeons (AAOS) recommends that orthopaedic surgeons be proactive in the prevention and treatment of osteoporosis. While treating fragility fractures, orthopaedic surgeons are uniquely positioned to initiate counseling and treatment, particularly for patients with poor bone quality noted at the time of surgery or those who have sustained a fragility fracture in the setting of osteopenia.

Epidemiology and Genetics

The overall prevalence of osteoporosis in the United States is estimated to be 10.3%; 54 million older adults (>50 years of age) in the United States have either low bone mass or frank osteoporosis.[1] Approximately 30% of postmenopausal women in the United States have osteoporosis.[2] Epidemiologic studies maintain that approximately 20% of men and women older than 50 years have at least one vertebral compression deformity, with a prevalence that increases with age, particularly for women.[3] The overall age- and sex-adjusted incidence of vertebral fractures is approximately 117 per 100,000 person-years.[4] Osteoporotic vertebral compression fractures (VCFs) have been

Table 1

World Health Organization Definitions of Normal Bone Density, Osteopenia, and Osteoporosis[a]

Diagnosis	T-score
Normal	≥ –1
Low bone mass (osteopenia)	–1 to –2.5
Osteoporosis	≤ –2.5
Severe osteoporosis	≤ –2.5 with fragility fracture

[a]Based on bone mineral density measurement at the spine, hip, or forearm.

T-score = number of SDs below the mean in healthy young women.

Adapted from Ekman EF: The role of the orthopaedic surgeon in minimizing mortality and morbidity associated with fragility fractures. *J Am Acad Orthop Surg* 2010;18(5):278-285.

Table 2

Summary of National Osteoporosis Foundation Screening Recommendations for Patients Based on Age and Risk Factors

Bone Mineral Density Recommended

Women aged ≥65 years and men aged ≥70 years

Postmenopausal women and men aged 50 to 69 years based on risk factor profile

All patients with a fragility fracture

Vertebral Imaging Recommended

Women >70 years and men ≥80 years

Women aged 65 to 69 years and men aged 75 to 79 years if bone mineral density is ≤–1.5

Postmenopausal women and men aged 50 to 69 years with a low energy fracture, previous height loss ≥4 cm, prospective height loss ≥0.8 cm, or recent/long-term treatment with glucocorticoids

Adapted from Lehman RA Jr, Kang DG, Wagner SC: Management of osteoporosis in spine surgery. *J Am Acad Orthop Surg* 2015;23(4): 253-263.

found to be associated with a higher 5-year mortality rate than fractures involving the proximal femur.[5] The development of another spinal fragility fracture is five times more likely in patients who have one or more vertebral fractures than in patients without a history of osteoporotic spine fracture.[6] Factors that place men at a particularly high risk for sustaining an additional fracture include two or more vertebral fractures, morphometric variations in the fractured vertebral body, simultaneous fractures in the thoracic and lumbar regions, and fractures with severe vertebral body compression.[7]

Genetic studies have shown vertebral BMD and fracture risk may be heritable.[8] Increased attention has been placed on identifying genetic variants that might impart susceptibility to fragility fractures. Genome-wide meta-analyses of lumbar spine BMD have revealed associations between the *SLC1A3* and the *EPHB2* genes and vertebral insufficiency fractures.[9]

Pharmacologic Treatment

Screening and Timing

In addition to measuring BMD with a dual-energy x-ray absorptiometry (DEXA) scan (**Table 1**), some osteoporosis guidelines advocate screening with spinal imaging for fracture risk assessment to determine the need for initiation of pharmacologic treatment.[10] The 2014 National Osteoporosis Foundation guidelines suggest spine imaging should be considered for women aged 70 years or older and for men aged 80 years or older if their DEXA T-score at the lumbar spine or hip is –1.0 or less. Imaging should be performed in women aged 65 to 69 years and men aged 70 to 79 years with a BMD of –1.5 or less at the lumbar spine, femoral neck, or total hip. Postmenopausal women and men at least 50 years of age with a fragility fracture during adulthood, a height loss of 4 cm based on patient history, a prospectively measured height loss of 2 cm, and/or recent or ongoing long-term glucocorticoid treatment also should be evaluated with imaging[11] (**Table 2**). If a fracture is detected, treatment for osteoporosis should be initiated.

A fracture risk assessment tool known as FRAX was developed by the World Health Organization to calculate the 10-year probability of hip fracture or major osteoporotic fracture (ie, a clinically important spine, hip, forearm, or shoulder fracture) using established risk factors for osteoporosis as well as BMD measured at the femoral neck.[12] FRAX often is used to establish an intervention threshold in patients who have not yet had a fragility fracture. FRAX–based treatment guidelines have been determined using either a fixed threshold probability that can be applied to men and women irrespective of age or a threshold probability in which the fracture probability and treatment initiation recommendations are specific for age.[13] For the initiation of pharmacologic treatment, guidelines most often use a threshold probability of 20% for a major osteoporotic fracture or a 3% probability for a hip fracture.

However, substantial variations in guidelines remain concerning the recommended timing for osteoporosis treatment. At a minimum, treatment is advocated in individuals with prior fragility fractures, particularly those involving the spine or hip. In addition, pharmacologic treatment is generally indicated in patients with a T score of –2.5 or less.[14]

Therapies

Pharmacologic treatment of osteoporosis involves antiresorptive and anabolic therapies, with the benefit of increasing BMD and decreasing fracture risks. Diphosphonates, a first-line treatment, reduce the rate of bone remodeling and have been shown to decrease the risk of spine fragility fracture.[15] A 15-minute infusion of zoledronic acid administered once per year in women with low BMD, a history of vertebral fracture, or both has been shown to reduce the risk for subsequent vertebral fracture by 70% compared with placebo.[16]

Although widely used and generally considered safe, initiation of diphosphonate therapy warrants clear appreciation of the adverse side effects and complications. Oral diphosphonates infrequently can cause hypocalcemia, gastrointestinal irritation, and myalgia. Intravenous diphosphonate therapy can lead to flulike symptoms as well as an increased risk of atrial fibrillation.[17] Atypical subtrochanteric femur fractures have been associated with prolonged diphosphonate use. Osteonecrosis of the jaw is another well-documented complication known to occur in the setting of diphosphonate therapy.[18] The incidence of osteonecrosis is higher among patients with cancer who are taking higher doses of diphosphonates. Importantly, in 2011, the American Dental Association recommended that osteoporosis treatment does not need to be altered before dental procedures.[19]

The benefit-to-risk ratio of diphosphonate therapy is highly favorable for up to 5 years for women with osteoporosis, with fewer than 1 adverse event caused per 100 fractures prevented.[15,20] Similar treatment data for men with osteoporosis are limited. After discontinuation of the use of diphosphonates such as alendronate or zoledronic acid, there are residual benefits. Thus, taking a so-called drug holiday can minimize adverse side effects while still imparting benefits. A drug holiday can be considered after 5 years of alendronate therapy or after 3 years of zoledronic acid therapy for patients with a lower fracture risk. Therapy is typically reinitiated after no longer than a 5-year hiatus.[14] Interestingly, the residual benefits of zoledronic acid and alendronate therapy after a drug holiday are more protective for preventing nonvertebral fractures; however, there is an increase in osteoporotic VCFs after discontinuation.[21,22] Therefore, the risk-benefit analysis of patients at higher risk of vertebral fracture may favor continuity of diphosphonate use without a drug holiday.

Of note, these drug holiday recommendations do not apply to risedronate or ibandronate.

Denosumab, a monoclonal antibody that binds to the receptor activator of nuclear factor-κ B ligand (RANKL), decreases osteoclast differentiation and has an effect analogous to that of osteoprotegerin. Unlike diphosphonates, it can be used in patients with renal dysfunction. Denosumab has been shown to reduce vertebral fractures by 68% in women with osteoporosis.[23]

Teriparatide, a recombinant human parathyroid hormone, is an anabolic agent that stimulates bone formation. It is administered by daily self-injections and has been shown to reduce the risk of vertebral fractures by 65% in women with low BMD and a history of fracture. Teriparatide does not have the prolonged effects of diphosphonate therapy after discontinuation, so its cessation should generally be followed by substitution with an antiresorptive agent.[24] On the basis of a long-term, high-dose study in rodents, there is a black box warning about the risk of osteosarcoma in patients using teriparatide, although only one case has been reported in more than one million human users.[14]

In postmenopausal women, estrogen and selective estrogen-receptor modulators have a direct effect on osteoblasts and osteoclasts, mitigating bone resorption and contributing to the maintenance of bone formation, with a resultant decrease in fracture risk.[25] Raloxifene is a selective estrogen-receptor modulator that increases spine BMD and has been shown to decrease vertebral fractures by 30%.[26]

In addition to studying new potential pharmacologic treatments, further investigation is needed to determine optimal patient-specific drug selection, whether one agent alone or in combination with others is ideal, and how long treatment should be continued. Novel agents of interest in the treatment of osteoporosis include cathepsin K inhibitor, monoclonal antibodies against sclerostin, and parathyroid hormone-related protein analogues.[27] Abaloparatide, a selective activator of parathyroid hormone type-1 receptor has been shown to reduce the likelihood of new vertebral and nonvertebral fractures in postmenopausal women, with a lower risk of hypercalcemia compared with that of teriparatide.[28]

Osteoporotic Vertebral Fractures

History and Evaluation

The diagnosis of a fracture is made with a thorough clinical history, physical examination, and imaging studies. Patients may report a recent traumatic episode preceding focal back pain and symptoms exacerbated by standing or changing positions. In many situations, however, VCFs

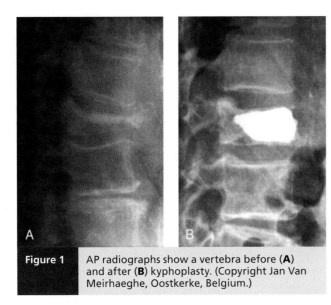

Figure 1 AP radiographs show a vertebra before (**A**) and after (**B**) kyphoplasty. (Copyright Jan Van Meirhaeghe, Oostkerke, Belgium.)

are clinically silent. Physical examination often reveals discrete tenderness to palpation over a spinous process. Examination findings should be correlated with the results of imaging studies, including plain radiographs, CT, or MRI if indicated.

MRI can reveal bony edema consistent with an acute fracture. This is characterized as increased signal within the vertebral body on T2-weighted and short tau inversion recovery MRI sequences and decreased signal (hypointensity) on T1-weighted MRIs. Bone scans, although less specific, also may be used to determine fracture acuity, with increased uptake from higher metabolic activity seen in new fractures. However, bone scans are likely to be positive for longer periods of time after fracture occurrence. As a result, MRI is considered the preferred imaging modality for assessing the acuity of a vertebral insufficiency fracture.

Nonsurgical Management

Nonsurgical, supportive care is the mainstay of treatment of an osteoporotic VCF. Most fractures heal on their own without complications or substantive long-term sequelae. Analgesics can be helpful for pain, with NSAIDs serving as a mainstay of treatment. Although not a widely used medication in the United States, the AAOS guideline for the treatment of symptomatic acute osteoporotic compression fractures has a recommendation for the use of calcitonin, citing studies that show its efficacy in alleviating pain.[29] Narcotics should be used cautiously on a short-term basis for analgesia. Although braces are frequently used as an adjunct to control pain, studies have not demonstrated that brace use accelerates fracture healing or affects the development of postfracture kyphosis.

Treatment of osteoporotic VCFs with a brace also has not been shown to influence long-term clinical outcome measures compared with treatment without a brace.[30]

Surgical Treatment

In recent years, there have been several high-profile investigations evaluating the efficacy and indications for cement augmentation of osteoporotic VCFs. Currently, two types of cement augmentation procedures exist: vertebroplasty and kyphoplasty. Vertebroplasty involves injection of bone cement into a fractured vertebral body to impart stability after the cement cures. Kyphoplasty uses an inflatable balloon to create a void and potentially increase vertebral body height, after which cement is injected (**Figure 1**). Cement augmentation may be indicated for patients hospitalized for pain and functional impairment after osteoporotic spine fractures because of the potential for rapid improvement in pain. By facilitating early mobilization and reducing the length of the hospital stay, surgical intervention in this setting has been shown to be a cost-effective approach.[31]

Contraindications to cement augmentation include asymptomatic fractures, clinical improvement with nonsurgical care, allergies to bone fillers or opacification agents (mixed in the cement to facilitate intraprocedural visualization), local infection, and use in patients with uncorrected coagulopathies. Relative contraindications to surgery include greater than 70% vertebral collapse (eg, vertebral plana), retropulsion of bone fragments into the spinal canal, and neurologic compromise.[32] Complications of cement augmentation include cement leakage, most commonly into the end plate or disk space, adjacent fractures, cement embolization (eg, to the lungs) and, rarely, neurologic impairment from extravasation into the spinal canal.

Citing two independent prospective randomized trials published in 2009 that showed no benefit of vertebroplasty when compared with a sham procedure,[33,34] the AAOS recommended against the use of vertebroplasty for the treatment of osteoporotic spinal compression fractures.[29] In the same guideline, the AAOS offered a limited recommendation for the use of kyphoplasty based on other prospective randomized trials comparing this procedure to more standard nonsurgical care. In a commentary, leadership of the North American Spine Society highlighted several shortcomings of the two 2009 trials, including a lack of clearly defined imaging criteria (such as bone edema detected on MRI) for inclusion in the study. As such, recommendations from the North American Spine Society advocated the use of either vertebroplasty or kyphoplasty as treatment of painful VCFs within 3 months of fracture onset.[35]

More recent trials have been published demonstrating the efficacy of cement augmentation procedures, including vertebroplasty, over nonsurgical management. These studies have demonstrated improved and sustained pain relief and diminished morbidity and mortality with cement augmentation procedures compared with standard nonsurgical management.[36-39] Age-adjusted life expectancy for patients who receive cement augmentation has been reported to be 85% longer than that of nonsurgically treated patients,[40] which likely is related to the decreased physical function in patients treated with standard nonsurgical management. It is important to realize, however, that some of this benefit may be the result of selection bias. Currently, it is generally accepted that cement augmentation is most beneficial for patients with acute pain (less than 3 months) and functional limitations after VCFs in whom appropriate nonsurgical management has been unsuccessful. The use of percutaneous cement augmentation also has been described to provide anterior column support for the surgical treatment of thoracolumbar burst fractures, when performed in conjunction with short segment posterior instrumented stabilization.

Considerations for Spine Surgery in the Setting of Osteoporosis

It is incumbent that orthopaedic surgeons understand the unique challenges associated with the surgical management of spinal disorders in patients with osteoporosis. Approximately 20% to 40% of the geriatric population has spinal hyperkyphosis, which is defined as excessive curvature of the thoracic spine. This condition can be associated with adverse health consequences, including impaired pulmonary and physical function and pain.[41] Osteoporosis is an independent risk factor for revision surgery after adult spinal deformity correction.[42]

Between 2001 and 2011, there was an approximate twofold increase in posterior fusion surgery for spinal deformity in the Medicare population. Surgical treatment typically involves instrumented fusion surgery, which relies on adequate bone quality at the bone-implant interface to permit and maintain correction. Pedicle screw pullout strength and cutout torque are directly proportional to BMD.[43] Osteoporosis contributes to instrumentation failure, pedicle and vertebral fractures, and proximal junctional kyphosis.[44]

Attention has been placed on identifying techniques that can improve fixation in patients with low BMD. Methods to improve the rigidity of fixation constructs include increasing the number of instrumented levels above and below the apex of the deformity and the addition of cross-links between rods. Cement augmentation in

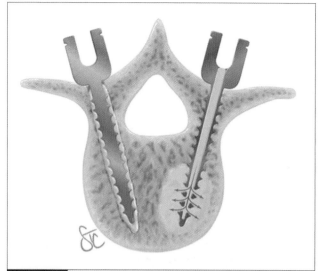

Figure 2 Illustration showing cement augmentation techniques used to improve screw purchase and decrease the risk of fracture or screw pullout. The screw tract can be filled with cement before screw placement (left) or cement can be injected through fenestrations in a cannulated screw (right). (Adapted from Choma TJ, Rechtine GR, McGuire RA, Brodke DS: Treating the aging spine. *J Am Acad Orthop Surg* 2015;23[12]:e91-e100.)

this setting also has gained attention, with the advantage of distributing stress around pedicle screws to decrease the risk of fracture or screw pullout[45] (**Figure 2**). Bone purchase can be improved by increasing screw diameter to enable greater contact with the cortices of the pedicle.

Alternative screw designs have been developed to improve fixation in osteoporotic bone. Manufacturers have designed expandable screws for greater trabecular purchase as well as hydroxyapatite-coated screws to enhance long-term ingrowth. Some intraoperative techniques may further enhance pedicle screw fixation in osteoporotic bone. Fixation strength can be improved by avoiding tapping or undertapping the pedicle screw tract.[46] As an alternative to the traditional transpedicular screw path, the cortical screw trajectory (using a dorsomedial to ventrolateral course) may offer the benefit of increased cortical purchase in osteoporotic bone[47] (**Figure 3**).

In adult spinal deformity surgery, administration of postoperative teriparatide has shown promise in improving volumetric bone density above the upper instrumented vertebra and in reducing the incidence of proximal junctional failure within the vertebral body.[48] Optimization of bone health with vitamin D and calcium supplementation, as well as the use of diphosphonates and teriparatide, are

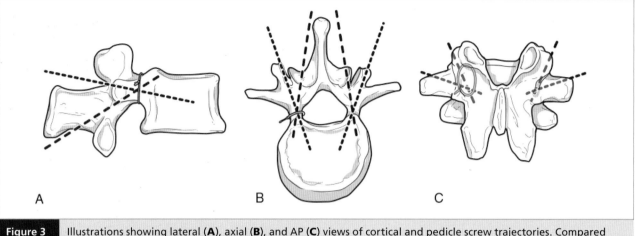

Figure 3 Illustrations showing lateral (**A**), axial (**B**), and AP (**C**) views of cortical and pedicle screw trajectories. Compared with the standard pedicle screw trajectory (dotted line), the cortical screw trajectory (dashed line) has a more medial starting point. The cortical screw trajectory is caudal to cephalad in the sagittal plane and medial to lateral in the axial plane.

important considerations for patients with low BMD undergoing spine surgery.

Summary

The involvement of orthopaedic surgeons in the prevention and treatment of vertebral fragility fractures is important for managing the increasing burden of osteoporosis of the spine. Weight-bearing exercises, fall prevention strategies, adequate calcium and vitamin D intake, appropriate screening, and timely initiation of pharmacologic therapies all play a role in decreasing the risks of these fractures. VCFs are generally treated with symptomatic support. Cement augmentation procedures may be considered in patients with acute fractures with debilitating pain and substantial functional impairment. For spinal surgeries in the setting of low BMD, alternative surgical techniques and implant designs can be considered to achieve adequate fixation.

Key Study Points

- Osteoporotic spinal fractures are associated with substantial morbidity and mortality, and they are increasing in prevalence within the aging US population.
- Patient education, adherence to screening guidelines, and the timely initiation of pharmacologic agents are key to treating patients with osteoporosis.
- Pharmacologic treatment is typically recommended in patients with a BMD T-score of –2.5 or less, a history of spine or hip fracture, or a FRAX score signaling increased fracture risk in the immediate future.
- VCFs are frequently treated successfully using nonsurgical techniques. In the event that nonsurgical management is unsuccessful and the patient has severe pain and/or functional limitations, cement augmentation using vertebroplasty or kyphoplasty remains an option within 3 months of fracture onset.
- Spine surgeons should be aware of the unique challenges associated with the placement of instrumentation in the osteoporotic spine and use available techniques to improve fixation and mitigate failure as deemed appropriate.

Annotated References

1. Wright NC, Looker AC, Saag KG, et al: The recent prevalence of osteoporosis and low bone mass in the United States based on bone mineral density at the femoral neck or lumbar spine. *J Bone Miner Res* 2014;29(11):2520-2526.

   The authors estimated the prevalence of osteoporosis and low bone mass based on BMD at the femoral neck and the lumbar spine in adults 50 years of age or older in the United States.

2. Davies KM, Stegman MR, Heaney RP, Recker RR: Prevalence and severity of vertebral fracture: The Saunders County Bone Quality Study. *Osteoporos Int* 1996;6(2):160-165.

3. Jackson SA, Tenenhouse A, Robertson L: Vertebral fracture definition from population-based data: Preliminary results from the Canadian Multicenter Osteoporosis Study (CaMos). *Osteoporos Int* 2000;11(8):680-687.

4. Cooper C, Atkinson EJ, O'Fallon WM, Melton LJ III: Incidence of clinically diagnosed vertebral fractures: A population-based study in Rochester, Minnesota, 1985-1989. *J Bone Miner Res* 1992;7(2):221-227.

5. Cooper C, Atkinson EJ, Jacobsen SJ, O'Fallon WM, Melton LJ III: Population-based study of survival after osteoporotic fractures. *Am J Epidemiol* 1993;137(9):1001-1005.

6. Lindsay R, Burge RT, Strauss DM: One year outcomes and costs following a vertebral fracture. *Osteoporos Int* 2005;16(1):78-85.

7. Karlsson MK, Kherad M, Hasserius R, et al: Characteristics of prevalent vertebral fractures predict new fractures in elderly men. *J Bone Joint Surg Am* 2016;98(5):379-385.

   This study evaluated characteristics of vertebral fractures in elderly men that may predict subsequent fractures. The authors found that older men with a prevalent fracture have three times the increased risk of sustaining new fractures compared with men without a vertebral fracture. Level of evidence: II.

8. Liu CT, Karasik D, Zhou Y, et al: Heritability of prevalent vertebral fracture and volumetric bone mineral density and geometry at the lumbar spine in three generations of the Framingham study. *J Bone Miner Res* 2012;27(4):954-958.

   This study investigated the genetic contributions to vertebral fracture, vertebral volumetric bone density, and geometry by using quantitative CT scans. It estimated the extent of heritability in adults of European ancestry from three generations of Framingham Heart Study families. Level of evidence: III.

9. Nielson CM, Liu CT, Smith AV, et al: Novel genetic variants associated with increased vertebral volumetric BMD, reduced vertebral fracture risk, and increased expression of SLC1A3 and EPHB2. *J Bone Miner Res* 2016; 31(12):2085-2097.

   This study is the first genome-wide association meta-analysis of lumbar spine volumetric BMD measured by quantitative CT. Genes *SCL1A3* and *EPHB2* were linked to clinically relevant vertebral osteoporosis phenotypes. Level of evidence: III.

10. Papaioannou A, Morin S, Cheung AM, et al; Scientific Advisory Council of Osteoporosis Canada: 2010 clinical practice guidelines for the diagnosis and management of osteoporosis in Canada: Summary. *CMAJ* 2010;182(17):1864-1873.

11. Cosman F, de Beur SJ, LeBoff MS, et al; National Osteoporosis Foundation: Clinician's Guide to Prevention and Treatment of Osteoporosis. *Osteoporos Int* 2014;25(10):2359-2381.

    This guide was developed by a committee of the National Osteoporosis Foundation in collaboration with multispecialty counsel of experts in the field of bone health. It discusses universal recommendations, diagnostic assessment, patient monitoring, and pharmacologic treatment recommendations.

12. Middleton RG, Shabani F, Uzoigwe CE, Shoaib A, Moqsith M, Venkatesan M: FRAX and the assessment of the risk of developing a fragility fracture. *J Bone Joint Surg Br* 2012;94(10):1313-1320.

    The authors describe FRAX, which was developed by the World Health Organization. This tool uses selected risk factors to calculate a quantitative, patient-specific, 10-year risk of sustaining a fragility fracture.

13. Kanis JA, Harvey NC, Cooper C, Johansson H, Odén A, McCloskey EV; Advisory Board of the National Osteoporosis Guideline Group: A systematic review of intervention thresholds based on FRAX: A report prepared for the National Osteoporosis Guideline Group and the International Osteoporosis Foundation. *Arch Osteoporos* 2016;11(1):25.

    This systematic review identified assessment guidelines for osteoporosis that incorporate FRAX. The various interventional thresholds are explored. Level of evidence: III.

14. Black DM, Rosen CJ: Postmenopausal osteoporosis. *N Engl J Med* 2016;374(21):2096-2097.

    This review of postmenopausal osteoporosis discusses treatment guidelines for pharmacologic agents, their benefits, associated complications, and the literature surrounding antiresorptive drug holidays.

15. Crandall CJ, Newberry SJ, Diamant A, et al: Comparative effectiveness of pharmacologic treatments to prevent fractures: An updated systematic review. *Ann Intern Med* 2014;161(10):711-723.

    The authors present a systematic review of the benefits and harms of pharmacologic treatments used to prevent fractures in at-risk adults. Level of evidence: III.

16. Black DM, Delmas PD, Eastell R, et al; HORIZON Pivotal Fracture Trial: Once-yearly zoledronic acid for

treatment of postmenopausal osteoporosis. *N Engl J Med* 2007;356(18):1809-1822.

17. Lyles KW, Colón-Emeric CS, Magaziner JS, et al; for the HORIZON Recurrent Fracture Trial: Zoledronic acid in reducing clinical fracture and mortality after hip fracture. *N Engl J Med* 2007;357(18):1799-1809.

18. Khan AA, Morrison A, Hanley DA, et al; International Task Force on Osteonecrosis of the Jaw: Diagnosis and management of osteonecrosis of the jaw: A systematic review and international consensus. *J Bone Miner Res* 2015;30(1):3-23.

    This article is a systematic review of the literature on the pathophysiology, diagnosis, and treatment of osteonecrosis of the jaw, including a discussion on prevention strategies. Level of evidence: III.

19. Hellstein JW, Adler RA, Edwards B, et al; American Dental Association Council on Scientific Affairs Expert Panel on Antiresorptive Agents: Managing the care of patients receiving antiresorptive therapy for prevention and treatment of osteoporosis: Executive summary of recommendations from the American Dental Association Council on Scientific Affairs. *J Am Dent Assoc* 2011;142(11):1243-1251.

    This review estimates the prevalence of antiresorptive agent-induced osteonecrosis of the jaw to be approximately 0.10%, and concludes that the benefit provided by antiresorptive therapy outweighs the risk of developing this rare complication.

20. Gedmintas L, Solomon DH, Kim SC: Bisphosphonates and risk of subtrochanteric, femoral shaft, and atypical femur fracture: A systematic review and meta-analysis. *J Bone Miner Res* 2013;28(8):1729-1737.

    This systematic review and meta-analysis suggests an increased risk of subtrochanteric, femoral shaft, and atypical femoral fractures in patients undergoing diphosphonate therapy. Level of evidence: III.

21. Black DM, Reid IR, Boonen S, et al: The effect of 3 versus 6 years of zoledronic acid treatment of osteoporosis: A randomized extension to the HORIZON-Pivotal Fracture Trial (PFT). *J Bone Miner Res* 2012;27(2):243-254.

    This study is an extension of a randomized controlled trial on zoledronic acid to investigate the long-term effects (6 years) of this drug on BMD and fracture risk. There was a small difference in bone density in those who continued therapy versus those who stopped the drug after 3 years. The authors concluded that, given zoledronic acid's residual effects, many patients may discontinue therapy for up to 3 years. Level of evidence: I.

22. Black DM, Schwartz AV, Ensrud KE, et al; FLEX Research Group: Effects of continuing or stopping alendronate after 5 years of treatment: The Fracture Intervention Trial Long-term Extension (FLEX). A randomized trial. *JAMA* 2006;296(24):2927-2938.

23. Cummings SR, San Martin J, McClung MR, et al; FREE-DOM Trial: Denosumab for prevention of fractures in postmenopausal women with osteoporosis. *N Engl J Med* 2009;361(8):756-765.

24. Black DM, Bilezikian JP, Ensrud KE, et al; PaTH Study Investigators: One year of alendronate after one year of parathyroid hormone (1-84) for osteoporosis. *N Engl J Med* 2005;353(6):555-565.

25. Cauley JA, Robbins J, Chen Z, et al; Women's Health Initiative Investigators: Effects of estrogen plus progestin on risk of fracture and bone mineral density: The Women's Health Initiative randomized trial. *JAMA* 2003;290(13):1729-1738.

26. Ettinger B, Black DM, Mitlak BH, et al; Multiple Outcomes of Raloxifene Evaluation (MORE) Investigators: Reduction of vertebral fracture risk in postmenopausal women with osteoporosis treated with raloxifene: Results from a 3-year randomized clinical trial. *JAMA* 1999;282(7):637-645.

27. Chan CK, Mason A, Cooper C, Dennison E: Novel advances in the treatment of osteoporosis. *Br Med Bull* 2016;119(1):129-142.

    The authors of this review searched for randomized controlled trials of new therapies for osteoporosis. Cathepsin K inhibitor, monoclonal antibodies against sclerostin, and parathyroid hormone–related protein analog were cited as promising osteoporosis therapies. Level of evidence: III.

28. Miller PD, Hattersley G, Riis BJ, et al; ACTIVE Study Investigators: Effect of abaloparatide vs placebo on new vertebral fractures in postmenopausal women with osteoporosis: A randomized clinical trial. *JAMA* 2016;316(7):722-733.

    The authors sought to determine the efficacy and safety of abaloparatide versus placebo for the prevention of new vertebral fracture in postmenopausal women. They found the study drug reduced the risk of new vertebral and nonvertebral fractures over an 18-month period. Level of evidence: I.

29. American Academy of Orthopaedic Surgeons: *The Treatment of Symptomatic Osteoporotic Spinal Compression Fractures: Guideline and Evidence Report*. Rosemont, IL, American Academy of Orthopaedic Surgeons, September 24, 2010. http://www.aaos.org/Research/guidelines/SCF-guideline.pdf.

30. Kim HJ, Yi JM, Cho HG, et al: Comparative study of the treatment outcomes of osteoporotic compression fractures without neurologic injury using a rigid brace, a soft brace, and no brace: A prospective randomized controlled non-inferiority trial. *J Bone Joint Surg Am* 2014;96(23):1959-1966.

    This prospective randomized controlled trial found that the Oswestry Disability Index scores of patients treated for compression fractures without a brace were not inferior to the scores of those treated with soft or rigid braces. Level of evidence: I.

31. Svedbom A, Alvares L, Cooper C, Marsh D, Ström O: Balloon kyphoplasty compared to vertebroplasty and nonsurgical management in patients hospitalised with acute osteoporotic vertebral compression fracture: A UK cost-effectiveness analysis. *Osteoporos Int* 2013;24(1):355-367.

This study uses a Markov simulation model to evaluate the cost-effectiveness of kyphoplasty for the treatment of patients hospitalized with acute VCFs in the United Kingdom. It was concluded that kyphoplasty may be a cost-effective intervention in this setting, compared with vertebroplasty and nonsurgical management.

32. Savage JW, Schroeder GD, Anderson PA: Vertebroplasty and kyphoplasty for the treatment of osteoporotic vertebral compression fractures. *J Am Acad Orthop Surg* 2014;22(10):653-664.

This is a review article of the published literature discussing vertebroplasty and kyphoplasty for the treatment of osteoporotic VCFs.

33. Kallmes DF, Comstock BA, Heagerty PJ, et al: A randomized trial of vertebroplasty for osteoporotic spinal fractures. *N Engl J Med* 2009;361(6):569-579.

34. Buchbinder R, Osborne RH, Ebeling PR, et al: A randomized trial of vertebroplasty for painful osteoporotic vertebral fractures. *N Engl J Med* 2009;361(6):557-568.

35. Bono CM, Heggeness M, Mick C, Resnick D, Watters WC III: North American Spine Society: Newly released vertebroplasty randomized controlled trials: a tale of two trials. *Spine J* 2010;10(3):238-240.

36. Klazen CA, Lohle PN, de Vries J, et al: Vertebroplasty versus conservative treatment in acute osteoporotic vertebral compression fractures (Vertos II): An open-label randomised trial. *Lancet* 2010;376(9746):1085-1092.

37. Edidin AA, Ong KL, Lau E, Kurtz SM: Morbidity and mortality after vertebral fractures: Comparison of vertebral augmentation and nonoperative management in the Medicare population. *Spine (Phila Pa 1976)* 2015;40(15):1228-1241.

This study in the Medicare population found that patients who underwent vertebral augmentation surgery had lower mortality and overall morbidity than patients treated nonsurgically.

38. Lange A, Kasperk C, Alvares L, Sauermann S, Braun S: Survival and cost comparison of kyphoplasty and percutaneous vertebroplasty using German claims data. *Spine (Phila Pa 1976)* 2014;39(4):318-326.

This observational study examined overall survival and treatment costs for osteoporotic VCFs and suggests a higher overall survival rate for patients undergoing surgical versus nonsurgical treatment. Level of evidence: III.

39. Rousing R, Hansen KL, Andersen MO, Jespersen SM, Thomsen K, Lauritsen JM: Twelve-months follow-up in forty-nine patients with acute/semiacute osteoporotic vertebral fractures treated conservatively or with percutaneous vertebroplasty: A clinical randomized study. *Spine (Phila Pa 1976)* 2010;35(5):478-482.

40. Edidin AA, Ong KL, Lau E, Kurtz SM: Life expectancy following diagnosis of a vertebral compression fracture. *Osteoporos Int* 2013;24(2):451-458.

This study evaluated the life expectancy of patients with VCFs as a function of their treatment. A longer adjusted life expectancy was found for those treated surgically versus those treated nonsurgically. Level of evidence: III.

41. Ailon T, Shaffrey CI, Lenke LG, Harrop JS, Smith JS: Progressive spinal kyphosis in the aging population. *Neurosurgery* 2015;77(suppl 4):S164-S172.

This is a review of the literature on thoracic kyphosis, its associated adverse health consequences, and its implications on adult spinal deformity. Level of evidence: III.

42. Puvanesarajah V, Shen FH, Cancienne JM, et al: Risk factors for revision surgery following primary adult spinal deformity surgery in patients 65 years and older. *J Neurosurg Spine* 2016;25(4):486-493.

This study demonstrates that osteoporosis increases the risk of revision surgery for elderly patients with adult spinal deformity. Level of evidence: III.

43. Paxinos O, Tsitsopoulos PP, Zindrick MR, et al: Evaluation of pullout strength and failure mechanism of posterior instrumentation in normal and osteopenic thoracic vertebrae. *J Neurosurg Spine* 2010;13(4):469-476.

44. DeWald CJ, Stanley T: Instrumentation-related complications of multilevel fusions for adult spinal deformity patients over age 65: Surgical considerations and treatment options in patients with poor bone quality. *Spine (Phila Pa 1976)* 2006;31(19suppl):S144-S151.

45. Pfeifer BA, Krag MH, Johnson C: Repair of failed transpedicle screw fixation: A biomechanical study comparing polymethylmethacrylate, milled bone, and matchstick bone reconstruction. *Spine (Phila Pa 1976)* 1994;19(3):350-353.

46. Goldstein CL, Brodke DS, Choma TJ: Surgical management of spinal conditions in the elderly osteoporotic spine. *Neurosurgery* 2015;77(suppl 4):S98-S107.

This review article discusses the effects of osteoporosis on spinal instrumentation and the evidence that supports the use of various techniques used to address this challenge.

47. Sansur CA, Caffes NM, Ibrahimi DM, et al: Biomechanical fixation properties of cortical versus transpedicular screws in the osteoporotic lumbar spine: An in vitro human cadaveric model. *J Neurosurg Spine* 2016;25(4):467-476.

The authors of this biomechanical cadaver study evaluated the efficacy of cortical spinal fixation as a surgical

8: Special Populations in Spine Care

alternative to transpedicular fixation in the osteoporotic lumbar spine under physiologic loading. Level of evidence: II.

48. Yagi M, Ohne H, Konomi T, et al: Teriparatide improves volumetric bone mineral density and fine bone structure in the UIV+1 vertebra, and reduces bone failure type PJK after surgery for adult spinal deformity. *Osteoporos Int* 2016.

This prospective study evaluated the effect of teriparatide for preventing vertebral failure-type proximal junctional kyphosis after surgery for adult spinal deformity. Level of evidence: II.

Chapter 40

Injured Workers and Disability Assessment

Adam LaBore, MD

Abstract

The core of orthopaedic practice is the restoration of function. Physicians and surgeons are in a position of responsibility for identifying, treating, and determining the resolution of injury. Orthopaedic care, with respect to occupational injury, requires a physician's attention to a greater number of details unrelated to the direct care of the injured than encountered in any other health-care arena. The context of legislated compensation of the injured adds to this complexity. Physicians who treat injured workers must maintain the highest ethical standards to help guide decision making.

Keywords: cost; ethics; injury prevention; return to work; workplace injury

Introduction

Orthopaedic care is designed to restore function. Orthopaedic specialists are responsible for the identification and treatment of injury. In the setting of occupational injury, orthopaedic care requires physicians to focus on a greater number of details unrelated to the direct care of the patient than is typical. To help guide decision making, physicians who treat injured workers must maintain the highest ethical standards.

Workplace Injury Treatment and Decision Making

The first goal of workplace injury treatment is to provide prompt diagnosis and an appropriate management

strategy for the injured worker. Access to expert care for an injury should be provided in a timely manner.

After an initial diagnosis has been made, a treatment plan is formulated. During the period of treatment, injured workers should rarely be restricted from all work. Rather, the physician specifically restricts those work and life activities that would hamper the worker's recovery.

Irrespective of whether surgical or nonsurgical treatment is deployed, the worker must be prepared for the resumption of work demands as recovery proceeds and function returns. This often can be accomplished in the context of natural recovery, well-directed physical therapy, and a stepwise return to normal occupational demands. If recovery of function and/or tolerance of duty demands do not progress along the expected timeline of injury recovery, formal work conditioning and/or work hardening may be ordered. Maximum medical improvement (MMI) has been reached if medical treatment can no longer predictably improve recovery from injury. If MMI has been achieved but full function and/or tolerance of duty demands has not, a functional capacity evaluation can help formally quantify what a worker is unable to do, instead of what he or she is unwilling to do.

MMI refers only to the likelihood that further medical intervention will help the injured worker's recovery of function. MMI does not imply the absence of need for further medical treatment; instead, this is the appropriate time to transfer care from the physician supervising the injury recovery to a primary care physician and/or specialist to oversee chronic care as indicated. MMI is achieved when subsequently scheduled medical care with the specialist treating the particular injury is no longer indicated.

After MMI has been reached, a final disposition with respect to work return must be determined for the injured individual. The most straightforward, common pathway is one of complete recovery and resumption of preinjury employment and function. Whether or not recovery of function allows the resumption of job

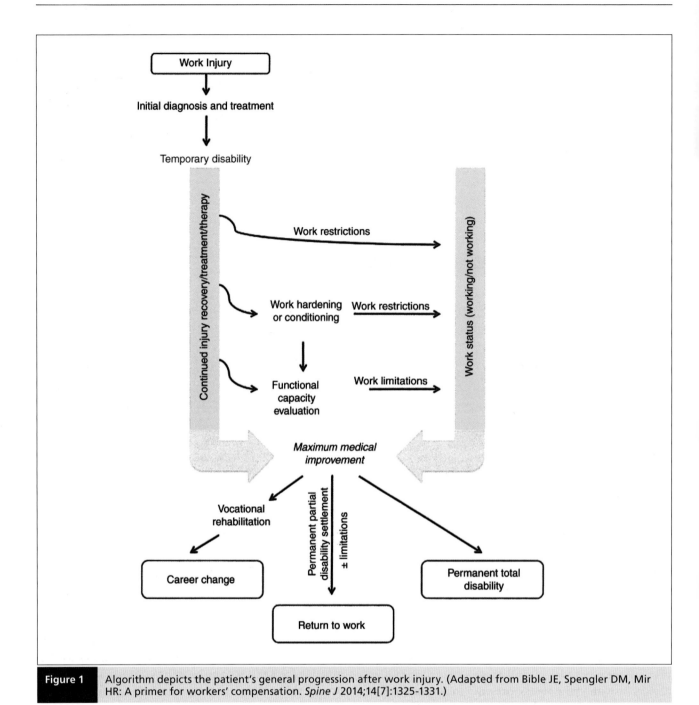

Figure 1 Algorithm depicts the patient's general progression after work injury. (Adapted from Bible JE, Spengler DM, Mir HR: A primer for workers' compensation. *Spine J* 2014;14[7]:1325-1331.)

demands, the patient may have residual impairment. In this situation, a permanent partial impairment rating is determined. When the injured worker's maximum recovery is insufficient for the demands of his or her occupation, vocational rehabilitation is appropriate, possibly resulting in a career change. When injuries result in permanent disability to the extent that the injured worker is unable to return to the workforce, a determination of permanent total disability can be made[1] (**Figure 1**).

Treatment, Recovery, and the Prevention of Future Injury

Understanding the workplace and workforce factors that influence injury prevention allows the treating physician to make meaningful recommendations to the injured worker, and possibly to the employer. In addition, well-conceived practical recommendations give employers the opportunity to intervene at a workforce level, potentially reducing the prospect of injury to others.

Table 1

Evidentiary Support for Modifiable Workplace Factors

Strong	Moderate	Weak
Lack of social support	Non–full-time work	Increased absenteeism tolerance
Job strain	Poor-quality leadership	Reorganizational stress
Increased physical demands	Lack of job control	Increased time to treatment
Low job satisfaction	Lack of fairness	
Lack of supervisory support	Lack of managerial involvement	
Increased psychologic demands		
Lack of worker control		

Data from White MI: Modifiable workplace risk factors contributing to workplace absence across health conditions: A stakeholder-centered best-evidence synthesis of systematic reviews. *Work* 2013;45(4):475-492.

Table 2

Evidentiary Support for Nonmodifiable Workplace Factors

Strong	Moderate	Weak	Inconsistent	Insufficient
NA	Lower occupational level	Longer length of employment	Company size	Lower job grade
	Existence of a workers' compensation claim		Compensation at high and low rates	Loss of benefits or financial disincentives to work
				Unstable employment
				Healthcare system factors
				Negative social factors

NA = not available.

Data adapted from White MI, Wagner SL, Schultz IZ, et al: Non-modifiable worker and workplace risk factors contributing to workplace absence: A stakeholder-centered synthesis of systematic reviews. *Work* 2015;52(2):353-373.

Evidence to date supports workplace intervention in the reduction of time lost because of musculoskeletal injury, including work-related injury involving the spine and back. Increased physical demands and decreased physical functioning both have been found to increase the risk of work absence.[2] Although the recommendations may be intuitive to the treating physician, the use of supporting evidence provides important justification for intervention. When a worker with spine injury presents for evaluation, the prescribed treatment and recommended modifications to the worker and the workplace impart cost to all stakeholders. Modifiable factors influencing return to work include those related to diagnosis and treatment, managing expectations, worker mood and depression, and workplace factors[2] (**Table 1**). Nonmodifiable risk factors influencing work return include demands of the occupation, severity of the injury, and the extent of recovery[3] (**Table 2**). For physicians, the first step of an encounter with an injured worker is to establish a diagnosis. A more specific diagnosis results in a more efficient treatment plan. Equally important to expertise in diagnosis and treatment is communicating appropriate expectations regarding recovery of function and resumption of occupational duties. As part of a comprehensive treatment plan, treating physicians also can recommend interventions to treat factors that are not injury specific. If a worker's abilities do not match the duties demanded by the assigned job, treatment recommendations should consider worker and workplace factors influencing recovery and resumption of those duties. One report identified the potential role of formal functional capacity evaluations as part of a prevention strategy.[4] Treating physicians should consider recommendations that improve worker physical conditioning, ergonomics intervention, and screening for psychosocial influences on injury and recovery, when appropriate.

In formulating treatment recommendations and setting realistic expectations, the factors influencing return to work following surgical treatment of spinal injury must be considered. Recent studies have reported the predictability of return to work after lumbar surgery.

A 2016 study reported on 3-month return to work after lumbar diskectomy.[5] Younger age, male sex, higher

8: Special Populations in Spine Care

Table 3

Comparison of Patients 3 Months After Lumbar Diskectomy

Variable	Working at 3 Months (n = 85)	Not Working at 3 Months (n = 42)	P Value
Age (y)[a]	44.45 ± 10.84	50.45 ± 13.60	0.008[b]
Male sex	47 (55.3%)	12 (28.6%)	0.005[b]
Body mass index (kg/m²)[a]	27.76 ± 5.54	28.25 ± 21.53	0.6283
Preoperative SF-36 score[a]	43.96 ± 23.54	30.32 ± 21.53	0.002[b]
Preoperative Oswestry Disability Index score[a]	43.82 ± 17.16	52.60 ± 19.13	0.01[b]
Diabetes	1 (1.2%)	2 (4.8%)	0.254
Smoker	14 (16.5%)	14 (33.3%)	0.031[b]
Systemic illness	7 (8.2%)	3 (7.1%)	1.00
Workers' compensation	0	1 (2.4%)	0.331
Working preoperatively	78 (91.8%)	11 (26.2%)	<0.0001[b]

SF-36 = Medical Outcomes Study 36-Item Short Form.

[a] Data are the mean ± SD.

[b] Data are significant.

Data from Than KD, Curran JN, Resnick DK, Shaffrey CI, Ghogawala Z, Mummaneni PV: How to predict return to work after lumbar discectomy: Answers from the NeuroPoint-SD registry. *J Neurosurg Spine* 2016;25(2):181-186.

Table 4

Regression-Estimated Likelihood That Patients Will Meet Job Requirements Following TLIF or ACDF

Preoperative Job Requirement	TLIF	ACDF, Patient Age 18 to 39 years	ACDF, Patient Age 40 to 49 years	ACDF, Patient Age ≥50 years
Sedentary/light	78% ± 14%	97% ± 3%	91% ± 6%	87% ± 10%
Medium	34% ± 8%	72% ± 9%	47% ± 11%	37% ± 11%
Heavy/very heavy	26% ± 8%	46% ± 12%	23% ± 9%	16% ± 8%

ACDF = anterior cervical decompression and fusion, TLIF = transforaminal lumbar interbody fusion.

Data are the likelihood ± standard error.

Data from Bohl DD, Ahn J, Collins M, et al: Functional capacity evaluation following spinal fusion surgery. *Spine (Phila Pa 1976)* 2016;41(13): 1104-1110.

preoperative Medical Outcomes Study 36-Item Short Form scores and lower Oswestry Disability Index scores, nonsmoking status, and preoperative work were factors that led to higher return-to-work rates. When controlling for preoperative working status, age was the only factor identified as a significant predictor: younger workers were more likely to return to work (**Table 3**).

In addition, analyses of return to work within 3 months following elective lumbar spine surgery demonstrated lower return rates among those who were employed but not working at the time of surgery, on workers' compensation, and on liability insurance. Other negative predictors included unfavorable baseline Oswestry Disability Index and Numeric Rating Scale scores for back pain, female sex, African American race, a history of diabetes mellitus, and higher American Society of Anesthesiologists grades.[6] Individuals with a higher educational level were more likely to return to work by 3 months compared with individuals with less than a high school education.

A prospective review examined the outcomes of functional capacity evaluation in patients following anterior cervical diskectomy and fusion or transforaminal lumbar interbody fusion.[7] Most patients were unable to resume the occupational demands they had before surgery. In addition, after fusion, approximately 20% were able to perform heavy-duty work, and 50% were able to perform medium-duty work (**Table 4**). Another study reported on the association of preoperative pain, disability, and depression with the extent of postoperative improvement and the capacity to return to work (independent of age); the presence of depression was found to be a particularly predictive factor.[8]

Cost of Injury and Treatment

Treating physicians should be able to identify the factors influencing the cost of spine care. Duration of active treatment, the direct cost of treatment, and lost work productivity are obvious factors to consider in the calculation of the cost of spine injury care. All stakeholders should understand the factors influencing these cost factors. The treating physician is pivotal in identifying, clarifying, and communicating these factors. In the context of evaluating and treating injured workers, a physician may want to perform earlier diagnostic testing, although there is no supporting evidence that the testing will immediately aid diagnosis, treatment, and/or prognosis. The automatic ordering of advanced imaging adds direct costs, risks direct influence on recommendations for intervention without immediate indication, and can unnecessarily extend the disabled state.[9] A population-based cohort study examined factors associated with early MRI performed in 1,830 patients with acute, nonspecific, uncomplicated, occupation-related low back pain.[9] Male sex, initial visit with a surgeon versus primary care physician or chiropractor, heightened work fear-avoidance, and greater severity of injury were associated with increased early use of MRI.

As with all medical treatment decision making, patient-centered surgical care for the injured worker requires individualized application of established surgical indications. A 2013 study examined cases derived from the Louisiana Workers' Compensation Corporation for the relationship between timing of surgery and overall healthcare cost.[10] Surgery did not correlate with higher total costs, and earlier progression of treatment to surgical intervention can be associated with lower cost and claim durations. Importantly, this association was applied in the context of "surgeries targeting a specific clinical indication," as opposed to tailoring treatment to the priorities of expedited case resolution.

A retrospective cohort study examined the influence of biopsychosocial variables on lumbar diskectomy costs in 266 workers' compensation patients in Utah.[11] Consistent with previously published data, variables including increased age, prior surgery, number of medical comorbidities, alcohol use, and lower education level were associated with increased total costs. These data, contextualized to the specifics of surgical intervention as part of treating compensable injury, allow anticipation of increased cost when certain factors are present. These reports are consistent with previously published data, and represent recent additions to understanding the care of injured workers with spinal disorders.

Medical Ethics and the Treatment of Work Injury

Ideal care for the injured worker in the United States intersects predictable costs, progressive innovation, adaptability to the continually evolving healthcare landscape, and mindfulness regarding ethical considerations. In this context, the four classic pillars of medical ethics—autonomy, justice, beneficence, and nonmaleficence—must be considered. Understanding these concepts and using them in the context of decision making minimizes risks to stakeholders during treatment of the injured worker.

Autonomy has been defined as patient freedom in making independent, informed decisions regarding personal health care. This freedom depends on being fully informed about treatment options, the risks and anticipated benefits of treatment, and the absence of coercion or biased provider influence. Often, informed decision making is executed in the context of stressors that impede objective reflection by patients, which fosters dependence on providers to guide optimal decision making. Physicians are responsible for providing expertise to facilitate framing this aspect of decision making for patients. For example, the physician can provide guidance to a patient regarding the factors influencing surgical versus nonsurgical treatment of acute lumbar disk herniation, short- and long-term considerations, and the risks associated with each option.

Justice, with respect to bioethics, including injury-related spine care, requires the same high level of awareness and integrity on the part of healthcare providers. Those positioned at the point of greatest influence in healthcare decision-making are most responsible for balancing patient-centered treatment options with how these options affect society. This balance occurs by impartially guiding the patient toward the treatment choices that provide the greatest personal benefit, but at minimal overall cost to the patient and society. A consideration of justice helps guide decisions away from surgical intervention or

8: Special Populations in Spine Care

prolonged treatment of symptoms when a lack of evidence exists for achieving predictable functional gain.

Beneficence underlies the concept of identifying treatment options that prioritize patient benefits. In the context of injury and recovery, beneficence can be mistaken as straightforward, and tends toward the path of least resistance (that is, patient comfort). However, restoration of ability is a maxim of treatment benefit for an injured worker. When appropriate, an injured worker may have to undergo substantial discomfort to achieve functional restoration. This discomfort is analogous to difficult athletic training. The injured worker may be adverse to this endeavor (such as rehabilitation after spine injury) and should be educated regarding the importance of this aspect of treatment.

Nonmaleficence is a more nuanced concept than beneficence. Nonmaleficence demands that healthcare providers make every effort to avoid harm to the patient or any part of society. Ostensibly, this means doing no harm, and in practice it means identifying treatment options that minimize potential negative effects on patients and society. For example, it is necessary to consider whether the risks associated with a particular surgical intervention yields predictably advantageous functional outcomes compared with nonsurgical care. These concepts are complicated and demand career-long consideration of all aspects of patient care.[12.]

Summary

Spine care for an injured worker is demanding, and a timely and precise diagnosis is required. Clearly communicating the diagnosis, treatment rationale, and expectations lay the groundwork for successful and expedient outcomes. Understanding the factors that influence return to work promotes efficacy in decision making and helps physicians avoid undue prolongation of the patient's injured state.

Key Study Points

- A complete understanding of treatment and transfer of care is necessary after a work-related spine injury.
- A variety of measures are available to prevent injury in the workplace.
- Many factors influence the cost of injury, both to the worker and society.
- Modifiable and nonmodifiable factors affecting return to work include those related to diagnosis and treatment, managing expectations, worker mood and depression, and workplace issues.
- The medical ethics involved in treating injured workers are classified as part of autonomy, justice, beneficence, and nonmaleficence.

Annotated References

1. Bible JE, Spengler DM, Mir HR: A primer for workers' compensation. *Spine J* 2014;14(7):1325-1331.

   The authors discuss why workers' compensation is necessary, the general course of treatment after work injury, the role of physicians in no-fault workers' compensation cases, the need for independent medical evaluations, the use of impairment ratings, and causation.

2. White M, Wagner S, Schultz IZ, et al: Modifiable workplace risk factors contributing to workplace absence across health conditions: A stakeholder-centered best-evidence synthesis of systematic reviews. *Work* 2013;45(4):475-492.

   The authors identify modifiable factors (according to strength of existing evidence) that contribute to risk of absence from work because of health conditions. Level of evidence: IV.

3. White MI, Wagner SL, Schultz IZ, et al: Non-modifiable worker and workplace risk factors contributing to workplace absence: A stakeholder-centred synthesis of systematic reviews. *Work* 2015;52(2):353-373.

   Based on the strength of existing evidence, the authors identify nonmodifiable factors related to health conditions that contribute to the risk of absence from work. Level of evidence: IV.

4. Legge J: The evolving role of physiotherapists in pre-employment screening for workplace injury prevention: Are functional capacity evaluations the answer? *Phys Ther Rev* 2013;18(5):350-357.

   This preliminary report examined the role of functional capacity evaluation in screening job applicants to reduce workplace injury. Level of evidence: V.

5. Than KD, Curran JN, Resnick DK, Shaffrey CI, Ghogawala Z, Mummaneni PV: How to predict return to work

after lumbar discectomy: Answers from the Neuro-Point-SD registry. *J Neurosurg Spine* 2016;25(2):181-186.

This study examined existing data regarding return to work predictability after lumbar diskectomy from the NeuroPoint-SD registry. Level of evidence: IV.

6. Asher AL, Chotai S, Devin CJ, et al; N2QOD Investigator Group: 148 predictive model for return to work after elective surgery for lumbar degenerative disease: An analysis from national neurosurgery quality outcomes database registry. *Neurosurgery* 2016;63(suppl 1):160.

This abstract reports on factors related to work capability and return after elective lumbar spine surgery. Level of evidence: IV.

7. Bohl DD, Ahn J, Collins M, et al: Functional capacity evaluation following spinal fusion surgery. *Spine (Phila Pa 1976)* 2016;41(13):1104-1110.

This study evaluated work ability after spinal fusion, including an assessment of return to preoperative capabilities. Level of evidence: III.

8. Parker SL, Godil SS, Zuckerman SL, Mendenhall SK, Devin CJ, McGirt MJ: Extent of preoperative depression is associated with return to work after lumbar fusion for spondylolisthesis. *World Neurosurg* 2015;83(4):608-613.

This study evaluated factors influencing delayed return to work after fusion surgery for lumbar spondylolisthesis. Preoperative depression was identified as an independent predictor of time to return to work. Level of evidence: IV.

9. Graves JM, Fulton-Kehoe D, Martin DP, Jarvik JG, Franklin GM: Factors associated with early magnetic resonance imaging utilization for acute occupational low back pain: A population-based study from Washington State workers' compensation. *Spine (Phila Pa 1976)* 2012;37(19):1708-1718.

This study examines the influence of early MRI on the nature and cost of care for workers undergoing treatment for uncomplicated occupational low back pain. Level of evidence: IV.

10. Lavin RA, Tao X, Yuspeh L, Bernacki EJ: Temporal relationship between lumbar spine surgeries, return to work, and workers' compensation costs in a cohort of injured workers. *J Occup Environ Med* 2013;55(5):539-543.

The relationship between time to indicated lumbar spine surgery and return to work in the Louisiana workers' compensation system is examined. Level of evidence: IV.

11. DeBerard MS, Wheeler AJ, Gundy JM, Stein DM, Colledge AL: Presurgical biopsychosocial variables predict medical, compensation, and aggregate costs of lumbar discectomy in Utah workers' compensation patients. *Spine J* 2011;11(5):395-401.

This retrospective cohort study examines the influence of biopsychosocial variables on lumbar diskectomy costs in 266 Utah workers' compensation patients. Level of evidence: IV.

12. Code of Medical Ethics and Professionalism for Orthopaedic Surgeons. American Academy of Orthopaedic Surgeons. Revised 2011. Available at: http://www.aaos.org/uploadedFiles/PreProduction/About/Opinion_Statements/ethics/Code%20of%20Ethics%202013%20color%20logo.pdf. Accessed March 13, 3017.

The American Academy of Orthopaedic Surgeons provides an updated code with a framework for approaching orthopaedic practice from a societal level.

8: Special Populations in Spine Care

Index

Index

Index

Index

prevention of, 521
return to play after, 524
spinal, 519–531
spinal cord, 443
thoracolumbar, 526t
Sprains/strains, treatments, 169
Spurling test, 67
SRS-Schwab Adult Spinal Deformity Classification, 336, 337t
Stagnara wake-up test, 92
Stakeholder, in interdisciplinary care, 129, 129t, 130t–132t, 134t
Staphylococcus aureus, 481–482, 485
STarT Back Tool, 159
Stem cells in discogenic pain, 204
Stenosis. *See also* Spinal canal stenosis
degenerative spine deformity and, 338
dural sac, 255f
epidural steroid injections in, 198
lumbar, 46f, 199t
osteopathic treatments, 169
thoracic spine, 229, 236–238
Steroid injections, 195–197, 285. *See also* Epidural steroid injections (ESI)
Stingers, sports-related, 522t, 523
Straight-leg raise test, 376
Strain-counterstrain techniques, 171
Stress reduction, mindfulness-based, 114
Stretch reflexes, 23, 25f, 66t
Stretchers, for field-of-play injuries, 521
Stroke, craniocervical dissociation and, 398
Subaxial Cervical Spine Injury Classification (SLIC), 388, 405
Subaxial cervical trauma, 395–418
Subaxial subluxation, 497
Suboccipital craniotomy, 497
Substantia gelatinosa, 23
Superior gluteal nerve, 65f
Supplements, spine care and, 183
Surgical site infections (SSIs), 314
Surgical Timing in Acute Spinal Cord Injury Study, 389
Sweating, absence of, 22
Swedish massage, for spine pain, 180
Symphysis pubis tenderness, 68
Syndesmophytes, 498
Syringomyelia, 295
Systemic hypothermia, 389

T

Tai chi, for spine disorders, 184
Tanner-Whitehouse method, 311
Tapotement therapy, 180
Taxpayer, as stakeholder in patient care, 129, 132t, 135t
Team approach, in interdisciplinary care, 128–129, 138t
Tectorial membrane, 6, 396
Temperature, nerve conduction studies and, 90

Teriparatide, 350, 535
Tethered cord, 295
Tetraplegia
after SCI, 450–451
definition of, 23, 25
incomplete, 383
Texas Back Institute (TBI), 137
Thecal sac, contrast material in, 77
Therapeutic exercise, 151–165
Thermal injuries, MEP monitoring, 95
Thermal neurolysis for discogenic pain, 201
Thermoregulation, fascia and, 180
Thigh thrust test, 69
Third-party payers, 129, 132t, 135t
Thoracic curve, radiographs, 310f, 312f
Thoracic disk disease, 236
Thoracic disk herniation
anterior surgical approaches, 231–233
clinical presentation, 230–231
imaging, 231
posterolateral surgical approaches, 233–236
surgical removal of, 232f
transfacet pedicle-sparing technique, 234
transpedicular approach, 234
treatment, 231
Thoracic diskectomy, 235, 235f
Thoracic insufficiency syndrome, 294
Thoracic kyphosis, 343, 499–500
Thoracic pain, whiplash injuries and, 434
Thoracic radiculopathy, 230–231
Thoracic scoliosis, 342
Thoracic spine
anatomy of, 8–9, 229–230
degenerative disease of, 229–241
disk herniation, 526t
fractures, 526t
kyphotic alignment, 229–230
nerves, 20
schwannomas, 474
sports-related injuries, 524–526
surgical approaches, 230f
T3-T4 flexion distraction fracture, 386f
vertebrae, 3
Thoracic stenosis, 229, 236–238
Thoracolumbar fascia, 180
Thoracolumbar Injury Classification and Severity Scale (TLICS), 420, 421f
Thoracolumbar spine
anterior approach to, 423
burst fractures, 422–423, 423f
compression fractures, 422
distraction injuries, 423–424
fractures, 422
posterior approach to, 422–423
posterior midline approach, 32–33
return to play after injuries, 528
sagittal plane angles, 358f

sports-related injuries to, 526t, 528
translational injuries, 424, 425f
trauma classifications, 420–424
traumatic injury, 419–432
complications, 429–430
initial imaging in, 386–387
Thoracotomy, 232–233
Thrust technique, 170f
Tibialis anterior muscles, 20, 94f, 95, 96f
Tissue dysfunction, MDT definition, 160
Tissue texture changes, 168–169
Tocilizumab for RA, 496
Tofacitinib for RA, 496
Torg ratio, 524
Total disk arthroplasty (TDA), 214, 508
Touch, assessment after SCI, 384
Traction, intraoperative, 320
Training, interdisciplinary systems and, 138t
Trampoline injuries, 521
Tranexamic acid, 320, 345–346
Transcranial motor-evoked potentials, intraoperative, 320, 345
Transcranial stimulation, 95
Transdisciplinary care
care access and, 118–119
case examples, 119–120
for cervical spine disorders, 113–125
clinical assessments, 119
monodisciplinary care *versus*, 116
patient integration with teams, 117f
patient needs and, 116
planning and coordination, 119
spheres of, 117f
team and patient integration, 117f
team foundations, 117–119
triage and, 118–119
Transforaminal lumbar interbody fusion (TLIF), 34–35, 267, 546t, 547
Translation per degree of rotation (TPDR), 48, 52
Transthoracic surgical approach, 230f
Transverse atlantal ligament (TAL) rupture, 399–400
Transverse pedicle angle (TPA), 9
Trapezius muscle innervation, 95
Traumatic injuries
bracing in, 388
cervical spine, 395–418
external immobilization in, 388
imaging assessment for, 385–386
spinal, 50
spinal deformity and, 336
spondylolisthesis, 372
therapeutic modalities, 387–389
thoracolumbar, 419–432
vehicular, 395
Treatment-based classification systems (TBCs)
classification using, 151–152, 157–158

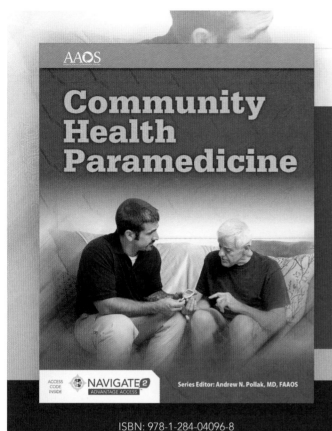
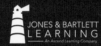

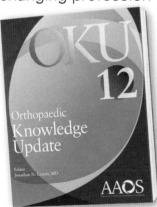
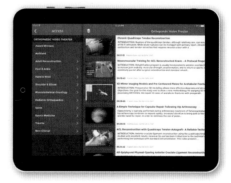

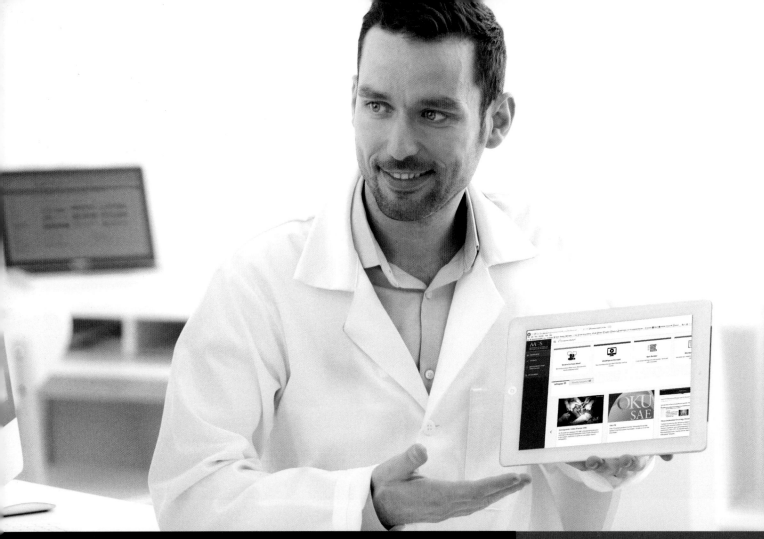

I learn by interactive experience

Energize your education with our new online learning platform

AAOS delivers complete learning experiences and exciting new learning formats to meet my educational needs.
The new AAOS online learning platform delivers more personalized and practice-relevant educational experiences – all in one place! I can explore a variety of interactive education experiences with video, self-assessment and self-paced activities.

- Challenge your knowledge with the all-new Orthopaedic Knowledge Update 12 Self-Assessment Examination

- Access new Annual Meeting Tracks for generalists or specialists in 5 orthopaedic specialty areas!

- Self-directed Musculoskeletal Oncology Review Course, and much more!

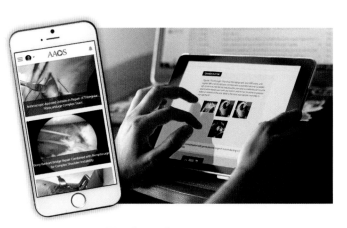

Explore **learn.aaos.org** and give us your feedback!

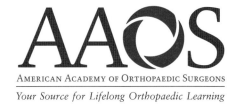

AMERICAN ACADEMY OF ORTHOPAEDIC SURGEONS
Your Source for Lifelong Orthopaedic Learning